ADVANCES IN

Pediatrics

Editor-in-Chief
Michael S. Kappy, MD, PhD

Professor of Pediatrics, University of Colorado
School of Medicine, Children's Hospital Colorado,
Aurora, Colorado

ELSEVIER

PHILADELPHIA   LONDON   TORONTO   MONTREAL   SYDNEY   TOKYO

ADVANCES IN
Pediatrics

VOLUMES 1 THROUGH 61 (OUT OF PRINT)

Senior Director, Content Strategy & Continuity: Adrianne Brigido
Editor: Kerry Holland
Developmental Editor: Donald Mumford

Printed in the United States of America.

Editorial Office:
Elsevier
1600 John F. Kennedy Blvd,
Suite 1800
Philadelphia, PA 19103-2899

International Standard Serial Number: 0065-3101
International Standard Book Number: 13: 978-0-323-44680-8

ADVANCES IN
Pediatrics

Editor-in-Chief

MICHAEL S. KAPPY, MD, PhD, Professor of Pediatrics, University of Colorado School of Medicine, Children's Hospital Colorado, Aurora, Colorado

Associate Editors

LESLIE L. BARTON, MD, Professor Emerita, Department of Pediatrics, Steele Memorial Children's Research Center, University of Arizona, Tucson, Arizona

CAROL D. BERKOWITZ, MD, Executive Vice Chair, Department of Pediatrics, Harbor-UCLA Medical Center; Distinguished Professor of Pediatrics, David Geffen School of Medicine at UCLA, Torrance, California

JANE CARVER, PhD, MS, MPH, Professor, Department of Pediatrics and Molecular Medicine, University of South Florida College of Medicine, Tampa, Florida

MORITZ ZIEGLER, MD, Retired Surgeon-in-Chief, Pediatric Surgery, Children's Hospital Colorado, Retired, Professor of Surgery, University of Colorado School of Medicine, Aurora, Colorado

CONTRIBUTORS

WILLIAM C. ANDERSON III, MD, Assistant Professor, Pediatric Allergy and Immunology, University of Colorado School of Medicine, Children's Hospital Colorado, Aurora, Colorado

EDWIN J. ASTURIAS, MD, FAAP, Associate Professor of Pediatrics, Section of Pediatric Infectious Disease, University of Colorado School of Medicine; Assistant Professor of Epidemiology, Colorado School of Public Health, Aurora, Colorado

STEPHEN BERMAN, MD, FAAP, Professor of Pediatrics and Epidemiology, University of Colorado School of Medicine and Colorado School of Public Health; Director, Center for Global Health in the Colorado School of Public Health; Endowed Chair in Academic General Pediatrics at Children's Hospital Colorado, Aurora, Colorado

MARK BORCHERT, MD, Associate Professor of Clinical Ophthalmology and Neurology, University of Southern California Keck School of Medicine; The Vision Center, Children's Hospital Los Angeles; The Saban Research Institute, Children's Hospital Los Angeles, Los Angeles, California

JOHN BRETT, PhD, Associate Professor, Department of Anthropology, College of Liberal Arts and Sciences, University of Colorado-Denver, Denver, Colorado

MONICA BUCCI, MD, Center for Youth Wellness, San Francisco, California

SHEANA BULL, PhD, Chair and Professor, Department of Community and Behavioral Health, Colorado School of Public Health, Aurora, Colorado

ELIZA BUYERS, MD, FACOG, Clinical Instructor of Obstetrics and Gynecology, Section of Pediatric and Adolescent Gynecology, University of Colorado School of Medicine, Aurora, Colorado

SUSAN E. CARLSON, PhD, AJ Rice Professor of Nutrition, Department of Dietetics and Nutrition, University of Kansas Medical Center, Kansas City, Kansas

MARCO CELADA, MD, Clinical Instructor, Department of Pediatrics, University of Colorado School of Medicine, Aurora, Colorado

MELISSA CHAMBERS, MD, Phoenix Children's Hospital, Phoenix, Arizona

REETI CHAWLA, MD, Phoenix Children's Hospital, Phoenix, Arizona

MICHAEL COHEN-WOLKOWIEZ, MD, PhD, Duke Clinical Research Institute, Duke University Medical Center; Department of Pediatrics, Children's Health Center, College of Medicine, Duke University, Durham, North Carolina

JOHN COLOMBO, PhD, Department of Neurology, University of Kansas Medical Center, Kansas City, Kansas; Professor, Department of Psychology, Life Span Institute, University of Kansas, Lawrence, Kansas

MAUREEN CUNNINGHAM, MD, MPH, Assistant Professor, Department of Pediatrics, University of Colorado School of Medicine, Aurora, Colorado

SHANLEE DAVIS, MD, Research Fellow, Department of Pediatrics, University of Colorado School of Medicine; Pediatric Endocrinology, Children's Hospital Colorado, Aurora, Colorado

GRETCHEN DOMEK, MD, MPhil, Assistant Professor, Department of Pediatrics, University of Colorado School of Medicine, Aurora, Colorado

MARY E. FALLAT, MD, Hirikati S. Nagaraj Professor and Division Director of Pediatric Surgery, Hiram C. Polk Jr Department of Surgery, Surgeon-in-Chief, Kosair Children's Hospital, University of Louisville, Louisville, Kentucky

MONICA J. FEDERICO, MD, Associate Professor, Department of Pediatrics, University of Colorado School of Medicine, Children's Hospital Colorado, Aurora, Colorado

MICHAEL FREEMARK, MD, Atkins Professor and Chief, Division of Pediatric Endocrinology, Duke University Medical Center, Durham, North Carolina

LAURA C. FULGINITI, PhD, Forensic Anthropologist, Maricopa County Office of the Medical Examiner, Phoenix, Arizona

RACHELLE GANDICA, MD, Assistant Professor of Pediatric Endocrinology, Naomi Berrie Diabetes Center, Columbia University Medical Center, New York, New York

MITCHELL E. GEFFNER, MD, Professor of Pediatrics, University of Southern California Keck School of Medicine; Center for Endocrinology, Diabetes, and Metabolism, Children's Hospital Los Angeles; The Saban Research Institute, Children's Hospital Los Angeles, Los Angeles, California

GRIFIN GOLDSMITH, MPH, Children's Health Fund, New York, New York

EDWARD GOLDSON, MD, Professor, Department of Pediatrics, Children's Hospital Colorado, University of Colorado School of Medicine, Aurora, Colorado

DANIEL GONZALEZ, PharmD, PhD, Division of Pharmacotherapy and Experimental Therapeutics, UNC Eshelman School of Pharmacy, University of North Carolina at Chapel Hill, Chapel Hill, North Carolina

DELANEY GRACY, MD, MPH, Children's Health Fund, New York, New York

ROY GRANT, MA, Children's Health Fund, New York, New York

KATHLEEN GRAZIANO, MD, Director, Reproductive Anomalies/DSD Clinic, Phoenix Children's Hospital, Phoenix, Arizona

ANDREA M. HAQQ, MD, Associate Professor, Division of Pediatric Endocrinology, University of Alberta, Edmonton, Alberta, Canada

NADINE BURKE HARRIS, MD, MPH, FAAP, Center for Youth Wellness, San Francisco, California

GRETCHEN HEINRICHS, MD, DTMH, Assistant Professor of Obstetrics and Gynecology, University of Colorado School of Medicine and Denver Health, Aurora, Colorado

HEATHER E. HOCH, MD, Pulmonary Fellow, Department of Pediatrics, University of Colorado School of Medicine, Children's Hospital Colorado, Aurora, Colorado

KAM LUN HON, MBBS, MD, FAAP, FCCM, Professor, Department of Paediatrics, Prince of Wales Hospital, Chinese University of Hong Kong, Shatin, Hong Kong

SUSAN HOWELL, MS, CGC, MBA, Senior Instructor, Department of Pediatrics, University of Colorado School of Medicine; Genetic Counselor, Developmental Pediatrics, Children's Hospital Colorado, Aurora, Colorado

KRYSTAL A. IRIZARRY, MD, Medical Instructor, Division of Pediatric Endocrinology, Duke University Medical Center, Durham, North Carolina

DENNIS JOHNSON, MPS, Children's Health Fund, New York, New York

CHIRAG KAPADIA, MD, Phoenix Children's Hospital, Phoenix, Arizona

MICHAEL S. KAPPY, MD, PhD, Department of Pediatrics, University of Colorado School of Medicine, Children's Hospital Colorado, Aurora, Colorado

LYNDSAY KRISHER, MPH, Guatemala Project Specialist, Center for Global Health, Colorado School of Public Health, Aurora, Colorado

ALEXANDER K.C. LEUNG, MBBS, FRCPC, FRCP (UK & Irel), FRCPCH, FAAP, Clinical Professor, Department of Pediatrics, University of Calgary, Alberta Children's Hospital, Calgary, Alberta, Canada

ELMER S. LIGHTNER, MD, Professor Emeritus of Pediatrics, University of Arizona College of Medicine, Tucson, Arizona

CLAUDIA LUNA-ASTURIAS, MSW, Adjunct Faculty, Physician Assistant Program and Clinical Instructor, Department of Pediatrics, University of Colorado School of Medicine, Aurora, Colorado

SARA SILVÉRIO MARQUES, DrPH, MPH, Center for Youth Wellness, San Francisco, California

KELLY MCCONNELL, MD, Fellow, Center for Global Health, Colorado School of Public Health and Department of Pediatrics, University of Colorado School of Medicine, Aurora, Colorado

DEBORAH K. MCCURDY, MD, Program Director of Rheumatology, Clinical Professor of Pediatrics, Division of Allergy/Immunology/Rheumatology, Department of Pediatrics, David Geffen School of Medicine, University of California Los Angeles, Los Angeles, California

ELIZABETH J. MCFARLAND, MD, Professor of Pediatrics, Section of Infectious Diseases, Department of Pediatrics, Children's Hospital Colorado, University of Colorado School of Medicine, Aurora, Colorado

MARK MILLER, MD, Fellow, Division of Pediatric Endocrinology, Duke University Medical Center, Durham, North Carolina

GRANT MORROW III, MD, Medical Director, Research Institute at Nationwide Children's Hospital, Professor Emeritus of Pediatrics, The Ohio State University, Columbus, Ohio

LEE S. NEWMAN, MD, MA, FCCP, FACOEM, Director, Center for Health, Work and Environment, Colorado School of Public Health, Aurora, Colorado

NATALIE J. NOKOFF, MD, Fellow, Division of Pediatric Endocrinology, Department of Pediatrics, University of Colorado School of Medicine, Aurora, Colorado

DEBORA OH, PhD, MSc, Center for Youth Wellness, San Francisco, California

YEN H. PHAM, MD, Assistant Professor, Pediatric Gastroenterology, Hepatology and Nutrition, Texas Children's Hospital, Baylor College of Medicine, Houston, Texas

JANIEL PIMENTEL, MD, Phoenix Children's Hospital, Phoenix, Arizona

MOLLY J. RICHARDS, MD, Assistant Professor of Pediatrics, Section of Adolescent Medicine, Children's Hospital Colorado, University of Colorado School of Medicine, Aurora, Colorado

PHILIP ROSENTHAL, MD, Professor of Pediatrics and Surgery; Director, Pediatric Clinical Research; Director, Pediatric Hepatology and Liver Transplant Research; Director, Pediatric Hepatology, UCSF Benioff Children's Hospital, University of California San Francisco, San Francisco, California

JUDY ROSS, MD, Professor, Department of Pediatrics, Thomas Jefferson University School of Medicine, Philadelphia, Pennsylvania; Pediatric Endocrinology, Nemours A.I. DuPont Hospital for Children, Wilmington, Delaware

ANNA RYABETS-LIENHARD, DO, Assistant Professor of Pediatrics, University of Southern California Keck School of Medicine; Center for Endocrinology, Diabetes, and Metabolism, Children's Hospital Los Angeles, Los Angeles, California

MADHIA SHAHID, MD, Phoenix Children's Hospital, Phoenix, Arizona

ELIZABETH SHICK, DDS, MPH, Assistant Professor of Pediatric Dentistry, University of Colorado School of Dental Medicine, Aurora, Colorado

DANIEL E. SHUMER, MD, MPH, Assistant Professor in Pediatrics, Division of Pediatric Endocrinology, Department of Pediatrics and Communicable Diseases, University of Michigan Health Systems, University of Michigan, Ann Arbor, Michigan

CHRISTIANA SMITH, MD, Instructor of Pediatrics, Section of Infectious Diseases, Department of Pediatrics, Children's Hospital Colorado, University of Colorado School of Medicine, Aurora, Colorado

NORMAN P. SPACK, MD, Senior Associate, Endocrine Division, Boston Children's Hospital, Associate Clinical Professor of Pediatrics, Harvard Medical School, Boston, Massachusetts

JOSEPH D. SPAHN, MD, Professor, Pediatric Allergy and Immunology, University of Colorado School of Medicine, Children's Hospital Colorado, Aurora, Colorado

CARLY STEWART, MHA, The Vision Center, Children's Hospital Los Angeles, Los Angeles, California

STANLEY J. SZEFLER, MD, Professor of Pediatrics, University of Colorado School of Medicine, Children's Hospital Colorado, Aurora, Colorado

TANEA TANDA, BS, Professional Research Associate, Department of Pediatrics, University of Colorado School of Medicine; Developmental Pediatrics, Children's Hospital Colorado, Aurora, Colorado

NICOLE TARTAGLIA, MD, MS, Associate Professor, Department of Pediatrics, University of Colorado School of Medicine; Developmental Pediatrics, Children's Hospital Colorado, Aurora, Colorado

LILIANA TENNEY, MPH, Instructor, Center for Health, Work and Environment, Colorado School of Public Health, Aurora, Colorado

LAURA A. WANG, MIPH, Duke Clinical Research Institute, Duke University Medical Center, Durham, North Carolina

REBECCA WILSON, PsyD, Associate Clinical Professor, Developmental Pediatrics, Children's Hospital Colorado, Aurora, Colorado

PHILIP ZEITLER, MD, PhD, Professor, Department of Pediatrics, University of Colorado School of Medicine; Chair, Pediatric Endocrinology, Children's Hospital Colorado, Aurora, Colorado

ADVANCES IN
Pediatrics

CONTENTS VOLUME 63 • 2016

Prader Willi Syndrome: Genetics, Metabolomics, Hormonal Function, and New Approaches to Therapy

Krystal A. Irizarry, Mark Miller, Michael Freemark, and
Andrea M. Haqq

Advances in the Care of Transgender Children and Adolescents

Daniel E. Shumer, Natalie J. Nokoff, and Norman P. Spack

Asthma Management for Children: Risk Identification and Prevention

Monica J. Federico, Heather E. Hoch, William C. Anderson III, Joseph D. Spahn, and Stanley J. Szefler

The Optic Nerve Hypoplasia Spectrum: Review of the Literature and Clinical Guidelines
Anna Ryabets-Lienhard, Carly Stewart, Mark Borchert, and Mitchell E. Geffner

Update on Pediatric Human Immunodeficiency Virus Infection: Paradigms in Treatment and Prevention
Christiana Smith and Elizabeth J. McFarland

Chronic Hepatitis C Infection in Children
Yen H. Pham and Philip Rosenthal

Update on Youth-Onset Type 2 Diabetes: Lessons Learned from the Treatment Options for Type 2 Diabetes in Adolescents and Youth Clinical Trial
Rachelle Gandica and Phil Zeitler

Comorbidities of Thyroid Disease in Children
Janiel Pimentel, Melissa Chambers, Madhia Shahid,
Reeti Chawla, and Chirag Kapadia

Advances in Pediatric Pharmacology, Therapeutics, and Toxicology

Laura A. Wang, Michael Cohen-Wolkowiez, and
Daniel Gonzalez

Attention-Deficit/Hyperactivity Disorder
Alexander K.C. Leung and Kam Lun Hon

Updates in Pediatric Rheumatology
Deborah K. McCurdy

Advances in Autism—2016
Edward Goldson

The Center for Human Development in Guatemala: An Innovative Model for Global Population Health
Edwin J. Asturias, Gretchen Heinrichs, Gretchen Domek,
John Brett, Elizabeth Shick, Maureen Cunningham,
Sheana Bull, Marco Celada, Lee S. Newman, Liliana Tenney,
Lyndsay Krisher, Claudia Luna-Asturias, Kelly McConnell, and
Stephen Berman

Better Transportation to Health Care Will Improve Child Health and Lower Costs
Roy Grant, Grifin Goldsmith, Delaney Gracy, and Dennis Johnson

Toxic Stress in Children and Adolescents
Monica Bucci, Sara Silvério Marques, Debora Oh, and Nadine Burke Harris

Update on Adolescent Contraception
Molly J. Richards and Eliza Buyers

Docosahexaenoic Acid and Arachidonic Acid Nutrition in Early Development
Susan E. Carlson and John Colombo

Using Shared Decision-Making Tools to Improve Care for Patients with Disorders of Sex Development
Kathleen Graziano and Mary E. Fallat

Advances in Pediatrics 63 (2016) xxv–xxvi

ADVANCES IN PEDIATRICS

Introduction

Michael S. Kappy, MD, PhD

The editors have assembled one of the most inclusive issues in the past 10 years.

We have our annual "Foundations of Pediatrics" article, honoring Vincent Fulginiti, MD, an icon in pediatric infectious disease and education, cowritten by his daughter, Laura Fulginiti, PhD, and colleagues, Grant Morrow III, MD and Elmer Lightner, MD.

Five interdisciplinary update articles in the care of children are presented:

Klinefelter syndrome by Davis and colleagues
Prader-Willi syndrome by Irizarry and colleagues
Transgender children and adolescents by Shumer and colleagues
Asthma by Federico and colleagues
Children with optic nerve hypoplasia syndrome by Ryabets, Lienhard and colleagues

Updates in infectious disease are provided by Smith and McFarland on HIV infections in children and on chronic hepatitis C infections by Pham and Rosenthal.

An update from the TODAY study on the treatment of type 2 diabetes in children is provided by Gandica and Zeitler, and advances in recognizing comorbidities in children with thyroid disorders are covered by Pimentel and colleagues.

Our biannual review of pharmacology, therapeutics, and toxicology is presented by Wang and Gonzales, and updates in the treatment of attention-deficit hyperactivity disorder (Leung and Hon), rheumatology (McCurdy), and autism (Goldson) are given.

General and global pediatric updates are supplied in the articles by Asturias and colleagues regarding an innovative health care program in Guatemala, a description of the difficulties in obtaining health care due to transportation issues (Grant and colleagues), toxic stress in children and adolescents (Bucci and colleagues), an update on adolescent contraception (Richards and Buyers), and the role of docosahexaenoic acid and arachidonic acid in infant nutrition (Carlson and Columbo).

Drs Graziano and Fallat present an approach to the surgical options for children with disorders of sexual development, an exciting, emerging surgical field.

0065-3101/16/$ – see front matter
http://dx.doi.org/10.1016/j.yapd.2016.06.001

As in the past, the editors invite suggestions for future articles as well as comments about the articles in this issue. These can be directed to:

Michael S. Kappy, MD, PhD
Department of Pediatrics
University of Colorado School of Medicine
Children's Hospital Colorado
13123 East 16th Avenue, B-265
Aurora, CO 80045, USA

E-mail address: michael.kappy@childrenscolorado.org

Advances in Pediatrics 63 (2016) 1–13

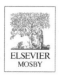

ADVANCES IN PEDIATRICS

Vincent A. Fulginiti, MD (1931–2013)
A Visionary Leader in Pediatric Education, Research, and Bioethics

Laura C. Fulginiti, PhD[a],*, Grant Morrow III, MD[b],
Elmer S. Lightner, MD[c]

[a]Maricopa County Office of the Medical Examiner, 701 West Jefferson Street, Phoenix, AZ 85007, USA; [b]Research Institute at Nationwide Children's Hospital, The Ohio State University, 700 Children's Drive, Columbus, OH 43205-2696, USA; [c]University of Arizona College of Medicine, 1501 North Campbell Avenue, Tucson, AZ 85724, USA

Keywords
• Vincent A. Fulginiti • Mentor • Pediatrics

Key points
• Vincent A. Fulginiti, MD was internationally recognized as a Pediatric Infectious Disease expert.
• Vincent A. Fulginiti, MD was a leader in medical education and a mentor to many.
• Vincent A. Fulginiti, MD published extensively in the fields of pediatric infectious disease, medical education and medical ethics.
• Vincent A. Fulginiti, MD maintained the highest level of personal and professional ethics and was beloved by his family, his friends and his faculty.

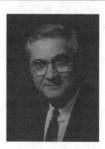

How to describe a man who was mentor to many, editor supreme, ... husband, father, grandfather...and overall a powerful influence on

*Corresponding author. E-mail address: fulginitil@mail.maricopa.gov

0065-3101/16/$ – see front matter
http://dx.doi.org/10.1016/j.yapd.2016.04.012

pediatric education…in the world? One could simply recite his biography and accomplishments but that would simply be the facts; underlying them is a force in pediatrics felt even today by his disciples throughout the world…. [1].

LAURA C. FULGINITI, PHD

So begins an *Advances in Pediatrics* article I found while researching the style of this feature. Those words refer to Waldo Nelson, MD, and they were written in tribute by Vincent A. Fulginiti, MD. Ironic that the words he chose to describe his mentor could also be ascribed to him? I think not. Vince modeled himself after admired individuals (Dr Nelson headed the list) and Dr Nelson helped mold the man he became.

Vince was born on August 8, 1931, at Methodist Hospital in the Italian enclave of South Philadelphia. His dad, John Vincent, and uncle, Samuel Vincent, married the Paravati sisters, Rose and Antoinette. Hard workers all, they were the children of immigrants from the Reggio Calabria region of southern Italy. The Fulginiti family was from the mountain village Gasparina and the Paravati family hailed from the neighboring village of Petrizzi. Somehow the name Fulginiti made it through the immigration process at Ellis Island and the names of family members can be seen on the commemorative stela at the park. Paravati, on the other hand, was converted to Perry by Grandfather Paravati for a $50 fee based on the belief that it would make the family seem more American.

Vince had 1 sister, Elizabeth (Betty), who was 4 years younger. Betty provided Vince with love and support throughout his life and they remained close until his death. Because he was the firstborn son, he was provided with a college education whereas Betty was not, even though they were both excellent students. He always respected her for making way for him and was saddened that she was forced to do so. Vince became a champion of women during his career, insisting that they be promoted and paid as equals to men. I suspect that this was in some part due to his personal situation. Vince describes his childhood as "happy," filled with schoolwork and fun. In his words, he "succeeded in school which made life easier for me" (Vincent A. Fulginiti, personal communication, 1994). His father was a softie and his mother was a disciplinarian. He attributes his success to his Grandfather Perry's admonition to gain an education and to his mother Rose's ability to make him stick to it. His parents were co-owners of a grocery store with his Uncle Sam, so food was available even during the restrictions of World War II. Vince describes playing stickball in the streets, riding the trolley to Market Street for his mom (by age 8!), working in the store, and going to Catholic mass in the neighborhood. Attending mass persisted until his teens when he diverted away from the Church as he became more interested in science. His one childhood regret was his parents refused to speak Italian with him on the advice of his Grandfather Perry, who wanted the family to sound more American.

Vince attended South Philadelphia High School from 1946 to 1949. His high school years were filled with his friends, trips to the New Jersey shore, working in the grocery store, and "studying to be the top student" (Vincent A. Fulginiti, personal communication, 1994). He received a full scholarship to Temple University, where he met individuals from all different backgrounds. According to him, college was "daunting" because many of his classmates were smarter than he was. Vince earned a doctor of medicine degree from Temple in 1957 followed by a master of science degree in 1961. After medical school, Vince completed an internship at Philadelphia General Hospital and then a pediatric residency at St. Christopher's Hospital for Children. He was chief resident with Dr Ray Helfer during 1960 and 1961.

In the early years of his medical career, Vince thought he wanted to be a surgeon but changed his mind and chose pediatrics. His particular interest, infectious disease, was sustained throughout his career and resulted in numerous publications. One of my favorite memories involves the day I came home from school with a sore throat and he did a cursory examination. He was forever minimizing family perceived life-threatening injuries, like the time I had purple spots on my toe and he told me I had purple spotted toe disease and then slowed down and went back for a second look. Apparently, I had some rare version of *Streptococcus* and he became really animated and wanted to take a photograph of it.

My parents met in the hallway at Philadelphia General Hospital in a manner that varies depending on who is telling the story. Their first date was at the opera, to which they rode in a veritable chariot: a borrowed flower truck. Shirley was raised in Westfield, a small town in upstate Pennsylvania near the border with New York State. She had moved to Philadelphia to become a registered nurse. They were married in June 1957 at Old Swedes' Church in Philadelphia. Their first son, John Vincent, was born in 1959 followed by Jeffrey Thomas (b 1961), Laura Carr (b 1962), and Paul Anthony (b 1966). John and Jeff were born during Vince's tenure in Philadelphia, and Laura and Paul were born in Denver, where Vince and Shirley moved to in 1961. Vince had transferred to the University of Colorado so he could complete a fellowship with C. Henry Kempe, MD, and where he joined the faculty as an assistant professor of pediatrics.

At the University of Colorado Health Sciences Center, Vince was responsible for teaching medical students, conducting research, and attending to patient care. In 1969 Vince and Shirley were recruited to Tucson, Arizona, where the University of Arizona was building a new medical school. Dean Monte Duval asked Vince, at age 38, to be the founding department head for pediatrics, a role he described in 1992 as "the most important promotion I ever had" (Vincent A. Fulginiti, personal communication, 1994). Prior to assuming that role he loaded his entire family onto the SS Rotterdam for a transatlantic voyage to the Netherlands, where he conducted research at the Radiobiological Institute in Ryswick. We lived in a large apartment on the banks of a canal, attended the American school, and were introduced to all things Dutch, including wooden shoes, ice skates, Sinterklaas, and Zwarte Piete. The research stint in the Netherlands led to multiple publications on infectious diseases, book chapters, and an edited volume (see Further readings). Vince's lifelong involvement in research included an encyclopedic and first-hand knowledge of the virology of smallpox and other viruses and their treatment. This expertise led to numerous lectures after the terrorist attacks of September 11, 2001, when there was increased concern that the viruses could be weaponized.

Vince worked as the department chair of pediatrics at the University of Arizona Health Sciences Center for 16 years and was responsible for growing the department. His achievements during that time revolved around general pediatrics, pediatric infectious diseases, immunization and immunology, medical curriculum, health care ethics, and faculty development. His efforts included delineation of the underlying immunologic mechanisms involved in adverse reactions to smallpox vaccine. He was involved in the analysis of the abnormal reactions to killed measles virus vaccine (atypical measles) and to killed respiratory syncytial virus vaccine. During this time he was asked to provide testimony in the Salk versus Sabin vaccine trial. He made multiple contributions to the development, deployment, and assessment of a variety of viral vaccines and had a rare understanding and passion about viruses and their respective treatments. He was involved in the care of one of the first immunosuppressed children confined in a sterile bubble at the University of Arizona. Vince was heavily involved in the development of curricula for the medical students, residents, and fellows. He was a hands-on mentor who took every opportunity to educate no matter his audience. Everyone has a personal story about his mentorship and is happy to share it. Years ago I was working as the anthropology section chair on a committee for the American Academy of Forensic Sciences. The chair of the pathology/biology section was Dr Scott Denton, a forensic pathologist in Ohio. He stopped me after the meeting and introduced himself. He reminded me that he had been a resident at the University of Arizona and told me that his favorite memory of Vince was when he lectured to the residents about the importance of wearing a white shirt and tie when meeting with patients. Scott described how this went over like a lead balloon because it was the 1970s and all the residents were antiestablishment hippies. Then he laughed ruefully and later said, "You know, your dad was right. I wore one every day in Chicago at the Medical Examiner's Office and it served me well" (Scott Denton, personal communication, 2015). As a side note, Scott was wearing a white shirt with a tie when he told me this story and truthfully I have never seen him in "civvies."

John Fulginiti told a similar story at the memorial service for Vince: "I deliberately chose to wear a pink shirt to the public memorial event to celebrate my Dad's life. I assure you for my Dad the choice was very clear; you wear a white shirt with a suit. During one of the most poignant conversations I ever had with my dad, we discussed a news article about how the President of the United States had worn the 'wrong' color suit; he was being severely criticized for horrendous unprofessional behavior. I was idealistically annoyed that the President would be challenged over his suit color. My Dad was always a teacher and, as often happened with situations like this one; he turned it into a learning opportunity. During that specific conversation, my Dad and I spoke about topics such as responsibility, authority, leadership, respect, choices, professionalism, standing your ground, giving ground, tolerance, patience, expectations, and rules. My Dad believed his position and I believed mine and there was no real resolution. At the time, my part of the conversation ended with the statement, 'Just for that, I am going to wear a pink tuxedo to your funeral!' For the memorial event, I chose a black suit…, with a pink shirt".

Vince also was involved in early comprehension of the infectious complications of liver transplantation in children. He served as the chair of the American Academy of Pediatrics *Red Book* and was appointed to the National Vaccine Advisory Committee of the Public Health Service. He was a prolific writer, publishing more than 200 articles, many coauthored with the Department of Pediatrics faculty at the University of Arizona. He also published 4 edited volumes during his lifetime, 1 of which was a major text on the methods of analyzing clinical problem solving. His evolving interests led to the development of an interactive computer-based program in pediatric clinical problem solving at the University of Arizona. He spearheaded the development of digital multimedia and Web sites for evidence-based patient care and medical education.

When computers first became publicly available, Vince adopted the technology immediately and never looked back. He was a gadget guy; he loved new electronic gizmos and the computer changed the way he thought, the way he wrote, and the way he envisioned the world. He initiated the development of offices of education and computer laboratories for students in all 3 major academic institutions with which he was affiliated. During his tenure at the University of Arizona, Vince served as the assistant dean and then acting dean at the College of Medicine. He became the editor for the *American Journal of Diseases of Children*, a post he retained for 11 years. He hired Joanne Quane and me to work as his editorial assistants. Those years taught me a lot about Vince. He had boundless energy, his thought processes were lightning-quick, and he was extremely decisive. He was always moving forward, no matter the obstacles. He had access to a vast network of expert contacts that he could tap to review every aspect of pediatric medicine.

His interest in the administrative side of medical school led to an appointment by Neal Vanselow to the deanship at Tulane University School of Medicine. There, his appreciation for computing became an integral part of his administration. The staff at Tulane did not have e-mail when he became dean and it was one of the first things he attended to on arrival. He could not imagine conducting business without it. Like his mentor Monty Duval, Vince recruited professional colleagues to join him at Tulane to build and develop the School of Medicine. As he left Tulane, one of those colleagues, James (Jim) Corrigan, remained to fill his post as dean. Leadership produces leadership.

This leads me to a little aside. I recently cleared out the books in Vince's library and I discovered that whenever he and Shirley moved they bought each other all manner of tomes regarding the new place of residence. I found guide-books, novels, cookbooks, and historical volumes from Colorado, Arizona, Louisiana, and Europe (the Netherlands). If a book was written about a place they were living or that they planned to travel to, then they likely had a copy of it in their library. Vince loved to cook so the cookbooks were especially useful.

Vince was also known for his doodles, many of which were created during contentious or lively departmental meetings. He once told John that the complexity of the doodles reflected the complexity and vigor of the conversation during the meeting rather than boredom or inattention, as the faculty supposed. A collection of his work was secreted away by the faculty who presented it to him in book form when he moved from Tucson to New Orleans. After he died, I was going through his personal drawings and that collection is as relevant now as it was then.

After New Orleans, Vince was appointed chancellor of the University of Colorado Health Sciences Center. He became involved in establishing the University of Colorado as a leader in modern health education and patient care and in the analysis of the major issues facing academic health centers in the modern clinical/research/educational milieu. He had a quick, incisive mind that could foresee issues that would confront large academic health centers, and this enabled him to position his institution favorably for the changes to come. He and Shirley had a lifelong interest in biomedical ethics and this passion was fueled by summers at the Given Institute in Aspen, Colorado. Vince established the first encompassing health center ethics program as opposed to programs contained within a single health professional school. He published extensively on medical ethics and the hard choices he could see down the road. He wrote about, testified in support of, and personally honored the highest code of ethics for all physicians.

During his long and varied career, Vince received multiple awards including a Temple University scholarship; the Markle Scholarship; the Western Society for Pediatric Research Ross Award and Teaching Ross Award; multiple teaching excellence awards at each university with which he was affiliated; the American Academy of Pediatrics Jacobi Award; the St. Geme Award for Academic Leadership by the Federation of Pediatric Organizations and Research Societies; multiple alumni of the year awards; the Student Buffalo Award for Outstanding Service to Students at the University of Colorado Health Sciences Center (shared with Shirley, cited for bringing "soul" to the campus); the 1st Annual Veritas Award for "sustained commitment to the educational mission of the Humanities in health care" from the University of Colorado Health Sciences Center Program in Health Care Ethics, Humanities and Law; and the Joseph A. Sewall Award for Leadership and Vision (University of Colorado Health Sciences Center). Vince was humbled by the accolades and proud to be the recipient of such prestigious honors.

The crowning achievement of Vince and Shirley's career followed from the foresight to move the University of Colorado Health Sciences Center from downtown Denver to Aurora. This decision forever changed the institution and health care in Colorado and has served as a model for the rest of the country. The decision came at a time when the military was downsizing and large military complexes were being reduced in size or closed. Fitzsimons Army Base was one such entity, occupying a huge tract of land in the city of Aurora and scheduled to close by 1999. Vince, as chancellor of the University of Colorado Health Sciences Center, recognized that expansion in Denver was not feasible and looked to Fitzsimons as an opportunity to grow the campus. In the early 1990s, Vince toured the proposed site with some of his staff. They tell funny stories about standing bemusedly in the middle of acres of brush with Vince describing how the new complex would look. Vince convinced everyone that the move was imperative and ultimately created a coalition to back his idea. The Army wanted to preserve their hospital, the city officials of Aurora could envision the benefit to their city long term, and the University of Colorado administration could foresee a sprawling medical campus. As city councilwoman Edna Mosley said in 1996, "It's a natural. It's a win-win situation." [2].

Over time, the campus development moved off blueprints onto the acreage in Aurora. The complex is now a comprehensive medical mecca, the Anschutz Medical Campus, that houses Children's Hospital Colorado; the University of Colorado Hospital; nursing, pharmacy, and medical schools; graduate schools; and, the point of pride for the Fulginiti family, the Fulginiti Pavilion for Ethics and Humanities [3]. This Japanese architecture inspired building sits at the north end of a courtyard bounded fittingly by many buildings dedicated to various medical education pursuits. "The Fulginiti," as it has come to be called, is regularly the site of lectures, music, and art in an effort to cultivate the creative side of future health care providers and members of the community. There are an art gallery, meeting rooms, a large auditorium, and the Gossard Forum, which was deliberately designed in the round for maximum engagement of participants. Vince imagined the Gossard Forum as a special location for ongoing ethical debate in medicine. The art gallery has hosted truly unique and provocative works, including, recently, a collection of photographs depicting skeletons of individuals from an old hospital in Pueblo, Colorado. I had the good fortune to analyze these skeletons with my first mentor J. Michael Hoffman, MD, PhD, when I was a young forensic anthropologist. Odd how the winds of fortune blow; I was not involved in any way in the selection of this artwork for the Pavilion gallery.

The Pavilion represents the culmination of all of Vince and Shirley's varied interests. They loved the opera, theater, books, and travel. They were forever seeking new information and traveling to new and different places. Vince's mantra in life was "Do it." He vehemently spoke these words to me when I told him I had been asked to take a seat on the board of directors for the American Academy of Forensic Sciences. The words did not even make it out of my mouth before he said, "Do it." No questions, no hesitations. There is a sculpture suspended over the grand piano in the atrium of the Pavilion. Entitled "Bright Idea," it is composed of a series of white bubbles seemingly floating upwards towards the ceiling. The concept for Bright Idea is "the process of how thoughts happen; how we bounce ideas back and forth in our head (represented by the crescent shapes); how we talk with other people about them. Often, our ideas have holes in them, are missing parts, and are misshapen. But we keep thinking, processing information, and distilling input until everything filters down into the big and bright idea" [4]. This piece was commissioned in honor of Vince's vision by his friends. They each describe him using the same words: visionary, teacher, maverick, Renaissance man.

John and Paul Fulginiti describe Vince using many of the same terms. They encapsulate the qualities that Vince possessed and that he passed to us, to his grandsons, and to the many students and young faculty he mentored. John says, "Some of my Dad's proudest moments included celebrating my accomplishments such as good grades; he supported me as I tried new things such as joining the high school football team, becoming the editor of my high school newspaper, and getting my first job. Dad wrote me an extensive letter about life lessons while I was in Nicaragua as a member of the Tucson Chapter of Amigos de las Américas service organization. He was particularly proud when I had a major accomplishment in my education and professional career. Dad insisted on being the first person to shake my hand when I earned my doctorate. During one particular discussion about the future, I told him I had decided to work as an educator and I wanted to be a higher education administrator. I believe he never forgot that was my goal. When I became a university assistant dean, one of my colleagues (who knew my father very well), told me Dad's eyes twinkled when he announced my new position" (John V. Fulginiti, personal communication, 2015).

Paul says, "My father was always available, even before cell phones and tweets. These days we are so connected, it is easy to stay in touch multiple times a day. Looking back now, I realize my Dad created that for his children years before the Internet. He would make our lunch, and on the brown paper bags he would draw related pictures of favorite characters, full color, keeping us together. If he traveled, we each received gifts and would run to the door to greet him. I remember now taking an art class on Saturdays. This was a big deal back in the days of a local art store—maybe 20 people would gather in the back of the store. We still have the original paintings from then hanging on our walls. Later, we shared spread sheets and organizational charts, research. We shared a love of books and authors, many on shelves in my home now. My Dad surrounded us with love, and protected our dreams. I do wish he could be here now, but truth be told, he is with me always" (Paul A. Fulginiti, personal communication, 2015).

For me, I will remember him for his laugh, his energy, and his determination. He was always there for me, encouraging me, supporting me, loving me. As with John, he put the doctoral hood on me in a quiet street prior to the commencement ceremony when I received my PhD. He walked me down the aisle and he held my son in quiet reflection. Nothing made him happier than being surrounded by his family.

When Vince was diagnosed with cancer he faced it head-on, and rather than opting for a quiet death, he did "not go gentle into that good night" [5]. He wanted to continue his legacy of education and pushing the frontiers of research. So even though he knew it was likely futile, he agreed to take part in experimental drug studies, in the hope that maybe someone else would benefit from his experience. His bravery and pragmatism were a direct reflection of how he lived his life. To the end, he was a model for, and inspiration to, all who knew him.

GRANT MORROW III, MD

In the initial section of this tribute to the life of Vincent Fulginiti, his daughter discusses the accomplishments and enormous successes Vince achieved during his academic career. Drs Morrow and Lightner focus their comments and observations on what Vince did in the way of changing their careers in positive ways. For many of us his talents in mentoring people had more long-term impacts and mesh with what Laura described from a family point of view.

Vincent Fulginiti was an amazingly effective leader in the academic medical world and it was an extremely fortunate honor for both of us to have worked under him but, even more, to have been mentored by him in both of our careers. He would always take the ethical pathway when he had to make difficult decisions and, in fact, would maintain the high road even if it meant that it would cost him his job. His faculty knew and admired this trait and it was a major reason that he was so highly respected.

Although we did not know Vince at the time we were both trained, we were amazed to learn that all 3 of us spent our medical educations in Philadelphia and were at many of the same great institutions in the same cities. Vince grew up in South Philadelphia; received his bachelor of arts, master of science, and doctor of medicine degrees from Temple University; interned at Philadelphia General Hospital; and completed his residency at St. Christopher's Hospital for Children in Philadelphia. His major mentor was Dr Waldo E. Nelson, who was famous for the classic, "*Nelson Textbook of Pediatrics.*" This fact certainly was one of the linchpins that helped Vince succeed in his spectacular career. Both Dr Lightner and I received our doctor of medicine degrees from the University of Pennsylvania in Philadelphia and spent time as medical students at the University of Pennsylvania and as residents at Children's Hospital of Philadelphia, when at the same time Vince was an intern at Philadelphia General Hospital.

Vince also spent the early years of his academic career at the University of Colorado Medical Center from 1961 through 1968. From there he became department chair of pediatrics at the University of Arizona in 1969. Vince was an infectious disease fellow at the University of Colorado Medical Center at the same time that I was a rotating intern at Denver General Hospital, which was staffed by faculty from the University of Colorado.

When one gets to a certain age and reminisces about the important accomplishments and key associates in one's life, it is amazing how often there are similarities that surprisingly are discovered between the important teachers and their pupils. Vincent A. Fulginiti became one of those amazing individuals in both of our lives.

I was invited to visit the new medical school at the University of Arizona in 1969. Few faculty had been recruited and the first class of medical students had just been admitted. For a variety of reasons, a move at that time was not possible but I was so impressed with Vince's sincerity and commitment to building a first rate training program. Fortunately, Vince persisted and asked me to revisit in 1971. This time it worked, and I and my pediatrician wife, Janet Orttung, decided to move to Tucson due, in large part, to the fact that Vince was able to create an ambulatory job for her. The other major reason was that Shirley Fulginiti effectively helped in the recruitment as well as involving us in events once we were in Tucson such that both of us felt a comforting family atmosphere in both the department and the community.

We settled in quickly as did our children. Janet became 1 of the first 4 residents in the psychiatry program 2 years later and built her career as a child psychiatrist.

One of the important changes for me happened when Vince asked me to function as the temporary chair during his well-earned sabbatical year abroad. It was a complete time off for him, and I had to learn how to make a department function. Faculty members who called him to resolve a problem were told to call me. This period of time was essential in learning how to manage a young developing department of pediatrics and made my 1978 move to Columbus Children's Hospital much easier. I could not have survived in Columbus without Vince's mentoring.

Vince was always willing to talk with faculty and the times that we met to discuss issues were serious but often he would laugh at things to lighten up the meeting. It is somewhat hard to describe his laugh because it was somewhere between a guffaw and a nasal snort but it was always obviously a laugh. He carried over this discussion technique in his departmental meetings. One of the issues that bothered him was that the 2 pediatric wards, if not completely full, would have adults sometimes transferred to the pediatric beds. Vince was strongly opposed to this practice because he felt that it compromised the care. He always placed patient care and teaching on the wards as essential, first-order priorities.

His decisions always came down on the side of taking the ethically correct pathway, as seen in his later career when he resigned rather than take a position that he felt was ethically compromised. Once Vince retired, his only flaw was that at an advanced age he took up golf. Fortunately he took it up as a hobby and not a way of life, as many of us have.

ELMER S. LIGHTNER, MD

Laura Fulginiti, PhD, and Grant Morrow III, MD, have written eloquently of Dr Fulginiti's major contributions to us all. They have beautifully summarized his career and life in a detailed overview. My portion is shorter, and the focus is on his mentoring and guidance in developing my professional career.

I met Vince when he was an intern and I was a fourth-year medical student at Philadelphia General Hospital in 1958. We initiated a friendship that lasted until his death in 2013. In 1958, I had no idea what a major role he would play in my life. After graduating from the University of Pennsylvania School of Medicine, I completed my pediatric residency at the Children's Hospital of Philadelphia (1961). After 2 years in the Army, I entered a private practice of pediatrics in Tucson, Arizona (1963). During the years 1963 to 1968, Vince was at the University of Colorado and Grant Morrow was at the University of Pennsylvania. In 1969, Vince was named chair of the Department of Pediatrics at the new medical school in Tucson, Arizona. He had many tasks, but a first priority was to develop a pediatric student clerkship for the entering junior class. At this time, the full-time faculty was small; community pediatricians were needed to do monthly clinical teaching rotations. He asked me to assist him in developing the associate clinical faculty schedule for 1970 to 1971. We accomplished this. In July of 1970 I taught the first junior students in their clinical pediatric ward rotation. I enjoyed teaching tremendously and continued to teach on an intermittent basis. In early 1971 I was asked to join the full-time faculty (Dr Morrow joined in December 1971). Vince knew of my interest in endocrinology and his plan was to have me initially work 50% of my time in general pediatrics and 50% developing a pediatric endocrine service. This rare opportunity was available for me because Vince had prior knowledge of the pediatric endocrine program at the University of Colorado. The section was headed by Dr Henry Silver, a nationally recognized pediatric endocrinologist and educator, who had no formal pediatric endocrinology training (ie, no fellowship) but developed a successful endocrine program. Vince took the risk of offering me the same opportunity (without the same national recognition that Dr Silver had achieved). Within 2 years I was practicing endocrinology 100% of the time.

Before I discuss Vince's skill in mentoring a "townie," I digress with a few words about his goals for the new pediatric department. First, he wanted the department to be fully integrated with the community pediatricians. Second, he wanted to develop a superb educational experience for the students, residents, and, later, fellows. Third, he wanted the department to grow steadily in teaching, service, and research. Faculty growth occurred rapidly. Vince and his wife Shirley were excellent recruiters. Here was an opportunity for young pediatric subspecialists to join a new and exciting program. Community pediatricians served as valued teachers and clinicians from the first day of his arrival. Although this may have been a practical necessity at first, it was Vince's master plan to have the medical school faculty and practicing pediatricians work together to develop a superb education experience for students and residents. It takes a special person to accomplish this blend of goals and Vince was successful. With the cooperation of Tucson Medical Center (TMC) administration, the inpatient services at both TMC and the University Medical Center (UMC) were combined for educational purposes. In practical terms, this meant that students and residents were taught by both practicing pediatricians who primarily admitted to TMC and by full-time faculty who admitted patients primarily to the UMC. Pediatric subspecialists from the medical school were available for consultation at TMC at all times. In addition to the inpatient experience, pediatric residents spent time in the offices of the community pediatricians. A broad educational experience was provided and the classic town/gown battle was avoided.

In October 1971, when I joined the full-time faculty, there were approximately 10 full-time faculty and 1 or 2 pediatric residents. When Vince stepped down from the chairmanship in 1985, there were 33 to 34 full-time faculty, more than 35 associate faculty, 36 pediatric residents, and several fellowship programs. Major factors in such rapid growth can be attributed to Vince's interpersonal skills, academic enthusiasm, and plans for the future. His humanness was visible to all. Once when a member of my family was seriously ill and hospitalized he said, "take the time you need to resolve this important personal issue." People love to work for this kind of department chair. As the educational programs of the department evolved, the junior clinical clerkship in pediatrics was consistently voted by the medical students as the best educational experience in the clerkship. His dedication to teaching was transmitted to the entire faculty.

Back to personal mentoring: in October 1971, a major change occurred in my life. Instead of being a practicing pediatrician, I was now a full-time member of the academic pediatric department. I was asked to develop the section of pediatric endocrinology. Knowing I had Vince's full support was absolutely crucial. His expectations of me were clearly stated and he gave me the opportunity to proceed and grow without micromanagement.

I was provided with

1. Phone time to consult with other pediatric endocrinologists
2. Time and financial support to attend endocrine meetings and review courses
3. Invited pediatric endocrinologists to visit Tucson
4. Visited other pediatric endocrine programs and attend their clinics

Vince's door was always open for discussion and guidance. Other faculty were also supportive (especially Drs George Comerci and Grant Morrow). I was guided (sometimes painfully) to do clinical research; present at local, state, and national meetings; and join national endocrine societies. Within the department, he gave me increasing responsibilities in clinical service, teaching, research, and administration. With increasing responsibilities came new problems and issues. He gave me constant encouragement. At the time I did not recognize the true value and quality of such a skilled mentor. In fact, most of the time I did not know I was being "mentored." Sometimes only in reflection do we truly recognize the value of such a person. His mentoring was done with respect and kindness and in a positive manner. Without Vince's willingness to take a risk hiring me and his constant mentoring, the academic fulfillment I so valued and obtained would not have been possible. The wisest decision in my professional career was moving from private practice to academic medicine. Vince took a chance and gave me that opportunity.

Vince—allow me 1 small "complaint." I was never advised, during recruitment, of the publish-or-perish pathway. Had I known that, I might have remained in private practice. Because it all worked out, okay, you are forgiven.

In summary, when one reads about Dr Fulginiti's career and life, it is apparent that he was a gentleman; a loving husband, father, and grandfather; a pediatrician; a teacher; a scholar; a mentor to many; and a servant to society. The field of pediatrics, pediatric institutions, and the many, many children he helped, but mostly his family, will miss him greatly.

Acknowledgments

L.C. Fulginiti would like to thank her brothers John and Paul Fulginiti for their thoughtful contributions toward and helpful editing of this article, her mother Shirley Fulginiti for her memories and comments, and her husband Dan Martin for his support and judicious review. Dr E.S. Lightner would like to thank L.C. Fulginiti for her support.

References

[1] Fulginiti VA. Waldo Nelson (1898-1997): a giant in pediatrics. Adv Pediatr 2011;58:1–10.
[2] Robey R. CU med center seeks fitz move. The Denver Post 1996.
[3] Available at: http://www.ucdenver.edu/academics/colleges/medicalschool/administration/alumni/CUMedToday/Peaks/Pages/Fulginiti-Pavilion.aspx. Accessed August 10, 2015.
[4] Program, Dedication of "Bright Idea" at the Fulginiti Pavilion, CU 2014.
[5] Thomas D. Do not go gentle into that good night. New York: New Directions; 1952 [From The Poems of Dylan Thomas].

Further readings

Fulginiti VA. Virus and virus vaccine-induced immunological injury. In: Samter M, editor. Immunological disease, vol. 1. Little Brown & Co; 1978.
Fulginiti VA. A new pertussis vaccine: hope for the future? J Infect Dis 1983;148:146–7.
Fulginiti VA. Pertussis, disease, vaccine and controversy. J Am Med Assoc 1984;251:251.
Fulginiti VA. Interprofessional education: the right issue at the right time. In: Holmes DF, Osterweis M, editors. Catalysts in interdisciplinary education: innovation by academic health centers. Washington, DC: Association of Academic Health Centers; 1999.
Fulginiti VA. The risks of smallpox vaccination [letter]. J Am Med Assoc 2003;290:1452.
Fulginiti VA, Brunell PA. Special report: aspirin and reye syndrome. Pediatrics 1982;69:810–2.
Fulginiti VA, Leland OS, Kempe CH. Evaluation of measles immunization methods. Am J Dis Child 1963;105:5–11.
Fulginiti VA, Eller JJ, Downie AW, et al. Altered reactivity to measles virus: Atypical measles in children previously immunized with inactivated (killed) measles vaccines. J Amer Med Assoc 1967;202:1075–80.
Fulginiti VA, Kempe CH, Hathaway WE, et al. Progressive vaccinia in immunologically-deficient individuals. Birth Defects 1968;68:129ff.
Kempe CH, Fulginiti VA, Minamitani M, et al. Smallpox vaccination of eczema patients with a strain of attenuated live vaccinia (CVI-78). Pediatrics 1968;42:980–5.

Advances in Pediatrics 63 (2016) 15–46

ADVANCES IN PEDIATRICS

ELSEVIER
MOSBY

Advances in the Interdisciplinary Care of Children with Klinefelter Syndrome

Shanlee Davis, MD[a,b], Susan Howell, MS, CGC, MBA[a,c],
Rebecca Wilson, PsyD[c], Tanea Tanda, BS[a,c], Judy Ross, MD[d,e],
Philip Zeitler, MD, PhD[a,b], Nicole Tartaglia, MD, MS[a,c,*]

[a]Department of Pediatrics, University of Colorado School of Medicine, 13123 East 16th Avenue, Aurora, CO 80045, USA; [b]Department of Endocrinology, Children's Hospital Colorado, University of Colorado School of Medicine, 13123 East 16th Avenue B265, Aurora, CO 80045, USA; [c]Developmental Pediatrics, Children's Hospital Colorado, University of Colorado School of Medicine, 13123 East 16th Avenue B140, Aurora, CO 80045, USA; [d]Department of Pediatrics, Thomas Jefferson University School of Medicine, 833 Chestnut Street, Philadelphia, PA 19107, USA; [e]Pediatric Endocrinology, Nemours A.I. DuPont Hospital for Children, 1600 Rockland Road, Wilmington, DE 19803, USA

Keywords
• Klinefelter syndrome • 47,XXY • Sex chromosome aneuploidy

Key points

• Klinefelter syndrome is a common but underdiagnosed genetic condition with significant phenotypic variability in childhood.

• The pediatrician needs to be aware of the increased risk for neuro-developmental, psychological, and medical conditions that are associated with an additional X-chromosome.

• Over the next decade, we anticipate a sharp increase in diagnosis rates with advances in genetics, particularly prenatal and neonatal diagnoses.

K linefelter syndrome (KS) is a common genetic disorder characterized by an additional X-chromosome in male individuals leading to a karyotype of 47,XXY. The clinical syndrome was first described nearly 75 years ago in several male individuals with small testes, tall stature, gynecomastia, and azoospermia [1]. Our construct of what KS entails has greatly changed

*Corresponding author. Department of Pediatrics, Children's Hospital Colorado, University of Colorado School of Medicine, 13123 East 16th Avenue B140, Aurora, CO 80045. *E-mail address:* Nicole.tartaglia@childrenscolorado.org

0065-3101/16/$ – see front matter
http://dx.doi.org/10.1016/j.yapd.2016.04.020

since then with identification of the genetic etiology in 1959, epidemiologic studies of birth cohorts in the 1980s, the development of rodent models, and many observational and interventional clinical studies in boys and men with KS [2–4]. Characterization of the neuropsychological profile, along with earlier diagnosis, facilitates earlier developmental evaluation and intervention services [5]. Optimizing testosterone treatment may prevent some of the physical manifestations of the "classic KS phenotype" [6]. Advanced reproductive technology (ART) has made it possible for nearly half of men with KS previously deemed infertile to have an opportunity to have a biological child [7,8]. Despite these scientific advances, the underlying molecular mechanisms underlying primary testicular failure and the phenotypic heterogeneity of physical and neurocognitive features observed in KS remains elusive. In this review, we will provide the pediatrician with an update on what is known about the clinical manifestations and current treatment recommendations for boys and men with KS. Table 1 provides a summary of current treatment recommendations.

EPIDEMIOLOGY AND DIAGNOSIS

KS is the most common sex chromosomal aneuploidy, with estimated prevalence rates ranging between 1 in 448 to 1 in 917 male births [9–14]. A comparative analysis of newborn karyotyping studies published in the 1960s to 1970s and studies published in the 1970s to 1980s reported an increase in the prevalence of KS [14]. An increasing prevalence of KS could theoretically be explained by increasing maternal age, environmentally derived increase of errors in paternal meiosis I, and decreasing rate of elective termination for prenatally diagnosed KS, although this increasing prevalence needs to be confirmed and further evaluated [12,14,15]. Epidemiologic studies of sex chromosome aneuploidies have been limited to industrialized nationals, and to our knowledge, there have been no reports of ethnic differences in KS prevalence.

Currently, there is a significant discrepancy between the known prevalence of KS based on newborn screening studies and the rate of clinical diagnosis. It is estimated that only 25% to 35% of male individuals with KS are diagnosed in their lifetime, with the remaining 65% to 75% left undiagnosed. A study in the United Kingdom estimated that of all expected cases, approximately 10% of diagnoses are made in the prenatal period, 6% in childhood or adolescence, and 19% in adulthood [16]. The small number of children who are diagnosed before puberty are typically identified due to underdeveloped genitalia, hypotonia, developmental delays, or learning and behavior problems. Diagnoses made in adolescence are secondary to small testicular size, gynecomastia, or rarely, incomplete puberty. Adults are most commonly diagnosed for infertility; however, may present for symptoms of hypogonadism [13]. The low rate of diagnosis in the pediatric population is due to a combination of factors, including subtle or underrecognized features that overlap with typical children and genetic testing practices of most pediatricians that do not cover the most common neurodevelopmental features in KS, such as reading disabilities or

Table 1
Pediatric evaluation and treatment recommendations for XXY/KS

Neurodevelopmental/ psychological risk	Recommendation for follow-up and further evaluation

Developmental delay (age 0–3 y)	• Developmental and ASD screening by PCP per AAP recommendations, and
	• Referral for comprehensive developmental assessments for all children, with evaluation of cognitive, speech-language, motor, social, and adaptive functioning domains using standardized measures.
	  ○ If prenatal diagnosis: evaluations at 9–15 mo, 18–24 mo, and 30–36 mo; sooner or more frequent if any developmental concerns.
	  ○ If postnatal diagnosis: evaluation at diagnosis, and then at ages recommended above.
	• If indicated, initiation of early interventions including developmental, speech, occupational, physical, or behavioral therapies.

Learning disabilities	• Monitoring of learning and academic performance from preschool throughout education. • Psychological evaluations to assess cognitive functioning, learning disabilities (reading and/or math) at key times during education and transitions: early elementary, late elementary, middle school, high school, transition to postsecondary programming/education. • Special education supports (504 plans or Individual Education Plans) as needed. • Evidence-based interventions for learning disabilities if identified. • Consideration of additional academic supports, tutoring, options for schools/educational settings. • Education of parents/caretakers about EF and manifestations of symptoms of EF deficits.
ADHD/EF problems	• Screening by school system and PCP with input from family and school, as presentation may vary in different environments. Recognition that ADHD-inattentive symptoms are more common in XXY. • Formal evaluation of EF and attention by psychologist or neuropsychologist beginning at 7–8 y of age, and at key times during education: late elementary, middle school, high school, transition to postsecondary programming. • Implementation of educational strategies and supports for EF and ADHD symptoms at school and home if present. • Consideration of medication treatment for attention disorders/ADHD if present.

Speech-language disorders	• Assessment with an experienced pediatric speech and language pathologist with evaluation of expressive-receptive language abilities, higher-order language skills, pragmatic/social use of language, and disorders of speech production (developmental dyspraxia/apraxia) or hypernasality due to possible VPI.
	  ○ Recommended yearly from birth to 4 y, then every 2–3 y depending on presence or severity of impairment.
	  ○ Referral to ear, nose, and throat physician if concerns of hypernasality, VPI
	• Speech-language therapy through early intervention, school system, and/or privately if indicated.
	• Consideration of role of speech difficulties in behavior/frustration.

(continued on next page)

Table 1
(continued)

Neurodevelopmental/ psychological risk	Recommendation for follow-up and further evaluation
Motor skills	• Beyond age 3, monitoring of fine and gross motor skills, balance, coordination, motor planning. OT and/or PT interventions if motor deficits causing difficulties with handwriting, play or recreational activities, dressing, eating, or other self-care skills.
Social skills difficulties	• Social development and ASD screening by PCP per AAP recommendations, and • Evaluation by developmental pediatrician, child psychiatrist and/or psychologist for evaluation if concerns of social functioning or ASD. • Consideration of whether social immaturity and/or language deficits contribute to social difficulties. • Therapy/counseling, school supports and/or medication treatment if indicated. • Consideration of social skills therapy/groups in academic setting or privately. • Involvement in clubs/activities of interest where peers share interests. • If ASD, evidence-based and individualized Applied Behavior Analysis therapies, such as ESDM.
Emotional/behavioral difficulties, anxiety	• Evaluation by developmental pediatrician, child psychiatrist, and/or psychologist for evaluation and treatment if concerns. • Involvement of school psychology/counseling team, incorporation of behavioral supports in school environment, consideration of contributions of bullying. • Consideration of behavioral responses relative to developmental level instead of chronological age. • Adaptations should be made in therapy approach if language deficits are present, parental involvement in therapy. • Consideration of medication treatment as indicated for anxiety, emotional lability, depression, mood dysregulation, irritability. • Consideration of OT/sensory-based approaches to address self-regulation, especially in younger ages or if difficulties with self-expression during therapy. • Consideration of complementary therapies, including equine therapy, art/music therapy, yoga.
Adaptive functioning problems	• Evaluation of adaptive functioning using standardized measures, including domains of self-care, communication, social, community use, safety and self-direction should be included as part of the psychological or educational evaluations recommended above. • Consideration of OT or other therapies for support throughout childhood and adolescence.

Medical features/risks	Recommendation for follow-up and further evaluation
Cardiovascular	
Congenital anomalies	• Cardiology consultation and/or echocardiogram/electrocardiogram for all new diagnoses or after birth in a prenatal diagnosis.
Dyslipidemia	• Cholesterol screening with lipid panel at age 9–11 and then again after puberty per AAP. 　○ Sooner and/or more frequent if family history and/or noted abnormalities.
Abdominal obesity, fatty liver disease, insulin resistance, metabolic syndrome	• Anticipatory guidance for establishing a healthy diet and active lifestyle in childhood. • If obesity is present, screening should include alanine aminotransferase and HbA1C. Referral to weight management programs if indicated.
Dental	
Enamel defects/caries Taurodontism	• Dental evaluation beginning at age 1, followed by dental visits twice per year or per dentist recommendation.
Endocrinologic	
Hypogonadism/ testosterone deficiency	• Consider consultation with Pediatric Endocrinology at approximately 2 mo of age. • Pubertal examination with every annual physical examination. • Referral to Pediatric Endocrinology at first sign of puberty or by age 10 y. • Monitoring of serum gonadotropins and testosterone every 6 mo when pubertal. • Consideration of testosterone supplementation based on provider assessment and family preference. The goal of treatment is to replace deficient endogenous testosterone production and support development of secondary sex characteristics, bone health, metabolic function, psychosocial health, and prevent consequences of hypogonadism, including gynecomastia and tall stature. Overtreatment should be avoided.
Gynecomastia	• Palpation for breast tissue with every annual physical examination. • Early referral to Endocrinology for any gynecomastia. Consideration of treatment with testosterone, aromatase inhibitors, and antiestrogens, and/or surgical resection if medical management fails.
Subfertility	• Consider semen analysis in adolescence if developmentally appropriate. • Consider referral to reproductive urologist with experience in testicular sperm extraction in KS if desired. • Ensure adequate dietary intake of calcium and vitamin D.
Osteopenia/ osteoporosis	• Consider measurement of vitamin D stores and replacement if deficient. • No current role for routine bone density measurement in pediatrics.

(continued on next page)

Table 1
(continued)

Medical features/risks	Recommendation for follow-up and further evaluation
Genetics	• If a prenatal diagnosis, postnatal confirmatory genetic testing is recommended, including florescence in situ hybridization testing for mosaicism. • Consultation with genetic counselor and/or clinical genetics on diagnosis. • Consultation in early adulthood; consider preimplantation genetic testing if paternity is pursued.
Genitourinary Undescended testes, inguinal hernia, hypospadias	• Referral to Urology if present. • Consider testicular tissue biopsy and preservation if surgery is indicated.
Microphallus	• Referral to Pediatric endocrinology or Urology if present in infancy. Short course of testosterone can be discussed.
Gastrointestinal/feeding Newborn feeding difficulties	• Lactation specialist, feeding therapy through occupational or speech therapist if indicated. • Weight/growth monitoring by PCP.
Reflux/constipation/abdominal complaints	• Evaluation and treatment with primary care provider if present. Referral to gastrointestinal consult if indicated. Consideration of eosinophilic esophagitis.
Hematology/oncology Hypercoagulability	• Awareness of increased hypercoagulable risk and symptoms (deep vein thrombosis, pulmonary embolism). • Prophylaxis in high-risk clinical situations (eg, orthopedic surgery, central lines). • Hypercoagulability evaluation and/or referral to Hematology if blood clot diagnosed.
Malignancy risk	• Palpation for breast tissue with every annual physical examination. Evaluation of any discrete masses. • CXR to rule out mediastinal mass if symptoms of cough, dyspnea, or chest pain. Immediate evaluation/endocrine referral for precocious puberty. Evaluation to include serum β-HCG and alpha-fetoprotein.
Immunology Autoimmune diseases	• Discussion and monitoring of symptoms of autoimmune disease with PCP. • Thyroid function screening every 1–2 y starting at age 10, sooner or more frequent if symptoms of hypothyroidism or hyperthyroidism are present.

Musculoskeletal	
Pes planus (flat feet)/ ankle pronation	• Referral to PT or orthopedics for consideration of orthotics if causing pain, limiting activities, or affecting motor coordination or motor skills.
Tall stature	• Considerations of adaptations if needed at home and school (ie, larger chairs/desks).Recognition that tall stature can lead to expectations of more mature behavioral functioning, when social maturity in KS may be average or slightly delayed relative to peers.
Neurologic	
Seizures	• Neurologic history, including questions about staring spells or atypical movements. Neurology consultation and/or EEG and brain MRI may be indicated. Anticonvulsant medication(s) if indicated.
Tremor	• Monitoring for intention and/or postural tremor, most commonly in upper extremities. Referral to Neurology and consideration of medication as needed or for daily use if interfering with school (handwriting), work tasks, daily living skills (dressing, eating).
Pulmonary	
Allergies/reactive airways/respiratory infections	• Management through PCP, referral if needed.
Sleep apnea	• Sleep study if symptoms of sleep apnea present (ie, daytime fatigue, short sleep latency, difficulty with morning awakening, snoring, apnea).

Abbreviations: AAP, American Academy of Pediatrics; ADHD, attention-deficit/hyperactivity disorder; ASD, autism spectrum disorder; CXR, chest radiograph; EEG, electroencephalogram; EF, executive function; ESDM, early start denver model; KS, Klinefelter syndrome; OT, occupational therapy; PCP, primary care practitioner; PT, physical therapy; VPI, velopharyngeal insufficiency.

speech-language disorders. Additionally, although most boys with KS will have mild to moderate neurodevelopmental and/or learning difficulties, there is phenotypic heterogeneity and approximately a quarter of boys with KS do not exhibit these challenges [5]. Finally, there appears to be a delay in diagnosis relative to when parents first expressed concern about their child to their physician, particularly for concerns of development [17]. When initial parental concerns were due to developmental delays, there was on average 4.8 years before genetic testing confirmed KS. The delay in diagnosis was only 2 years when parental concern was pubertal development, microorchidism, or gynecomastia; however, the average age of diagnosis in that cohort was still older than 20 years [17]. Therefore, recognition of features of KS by the pediatrician can result in increased diagnosis rate and more appropriate care.

The diagnosis of KS is made with prenatal or postnatal karyotype or DNA microarray. Historically, prenatal screening by ultrasound and/or maternal serum biochemical markers dramatically increased identification of pregnancies at risk for autosomal aneuploidies, yet KS pregnancies have failed to correlate with these screening markers. However, new prenatal genetic screening technology, referred to as noninvasive prenatal testing (NIPT), analyzes cell-free fetal DNA circulating in maternal blood. This low-risk screening modality is typically performed in the first trimester and can detect sex chromosome aneuploidies (SCA). Although sensitivity and specificity of NIPT is high for the detection of autosomal trisomies, there is a lower accuracy for SCA. In a recent study by Meck and colleagues [18], NIPT specific to XXY was shown to have a positive predictive value of only 67% (confidence interval 22.3%–95.7%). Moreover, a 2014 study by Wang and colleagues [19] identified that 8% of NIPTs positive for SCA were due to an abnormal maternal karyotype. Thus, in cases of NIPT positive for SCA, both follow-up diagnostic testing (by prenatal chorionic-villous sampling, amniocentesis, and/or postnatal blood testing) and maternal karyotyping are recommended. Although a relatively high rate of false positives remain, NIPT creates a landmark opportunity to dramatically increase prenatal ascertainment of KS, with estimates citing the diagnosis rate for infants would increase tenfold if NIPT were to be standard screening for all pregnancies. There has also been discussion about including Fragile X on standard newborn screen, which would also identify some cases of KS [20]. With the possible increasing prevalence and significantly increasing childhood ascertainment rate, the pediatrician will likely care for more infants and children with a known diagnosis of KS.

GENETICS

KS was confirmed to be attributed to the presence of a supernumerary X-chromosome resulting in a karyotype of 47,XXY by Drs Jacobs and Strong in 1959 [21]. The supernumerary X-chromosome is acquired randomly predominantly through meiotic nondisjunction events during maternal or paternal gametogenesis or secondarily through postzygotic nondisjunction during early embryonic mitotic divisions [22]. The supernumerary X-chromosome is inherited from the mother in approximately 50% of cases, and from the father in the other 50% [23]. Up to half of cases with maternally derived supernumerary X cases are due to errors in meiosis I and become more common with increasing maternal age, whereas maternal meiosis II nondisjunction errors and paternal errors are not associated with parental age. The 2008 study by Morris and colleagues [14] describing an increase in the prevalence of KS proposes that environmental factors have led to increased paternal meiosis I errors; however, this finding remains controversial.

Mosaicism

Although approximately 90% of KS cases are nonmosaic 47,XXY, mosaicism is identified in approximately 7% of cases, and the other 3% are made up of rare variants [13]. Mosaic forms of KS are identified when the XXY cell line is found in the presence of another cell line, such as 46,XY or other karyotypes (ie, 47,XYY or 47,XXX). The phenotypic variability of mosaic KS is dependent on the karyotype and percentage of the additional cell lines. In cases of XXY/XY mosaicism, phenotypic symptoms may present more mildly and many cases fail to be identified. In cases of XXY mosaicism with abnormal karyotypes, such as XXY/XXYY or XXY/XXXY, phenotypic presentation may be more severe. Routine karyotype studies analyze approximately 20 cells; however, in the case of possible mosaicism, additional testing should be pursued by florescence in situ hybridization of the X and Y chromosomes to analyze a larger number of interphase nuclei. A significant limitation to testing for mosaicism is that peripheral blood may not accurately reflect levels of mosaicism across different tissue types, so phenotypic interpretation continues to be heavily dependent on clinical evaluation.

Since the original 1959 report of KS being caused by a single extra X-chromosome, several other rare sex chromosome variations in male individuals have been identified and characterized by the presence of 2 or more extra X and Y chromosomes, including 48,XXYY, 48,XXXY, and 49,XXXXY syndromes, occurring in 1:18,000 to 1:100,000 male births. Although these syndromes have been labeled as "variants" of KS because of shared features, including hypergonadotropic hypogonadism and tall stature, these syndromes are characterized by a more severe phenotype, including additional physical findings, congenital malformations, medical problems, and psychological features [24,25].

The mechanisms of how the presence of supernumerary X-chromosome(s) impact phenotypic features and variability observed in KS continue to be poorly understood. Studies continue to investigate the most implicated mechanisms, including gene dosage, skewed X-inactivation, genetic polymorphisms, and parental origin of the supernumerary X-chromosome. Many of these potential mechanisms suggest an important role of epigenetic processes in KS.

Gene dosage and expression

Gene dosage compensation is the mechanism of equalizing gene expression between male (XY) and female (XX) individuals due to the different number of genes contained on the sex chromosomes. This genetic equalization is achieved through a process of X-inactivation, in which one of the X-chromosomes in every female cell is randomly silenced, leaving only 1 X-chromosome transcriptionally active. In cases of X-chromosome aneuploidy, each X-chromosome in excess of 1 is inactivated by this same mechanism. However, 2 homologous regions of the sex chromosomes, known as pseudoautosomal regions (PAR1 and PAR2), as well as an additional 5% to 15% of X-chromosome genes, escape inactivation and are expressed from both X-chromosomes [26,27]. An extra copy of these "escapee" genes are therefore transcriptionally active in male individuals with KS, and overexpression then leads to excess mRNA and gene product, subsequently affecting the cellular and developmental pathways affected by these genes. The observation that clinical phenotype progressively deviates as the number of supernumerary sex chromosomes increases further supports this theory. This overexpression of escapee genes continues to be heavily studied as a likely mechanism leading to the phenotype and impacting phenotypic variability in KS.

An example of such an X-linked escapee gene is the short stature homeobox gene (SHOX), which has demonstrated a gene dosage impact in SCAs. SHOX is located within the pseudoautosomal region (PAR1) of the X-chromosome and encodes a transcription factor expressed in the developing skeleton impacting height. Short stature seen in Turner syndrome (45,X) has been established to result from haploinsufficiency of SHOX. Although tall stature in KS partially results from slower closure of epiphyseal plates secondary to hypogonadism, SHOX overexpression has also been implicated in the accelerated growth velocity and increased height observed in sex chromosome trisomies [28].

Further studies have analyzed differential genetic expression patterns in men with KS compared with male and female controls with the hope of elucidating differences in gene expression and regulation. In 2007, Vawter and colleagues [29] compared 11 men with KS with 6 XY male individuals by whole genome expression array and identified differential expression of 129 genes, 14 of which were X-linked genes and many of which showed correlation with verbal cognition. Additional studies evaluating genetic expression differences in brain, testes, and blood further suggest that autosomal genes are also differentially expressed in KS [30–32]. More recently, Zitzmann and colleagues [33] compared gene expression patterns of 132 male individuals with KS with male and female controls. This study identified differential gene expression in 36 total genes (21 X-linked and 15 autosomal) compared with male controls and 86 total genes compared with female controls (46 Y-linked, 10 X-linked, and 30 autosomal). Several of these identified X-linked genes are known to escape X-inactivation and are involved in pathways associated with phenotypic physical findings commonly seen in KS and therefore considered likely candidates to the pathophysiology of KS. Understanding the role of differential gene expression differences in KS is made more complex by the recent finding of increased copy number variations of X-chromosome genes in KS compared with typical male and female individuals, most of which were duplications and falling within areas that escape X-inactivation [34]. Further work is needed to investigate regulatory mechanisms influencing differential gene expression, not only in escapee genes, but also across the entire genome as it relates to KS.

Skewed X-inactivation

Another genetic mechanism possibly leading to phenotypic variation in KS is skewed X-inactivation. Typically, X-inactivation is a random process resulting in a ratio of active to inactive X-chromosome alleles (outside of the PARs) of approximately 50%. Skewed X-inactivation, defined as greater than 80% methylation of 1 allele, results from preferential inactivation of a specific X-chromosome. Studies analyzing skewed X-inactivation in patients with KS have ranged in finding fewer than 10% to more than 40% of subjects with skewing, and conflicting results regarding association of phenotypic features with skewing [35–37].

In 2014, the evaluation of Skakkebaek and colleagues [38] of 73 male individuals with KS found no association between skewed X-inactivation and cognition or psychological phenotypic variation. They did however find a significant correlation between skewed X-inactivation and smaller gray matter volume in the left insula of the brain. The insular cortex area of the brain plays an important role in social, emotional, and mental processing, all of which are variably affected in KS [39]. Caution should be taken for interpretation of results from any study of X-inactivation, however, as X-inactivation is typically measured in peripheral blood but can vary between tissues. Further, effects of skewed X-inactivation itself remain dependent on the polymorphisms and activity of the genes expressed from the more active chromosome, which varies between individuals.

Parental origin

Several studies have analyzed phenotypic variability in KS based on parental origin of the supernumerary X-chromosome and possible differential expression of maternal versus paternal alleles. To date, these results have been inconsistent. Although most studies are unable to establish a significant correlation between parental origin and phenotypic variability [36,38,40,41], some studies have demonstrated a higher incidence of findings when the supernumerary X-chromosome was paternally derived, including developmental problems, altered steroidogenesis, increased hematocrit, later puberty, insulin resistance, and cardiac findings of a shorter QTc time [33,42,43].

Gene polymorphisms

Another gene of interest in KS is the androgen receptor gene (AR), which is located on the X-chromosome and contains a highly polymorphic CAG trinucleotide repeat, with a normal range of 9 to 37 CAG repeats [36,44,45]. Studies have correlated the CAG repeat length with physiologic androgen effects, in which receptor activity is inversely related to the length of CAG repeat [36]. Several studies have demonstrated the CAG repeat length to be correlated with variable characteristics of the KS phenotype. Studies have reported a correlation of long CAG repeat length (low receptor activity) with height, arm span, likelihood for gynecomastia, small testes, HDL cholesterol, hematocrit, and later reactivation of pituitary-testicular axis, all of which are more characteristic of a more "severe" KS phenotype [36,41,46]. Additional studies have also demonstrated correlations of short CAG repeat length (high receptor activity) to longer penile length, higher bone density, and higher likelihood of having a stable partnership or professional employment [36,43,47]. Not all studies have supported phenotypic correlations with CAG repeat number, however, including a study of 73 men with KS in which there was no correlation with psychological phenotypic variation [38], and a study of 50 boys with KS in which there was no relationship with cognitive or motor development [48].

Genetic counseling

Genetic counseling in KS is important in multiple settings, including in the setting of a prenatal diagnosis, pediatric/adolescent cases with a new diagnosis, and in adulthood. For parents with an intrauterine diagnosis of KS, it is important for them to know there is no increased risk for miscarriage [49]. Prenatal or pediatric counseling should provide a comprehensive depiction of the phenotypic variability in KS, as well as include recommendations for developmental assessments/interventions, neuropsychological assessments/academic supports, social and emotional assessments/supports, indicated medical evaluations, including endocrinology evaluation for testosterone replacement, current reproductive options, timing and approach to disclosure, and information regarding both local and national support groups [50].

Counseling regarding fertility and options for fathering children in KS has changed significantly in the past decade with advancing reproductive technology. Historically the presence of infertility in KS was considered universal, and azoospermia continues to be present in the vast majority of men with KS. However, research has supported that up to 8% of men with KS have a small number of sperm in ejaculate [51,52], and there are rare case reports of spontaneous pregnancies. Much more promising is the current success rate of 50% to 60% in fathering biological children using advance reproductive techniques including microsurgical dissection of sperm from the testicle followed by in vitro fertilization, described in more detail in the endocrinology section later in this article. Although reported outcomes of children fathered from men with KS have been reassuring overall and most children have normal karyotypes, there have been slightly increased rates of children with KS and autosomal abnormalities reported. Preimplantation genetic diagnosis is available [53]. Due to a relatively young field, these risks require additional research. Regardless, it is important that counseling in all cases of KS emphasizes updated information about successes in the field of fertility, as this is a significant area of concern for parents, adolescents, and adults with KS [54–56]. It is also important to provide counseling related to other options for fatherhood chosen by many men with KS, including sperm donation and adoption.

Disclosure

With the advances in prenatal screening and increasing attention about KS in the medical literature, rates and ages of ascertainment are bound to improve. As such, pediatricians are often consulted by parents regarding decisions on when and how to disclose the diagnosis to the child. Research into other types of parent-to-child disclosures have identified barriers to communication causing possible avoidance of disclosure, including parents having difficulty understanding and/or being emotionally upset by the information, as well as being uncertain when and how to explain the information to the child and the child's ability to understand [57–59]. A recent study by Dennis and colleagues [60] evaluated the disclosure process of an SCA diagnosis from both parents and individuals, including 68 parents of male individuals with XXY and 58 individuals with XXY. Study results identified important common themes and experiences, which led to formulation of recommendations supporting that the disclosure process include discussing the diagnosis gradually, honestly, and simply with age-appropriate terms and a positive attitude. Results further supported telling the child early, such as during childhood or before puberty, possibly prompted by when the child starts asking questions or if interventions are being pursued. Parents and individuals participating in this study encouraged the disclosure process to incorporate elements of support, including pointing out the child's strengths, encouraging the child to ask questions, recognizing the common prevalence of the condition, and acknowledging research advancements and future possibilities [61]. Resources for parents about disclosure are available at www.genetic.org.

DEVELOPMENT, BEHAVIOR AND PSYCHOLOGY

Early development

There is significant variability in the developmental profiles of boys with KS; however, there is an elevated risk for mild to moderate developmental delays for which monitoring is important so interventions can be implemented if needed. Prospective studies of infants with KS diagnosed by newborn screening identified speech-language delays in 75% and motor skills delays in 50% [62–65]. Average age of milestones, including first words and first steps, are each approximately 2 to 3 months later compared with typical XY peers. Although these delays are milder in comparison with other genetic disorders, such as Fragile X or Down syndrome, speech and motor deficits do not generally resolve without therapies, and thus early intervention is recommended on identification of a delay in 1 or more developmental domains. In 25% to 50% of cases, early development progresses typically without significant developmental concerns or apparent need for intervention.

In young boys with speech delays, language testing most often shows a pattern, with receptive language skills higher than expressive skills [62,66,67]. An increased frequency of difficulties with oromotor planning and coordination called apraxia or dyspraxia of speech has also been described and can contribute to the expressive language delays in XXY [68]. Language difficulties can take a toll early in the development of self-expression and can impact tolerance for frustration, regulation of interpersonal challenges, and are often cited as likely contributory factors to behavioral concerns [69]. Speech-language evaluation of the young child with KS should occur yearly for the first 3 years of life or on diagnosis, and should include assessment of all language domains as well as evaluation for features of apraxia so that appropriate therapy techniques can be implemented.

Motor delays are present in approximately 50% of boys with KS, and hypotonia is commonly associated [48,70]. Other common features such as mild hypermobility, pes planus with ankle pronation, and/or genu valgum can further affect motor development. Motor domains, including dexterity, coordination, and graphomotor skills, are commonly areas of weakness, which can then lead to difficulties with handwriting and self-care skills, such as dressing, tying shoes, and eating (Martin S, Cordeiro L, Richarson P, et al. The association of motor skills and adaptive functioning in XXY/Klinefelter and XXYY syndromes. Manuscript Pending Review.) [48,70]. Physical and/or occupational therapy can be helpful for addressing motor and self-care difficulties. Orthotics are often prescribed for pes planus to support motor development and prevent lower extremity pain.

Cognitive, language, and learning profiles

Early studies of KS that reported increased rates of intellectual disability were flawed by ascertainment bias as they sampled populations from mental health settings and long-term care facilities rather than a broader representative sample [71–74]. Since that time, our understanding of the cognitive profile in KS has evolved, and studies have established that the average full-scale IQ ranges from 90 to 100, with expected variability around the mean from low to above average following a standard distribution [3,5,75]. In this respect, many individuals with KS will not be significantly impacted by cognitive concerns and will achieve success in academic, personal, and career endeavors. On the other hand, statistically significant discrepancies have been shown relative to the general population and biological sibling controls. The overall mean for individuals with KS falls in the 90s and 5 to 10 points lower than the population and sibling controls [66,76–78]. In most studies, Verbal IQ scores are found to be lower than Performance/Nonverbal IQ scores, and it is these deficits in the verbal conceptual domain that account for the downward skewing of Full-Scale IQ [75]. In this respect, nonverbal, visual perceptual, and spatial reasoning abilities are often an area of strength relative to verbal reasoning weaknesses.

Weaknesses in verbal skills align with speech-language profiles that commonly show difficulties in many language-related domains, and language disorders can be identified in 50% to 75% of boys with KS through adolescence [66,67,79]. Generally, basic receptive and expressive vocabulary skills are intact. As language skills advance and become more complex, higher-level language deficits are common, including poor grasp of verbal concepts, verbal processing difficulties, slow verbal processing speed, decreased verbal fluency, word retrieval problems, social communication difficulties, and difficulty with open-ended narrative construction [62,66,77,79–82]. Understanding the behavior of male individuals with KS in the context of their language abilities is important, both in terms of processing language and formulating verbal responses. For example, slower verbal processing can make highly verbal situations, such as classroom lectures or interpersonal interactions, more challenging or anxiety-provoking, and difficulty with word retrieval and/or language formulation can then affect speed and content of verbal responses in both educational and social settings. Speech-language therapy can continue to play an important role beyond early language development, and speech-language evaluation is recommended for all children and teens with KS displaying behavioral, social, or educational difficulties to determine if therapies addressing higher-level language skills and social/pragmatic language may be helpful.

In the school-aged years, boys with KS are at higher risk than the general population for language-based learning disabilities, including dyslexia [83,84]. Occurrence ranges between 50% and 80% [62,66,78], and family history of learning disability increases this risk [85]. More broadly, approximately 80% of boys with KS require some form of specialized support in school for language-based learning or reading concerns [62]. This is typically provided in the form of an Individualized Education Plan (IEP) or 504 plan, and it is strongly recommended that providers take an assertive stance with regard to advocating for intervention and educational supports. Lapses in support and intervention tend to create significant delays that are difficult to remediate. Evidence-based treatment approaches for reading disorders such as Linda-Mood-Bell or Orton-Gillingham are recommended, either through special education and/or private reading therapy. The high prevalence of learning disabilities in KS justifies periodic neuropsychological evaluation for all children with KS, starting in early grade school when early literacy is developing and deficits are simpler to address. Reassessment of cognitive and academic skills approximately every 3 years is then recommended, as deficits may not arise in some individuals until material becomes more complex and abstract with age. If lack of a formal learning disability diagnosis disqualifies a student from an IEP or educational supports, then advocating for services under the medical/health condition of KS with associated learning and executive functioning deficits is often successful to provide additional support.

Neuropsychological studies in KS have also consistently identified an increased risk for deficits in executive function (EF), including attention, working memory, cognitive flexibility, task initiation, fluency, and inhibition [86–90]. Executive dysfunction can have broad effects across home, school, and occupational settings, where additional supports in initiating, organizing, and executing tasks and assignments are often needed. Recent research in KS has also linked decreased EF and inhibition to increased behavioral difficulties, including aggression, rule-breaking behavior, and thought problems [91]. Neuropsychological and educational assessment in KS should include direct evaluation of EF, and parents and teachers should be educated about behavioral manifestations of EF difficulties, as well as effective interventions and supports, which should be included as part of a comprehensive educational plan.

There is an increased risk for attentional problems, and attention-deficit/hyperactivity disorder (ADHD) diagnosis rates range from 36% to 63% [48,92,93]. Distractibility and inattentive symptoms are more common than hyperactivity and impulsivity. It is important for children with KS who have attentional difficulties to have a neuropsychological evaluation that includes assessment of attention and EF, as well as other comorbidities that might present as inattention, such as learning disability, language disorder, or anxiety [77,94,95]. There is a positive response to treatment of ADHD symptoms with stimulant or nonstimulant ADHD medication in approximately 75% of patients, and thus a trial of medication(s) should be recommended as per standard ADHD treatment guidelines. However, as with other neurodevelopmental disorders, medications should be started at a lower dose and advanced conservatively while monitoring for side effects, and the contribution of comorbidities, such as anxiety or learning disabilities, should be considered if there is poor medication response or side effects. In complex or difficult cases, referral to developmental pediatrics or child psychiatry for medication management is recommended.

Behavior/social-emotional development

Studies report a range of behavioral features and psychological risks that can be associated with KS, including behavioral difficulties, social-emotional immaturity, low frustration tolerance, decreased self-esteem, and emotional sensitivity, along with higher rates of anxiety and depressive concerns [5,56,69,91,96–99]. As with other associated features, there is broad variability in the presence and severity of these symptoms between individuals with KS. Behavioral and emotional concerns should be screened for routinely, with referrals made for further psychological evaluation and therapy/counseling as needed. Counselors and therapists often have to modify therapeutic approaches due to the presence of language disorders and difficulties with self-expression, and thus identifying a therapist with experience working with children with delays or disabilities is helpful. Occupational therapy approaches to teach sensory-based self-regulation strategies are often less verbal and can be very successful for patients with KS throughout childhood. Psychopharmacologic medication treatment should be considered in childhood through adulthood to address behavioral or emotional regulation, anxiety, or depression if these symptoms are affecting home, school, and/or social functioning.

Social difficulties and elevated rates of autism symptoms have also been described in KS [82]. Most studies have focused on describing autism symptoms, which have identified features such as decreased social attention, decreased empathic skills, difficulty interpreting facial expressions, and social communication difficulties [67,100–102]. Studies that have included direct diagnostic assessment for autism spectrum disorders (ASDs) are more limited, and report a rate of 27% in a Dutch cohort (n = 51) using a standardized diagnostic autism interview called the ADI-R [92], and a rate of 10% in an American cohort (n = 20) using a battery including the ADI-R and direct assessment via the Autism Diagnostic Observation Scales (ADOS) [5]. Two other studies that evaluated rates of previous clinical ASD diagnosis in their cohort with KS also reported approximately 10% with ASD [67,100]. Recent important studies comparing autism symptoms and neuroanatomy in XXY to a group with idiopathic autism demonstrated that although behavioral questionnaires indicated similar autism symptoms between the groups, there were significant neuroanatomical differences in XXY compared with idiopathic ASD, suggesting that autism symptoms in the respective groups may have, at least partially, different etiologies [102]. Taken together, these studies support that ASD is an important clinical consideration in KS.

Screening for ASD should begin in early childhood as per the American Academy of Pediatrics recommendations, with referral for ASD assessment if indicated by screening results or if there are other concerns for ASD or social development raised by parents, teachers, or other providers. During assessment of social or ASD concerns, it is important and sometimes nuanced to differentiate the atypical social development and decreased reciprocity of ASD from social-emotional immaturity and/or expressive language deficits common in KS that can both also impact social relationships with peers. Further, it is common for concerns about ASD to become more apparent in boys with KS, as social interactions become more complex beyond the first few years of life, and thus ASD evaluation should be included within a psychological evaluation for social or behavioral concerns. ASD diagnosis can be important so as to guide services and supports, as well as to help families, educators, and others better understand and support social development for the boy with KS.

Studies that drew subject participation from clinical settings have reported elevated rates of a number of more complex psychiatric conditions, including bipolar disorder and psychotic spectrum disorders, with symptoms of paranoia, delusional thinking, and hallucinations [92,101,103]. Hospitalization for disorders associated with psychosis is reported as small in KS, but increased over the general population [104]. Thus, providers should be aware of this increased risk and make referrals for psychiatric care if patients or parents bring up any concerns.

Although we have emphasized many different cognitive, behavioral, and social features that can be associated with KS, it is again important to emphasize the variability of the phenotype and the importance of also identifying areas of strengths and talent in each individual. Although therapies and supports for areas of difficulty may be needed, it is equally important to encourage constructive opportunities for development in areas of strength and interest for positive self-esteem and quality of life. Parents should be encouraged to balance therapies and interventions with playtime, recreational or community activities, clubs/organizations that interest the child, and other positive activities.

TESTICULAR DEVELOPMENT AND FUNCTION

One of the most commonly recognized features of KS is primary testicular insufficiency, which is present in the large majority of male individuals with KS by early adulthood. The molecular mechanisms underlying this nearly universal manifestation remain elusive; however, testicular development seems to be abnormal from very early in life [105]. The normal testis is made up of germ cells, Leydig cells, and Sertoli cells. From the limited studies reporting testicular biopsies in KS, germ cells are reduced in number from infancy and the deficit appears to be progressive, particularly after puberty, with only rare pockets of active spermatogonia seen in adulthood [106]. Evaluation of Leydig and Sertoli cell function largely relies on measurement of serum hormone concentrations. The Leydig cells produce testosterone, which has important local and systemic effects, and Sertoli cells produce inhibin B and anti-Müllerian hormone (AMH), both of which have important local effects but unknown systemic effects. Assessment of serum hormone concentrations, particularly testosterone, is limited by assay variability, insensitivity of the assays in the hormone ranges typical of prepubertal children, and the observation that serum measurements do not necessarily accurately reflect intratesticular hormone concentrations. Regulation of gonadal function is primarily via the hypothalamic-pituitary-gonadal axis in which luteinizing hormone (LH) and follicle-stimulating hormone (FSH) stimulate Leydig and Sertoli cells respectively. The hypothalamic-pituitary-gonadal axis is activated in boys during the first 2 to 3 months of life (often called the mini-puberty period of infancy), then again during puberty and remains active throughout the adult life span. There is overlap in testosterone levels in boys with and without KS; however, male individuals with KS on average seem to have lower serum testosterone (Fig. 1).

Infancy

Hypogonadism in KS may start as early as fetal life or early infancy [107]. Evidence to support this includes a higher prevalence of underdeveloped genitalia and cryptorchidism in infants, reduced germ cell number in testicular biopsies, smaller testicular size, and several studies suggesting a blunted testosterone

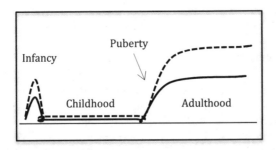

Fig. 1. T levels are abnormal throughout the lifespan in KS (*solid*) compared to normal male (*dashed*).

surge during the mini-puberty period of infancy [108–111]. Some endocrinologists measure testosterone, LH, and FSH at approximately 6 to 12 weeks of life during the mini-puberty period of infancy. However, the mini-puberty period in the healthy infant is vaguely defined, so it is not clear if this information has prognostic or management implications. Similarly, some providers will give testosterone during the first few months of life in infants with KS; however, there is currently insufficient evidence to support this practice [112]. Recent report of cognitive and behavioral benefits in male individuals with KS who had previously received testosterone has stimulated a great deal of interest from families [113,114]; however, these findings have to be replicated with prospective, randomized study designs. A randomized trial of intramuscular testosterone during the mini-puberty period of infancy is currently enrolling (NCT02408445).

Endocrine evaluation during infancy should include measurement of stretched penile length and documentation of bilateral descended testes. If micropenis is present (<1.9 cm from 0–6 months of life) or the family desires further discussion regarding endocrinologic manifestations in infancy, referral to a pediatric endocrinologist should be sought [115]. If cryptorchidism (persistent >6 months), inguinal hernia, or any other urogenital malformations are present, the infant should be referred for urology consultation.

Childhood
Before puberty in boys with KS, testicular volume is often less than 2 mL and penile growth throughout childhood has been noted to be slow [40,116]. The hypothalamic-pituitary-gonadal axis is quiescent in childhood; therefore, evaluation of LH, FSH, and testosterone concentrations are generally not clinically useful. However, 10% to 20% of boys with KS may have prepubertal elevation of FSH, low inhibin B, and/or elevated AMH reflecting abnormal Sertoli cell function [117]. Whether prepubertal Sertoli cell function is related to overall gonadal function in puberty and adulthood is yet to be determined. Results from a recently completed randomized controlled trial of oxandrolone (a non-aromatizable androgen) are expected soon. At this time, there are no recommendations for prepubertal hormonal evaluation or treatment.

Puberty
Most studies report a normal age of onset and tempo of early puberty in boys with KS [3,118].

Testes begin to enlarge but typically reach a peak volume of no more than 10 mL and then decrease down to smaller than 4 mL [119]. Serum testosterone may rise appropriately in boys with KS in early puberty, but often eventually plateaus or even declines when serially monitored [120]. FSH rises above the normal range on average a year after pubertal onset and LH approximately 2 years after pubertal onset. Endogenous testosterone usually supports virilization with penile enlargement and pubic hair development, although some young men with KS will not develop as much body or facial hair as would be expected for family. Fusion of the epiphyses may be delayed, contributing to tall stature. Gynecomastia probably occurs about as often as in pubertal boys without KS ($\sim 50\%$); however, may be more likely to persist in KS [121,122]. Physical examination should always include palpation for breast tissue, and if present warrants consideration of testosterone supplementation. The pathophysiology of gynecomastia is an abnormal testosterone-to-estrogen ratio; therefore, aromatase inhibitors have been used, however a randomized controlled trial in pubertal boys with physiologic gynecomastia (not KS) did not find benefit of anastrozole compared with placebo [123]. Estrogen receptor inhibitors (tamoxifen) have been reported in uncontrolled trials to reduce breast tissue size; however, it is unclear if this is superior to the outcome without medication and no studies have been done in boys with KS [124]. Surgery can be considered if gynecomastia fails to resolve with time and hormone manipulation; however, surgery does have perioperative risks and gynecomastia can recur postoperatively [125].

We recommend referral to an endocrinologist at approximately 10 years of age or at the first sign of puberty, whichever is earliest. This initial visit is largely educational and establishes rapport. Boys with KS who have clinical signs of puberty should be monitored with pubertal examination and laboratory evaluation with serum LH, FSH, and testosterone approximately every 6 months. Currently there are no universally accepted guidelines for when (or if) to start androgen replacement. One option is waiting until clear biochemical and/or clinical evidence of hypogonadism with elevated LH, low or falling testosterone, and presence of gynecomastia, poor muscle mass, fatigue, or incomplete virilization. Another approach is to initiating low-dose testosterone when LH has risen outside the normal range for pubertal development. A more aggressive option would be initiating testosterone in early puberty before any overt evidence of gonadal insufficiency. A randomized controlled trial that is currently enrolling hypothesizes psychosocial and motor benefits to low-dose testosterone treatment in early puberty (NCT01585831). Until more evidence is available from research studies, the preference of the patient and parents should be greatly considered in determining the timing of androgen replacement.

Although there are many testosterone formulations available, options for adolescents are generally limited to depot injections of testosterone or topical testosterone gel, as other formulations do not allow for small enough dosing increments or are not well tolerated by adolescent boys [7]. Injections have been used for decades, and most endocrinologists are familiar with their use. Injections can be given at home or in the primary care physician's office, and dosing is typically titrated based on symptomatology and psychic examination. Disadvantages of injections include the presence of peaks and troughs in serum testosterone and the inconvenience and/or pain of shots. Topical testosterone gels are newer and may not be covered by all insurance carriers. If starting with gel, the smallest increment of the lowest potency available is recommended as the starting dose, with the goal of achieving serum testosterone concentrations in the normal range for pubertal stage. Disadvantages of gels include the need for daily application, skin irritation, or sensory issues. Occasionally even the lowest available gel doses are too high for some pubertal boys, which may lead to elevated testosterone concentrations and subsequent rapid pubertal progression and/or premature fusion of the growth plates. Long-acting injections or testosterone pellets are being increasingly used in the United States; however, these are not recommended until late adolescence or adulthood when steady dose needs have been established.

Adulthood

The focus of this review precludes a comprehensive discussion on testicular function in adult men with KS. In brief, testicular size is universally small and usually firm, as the germ cells that should make up the bulk of the testis volume in adults are profoundly reduced in KS [122]. It is important to note, however, that the male genitalia otherwise has normal structure, size, and function. Nearly all untreated men with nonmosaic KS will have elevated LH and FSH, with low or low-normal testosterone and low or undetectable inhibin B and AMH [7]. Testosterone replacement should be offered to all men with evidence of hypergonadotropic hypogonadism, even if they are asymptomatic, as many manifestations of gonadal insufficiency may be subtle. The Endocrine Society has published guidelines for testosterone replacement in men with hypogonadism [126].

Azoospermia is nearly universal; however, the concept of "universal infertility" in KS has drastically changed with the ART technique of testicular sperm extraction (TESE) followed by intracytoplasmic sperm injection (ICSI) [8]. Using these techniques, small pockets of testicular tissue producing a few sperm can be identified during microsurgery, which are then extracted and injected through ICSI into a retrieved ovum, followed by in vitro fertilization. Currently, success rates of 50% to 75% are reported in adult men with KS seeking biological paternity using TESE and ICSI [127,128]. Studies have not found consistent predictors for which individuals will be more likely to have success with TESE, although mosaicism with a 46,XY cell line may have a more favorable outcome and older age (particularly more than 30 years), has been reported to have a less favorable outcome [129,130]. Many centers internationally have explored TESE for sperm cryopreservation from adolescents with KS, and current success rates do not consistently exceed those achieved in adulthood [127,131]. Based on this evidence and the relative newness of the field, we recommend that families are informed of the active and promising research in this field, and that consultation with a reproductive urologist is offered for all interested families, adolescents, or adults with KS seeking more information and options related to fertility. Invasive procedures for fertility preservation in childhood or adolescents are not currently routine practice outside of research protocols, although this may change as technology advances. Also important, several studies report similar fertility potential for male individuals with KS with previous exogenous testosterone exposure [127,128,130]; therefore, testosterone treatment should not be withheld from hypogonadal male individuals for future fertility concerns.

OTHER MEDICAL ISSUES
Insulin resistance and cardiovascular disorders

Adults with KS are known to have a high prevalence of disorders related to insulin resistance, including type 2 diabetes mellitus, dyslipidemia, and fatty liver disease [132]. Metabolic syndrome, a constellation of signs, including large waist circumference, dyslipidemia, elevated fasting blood glucose, and high blood pressure, is present in approximately 50% of men with KS [133–135]. The presence of these conditions correlates with abnormal body composition (particularly abdominal adiposity) and hypogonadism [135]. Together, type 2 diabetes and cardiovascular diseases yield a standardized mortality ratio of 5.8 in adults with KS [136].

Much less work has been done in children with KS; however, recent studies have found a high prevalence of metabolic syndrome features, as well as a high body fat percentage, in this population [137,138]. Importantly, features of metabolic syndrome in boys with KS appear to be independent of age or body mass index (BMI). Counseling regarding a healthy diet and regular exercise is imperative from an early age. We recommend cholesterol screening with a fasting lipid panel at age 9 to 11 years and after puberty is completed (consistent with American Academy of Pediatrics recommendations for all children), and sooner if additional risk factors are present [139]. Lipid panel should be repeated in puberty if the previous panel was abnormal or additional risk factors are present, such as obesity, untreated hypogonadism, or atypical antipsychotic use.

The risk of peripheral vascular disease and thromboembolic disease is increased in male individuals with KS, resulting in significantly increased mortality [136]. Venous stasis and recurrent leg ulcers are also quite common [140,141]. Although these conditions are more common with age, we have had several adolescents with KS who developed venous thrombus in at-risk situations, such as with a central venous catheter or surgery with immobilization. Consideration of prophylaxis measures should be considered if an adolescent or young adult is in a clinical situation that may predispose to clotting.

Bone health

Studies in adult men with KS report lower bone mineral density and a higher morbidity and mortality from hip and spine fractures [136,142]. It is speculated hypogonadism contributes to these findings; however, a mouse model suggests the additional X-chromosome itself results in abnormal bone structure [143]. A single study in 18 children and adolescents with KS reports normal bone mineral density [137]. In our anecdotal experience, we have not seen a high prevalence of pathologic fractures in children and adolescents with KS, and we do not recommend routine evaluation of bone mineral density. We do recommend attention to standard pediatric guidelines and ensuring adequate calcium and vitamin D intake, regular physical exercise, maintaining a normal BMI, and tobacco avoidance [144]. For postpubertal boys with KS, maintenance of sex steroid levels in the normal range likely helps bone density [145]. Chronic or unexplained back pain in an adolescent or adult with KS should raise concern for a vertebral compression fracture and appropriate evaluation undertaken.

Autoimmunity

Many case series and later epidemiologic studies have reported an increased prevalence of several autoimmune diseases in KS compared with 46,XY male individuals. A recent medical record linkage study of hospitalized men in England found significantly higher rates of several autoimmune diseases in men with KS, including rheumatoid arthritis (Relative Risk [RR] 3.3), lupus, multiple sclerosis (RR 18.1), Addison disease (RR 11.7), Sjögren syndrome (RR 19.3), autoimmune hypothyroidism (RR 2.7), and type 1 diabetes mellitus (RR 6.1) [146]. Although these are all significantly higher in adult men with KS compared with men in the general population, most of these autoimmune conditions are known to have a female predominance, and the risk of these autoimmune diseases is similar to women in the general population [147]. No studies have evaluated autoimmune diseases in children with KS. Although screening for primary hypothyroidism is often recommended in KS [148], evidence is lacking to recommend this in pediatrics. It is important to be aware of the increased prevalence of autoimmunity in KS and evaluate if suggestive symptoms are present.

Malignancy

An excellent review of the literature of malignancies in KS was published in 2013 [149]. Despite abundant case reports, there are few epidemiologic studies available. Because only a minority of male individuals with KS are diagnosed before adulthood, the natural history of malignancies in children with KS is really not known. The 3 cancers that are consistently found to be more prevalent in KS compared with male individuals in the general population are breast cancer, extragonadal germ cell tumors, and non-Hodgkin lymphoma. No routine screenings are recommended for any of these malignancies in childhood, but suspicious symptoms should be evaluated.

Breast cancer is approximately 20 times more common in men with KS compared with men without KS; however, it is still less common than in women [150]. Overall, breast cancer affects approximately 3% to 7% of men with KS [151,152], but is rare in adolescents. Self-examinations as well as regular physician examinations should be routine, and any palpable mass should be evaluated.

Extragonadal germ cell tumors are diagnosed in approximately 0.1% of male individuals with KS, representing a large increased risk compared with the general population. Unlike breast cancer, which does not typically present until adulthood, approximately half the reported cases of extragonadal germ cell tumors occur in pediatrics, with a peak age in adolescence [153]. Precocious puberty is the most common presenting symptom in boys younger than 10 years, whereas cough, dyspnea, or chest pain was most common in adolescents and adults given the most common tumor location is the mediastinum [154]. If these symptoms are present, extragonadal germ cell tumor should be suspected, and evaluation pursued with a chest radiograph to evaluate for a mediastinal mass as well as measurement of serum β-HCG and alpha-fetoprotein [149].

Finally, an association with non-Hodgkin lymphoma was reported in a large British cohort, particularly in boys with more than 3 sex chromosomes (48,XXYY); however, this was not found in other studies and requires further investigation [150]. There are many case reports of other hematological malignancies in male individuals with KS; however, epidemiologic studies do not show an increased incidence or mortality from leukemias or other lymphomas in KS [155]. It is important to keep in mind, however, that leukemia is the most common cancer in childhood, and therefore it would still be more likely for a boy with KS to develop leukemia than any of the other malignancies described previously.

Other medical conditions

Congenital anomalies are more prevalent in infants with KS than in the general population and lead to a higher mortality [136]. Congenital anomalies are much more common in boys with more than 3 sex chromosomes [156]. The most frequently reported anomalies include inguinal hernia, congenital heart disease, cleft palate and velopharyngeal insufficiency, and kidney malformations. Dental conditions, particularly taurodontism and frequent caries possibly from enamel defects, are common [24,157], and children with KS should have regular dental care.

Multiple case series have reported seizures in boys with KS, and a large epidemiologic study from Britain found a standardized mortality ratio from epilepsy of 7.2 in male individuals with KS compared with the general population [136]. Seizures are present in 15% of male individuals with 48,XXYY syndrome [24]. Seizures can present at any age. Tremor is also noted, particularly in male individuals with more than 3 sex chromosomes starting in adolescence [24,158].

Little is reported in the literature on atopy in KS; however, we appreciate a high prevalence of asthma and allergies in children with KS. In a study of 95 male individuals with 48XXYY syndrome, 55% and 60% had allergies and asthma, respectively [24]. Death from chronic lower respiratory disease, which would include asthma, was twice as likely in men with KS compared with the general population in Britain [136]. Further investigation is needed to explore whether this is a true association.

In summary, KS is a common but underdiagnosed genetic condition with significant phenotypic variability in childhood. The pediatrician needs to be aware of the increased risk for neurodevelopmental, psychological, and medical conditions that are associated with an additional X-chromosome. Over the next decade, we anticipate a sharp increase in diagnoses rates with advances in genetics, particularly prenatal and neonatal diagnoses. In the United States, more multidisciplinary clinics are being established to provide comprehensive care for children and adults with KS and other sex chromosome variations [95]. More research is needed to further define the natural history of KS in infancy and childhood with these unbiased populations, as well as understand genetic and environmental contributors to phenotypic variability and determine best practice screening and management guidelines for boys with KS.

References

[1] Klinefelter HF, Reifenstein EC, Albright F. Syndrome characterized by gynecomastia, aspermatogenesis without aleydigism, and increased excretion of follicle-stimulating hormone. J Clin Endocrinol 1942;2:615–27.

[2] Lue Y, Rao PN, Sinha Hikim AP, et al. XXY male mice: an experimental model for Klinefelter syndrome. Endocrinology 2001;142(4):1461–70.

[3] Robinson A, Bender BG, Linden MG, et al. Sex chromosome aneuploidy: the Denver Prospective Study. Birth Defects Orig Artic Ser 1990;26(4):59–115.

[4] Klinefelter HF. Klinefelter's syndrome: historical background and development. South Med J 1986;79(9):1089–93.

[5] Tartaglia N, Cordeiro L, Howell S, et al. The spectrum of the behavioral phenotype in boys and adolescents 47,XXY (Klinefelter syndrome). Pediatr Endocrinol Rev 2010;8(Suppl 1): 151–9.

[6] Rogol AD, Tartaglia N. Considerations for androgen therapy in children and adolescents with Klinefelter syndrome (47, XXY). Pediatr Endocrinol Rev 2010;8(Suppl 1):145–50.

[7] Davis SM, Rogol AD, Ross JL. Testis development and fertility potential in boys with Klinefelter syndrome. Endocrinol Metab Clin North Am 2015;44(4):843–65.

[8] Plotton I, Brosse A, Cuzin B, et al. Klinefelter syndrome and TESE-ICSI. Ann Endocrinol (Paris) 2014;75(2):118–25.

[9] Hook E. Chromosome abnormalities: prevalence, risks and recurrence. Prenatal diagnosis and screening. Edinburgh (Scotland): Churchill Livingstone; 1992. p. 351–92.

[10] Nielsen J. Sex chromosome abnormalities found among 34,910 newborn children: results from a 13-year incidence study in Arhus, Denmark. Birth Defects Orig Artic Ser 1990;26(4):209–23.

[11] Coffee B, Keith K, Albizua I, et al. Incidence of fragile X syndrome by newborn screening for methylated FMR1 DNA. Am J Hum Genet 2009;85(4):503–14.

[12] Herlihy AS, Halliday JL, Cock ML, et al. The prevalence and diagnosis rates of Klinefelter syndrome: an Australian comparison. Med J Aust 2011;194(1):24–8.

[13] Bojesen A, Juul S, Gravholt CH. Prenatal and postnatal prevalence of Klinefelter syndrome: a national registry study. J Clin Endocrinol Metab 2003;88(2):622–6.

[14] Morris JK, Alberman E, Scott C, et al. Is the prevalence of Klinefelter syndrome increasing? Eur J Hum Genet 2008;16(2):163–70.

[15] Boyd PA, Loane M, Garne E, et al. Sex chromosome trisomies in Europe: prevalence, prenatal detection and outcome of pregnancy. Eur J Hum Genet 2011;19(2):231–4.

[16] Abramsky L, Chapple J. 47,XXY (Klinefelter syndrome) and 47,XYY: estimated rates of and indication for postnatal diagnosis with implications for prenatal counselling. Prenat Diagn 1997;17(4):363–8.

[17] Visootsak J, Ayari N, Howell S, et al. Timing of diagnosis of 47,XXY and 48,XXYY: a survey of parent experiences. Am J Med Genet A 2013;161A(2):268–72.

[18] Meck JM, Kramer Dugan E, Matyakhina L, et al. Noninvasive prenatal screening for aneuploidy: positive predictive values based on cytogenetic findings. Am J Obstet Gynecol 2015;213(2):214.e1–5.

[19] Wang Y, Chen Y, Tian F, et al. Maternal mosaicism is a significant contributor to discordant sex chromosomal aneuploidies associated with noninvasive prenatal testing. Clin Chem 2014;60(1):251–9.

[20] Tassone F. Newborn screening for fragile X syndrome. JAMA Neurol 2014;71(3):355–9.

[21] Jacobs PA, Strong JA. A case of human intersexuality having a possible XXY sex-determining mechanism. Nature 1959;183(4657):302–3.

[22] MacDonald M, Hassold T, Harvey J, et al. The origin of 47,XXY and 47,XXX aneuploidy: heterogeneous mechanisms and role of aberrant recombination. Hum Mol Genet 1994;3(8):1365–71.

[23] Thomas NS, Hassold TJ. Aberrant recombination and the origin of Klinefelter syndrome. Hum Reprod Update 2003;9(4):309–17.

[24] Tartaglia N, Davis S, Hench A, et al. A new look at XXYY syndrome: medical and psychological features. Am J Med Genet A 2008;146A(12):1509–22.

[25] Peet J, Weaver DD, Vance GH. 49,XXXXY: a distinct phenotype. Three new cases and review. J Med Genet 1998;35(5):420–4.

[26] Berletch JB, Yang F, Disteche CM. Escape from X inactivation in mice and humans. Genome Biol 2010;11(6):213.

[27] Berletch JB, Yang F, Xu J, et al. Genes that escape from X inactivation. Hum Genet 2011;130(2):237–45.

[28] Ottesen AM, Aksglaede L, Garn I, et al. Increased number of sex chromosomes affects height in a nonlinear fashion: a study of 305 patients with sex chromosome aneuploidy. Am J Med Genet A 2010;152A(5):1206–12.

[29] Vawter MP, Harvey PD, DeLisi LE. Dysregulation of X-linked gene expression in Klinefelter's syndrome and association with verbal cognition. Am J Med Genet B Neuropsychiatr Genet 2007;144B(6):728–34.

[30] Huang J, Zhang L, Deng H, et al. Global transcriptome analysis of peripheral blood identifies the most significantly down-regulated genes associated with metabolism regulation in Klinefelter syndrome. Mol Reprod Dev 2015;82(1):17–25.

[31] Viana J, Pidsley R, Troakes C, et al. Epigenomic and transcriptomic signatures of a Klinefelter syndrome (47,XXY) karyotype in the brain. Epigenetics 2014;9(4):587–99.

[32] D'Aurora M, Ferlin A, Di Nicola M, et al. Deregulation of Sertoli and Leydig cells function in patients with Klinefelter syndrome as evidenced by testis transcriptome analysis. BMC Genomics 2015;16:1356.

[33] Zitzmann M, Bongers R, Werler S, et al. Gene expression patterns in relation to the clinical phenotype in Klinefelter syndrome. J Clin Endocrinol Metab 2015;100(3):E518–23.

[34] Rocca MS, Pecile V, Cleva L, et al. The Klinefelter syndrome is associated with high recurrence of copy number variations on the X chromosome with a potential role in the clinical phenotype. Andrology 2016;4(2):328–34.

[35] Tuttelmann F, Gromoll J. Novel genetic aspects of Klinefelter's syndrome. Mol Hum Reprod 2010;16(6):386–95.

[36] Zinn AR, Ramos P, Elder FF, et al. Androgen receptor CAGn repeat length influences phenotype of 47,XXY (Klinefelter) syndrome. J Clin Endocrinol Metab 2005;90(9):5041–6.

[37] Iitsuka Y, Bock A, Nguyen DD, et al. Evidence of skewed X-chromosome inactivation in 47,XXY and 48,XXYY Klinefelter patients. Am J Med Genet 2001;98(1):25–31.

[38] Skakkebaek A, Bojesen A, Kristensen MK, et al. Neuropsychology and brain morphology in Klinefelter syndrome—the impact of genetics. Andrology 2014;2(4):632–40.

[39] Nagai M, Kishi K, Kato S. Insular cortex and neuropsychiatric disorders: a review of recent literature. Eur Psychiatry 2007;22(6):387–94.

[40] Zeger MP, Zinn AR, Lahlou N, et al. Effect of ascertainment and genetic features on the phenotype of Klinefelter syndrome. J Pediatr 2008;152(5):716–22.

[41] Chang S, Skakkebaek A, Trolle C, et al. Anthropometry in Klinefelter syndrome—multifactorial influences due to CAG length, testosterone treatment and possibly intrauterine hypogonadism. J Clin Endocrinol Metab 2015;100(3):E508–17.

[42] Stemkens D, Roza T, Verrij L, et al. Is there an influence of X-chromosomal imprinting on the phenotype in Klinefelter syndrome? A clinical and molecular genetic study of 61 cases. Clin Genet 2006;70(1):43–8.

[43] Wikstrom A, Painter J, Raivio T, et al. Genetic features of the X chromosome affect pubertal development and testicular degeneration in adolescent boys with Klinefelter syndrome. Clin Endocrinol (Oxf) 2006;65(1):92–7.
[44] Choong CS, Wilson EM. Trinucleotide repeats in the human androgen receptor: a molecular basis for disease. J Mol Endocrinol 1998;21(3):235–57.
[45] Zitzmann M, Nieschlag E. The CAG repeat polymorphism within the androgen receptor gene and maleness. Int J Androl 2003;26(2):76–83.
[46] Bojesen A, Hertz JM, Gravholt CH. Genotype and phenotype in Klinefelter syndrome—impact of androgen receptor polymorphism and skewed X inactivation. Int J Androl 2011;34(6 Pt 2):e642–8.
[47] Zitzmann M, Depenbusch M, Gromoll J, et al. X-chromosome inactivation patterns and androgen receptor functionality influence phenotype and social characteristics as well as pharmacogenetics of testosterone therapy in Klinefelter patients. J Clin Endocrinol Metab 2004;89(12):6208–17.
[48] Ross JL, Roeltgen DP, Stefanatos G, et al. Cognitive and motor development during childhood in boys with Klinefelter syndrome. Am J Med Genet A 2008;146A(6):708–19.
[49] Hook EB, Topol BB, Cross PK. The natural history of cytogenetically abnormal fetuses detected at midtrimester amniocentesis which are not terminated electively: new data and estimates of the excess and relative risk of late fetal death associated with 47,+21 and some other abnormal karyotypes. Am J Hum Genet 1989;45(6):855–61.
[50] Dondorp W, de Wert G, Bombard Y, et al. Non-invasive prenatal testing for aneuploidy and beyond: challenges of responsible innovation in prenatal screening. Eur J Hum Genet 2015;23(11):1438–50.
[51] Lanfranco F, Kamischke A, Zitzmann M, et al. Klinefelter's syndrome. Lancet 2004;364(9430):273–83.
[52] Selice R, Di Mambro A, Garolla A, et al. Spermatogenesis in Klinefelter syndrome. J Endocrinol Invest 2010;33(11):789–93.
[53] Staessen C, Tournaye H, Van Assche E, et al. PGD in 47,XXY Klinefelter's syndrome patients. Hum Reprod Update 2003;9(4):319–30.
[54] Puck MH, Bender BG, Borelli JB, et al. Parents' adaptation to early diagnosis of sex chromosome anomalies. Am J Med Genet 1983;16(1):71–9.
[55] Gies I, Tournaye H, De Schepper J. Attitudes of parents of Klinefelter boys and pediatricians towards neonatal screening and fertility preservation techniques in Klinefelter syndrome. Eur J Pediatr 2015;175(3):399–404.
[56] Turriff A, Levy HP, Biesecker B. Prevalence and psychosocial correlates of depressive symptoms among adolescents and adults with Klinefelter syndrome. Genet Med 2011;13(11):966–72.
[57] Metcalfe A, Coad J, Plumridge GM, et al. Family communication between children and their parents about inherited genetic conditions: a meta-synthesis of the research. Eur J Hum Genet 2008;16(10):1193–200.
[58] Sutton EJ, Young J, McInerney-Leo A, et al. Truth-telling and Turner syndrome: the importance of diagnostic disclosure. J Pediatr 2006;148(1):102–7.
[59] Mac Dougall K, Becker G, Scheib JE, et al. Strategies for disclosure: how parents approach telling their children that they were conceived with donor gametes. Fertil Steril 2007;87(3):524–33.
[60] Dennis A, Howell S, Cordeiro L, et al. "How should I tell my child?" Disclosing the diagnosis of sex chromosome aneuploidies. J Genet Couns 2015;24(1):88–103.
[61] Tremblay I, Van Vliet G, Gonthier M, et al. Partnering with parents to disclose Klinefelter syndrome to their child. Acta Paediatr 2016;105(5):456–61.
[62] Bender B, Fry E, Pennington B, et al. Speech and language development in 41 children with sex chromosome anomalies. Pediatrics 1983;71(2):262–7.
[63] Linden MG, Bender BG. Fifty-one prenatally diagnosed children and adolescents with sex chromosome abnormalities. Am J Med Genet 2002;110(1):11–8.

[64] Robinson A, Bender BG, Linden MG. Summary of clinical findings in children and young adults with sex chromosome anomalies. Birth Defects Orig Artic Ser 1990;26(4):225–8.

[65] Ratcliffe SG. Speech and learning disorders in children with sex chromosome abnormalities. Dev Med Child Neurol 1982;24(1):80–4.

[66] Graham JM Jr, Bashir AS, Stark RE, et al. Oral and written language abilities of XXY boys: implications for anticipatory guidance. Pediatrics 1988;81(6):795–806.

[67] Bishop DV, Jacobs PA, Lachlan K, et al. Autism, language and communication in children with sex chromosome trisomies. Arch Dis Child 2011;96(10):954–9.

[68] Samango-Sprouse C, Rogol A. XXY the hidden disability and a prototype for an infantile presentation of developmental dyspraxia (IDD). Infants Young Child 2002;15(1):11–8.

[69] Bancroft J, Axworthy D, Ratcliffe S. The personality and psycho-sexual development of boys with 47 XXY chromosome constitution. J Child Psychol Psychiatry 1982;23(2): 169–80.

[70] Salbenblatt JA, Meyers DC, Bender BG, et al. Gross and fine motor development in 47,XXY and 47,XYY males. Pediatrics 1987;80(2):240–4.

[71] Eriksson B. Sex chromatin deviations among school children in special classes. A study of prevalence and an investigation of birth histories. J Ment Defic Res 1972;16(2):97–102.

[72] Singh DN, Osborne RA, Paul JR, et al. Cytogenetic survey of 504 mentally retarded individuals. J Ment Defic Res 1974;18(4):293–305.

[73] Bourgeois M, Benezech M. Cytogenic survey of 600 mentally retarded hospitalized patients [in French]. Encephale 1977;3(3):189–202.

[74] Johnston AW, Speed RM, Evans HJ. A chromosome survey of a population of mentally retarded persons. Birth Defects Orig Artic Ser 1974;10(10):30–5.

[75] Leggett V, Jacobs P, Nation K, et al. Neurocognitive outcomes of individuals with a sex chromosome trisomy: XXX, XYY, or XXY: a systematic review. Dev Med Child Neurol 2010;52(2):119–29.

[76] Ratcliffe SG, Masera N, Pan H, et al. Head circumference and IQ of children with sex chromosome abnormalities. Dev Med Child Neurol 1994;36(6):533–44.

[77] Rovet J, Netley C, Keenan M, et al. The psychoeducational profile of boys with Klinefelter syndrome. J Learn Disabil 1996;29(2):180–96.

[78] Bender B, Puck M, Salbenblatt J, et al. Cognitive development of children with sex chromosome abnormalities. San Diego (CA): College Hill Press; 1986.

[79] Netley C, Rovet J. Verbal deficits in children with 47,XXY and 47,XXX karyotypes: a descriptive and experimental study. Brain Lang 1982;17(1):58–72.

[80] Rovet J, Netley C, Bailey J, et al. Intelligence and achievement in children with extra X aneuploidy: a longitudinal perspective. Am J Med Genet 1995;60(5):356–63.

[81] Geschwind DH, Gregg J, Boone K, et al. Klinefelter's syndrome as a model of anomalous cerebral laterality: testing gene dosage in the X chromosome pseudoautosomal region using a DNA microarray. Dev Genet 1998;23(3):215–29.

[82] Bender BG, Linden MG, Robinson A. Verbal and spatial processing efficiency in 32 children with sex chromosome abnormalities. Pediatr Res 1989;25(6):577–9.

[83] Pennington BF, Bender B, Puck M, et al. Learning disabilities in children with sex chromosome anomalies. Child Dev 1982;53(5):1182–92.

[84] Bender BG, Linden MG, Robinson A. Neuropsychological impairment in 42 adolescents with sex chromosome abnormalities. Am J Med Genet 1993;48(3):169–73.

[85] Samango-Sprouse CA, Stapleton EJ, Mitchell FL, et al. Expanding the phenotypic profile of boys with 47, XXY: the impact of familial learning disabilities. Am J Med Genet A 2014;164A(6):1464–9.

[86] Boada R, Janusz J, Hutaff-Lee C, et al. The cognitive phenotype in Klinefelter syndrome: a review of the literature including genetic and hormonal factors. Dev Disabil Res Rev 2009;15(4):284–94.

[87] Boone KB, Swerdloff RS, Miller BL, et al. Neuropsychological profiles of adults with Klinefelter syndrome. J Int Neuropsychol Soc 2001;7(4):446–56.

[88] Lee NR, Wallace GL, Clasen LS, et al. Executive function in young males with Klinefelter (XXY) syndrome with and without comorbid attention-deficit/hyperactivity disorder. J Int Neuropsychol Soc 2011;17(3):522–30.

[89] van Rijn S, Swaab H, Magnee M, et al. Psychophysiological markers of vulnerability to psychopathology in men with an extra X chromosome (XXY). PLoS One 2011;6(5):e20292.

[90] Temple CM, Sanfilippo PM. Executive skills in Klinefelter's syndrome. Neuropsychologia 2003;41(11):1547–59.

[91] van Rijn S, Swaab H. Executive dysfunction and the relation with behavioral problems in children with 47,XXY and 47,XXX. Genes Brain Behav 2015;14(2):200–8.

[92] Bruining H, Swaab H, Kas M, et al. Psychiatric characteristics in a self-selected sample of boys with Klinefelter syndrome. Pediatrics 2009;123(5):e865–70.

[93] Tartaglia N, Davis S, Hansen R, et al. Abstract: Attention deficit hyperactivity disorder and autism spectrum disorders in males with XXY, XYY, and XXYY syndromes. J Intellect Disabil Res 2006;50(11):787.

[94] Tartaglia NR, Ayari N, Hutaff-Lee C, et al. Attention-deficit hyperactivity disorder symptoms in children and adolescents with sex chromosome aneuploidy: XXY, XXX, XYY, and XXYY. J Dev Behav Pediatr 2012;33(4):309–18.

[95] Tartaglia N, Howell S, Wilson R, et al. The eXtraordinarY Kids Clinic: an interdisciplinary model of care for children and adolescents with sex chromosome aneuploidy. J Multidiscip Healthc 2015;8:323–34.

[96] Bender B, Harmon RJ, Linden MG, et al. Psychosocial adaptation in 39 adolescents with sex chromosome abnormalities. Pediatrics 1995;96:302–8.

[97] Visootsak J, Graham JM Jr. Social function in multiple X and Y chromosome disorders: XXY, XYY, XXYY, XXXY. Dev Disabil Res Rev 2009;15(4):328–32.

[98] Close S, Fennoy I, Smaldone A, et al. Phenotype and adverse quality of life in boys with Klinefelter syndrome. J Pediatr 2015;167(3):650–7.

[99] van Rijn S, Stockmann L, Borghgraef M, et al. The social behavioral phenotype in boys and girls with an extra X chromosome (Klinefelter syndrome and Trisomy X): a comparison with autism spectrum disorder. J Autism Dev Disord 2014;44(2):310–20.

[100] Cordeiro L, Tartaglia N, Roeltgen D, et al. Social deficits in male children and adolescents with sex chromosome aneuploidy: a comparison of XXY, XYY, and XXYY syndromes. Res Dev Disabil 2012;33(4):1254–63.

[101] van Rijn S, Swaab H, Aleman A, et al. X chromosomal effects on social cognitive processing and emotion regulation: a study with Klinefelter men (47,XXY). Schizophr Res 2006;84(2–3):194–203.

[102] Goddard MN, Swaab H, Rombouts SA, et al. Neural systems for social cognition: gray matter volume abnormalities in boys at high genetic risk of autism symptoms, and a comparison with idiopathic autism spectrum disorder. Eur Arch Psychiatry Clin Neurosci 2015. [Epub ahead of print].

[103] DeLisi LE, Maurizio AM, Svetina C, et al. Klinefelter's syndrome (XXY) as a genetic model for psychotic disorders. Am J Med Genet B Neuropsychiatr Genet 2005;135B(1):15–23.

[104] Bojesen A, Juul S, Birkebaek NH, et al. Morbidity in Klinefelter syndrome: a Danish register study based on hospital discharge diagnoses. J Clin Endocrinol Metab 2006;91(4):1254–60.

[105] Mikamo K, Aguercif M, Hazeghi P. Martin-Du Pan R. Chromatin-positive Klinefelter's syndrome. A quantitative analysis of spermatogonial deficiency at 3, 4, and 12 months of age. Fertil Steril 1968;19(5):731–9.

[106] Wikstrom AM, Raivio T, Hadziselimovic F, et al. Klinefelter syndrome in adolescence: onset of puberty is associated with accelerated germ cell depletion. J Clin Endocrinol Metab 2004;89(5):2263–70.

[107] Fennoy I. Testosterone and the child (0-12 years) with Klinefelter syndrome (47XXY): a review. Acta Paediatr 2011;100(6):846–50.

[108] Lahlou N, Fennoy I, Ross JL, et al. Clinical and hormonal status of infants with nonmosaic XXY karyotype. Acta Paediatr 2011;100(6):824–9.

[109] Cabrol S, Ross JL, Fennoy I, et al. Assessment of Leydig and Sertoli cell functions in infants with nonmosaic Klinefelter syndrome: insulin-like peptide 3 levels are normal and positively correlated with LH levels. J Clin Endocrinol Metab 2011;96(4):E746–53.

[110] Lahlou N, Fennoy I, Carel JC, et al. Inhibin B and anti-Mullerian hormone, but not testosterone levels, are normal in infants with nonmosaic Klinefelter syndrome. J Clin Endocrinol Metab 2004;89(4):1864–8.

[111] Ross JL, Samango-Sprouse C, Lahlou N, et al. Early androgen deficiency in infants and young boys with 47,XXY Klinefelter syndrome. Horm Res 2005;64(1):39–45.

[112] Wosnitzer MS, Paduch DA. Endocrinological issues and hormonal manipulation in children and men with Klinefelter syndrome. Am J Med Genet C Semin Med Genet 2013;163C(1):16–26.

[113] Samango-Sprouse CA, Sadeghin T, Mitchell FL, et al. Positive effects of short course androgen therapy on the neurodevelopmental outcome in boys with 47,XXY syndrome at 36 and 72 months of age. Am J Med Genet A 2013;161A(3):501–8.

[114] Samango-Sprouse C, Stapleton EJ, Lawson P, et al. Positive effects of early androgen therapy on the behavioral phenotype of boys with 47,XXY. Am J Med Genet C Semin Med Genet 2015;169(2):150–7.

[115] Hatipoglu N, Kurtoglu S. Micropenis: etiology, diagnosis and treatment approaches. J Clin Res Pediatr Endocrinol 2013;5(4):217–23.

[116] Ratcliffe SG, Murray L, Teague P. Edinburgh study of growth and development of children with sex chromosome abnormalities. III. Birth Defects Orig Artic Ser 1986;22(3):73–118.

[117] Davis S, Lahlou N, Bardsley MZ, et al. Longitudinal study of boys with Klinefelter syndrome gives evidence of prepubertal testis defect. San Diego (CA): The Endocrine Society; 2015.

[118] Laron Z, Topper E. Klinefelter's syndrome in adolescence. Arch Dis Child 1982;57(11): 887–8.

[119] Salbenblatt JA, Bender BG, Puck MH, et al. Pituitary-gonadal function in Klinefelter syndrome before and during puberty. Pediatr Res 1985;19(1):82–6.

[120] Bastida MG, Rey RA, Bergada I, et al. Establishment of testicular endocrine function impairment during childhood and puberty in boys with Klinefelter syndrome. Clin Endocrinol 2007;67(6):863–70.

[121] Mieritz MG, Raket LL, Hagen CP, et al. A longitudinal study of growth, sex steroids, and IGF-1 in boys with physiological gynecomastia. J Clin Endocrinol Metab 2015;100(10): 3752–9.

[122] Pacenza N, Pasqualini T, Gottlieb S, et al. Clinical presentation of Klinefelter's syndrome: differences according to age. Int J Endocrinol 2012;2012:324835.

[123] Plourde PV, Reiter EO, Jou HC, et al. Safety and efficacy of anastrozole for the treatment of pubertal gynecomastia: a randomized, double-blind, placebo-controlled trial. J Clin Endocrinol Metab 2004;89(9):4428–33.

[124] Lapid O, van Wingerden JJ, Perlemuter L. Tamoxifen therapy for the management of pubertal gynecomastia: a systematic review. J Pediatr Endocrinol Metab 2013;26(9–10): 803–7.

[125] Fischer S, Hirsch T, Hirche C, et al. Surgical treatment of primary gynecomastia in children and adolescents. Pediatr Surg Int 2014;30(6):641–7.

[126] Bhasin S, Cunningham GR, Hayes FJ, et al. Testosterone therapy in men with androgen deficiency syndromes: an Endocrine Society clinical practice guideline. J Clin Endocrinol Metab 2010;95(6):2536–59.

[127] Plotton I, d'Estaing SG, Cuzin B, et al. Preliminary Results of a prospective study of testicular sperm extraction in young versus adult patients with nonmosaic 47,XXY Klinefelter syndrome. J Clin Endocrinol Metab 2015;100(3):961–7.

[128] Mehta A, Bolyakov A, Roosma J, et al. Successful testicular sperm retrieval in adolescents with Klinefelter syndrome treated with at least 1 year of topical testosterone and aromatase inhibitor. Fertil Steril 2013;100(4):970–4.

[129] Gies I, De Schepper J, Van Saen D, et al. Failure of a combined clinical- and hormonal-based strategy to detect early spermatogenesis and retrieve spermatogonial stem cells in 47,XXY boys by single testicular biopsy. Hum Reprod 2012;27(4):998–1004.

[130] Rohayem J, Fricke R, Czeloth K, et al. Age and markers of Leydig cell function, but not of Sertoli cell function predict the success of sperm retrieval in adolescents and adults with Klinefelter's syndrome. Andrology 2015;3(5):868–75.

[131] Nahata L, Yu RN, Paltiel HJ, et al. Sperm retrieval in adolescents and young adults with Klinefelter syndrome: a prospective, pilot study. J Pediatr 2015;170:260–5.e2.

[132] Jiang-Feng M, Hong-Li X, Xue-Yan W, et al. Prevalence and risk factors of diabetes in patients with Klinefelter syndrome: a longitudinal observational study. Fertil Steril 2012;98(5):1331–5.

[133] Gravholt CH, Jensen AS, Host C, et al. Body composition, metabolic syndrome and type 2 diabetes in Klinefelter syndrome. Acta Paediatr 2011;100(6):871–7.

[134] Bojesen A, Host C, Gravholt CH. Klinefelter's syndrome, type 2 diabetes and the metabolic syndrome: the impact of body composition. Mol Hum Reprod 2010;16(6):396–401.

[135] Bojesen A, Kristensen K, Birkebaek NH, et al. The metabolic syndrome is frequent in Klinefelter's syndrome and is associated with abdominal obesity and hypogonadism. Diabetes Care 2006;29(7):1591–8.

[136] Swerdlow AJ, Higgins CD, Schoemaker MJ, et al, United Kingdom Clinical Cytogenetics Group. Mortality in patients with Klinefelter syndrome in Britain: a cohort study. J Clin Endocrinol Metab 2005;90(12):6516–22.

[137] Aksglaede L, Molgaard C, Skakkebaek NE, et al. Normal bone mineral content but unfavourable muscle/fat ratio in Klinefelter syndrome. Arch Dis Child 2008;93(1):30–4.

[138] Bardsley MZ, Falkner B, Kowal K, et al. Insulin resistance and metabolic syndrome in prepubertal boys with Klinefelter syndrome. Acta Paediatr 2011;100(6):866–70.

[139] Daniels SR, Greer FR, Committee on Nutrition. Lipid screening and cardiovascular health in childhood. Pediatrics 2008;122(1):198–208.

[140] Seth A, Rajpal S, Penn RL. Klinefelter's syndrome and venous thrombosis. Am J Med Sci 2013;346(2):164–5.

[141] Salzano A, Arcopinto M, Marra AM, et al. Management of endocrine disease: Klinefelter syndrome, cardiovascular system and thromboembolic disease. Review of literature and clinical perspectives. Eur J Endocrinol 2016;175(1):R27–40.

[142] Bojesen A, Gravholt CH. Morbidity and mortality in Klinefelter syndrome (47,XXY). Acta Paediatr 2011;100(6):807–13.

[143] Liu PY, Kalak R, Lue Y, et al. Genetic and hormonal control of bone volume, architecture, and remodeling in XXY mice. J Bone Miner Res 2010;25(10):2148–54.

[144] Bachrach LK. Diagnosis and treatment of pediatric osteoporosis. Curr Opin Endocrinol Diabetes Obes 2014;21(6):454–60.

[145] Jo DG, Lee HS, Joo YM, et al. Effect of testosterone replacement therapy on bone mineral density in patients with Klinefelter syndrome. Yonsei Med J 2013;54(6):1331–5.

[146] Seminog OO, Seminog AB, Yeates D, et al. Associations between Klinefelter's syndrome and autoimmune diseases: English national record linkage studies. Autoimmunity 2015;48(2):125–8.

[147] Sawalha AH, Harley JB, Scofield RH. Autoimmunity and Klinefelter's syndrome: when men have two X chromosomes. J Autoimmun 2009;33(1):31–4.

[148] Radicioni AF, Ferlin A, Balercia G, et al. Consensus statement on diagnosis and clinical management of Klinefelter syndrome. J Endocrinol Invest 2010;33(11):839–50.

[149] De Sanctis V, Fiscina B, Soliman A, et al. Klinefelter syndrome and cancer: from childhood to adulthood. Pediatr Endocrinol Rev 2013;11(1):44–50.

[150] Swerdlow AJ, Schoemaker MJ, Higgins CD, et al. Cancer incidence and mortality in men with Klinefelter syndrome: a cohort study. J Natl Cancer Inst 2005;97(16):1204–10.
[151] Sasco AJ, Lowenfels AB, Pasker-de Jong P. Review article: epidemiology of male breast cancer. A meta-analysis of published case-control studies and discussion of selected aetiological factors. Int J Cancer 1993;53(4):538–49.
[152] Brinton LA. Breast cancer risk among patients with Klinefelter syndrome. Acta Paediatr 2011;100(6):814–8.
[153] Hasle H, Mellemgaard A, Nielsen J, et al. Cancer incidence in men with Klinefelter syndrome. Br J Cancer 1995;71(2):416–20.
[154] Volkl TM, Langer T, Aigner T, et al. Klinefelter syndrome and mediastinal germ cell tumors. Am J Med Genet A 2006;140(5):471–81.
[155] Keung YK, Buss D, Chauvenet A, et al. Hematologic malignancies and Klinefelter syndrome. A chance association? Cancer Genet Cytogenet 2002;139(1):9–13.
[156] Tartaglia N, Ayari N, Howell S, et al. 48,XXYY, 48,XXXY and 49,XXXXY syndromes: not just variants of Klinefelter syndrome. Acta Paediatr 2011;100(6):851–60.
[157] Schulman GS, Redford-Badwal D, Poole A, et al. Taurodontism and learning disabilities in patients with Klinefelter syndrome. Pediatr Dent 2005;27(5):389–94.
[158] Lote H, Fuller GN, Bain PG. 48, XXYY syndrome associated tremor. Pract Neurol 2013;13(4):249–53.

Advances in Pediatrics 63 (2016) 47–77

ADVANCES IN PEDIATRICS

Prader Willi Syndrome
Genetics, Metabolomics, Hormonal Function, and New Approaches to Therapy

Krystal A. Irizarry, MD[a], Mark Miller, MD[a],
Michael Freemark, MD[a], Andrea M. Haqq, MD[b],*

[a]Division of Pediatric Endocrinology, Duke University Medical Center, 3000 Erwin Road, Suite 200, Durham, NC 27705, USA; [b]Division of Pediatric Endocrinology, University of Alberta, 1C4 Walter C. Mackenzie Health Sciences Center, 8440 - 112 Street Northwest, Edmonton, Alberta T6G 2R7, Canada

Keywords

- Imprinting defect • Hyperphagia • Childhood obesity syndrome
- Growth hormone

Key points

- Prader Willi syndrome (PWS) has a unique phenotypic and metabolic profile and remains the most common cause of syndromic obesity.
- Diagnostic advances have resulted in early detection of PWS in infants and young children, allowing for early treatment and improved outcomes.
- Growth hormone (GH) therapy has been shown to have therapeutic benefits in PWS, and requires close monitoring for adverse events.
- Several top priority areas for GH research in PWS include determination of optimal timing and dosage of GH treatment initiation in early life, longer-term data on safety and efficacy of GH in PWS populations across international databases and registries, further evaluation of GH effects on behavior and cognition across development, longer-term data on appropriate monitoring for sleep-disordered breathing post-GH initiation, and randomized controlled trials to evaluate the effects of GH therapy in concert with other novel therapeutic strategies including bariatric surgery.

Disclosures: None.

Funding: The authors are supported in part by a grant from the Foundation for Prader-Willi Research (A.M. Haqq, M. Freemark), grant from the Canadian Institutes of Health Research MOP 119504 (A.M. Haqq), and NIH 5T32HD043029-12 (K.A. Irizarry) to the Duke Department of Pediatrics.

*Corresponding author. E-mail address: haqq@ualberta.ca

0065-3101/16/$ – see front matter
http://dx.doi.org/10.1016/j.yapd.2016.04.005

Learning objectives

1. Identify physical, hormonal, and biochemical features of Prader Willi syndrome (PWS).
2. Discuss the use of growth hormone therapy and risks and benefits of this and other treatments in PWS.
3. Review advances in therapeutic strategies for common comorbid conditions in PWS, including sleep disturbance, hyperphagia, and skin picking.

INTRODUCTION

Advances in clinical assessment, epidemiology, metabolomics, and genomics have provided new insights into the pathogenesis of obesity comorbidities, including insulin resistance, fatty liver disease, type 2 diabetes mellitus (T2DM), and cardiovascular disease; yet, we know very little about the factors causing people to become obese in the first place. In that regard, studies of genetic obesity models in humans and experimental animals are of critical value. Here we provide a review and update on Prader Willi syndrome (PWS), a unique genetic model of obesity associated with hypotonia, sarcopenia, cognitive dysfunction, hyperphagia, progressive fat deposition, and varying degrees of hypopituitarism.

GENETICS OF PRADER WILLI SYNDROME

Chromosomal localization

PWS is the most common syndromic obesity disorder, with a prevalence of 1 in 10,000 to 1 in 15,000 live births annually. Occurring equally in male and female individuals and detected in all races [1], it is characterized by infantile hypotonia and failure to thrive, followed by progressive obesity and hyperphagia in childhood. PWS results from lack of expression of paternally inherited genes in the region of chromosome 15q11.2-q13 [1]. Seventy percent of patients have a deletion of the paternally inherited region, whereas 25% have inherited 2 copies of the critical region on chromosome 15 from the mother; the latter is called maternal uniparental disomy. Five percent have abnormal imprinting or methylation that silences paternal genes in the PWS region.

Candidate genes

Chromosome 15q11.2 to 13 contains a number of genes that contribute to the PWS phenotype (Fig. 1).

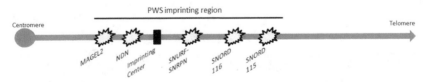

Fig. 1. Representation of chromosome 15q11 to 13.

Targeted knockout of individual genes in mice recapitulates some but not all of the clinical and biochemical features of PWS; the complete clinical picture likely requires deletion or deficiencies of 2 or more of the candidate genes.

Necdin gene

The *NDN* gene (see Fig. 1) encodes the protein necdin, which is preferentially expressed in the hypothalamus [2]. Experimental studies in mice have demonstrated at least 4 different phenotypes of necdin-null mutations. These have included respiratory defects similar to those found in children and adults with PWS. One necdin-deficient mouse model had respiratory failure secondary to abnormal central respiratory drive with frequent apnea and decreased respiratory response to hypoxia [2]. Another necdin knockout model showed reduced hypothalamic neuron populations within oxytocin-expressing neurons in the paraventricular nuclei and gonadotropin-releasing hormone (GnRH) neurons in the preoptic area [2]. It is theorized that the reduction in GnRH neurons might explain the reduced gonadal function in PWS [3]. Behavioral studies in these mouse models have identified increased skin scraping, similar to skin picking manifestations of PWS [2]. Last, necdin-deficient mouse models also had increased pain tolerance similar to patients with PWS, possibly due to necdin promotion of nerve-growth factors within sensory neurons [2].

MAGEL2 family member

The *MAGEL2* gene is located upstream of *NDN* (see Fig. 1), and encodes the protein MAGEL 2 protein, which like necdin is highly expressed in the hypothalamic supraoptic, paraventricular, and suprachiasmatic nuclei [2]. MAGEL2 knockout mice have decreased wakefulness as measured by decreased daytime running and motor activity that is associated with decreased levels of orexin, a sleep-regulating and appetite-regulating hormone [2]. MAGEL2 knockout mice also have postnatal growth retardation until week 6 of life, and then accelerated postnatal catch-up growth and adiposity [4]. In contrast to young children with PWS, MAGEL2 knockout mice are hypophagic; thus, their adiposity may result from diminished energy expenditure. Last, MAGEL2 knockout mouse models have demonstrated delayed pubertal onset and decreased fertility in females. The number of hypothalamic GnRH neurons is normal but the number of corpus lutea is diminished, suggesting decreased ovulation [2]. Male Magel2 knockouts have lower levels of testosterone but no defects in genital anatomy or sperm count [2]. Therefore, although the MAGEL2 knockout has similar wakefulness, growth, adiposity, and pubertal patterns to patients with PWS, these are not as severe and do not explain the complete human phenotype.

SNRPN Upstream Reading Frame

SNURF (SNRPN Upstream Reading Frame) is a small nuclear ribonucleoprotein complex involved in mRNA splicing in the brain. Mouse models lacking the *SNRPN* gene have variable phenotype with some exhibiting hypotonia and impaired feeding [2]. Early mortality has thus far precluded analysis of metabolic status and feeding behavior.

SNORD 116

The nucleolus contains diverse small RNAs (snoRNAs) that complex with small nucleolar ribonucleoproteins and mediate posttranscriptional, sequence-specific methylation that dictates mRNA folding and stability. Defects in certain snoRNAs have been implicated in neurologic, cardiovascular, and oncologic diseases [2]. SNORD 116 is expressed at high levels in appetite-controlling centers of the hypothalamus, including the arcuate, paraventricular, and ventromedial nuclei. SNORD 116 deletion in mice leads to anxiety, deficiency in motor learning, and growth retardation, mimicking in some ways the hypotonia and failure to thrive seen in infants with PWS [2]. Unlike other animal knockout models, SNORD 116 knockout mice are hyperghrelinemic and moderately hyperphagic [5]; however, under standard feeding conditions, they do not become obese.

As no single gene knockout can fully explain the PWS phenotype, it is thought that PWS represents a contiguous gene disorder requiring loss of expression of several genes to cause the complete phenotype.

CLINICAL MANIFESTATIONS OF PRADER WILLI SYNDROME

Although the exact genetic mechanisms leading to PWS remain unclear, the phenotype is well-described [6]. Clinical characteristics of PWS vary with age, and minor clinical manifestations are often nonspecific (Table 1). Previous scoring symptoms quantifying number of major and minor clinical manifestations were used for diagnosis of PWS [6]. With improved sensitivity and availability of genetic testing, criteria for identifying patients needing prompt genetic testing have been developed [7]. The most distinctive major clinical characteristics of PWS are infantile central hypotonia and failure to thrive, followed by

Table 1
Major and minor clinical manifestations of Prader Willi syndrome

Age	Major characteristics	Minor characteristics
Birth to 2 y	Neonatal central hypotonia (ie, floppy infant, poor suck) Failure to thrive in infancy Global developmental delay	Decreased fetal movement, weak cry Infantile lethargy
2 y–6 y	Excess and rapid weight gain with central obesity	Behavioral problems (obsessive compulsive disorder, manipulative, perseverating, stealing) Sleep apnea
12 y–adulthood	Hyperphagia and obsession with food Hypogonadotropic gonadism with genital hypoplasia, delayed or incomplete pubertal progression Cognitive impairment, learning delays	Short stature Behavioral disorders (temper tantrums, obsessive compulsive disorder) Skin picking

progressive hyperphagia and fat deposition in early childhood. The infantile hypotonia and failure to thrive are so severe they generally (but not always) require assisted feedings with nasal gavage or gastrostomy tube. Minor criteria include developmental delay and hypothalamic dysfunction, manifest as temperature dysregulation, increased pain tolerance, and central as well as obstructive sleep apnea. Hypothalamic dysfunction can also result in central hypothyroidism, central adrenal insufficiency, growth hormone (GH) deficiency, and hypogonadotropic hypogonadism (discussed later in this article). Many children with PWS also have behavioral disorders including anxiety and obsessive compulsive disorder that can be associated with chronic skin picking. The physical features and facies of PWS often become more pronounced with age (Fig. 2).

CONTROL OF FOOD INTAKE IN PRADER WILLI SYNDROME

Our group has published studies evaluating the developmental changes in appetite-regulating hormones, such as ghrelin in PWS versus control infants and children. In a cross-sectional study of 33 infants with PWS and 28 healthy controls, we determined that total serum ghrelin trended higher in the PWS group, but did not differ significantly from comparable controls of equivalent age, weight-for-age percentile, and z-score and sex. However, one-third of young patients with PWS (11/33) had ghrelin levels higher than the 95th percentile of ghrelin values in the healthy controls; thus, hyperghrelinemia was detected in one-third of patients with PWS at an early age in the absence of reported hyperphagia [8]. More variability in ghrelin concentrations was also

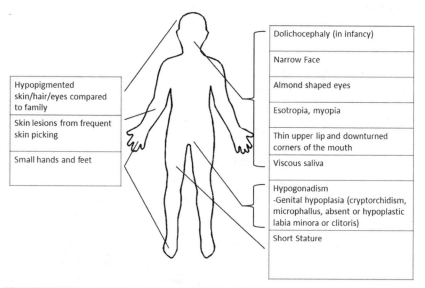

Fig. 2. Physical findings in PWS.

noted in young children with PWS compared with controls. Interestingly, 6 of the 11 young patients with PWS with relatively high ghrelin concentrations had weight-for-age z-score less than 0. We speculate that hyperghrelinemia in young children with PWS might be a response to failure to thrive or food restriction in infancy. A longitudinal assessment of total ghrelin in 9 young children with PWS showed no significant changes over 18 months. Total ghrelin in young children with PWS and control children was significantly higher than in older counterparts and the decline in ghrelin with age was more exaggerated in the control subjects than in the patients with PWS. Other researchers published similar findings to ours that there were no significant differences in plasma insulin or ghrelin levels between young patients with PWS and controls [9,10]. Similar to our study, Goldstone and colleagues [9] also reported significantly higher plasma leptin levels in young patients with PWS versus controls, suggesting a relative excess of fat to lean body mass. No relationship was found between eating behavior in patients with PWS and concentrations of any hormones or insulin resistance, independent of age. It is postulated that changes in central pathways controlling appetite regulation and food reward might be responsible for the development of hyperphagia in PWS. Careful prospective longitudinal studies of infants and young children with PWS compared with controls are needed to examine further the relationship among changes in appetite-regulating hormones, body composition, and eating behaviors.

In older children with PWS compared with obese controls (OC), our group and others have demonstrated significantly higher ghrelin levels, total adiponectin, high molecular weight (HMW) adiponectin and HMW adiponectin-leptin ratio and lower fasting insulin levels and HOMA-IR [8,11–13]. These findings are in the setting of equivalent leptin concentrations between PWS and OC, suggesting comparable degrees of adiposity. Lower levels of inflammatory cytokines, such as interleukin-6 and c-reactive protein have also been reported in PWS compared with OCs by our group [13]. Interestingly, we also found sex differences, with female patients with PWS showing more striking hyperghrelinemia, hyperadiponectinemia, and insulin sensitivity compared with male patients with PWS [12]. The effects of sex hormones and treatment with GH on these findings remain unclear.

Overall, these findings are consistent with a higher degree of insulin sensitivity in older patients with PWS. Moreover, high-density lipoprotein levels were lower and triglycerides higher in OCs, but not patients with PWS. No group differences in glucagonlike peptide-1 or aspartate aminotransferase or alanine aminotransferase were seen. Interestingly, we found a greater decline in ghrelin with age in controls versus patients with PWS. A negative relationship between ghrelin and body mass index (BMI) z-score was also found in the older patients with PWS and controls, but not in the younger cohort. Further studies are required to understand the pathophysiology of increased insulin sensitivity in PWS and to determine if their increased insulin sensitivity translates into protective clinical benefits long-term.

Finally, recent studies from our laboratory have assessed the acute effects of varying macronutrient content (high fat [HF] or high carbohydrate [HC] iso-caloric breakfast meals) in a randomized cross-over study of 14 patients with PWS and 14 age-matched and BMI-z–matched OCs [14]. Relative to OCs, children with PWS had lower fasting insulin and higher fasting ghrelin and ghre-lin/Peptide YY (PYY). Ghrelin levels were higher in PWS across all postprandial time-points. Carbohydrate was more potent than fat in suppress-ing ghrelin concentrations in PWS ($P = .028$); HC and HF were equipotent in OCs, but less potent than in PWS ($P = .011$). Interestingly, the rise in PYY following HF was attenuated in PWS ($P = .037$); thus, postprandial ghrelin/PYY remained higher throughout. In summary, we found that children with PWS had both fasting and postprandial hyperghrelinemia and an attenuated response to fat, yielding a high ghrelin-PYY ratio. We propose that the ratio of ghrelin-PYY might be a novel marker of orexigenic drive in PWS and child-hood obesity. Therapeutic approaches to either increase PYY or decrease ghre-lin in PWS might prove successful. Future longer-term randomized controlled trials of varying macronutrient composition will facilitate the development of optimal dietary therapies to attenuate hyperphagia, prevent weight gain, and promote weight loss in PWS.

HYPOTHALAMIC PITUITARY FUNCTION IN PRADER WILLI SYNDROME
Growth hormone deficiency and short stature
Mild prenatal growth retardation occurs commonly in PWS; 41% of infants have a birth weight less than 2.5 kg; birth length is either normal or slightly below normal. Short stature is almost always present by 1 year of age and con-tinues throughout childhood. The cause of the short stature is both GH defi-ciency and the lack of a sufficient pubertal growth spurt [15,16]. The average height of untreated men with PWS is 155 cm and of women with PWS 145 cm [17]. The GH deficiency seen in PWS is independent of obesity and manifests in low spontaneous and pharmacologically stimulated GH secretion and low serum concentrations of insulinlike growth factor 1 (IGF-1) in both children and adults [18–29]. This is unlike overnutrition in common obesity, which is associated with normal or increased IGF-1 levels. Body composition in individuals with PWS resembles that of classic GH deficiency, with decreased lean mass and increased adipose tissue mass compared with age-matched controls [30].

Recombinant GH therapy for PWS was approved in the United States in 2000 and in Europe in 2001; GH is still not approved in some countries, such as Canada. Generally agreed on exclusion criteria for therapy include se-vere obesity, uncontrolled diabetes mellitus, untreated severe obstructive sleep apnea, active cancer, or psychosis [31]. Recently, updated standardized growth charts for individuals with PWS not treated with GH (3–18 years) were devel-oped and can be used to monitor response to GH therapy or to assess nutri-tional status [32].

Presented in the following text is evidence supporting the use of GH in PWS in infants/toddlers, children, and adults. There does not seem to be a differential GH response based on genetic subtype of PWS [33,34].

Studies in infants/toddlers
Body fat content is increased and lean body mass is reduced in young infants and toddlers with PWS, even before progressive weight gain ensues [35,36]. This finding provides a rationale for initiating GH therapy at a young age. In a large randomized controlled GH trial in 91 prepubertal children with PWS, 42 infants and 49 children were randomized to GH treatment or no GH treatment [37]. During year 1, infants were randomized to GH (1 mg/m^2 per day) or no treatment; all infants were treated in the second year. Children older than 3 years were randomized to GH treatment (1 mg/m^2 per day) or no treatment for 2 years. The median height improved over 2 years in both the treated infant and childhood groups. Further, head circumference normalized during GH therapy. Although body fat percentage, body proportions, and lean body mass standard deviation score (SDS) improved in GH-treated children, they did not normalize fully. Interestingly, it was noted that GH prevented the reduction in lean body mass found in the untreated controls [37].

More recently, another randomized controlled GH trial was completed in 85 infants with PWS and prepubertal children older than 24 months with PWS. At baseline, mean fat percentage was elevated and 63% of infants and 73% of prepubertal children exhibited cardiovascular risk factors, such as hypertension or dyslipidemia. GH treatment improved height-SDS and BMI-SDS and reduced fat mass and % body fat, and increased the ratio of high-density lipoprotein (HDL):low-density lipoprotein (LDL) [38]. There were no effects on glucose homeostasis or plasma acylation stimulation protein (ASP). ASP is a hormone produced by adipocytes that is important in maintaining lipid homeostasis by increasing triglyceride storage and glucose uptake within adipose cells and reducing triglyceride lipolysis by inhibiting hormone-sensitive lipase.

Unique to the infant/toddler age, some investigators report that GH has benefits on cognition. GH prevented the deterioration of specific cognitive skills over a 2-year randomized controlled GH trial in 50 prepubertal children with PWS [33]: over 4 years of GH treatment, an improvement in abstract reasoning and visuospatial abilities were noted. Further longer-term controlled GH studies are required to assess the benefits of GH on cognition in early development in infants/toddlers with PWS.

Although GH has demonstrated many beneficial effects, there are notable risks of treatment. Some clinicians consider scoliosis to be a contraindication for GH treatment in PWS. However, a multicenter, randomized controlled GH study in infants and prepubertal and pubertal children (median age 4.7 [2.1–7.4] years) over 2 years demonstrated that both the onset and curve progression of scoliosis were no different between those on treatment than in controls [39]. A higher baseline IGF-1 SDS was associated with a lower severity of scoliosis, suggesting a protective effect of GH.

In smaller studies, GH therapy has been associated temporally with sudden death in PWS. The deaths have been concentrated in young children who have a history of respiratory obstruction/infection or severe obesity [40–48]. Deaths have generally occurred early in the course of GH therapy. The exact cause of the sudden deaths has not been determined. Possibilities include impaired ventilatory responsiveness to hypercapnia and hypoxia, increased lymphoid tissue or tonsillar hyperplasia, and/or adrenal insufficiency. It is nevertheless unclear if mortality in GH-treated patients with PWS exceeds expected mortality from PWS per se. Indeed, other studies support an opposing view that postulates a beneficial role for GH therapy in improved ventilation responsiveness to carbon dioxide and improved sleep quality in children with PWS [27,49,50].

Data in older children
In older children with PWS, GH treatment is now approved by the Food and Drug Administration and improves growth velocity and final height [51]. Additionally, body composition and bone mineral density are improved and resting energy expenditure (REE) is increased as a consequence of increases in skeletal muscle mass and enhanced rates of fatty acid oxidation [23,27,50–55]. Improvements in physical strength, respiratory muscle hypotonia, and peripheral chemoreceptor sensitivity to carbon dioxide have also been noted [27,28,50,51]. One study has also reported that GH treatment may improve overall sleep quality, with reduction in number of hypopnea and apnea events [50]. Finally, a few studies have found mild behavioral improvements, including reduction in depressive symptoms in those older than 11 years of age. In contrast, a long-term randomized controlled trial of GH in 42 children with PWS (3.5–14 years) showed no improvement in behavior problems (measured by a Developmental Behavior Checklist and a Children's Social Behavior Questionnaire).

Adaptive function (the ability to complete daily activities) was recently assessed in a 1-year to 2-year randomized controlled trial that then extended into 7 years of continuous GH treatment (1 mg/m^2 per day). The investigators showed a marked delay in adaptive functioning (Vineland Adaptive Behavior Scale) in infants and children with PWS, the severity of which increased with age and correlated inversely with IQ [56]. Those who began GH treatment in infancy had significantly improved adaptive functioning. No significant change in intelligence quotient has been demonstrated when GH therapy has been initiated later in childhood [50,57].

Fewer studies have examined the efficacy and safety of longer-term (beyond 2 years) GH treatment in children with PWS. The longest study to date followed 60 prepubertal children for 8 years on continuous GH treatment (1 mg/m^2 per day) [58]. Lean body mass (LBM) increased significantly during the first year and stabilized thereafter at a level above pretreatment baseline values ($P < .0001$). Percentage fat SDS and BMI SDS decreased significantly during the first year but then remained stable at values comparable to those at baseline ($P = .06$). The BMI-SDS, however, was significantly reduced at

8 years compared with baseline ($P<.0001$). Height SDS and head circumference SDS both completely normalized. IGF-1 SDS increased to +2.36 after the first year ($P<.0001$) and remained stable thereafter. No adverse outcomes on glucose homeostasis, lipids, blood pressure, or bone maturation were observed. Therefore, long-term GH therapy has positive effects on height and body composition that reduce the severity (but do not eliminate the risk) of childhood or adult obesity.

Data in adulthood

The use of GH in adults with PWS has been studied on a limited basis; doses have ranged from 0.2 to 1.6 mg daily. Sode-Carlsen and colleagues [59] evaluated the effects and safety of 2 years of GH therapy (average dose 0.61 mg daily) in 43 adults with PWS. Based on computed tomography findings, thigh muscle volume and LBM increased ($P<.001$) while abdominal subcutaneous fat volume and body fat mass decreased ($P<.01$). Fifteen of the patients had either diabetes (n = 4) or impaired glucose tolerance (IGT) (n = 11) at baseline. Among the 11 subjects with IGT, 3 progressed to overt diabetes, and 3 reverted to normal glucose tolerance. Höybye [60] studied 10 men with PWS after more than 5 years of GH treatment. The men who began treatment during childhood years were taller (178 ± 11 cm vs 156 ± 5 cm) and had lower fat mass and higher fat-free mass (FFM). Four individuals had type 2 diabetes that remained in good metabolic control. Two of these were treated with GH in childhood for 6 to 7 years' duration and 2 were treated in adulthood with GH duration 14 to 23 years. The investigators concluded that the decision to use GH needs to weigh both the benefits and potential side-effects in each patient [60].

Thus far, no consensus exists as to age of initiation of GH treatment. Infants as young as 2 to 4 months of age have been treated with GH, although no studies have systematically examined the risks and benefits of treatment in infancy. Currently, general consensus aims to treat before onset of obesity; thus, many begin treatment before 2 years of age [31]. Treatment should be initiated by an experienced clinician. Although further studies are still needed to determine optimal dosing in PWS, infants and children are generally started on a daily dose of 0.05 to 1 mg/m^2 per day or 0.1 to 0.15 mg/kg per week, with subsequent adjustments based on clinical response and IGF-1 levels (target +1 to +2 SDS). Adults can begin with a dose of 0.1 to 0.2 mg daily, with subsequent adjustments based on clinical response and IGF-1 levels (target 0 to +2 SDS). Until studies definitively address concerns regarding sleep apnea and growth hormone use, a pretreatment airway and sleep evaluation is recommended before, and possibly during, GH therapy. The dose of GH should be adjusted to maintain IGF-1 levels in the normal range (to prevent lymphoid or tonsillar hyperplasia). Children receiving GH therapy also should be monitored for potential side effects of GH, which can include headaches, glucose intolerance, and worsening scoliosis. Our suggested protocol for initiation of GH and monitoring of infants/children with PWS on therapy is shown in Fig. 3.

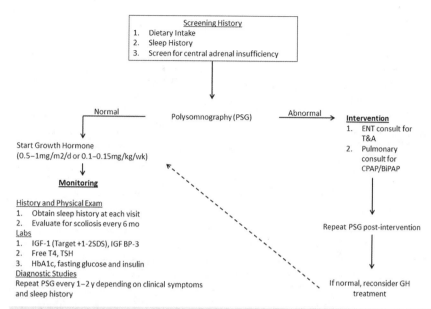

Fig. 3. Algorithm for initiation of GH therapy in infants and children. ENT, ear, nose, and throat; PSG, polysomnography. BiPAP, bilevel positive airway pressure; T&A, tonsillectomy and adenoidectomy.

Central adrenal insufficiency

Infants and children with PWS have hypothalamic dysfunction and, therefore, are at risk of central adrenal insufficiency. The prevalence of adrenal insufficiency remains unknown. Some studies that used metyrapone testing reported rates of central adrenal insufficiency as high as 60%; however, testing modalities vary considerably and more recent studies with low-dose adrenocorticotropic hormone (ACTH) stimulation suggest prevalence as low as 14.3% [61]. The identification and treatment of central adrenal insufficiency are critical, as it is suspected to be a potential cause of sudden death in some patients: small adrenal glands were found on autopsy in a subset of patients with PWS who had died suddenly in childhood [62]. Additionally, GH may decrease conversion of cortisone to cortisol by inhibiting 11-beta hydroxysteroid dehydrogenase type 1. The impact of GH therapy on baseline adrenal function and the adrenal response to stress in PWS remains unclear.

Although no consensus guidelines exist, we recommend an evaluation of the corticoadrenal axis in patients with PWS. To that end, the levels of ACTH and cortisol should be obtained at the time of diagnosis, before starting GH therapy (see Fig. 3) and during times of acute stress (ie, severe illness, before anesthesia or surgery) [63]. Parents should be provided a vial of parenteral hydrocortisone that can be used at times of high fever, vomiting, or trauma. Prophylactic stress dose glucocorticoid treatment should be administered (37.5–50 mg/m^2 per day) during times of acute illness or surgery [61,63,64].

Hypogonadism

Children with PWS classically have physical findings of hypogonadism. However, the degree of hypogonadism varies in severity: pubertal development is absent in some and delayed or arrested in others. Varying degrees of genital hypoplasia may be detected at birth. Girls may have small labia or hypoplastic clitoris [63]. Boys commonly have either unilateral or bilateral cryptorchidism, underdeveloped scrotum, and/or microphallus [63]. Boys may require orchiopexy, but some studies suggest use of human chorionic gonadotropin (HCG) to promote testicular descent and increase scrotal and penile size [65]. Long-term data regarding use of HCG in infants with PWS is currently insufficient, but hormone treatment may prevent need for surgery and general anesthesia.

The cause of hypogonadism remains unclear. Although it has generally been felt to be caused by hypogonadotropic hypogonadism, the evidence for this is conflicting and some argue there may be a component of primary gonadal insufficiency. Hirsch and colleagues [66] demonstrated increased gonadotropins with low inhibin B and low testosterone levels in teenage and adult male individuals suggestive of primary gonadal dysfunction. Female patients with PWS have delayed or absent maturation of ovarian follicles associated with delayed or arrested pubertal progression [67]. Despite this, they have normal or subnormal gonadotropin levels, suggesting central or hypothalamic hypogonadism. Breast development is highly variable with some studies demonstrating complete tanner V breast development and vaginal bleeding occurs in some but not all [66]. Interestingly, despite delayed or incomplete pubertal development, patients with PWS often have precocious adrenarche [63]. Compared with healthy children, children with PWS have higher serum DHEAS levels, possibly reflecting early maturation of the adrenal zona reticularis [68].

There are case reports of female patients with PWS giving birth to children with Angelman syndrome [69,70]. Therefore, we recommend family planning counseling for teenage and adult women with PWS.

Hypothyroidism

Up to one-third of children with PWS have been reported to have hypothyroidism due to hypothalamic pituitary dysfunction [63], with low or low-normal thyroid-stimulating hormone (TSH) and low total or free thyroxine (fT4). Because thyroid hormone is essential for appropriate neurodevelopment during the first 3 years of life, we recommended that thyroid function be assessed at 3, 6, and 12 months of age and then at least annually [63]. Hypothyroidism can impede GH synthesis and secretion; thus, GH testing in children with PWS should be conducted only after normal thyroid function is established. Conversely, GH treatment may affect thyroid function; it is critical that thyroid function be monitored during GH therapy.

Glucose homeostasis

Obesity is a strong risk factor for the development of type 2 diabetes (T2D). The prevalence of T2D in adults with PWS (7%–20%) exceeds greatly the prevalence in the general population (5%–7%) [71]. In one cohort of 66 adults with PWS, the mean onset of T2D was 20 years [71]. It is uncommon for prepubertal children with PWS to develop overt diabetes or glucose intolerance: a large population-based PWS cohort in France showed no cases of T2D and only 4% incidence of glucose intolerance at a mean age of 10.2 years [72].

In fact, fasting insulin and HOMA-IR in PWS are comparable to those in BMI–age-matched controls before age 5 years [9] and are significantly *lower* by age 11 [73]. In several studies, the lower fasting insulin and HOMA-IR were seen in adults with PWS [73,74]; however, a more recent smaller study failed to recapitulate these findings and suggested further investigation with hyperinsulinemic-euglycemic clamp [75].

It has been assumed that T2D in PWS develops as a consequence of morbid obesity and concomitant insulin resistance. However, recent studies suggest the relationship between morbid obesity and development of T2D is more complex and appears to differ in individuals with PWS versus those without PWS. For example, in children with PWS compared with BMI-matched controls, the insulin response to both a mixed meal and an oral glucose load is lower [14]. Additionally, first and second phase insulin secretion were significantly lower in adults with PWS compared with OCs during an intravenous glucose tolerance test (IVGTT) [76]. Finally, normal or increased sensitivity to exogenous insulin has been observed in individuals with PWS [77,78]. In a recent study by our group, patients with PWS had relatively lower fasting insulin levels and increased adiponectin levels compared with BMI-matched OCs despite having similar levels of leptin [12]. These findings suggest that children with PWS may be protected to some extent from obesity-associated insulin resistance [13].

The incretin system has been inadequately investigated as a cause of the relative hypoinsulinemia seen in PWS. Several case reports suggest favorable outcomes using glucagon-like peptide 1 (GLP-1) agonists/analogs with regard to weight loss, glycemic control, ghrelin reduction, and preprandial insulin secretion [79]. The paucity of side effects with GLP-1 pharmacotherapy in this group has led some to speculate those with PWS may have deficient GLP-1 signaling in the brain [80]. Fasting GLP-1 levels were no different between PWS and OCs [75,81], but levels have not been evaluated after stimulation with oral glucose tolerance test (OGTT). Fasting glucose-dependent insulinotropic polypeptide (GIP) levels are higher in those with PWS compared with OCs, but levels also have not been evaluated after enteral stimulation [82].

The explanation for beta-cell dysfunction in PWS remains elusive, but one hypothesis is that a decrease in vagal parasympathetic tone to the pancreas in individuals with PWS reduces insulin secretion [83]. Another hypothesis proposes that GH deficiency in PWS reduces beta cell insulin secretion and increases insulin sensitivity. We have also hypothesized that relative hyperadiponectinemia may promote fatty acid oxidation and thereby increase insulin sensitivity [12]. Exploration of the association among various genotypes in

PWS and the presence or absence of glucose intolerance and diabetes has not been fully explored.

Treatment of T2D in individuals with PWS requires weight reduction by dietary modification and, sometimes, addition of an oral agent such as metformin, or insulin therapy. The role of GLP-1 agonist therapy is promising, but has not yet been fully elucidated.

EXTRAHORMONAL COMORBIDITIES IN PRADER WILLI SYNDROME

Sleep disorders

Sleep disturbances are common in children with PWS. This may manifest as obstructive sleep apnea, central sleep apnea, and hypoventilation syndromes. Children with PWS may have abnormal arousal and cardiorespiratory response to hypercapnia [81]. Central sleep apnea occurs more commonly in infants with PWS (younger than 2 years), whereas obstructive sleep apnea is more frequent in children older than 2 years [84]. Central sleep apnea may result from hypothalamic dysfunction and/or abnormal responses to hypoxia and hypercapnia by chemoreceptors; obstructive sleep apnea reflects the combined effects of obesity and hypotonia [84]. GH may potentiate the risk of obstructive sleep apnea by increasing growth of adenotonsillar tissue (see more later in this article).

The effects of chronic sleep disturbance and hypoventilation on long-term neurocognitive outcomes remain unknown. Nevertheless, a sleep history should be obtained at each clinic visit; formal polysomnography should be performed if there is any evidence of sleep disturbance, including persistent snoring or excessive daytime sleepiness. Recent guidelines from the American Academy of Pediatrics recommend obtaining polysomnography before GH therapy and within 2 to 3 months following initiation of GH treatment with annual evaluation [65].

Some centers recommend low-flow nocturnal supplemental oxygen therapy for infants with PWS with central sleep apnea [84]. Older children with obstructive sleep apnea may respond to intranasal glucocorticoids or may require ear, nose, and throat referral for tonsillectomy/adenoidectomy [84] or initiation of continuous positive airway pressure.

Some children with PWS have narcolepsy [85,86]. Narcolepsy is associated with a reduction in neurons expressing hypocretin (orexin), a neurohormone secreted by the lateral hypothalamus [87]. Therefore, it has been theorized that sleep disturbances in PWS are caused by hypothalamic dysfunction. However, studies of the total number of hypocretin neurons in PWS have been conflicting [87,88]. Treatments of sleep disturbances, including narcolepsy, are discussed later in this review.

Behavioral problems and psychiatric disturbances

Children with PWS can have several behavioral problems in addition to disordered feeding [1]. In young children, these range from mild tantrums and stubbornness to more extreme property destruction or physical attacks of rage [89,90]. Older adolescents and adults may exhibit sadness, anxiety, and depression, leading to negative self-image and withdrawal [89,91]. In addition, children and adolescents may develop a form of obsessive-compulsive disorder. This may manifest as hoarding (food and nonfood items), repetitive rituals, and skin picking [89].

The pathogenesis of the various behavioral concerns is currently unclear, but recent findings implicate a role for the hormone oxytocin. Oxytocin is an anorexigenic neuropeptide secreted by the hypothalamic paraventricular nucleus; it is also thought to play a role in social cognition and obsessive-compulsive disorder. Reports have published decreased expression of the oxytocin receptor and decreased oxytocin neurons within the hypothalamic paraventricular neurons, and recent data have shown elevated oxytocin levels in PWS compared with healthy controls [92]. The increased oxytocin levels may reflect oxytocin resistance and help explain the obsessive-compulsive tendencies in PWS, but further studies are needed to determine causality. Recent studies showing increased oxytocin levels in PWS may reflect loss of regulatory feedback due to decreased oxytocin receptor expression [92].

METABOLIC STUDIES
Body composition in Prader Willi syndrome
Several studies looking at body composition in children with PWS by various methods (skinfold measurements, total body water, bioelectrical impedance analysis [BIA], deuterium dilution method) have demonstrated higher amounts of adipose tissue in children with PWS compared with obese children without PWS [93,94]. However, as each technique has its advantages and disadvantages [17], results have been inconsistent [18,19]. Our group has recently [19] used an abdominal MRI technique to compare changes in body composition between children with PWS and non-PWS BMI-z and age-matched controls. Preliminary results indicate that children with PWS have lower skeletal muscle mass compared with controls, but similar total adipose tissue volume in the abdominal region. In addition, a greater ratio of intramuscular adipose tissue/skeletal muscle was found in the PWS group, suggesting the possibility that PWS represents a unique congenital model of sarcopenia. Further studies are required to determine if this altered body composition phenotype in PWS might be associated with poor motor function throughout development.

Energy balance in Prader Willi syndrome
Evidence suggests that the distinctive weight gain in individuals with PWS may be caused by an alteration of the components of total energy expenditure (EE), such as REE, activity energy expenditure (AEE), and diet-induced thermogenesis (DIT) [95]. To date, the critical underlying EE and energy intake factors that regulate energy balance in PWS are not fully understood. REE is considered the main component of daily EE, accounting for 50% to 75% of total EE. Approximately 20% to 40% of EE is spent during AEE, and 10% to 15% on

DIT [96]. A major determinant of REE is the FFM. Total EE, measured by doubly labeled water, has been found to be decreased in individuals with PWS; most, but not all, of the decrease has been attributed to their small FFM and reduced physical activity [94]. Overall, studies also indicate that individuals with PWS have lower absolute REE or basal metabolic rate than matched controls [94,97–101]. However, when results were adjusted for the lower FFM in PWS (per unit of body surface area [function of weight and height] or per kilogram of LBM), differences were no longer apparent. DIT (the energy expended with the digestion and absorption of food) has been studied on a limited basis in individuals with PWS and the results have been inconclusive. Some studies showed lower values of DIT in obese individuals and individuals with PWS [102–105], whereas others showed increased values of DIT after a meal challenge [106] or no difference at all [75,107,108]. Therefore, obese individuals and individuals with PWS may exhibit subtle changes in DIT and further controlled studies are required to assess for this defect, which might have effects on metabolic health. Finally, the contribution of physical activity to total EE in individuals with PWS has been examined. These studies suggest that individuals with PWS are less active in general, but there is a wide range of activity levels, which is a function of individual characteristics. Also, physical activity is as energy burning and as metabolically beneficial in individuals with PWS as in healthy individuals [109–111]. Therefore, raising physical activity levels in individuals with PWS will increase their total EE, increase their LBM, and help in maintenance of body weight in general [112].

CURRENT STANDARD THERAPIES
Nutritional phases and hyperphagia
Three major nutritional phases with distinctive clinical characteristics have been defined in PWS (Fig. 4) [113]. In phase 1 (0–9 months), newborns exhibit low muscle tone (hypotonia) with weak and uncoordinated suck, resulting in low caloric intake. Typically, infants need gavage feeding or the use of special nipples to maintain body weight. By the age of 9 to 25 months, infants no longer need assisted feeding. In phase 2 (2.1–4.5 years), there is an increase in body weight without obvious food seeking or a change in dietary intake. At this stage, infants are likely to become obese if their caloric intake is not restricted. By the age of 4.5 to 8.0 years during phase 2b, a significant increase in appetite and a marked interest in food are noted. Yet children may stop eating voluntarily at this stage. However, if food intake is not strictly supervised during phase 3 (8 years to adulthood), which is characterized by chronic overeating (hyperphagia) and lack of satiety, individuals will gain excessive weight and manifest progressive obesity [113].

Food-related behaviors, such as sneaking and hoarding food, are serious problems for individuals with PWS. When given unlimited access to food, children and teenagers with PWS can consume massive amounts of food. Bray and colleagues [77] reported the average ad libitum energy intake of 6 unsupervised individuals with PWS ages 16 to 25 years to be 5167 ± 503 kcal per day.

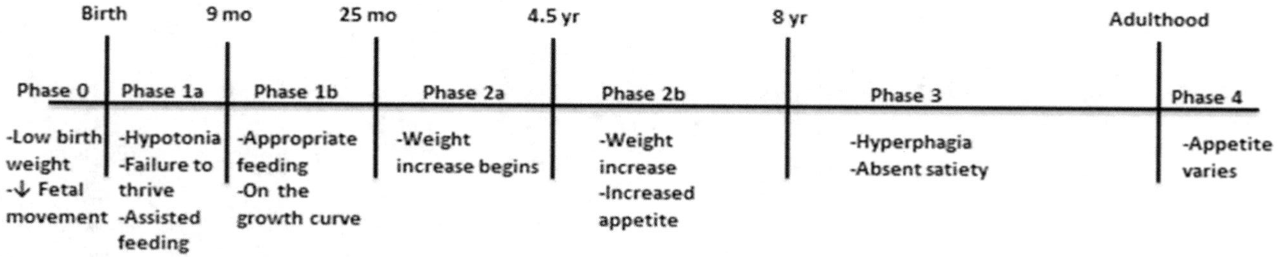

Fig. 4. Timeline of nutritional phases in PWS. (*Adapted from* Miller JL, Lynn CH, Driscoll DC, et al. Nutritional phases in Prader–Willi syndrome. Am J Med Genet Part A 2011;155(5):1040–9.)

Consumption of food considered inappropriate (such as dog and cat food, garbage) may be an additional concern. Families report that children with PWS may be obsessed with refrigerators and freezers, worry about food (if there is enough, where the next meal will come from) and are generally preoccupied with food and eating [114].

Nutritional management

Data generated on preschool and school-age children with PWS indicate that an energy-restricted diet of 7 kcal/cm per day will induce weight loss in PWS at any age [114,115]. In addition, diets providing 8 to 11 kcal/cm per day have been reported to allow for weight maintenance [114,115]. These energy goals translate into daily intakes of approximately 600 to 800 kcal for young children with PWS and 800 to 1300 kcal for older children and adults with PWS [115]. These energy goals are considerably lower than the caloric intake of normal children. Of note is that many group homes for individuals with PWS provide a diet consisting of 1000 kcal/day [116]. It is important to note that early dietary restriction in children with PWS may limit growth velocity and, possibly, final height. In this regard, GH therapy may be useful in promoting linear growth and improving body composition (increase lean mass and reduce fat mass).

The optimal macronutrient composition of the diet for individuals with PWS has not been determined. Some investigators suggest a diet consisting of approximately 25% protein, 50% carbohydrate, and 25% fat [115]. Based on limited data, others suggest that hunger may be attenuated by the use of a ketogenic diet or protein-sparing modified fast [117]; however, findings remain inconclusive. Indeed, various dietary interventions have been studied in children with PWS; these include low-calorie diets combined with specific behavior management [118–120], hypocaloric diets [114,121–123], hypocaloric protein-sparing diets [124,125], energy-restricted ketogenic diets [109,117], and balanced macronutrient diets devoid of simple sugar [126]. Each of these dietary interventions required long-term intervention/adherence and had only limited success. The dietary composition of macronutrients optimal for metabolic control (eg, maximizing degree and duration of ghrelin suppression and optimizing insulin sensitivity) in PWS remains to be determined and is the subject of our groups' ongoing work [14]. Finally, an accurate pictorial assessment tool for appetite, satiety, and degree of hyperphagia in PWS is also the subject of ongoing research in our group.

Due to potential for insufficient intake of essential vitamins and minerals during prolonged periods of caloric restriction, a daily multivitamin and calcium and vitamin D supplementation is often required.

Nutritional management should begin in toddlerhood to prevent excessive weight gain and obesity-related risks, such as type 2 diabetes and cardiovascular disease. Obesity typically emerges soon after the age of 2 years if dietary intake is not closely monitored. Early intervention may be helpful in preventing excessive weight gain [127]; control of dietary intake through behavior and environmental modification (eg, locking the refrigerator and cupboards) is required.

In general, nutrition education is essential to help individuals with PWS maintain healthy weights. Because infants with PWS rarely wake to feed during nutritional phase 1, a regular feeding schedule should be one of the first strategies implemented by parents and caregivers. Monitoring of caloric intake and monthly monitoring of height, weight, and head circumference for the first 6 months and quarterly for 12 to 24 months is advisable. Caloric intake should be increased gradually (by a maximum ~100–200 kcal/d) to avoid overshooting weight goals. Consistency with meal patterns and times for eating is important.

Care providers should be taught about portion sizes; these are best described using common measurements, such as cups, teaspoons, and fluid ounces or grams. It may be useful initially to record measurements for all daily food intake. Individualized menus should account for different family lifestyles and be planned with a nutritionist on an ongoing basis. Consideration of food preferences is important; individuals with PWS do have definite consistent preferences for sweets, and in most studies have exhibited a preference for calorie-dense over lower-calorie foods [128]. The child should play an active role in meal planning when possible. Vitamin and mineral intake also should be monitored (especially calcium and vitamin D), and supplements given as needed.

Finally, daily exercise should be part of the regular routine to enhance aerobic fitness and EE and sustain weight loss [129]. A reward system of points or verbal praise may provide motivation for weight loss. Additional nutritional education resources are available from the Prader-Willi Syndrome Association (United States).

Sex hormone replacement therapy

Male and female adolescents with PWS classically have incomplete or absent pubertal development; together with sarcopenia and low muscle tone, sedentary lifestyle, and GH deficiency [130], this places them at risk for osteopenia and fractures. Treatment with sex hormones may improve bone health, muscle mass, and overall well-being. However, recent studies have determined GH treatment will improve bone size and strength independent of sex steroid replacement [131]. Although experts agree that dosing and timing of sex hormone replacement should mirror normal pubertal timing, there is no consensus on a regimen or timing for pubertal induction [132]. Therapy must be individualized; thus, the management of sex hormone replacement therapy should be supervised by a pediatric endocrinologist.

Initial evaluation of teenage girls with incomplete or arrested puberty should include measurements of estradiol, gonadotropins, and inhibin B [66]. Those without contraindications may be treated with a low-dose estrogen patch; progesterone can be added after the onset of menses. Contraceptive counseling is warranted, as some women with PWS have been reported to give birth [133]. There have been no documented cases of male PWS paternity [63].

Testosterone has been reported to precipitate or exacerbate aggression in some adolescent males with PWS [132]. Teenagers should be treated initially with transdermal testosterone at low doses, with cautious dose titration as tolerated [132].

NEW APPROACHES TO THERAPY

Oxytocin for hyperphagia and behavioral disorders

Levels of the anorexigenic neuropeptide oxytocin have been shown to be higher in patients with PWS compared with healthy controls, suggesting dysregulated oxytocin feedback or responsiveness may play a role in hyperphagia and behavioral disturbances [92]. Oxytocin has been shown to decrease aggressive behavior in animal studies, and improve recognition of facial emotions in adolescents with autism [134]. Clinical trials in PWS investigating the effects of intranasal oxytocin on hyperphagia, skin picking, obsessions, and emotional states have yielded conflicting results, with single-dose trials showing improved trust in treated participants but multidose trials showing no benefits in clinical outcomes [134,135].

Co-enzyme Q10 and carnitine to increase energy expenditure

PWS is characterized by infantile hypotonia, sarcopenia, and decreased REE [63]. Some of these features are found in other disorders with low levels of co-enzyme Q10 (CoQ10), an electron carrier and essential component of the mitochondrial respiratory chain [136]. CoQ10 levels have been shown to be lower in children with PWS and obese children relative to healthy non-OCs [137]. Although CoQ10 is often used as an adjunct treatment in PWS with no known adverse effects, its efficacy in improving motor development and metabolic function is inconclusive [138]. However, individuals have reported improved daytime alertness with CoQ10 supplementation [139].

Carnitine deficiency, similar to CoQ10 deficiency, is associated with hypotonia, poor growth, and easy fatigability. Interestingly, unlike CoQ10, carnitine levels have been shown to be higher in PWS than in healthy controls, suggesting impaired carnitine utilization in PWS [139]. Data remain inconclusive as to any positive effects of carnitine supplementation. In a recent study, 20 subjects were treated with carnitine 25 mg/kg twice daily; 13 subjects reported improved exercise tolerance and daytime alertness and 7 subjects reported no benefits [139].

Modafinil for narcolepsy and daytime sleepiness

Excessive daytime sleepiness and increased napping can have a negative impact on quality of life [85]. Modafinil is a central stimulant that has been used in adults with narcolepsy and has recently been studied in adolescents with PWS with hypersomnia. In a pilot study, modafinil was well tolerated and reduced daytime sleepiness without serious side effects, such as headache, insomnia, anxiety, or nausea [85].

N-acetylcysteine for obsessive picking of the skin

As previously discussed, children with PWS and teens may have self-mutilation behaviors, such as skin-picking. This has been related to obsessive-compulsive disorder and can be severe, leading to skin infections and scarring. Areas most commonly affected are the face, hands, and legs and may be increased in areas of bug bites, scabs, or eczematous lesions. Animal models have implicated glutamate neurotransmission in obsessive-compulsive behaviors [140]. *N*-acetylcysteine (NAC) acts on the N-methyl-D-aspartate glutamate receptors to increase glutathione and has had potential efficacy in reducing nicotine-seeking and obsessive-compulsive behaviors in rat studies [141]. A recent pilot study evaluated the effect of NAC on skin-picking behavior in PWS [142]. Thirty-five children with PWS with skin-picking received an oral dose of 450 to 1200 mg NAC daily and were then followed for 12 weeks. In this pilot study, results showed complete resolution of skin picking in approximately 70% and reduction in skin picking in almost 30%. Future studies with long-term follow-up are still needed to determine efficacy. Although NAC is generally well-tolerated, side effects have included abdominal cramping, flatulence, and diarrhea.

Beloranib for hyperphagia

Of great interest to the PWS research community is a medical agent that can reduce hyperphagia. Beloranib is an irreversible inhibitor of methionine amino-peptidase 2 (MetAP2), an enzyme that removes N-terminal methionine residues from newly synthesized proteins. MetAP2 inhibitors were previously used in cancer therapy because of their ability to slow endothelial cell growth and reduce angiogenesis; they were found to reduce food intake, lower body weight, and decrease adipose tissue mass at doses lower than those needed to inhibit angiogenesis and tumor growth [143]. Although the exact mechanism of weight loss and decreased appetite is unclear, the MetAP2 inhibitors result in triglyceride lipolysis, fatty acid oxidation, ketogenesis, and suppression of food intake related to alterations in signaling of the extracellular signal-related kinase (ERK) stress kinase pathway [143]. Small randomized, double-blind, placebo-controlled 4-week trials of beloranib as a novel treatment for PWS (n = 17) have shown dose-dependent (placebo, 1.2 mg, 1.8 mg beloranib twice weekly) body weight/mass reductions despite concurrent 50% increase in total caloric intake during the study. Elevation in HDL and adiponectin and reduction in leptin, LDL and high sensitivity C-reactive protein were also observed during treatment [144]. A similar randomized, double-blind placebo-controlled 4-week trial of beloranib (1.8 mg twice weekly) in patients with hypothalamic obesity also showed beneficial weight loss and improvements in cardiometabolic profile and hyperphagia [145]. Future longer-term clinical trials of beloranib are warranted to assess for changes in body weight, hyperphagia-related behaviors, and overall longer-term side-effect profile. As of December 2015, beloranib PWS trials have been placed on a partial clinical hold due to the death of 2 patients receiving the drug. The causes of death in each case were pulmonary emboli, but it is not known if these events were caused by beloranib. Prior trials using the medication had reported thromboembolic events, and clinical research participants will be screened for thromboembolic disease.

Bariatric surgery

Although a medical cure for hyperphagia remains elusive both in PWS and the general population, bariatric surgery has found increasing success in the treatment of morbid obesity. Concerns were initially raised about the safety and long-term efficacy of surgical procedures, including truncal vagotomy, gastroplasty, and endoscopic balloon placement, and malabsorptive procedures, such as Roux-en-Y gastric bypass and biliopancreatic diversion, in the PWS population [97]. However, more recent data from several groups report beneficial effects of bariatric procedures in PWS. One group from Saudi Arabia reported findings in 24 subjects with PWS (4.9–18 years; preoperative BMI = 46.2 ± 12.2 kg/m^2) who underwent laparoscopic sleeve gastrectomy (LSG) [146]. BMI (kg/m^2) changes in yearly visits during 5 years of follow-up were as follows: -14.7 (year 1; n = 22), -15.0 (year 2; n = 18), -12.2 (year 3; n = 13), -12.7 (year 4; n = 11), and -10.7 (year 5; n = 7). Most subjects lost most of their weight within the first 2 years after surgery, with a plateau thereafter for another year, following by subsequent weight regain. The PWS group had 95% of comorbidities in remission or improved. No significant differences were seen in BMI change or growth rate or remission in obesity-related comorbidities between PWS and a non-PWS control group that underwent similar surgical procedures. No mortality or major morbidity were reported over the 5-year follow-up period. Interestingly, the families reported better control of hyperphagia and food-seeking behaviors postoperatively.

Another group from China reported their data on 3 children with PWS (15–23 years; mean BMI = 46.7 kg/m^2) [147]. Two patients underwent sleeve gastrectomy, and 1 underwent laparoscopic mini-gastric bypass. The mean weight loss and percentage of excessive weight loss at 2 years was 32.5% and 63.2%, respectively. The mean level of fasting acylated ghrelin decreased from 1134.2 pg/mL preoperatively to 519.8 pg/mL 1 year postoperatively. No major perioperative complications or mortality occurred. These investigators also noted all patients had subjectively reduced food-seeking behaviors and hyperphagia.

Removal of more than 75% of the stomach by sleeve gastrectomy is associated with favorable metabolic changes (reduction in ghrelin and increase in GLP-1) with minimal nutrient malabsorption. Future long-term studies of the use of LSG in patients with PWS are warranted. Careful analysis of degree of weight loss, resolution of comorbidities, and safety will be required to assess the overall success of bariatric procedures in the PWS population.

LONG-TERM CARE AND LIFE SPAN

Although much is known about PWS in childhood and early adulthood, less is known about PWS in later adulthood. There are limited survival data beyond the fifth to sixth decade, but recent surveillance data estimate that mortality rates have declined to less than 3% annually due to improved medical care [148]. Given the increasing life span of PWS, it is generally advised to provide routine health surveillance for earlier detection of adult illness [149]. The more frequently reported illnesses in older adults with PWS have included diabetes, cardiovascular disease with hypertension, osteoporosis, and sleep disorders [149]. The major causes of death are secondary to obesity and include respiratory failure with cor pulmonale, type 2 diabetes mellitus, and arteriosclerosis. Due to autonomic dysfunction manifesting as a high pain threshold and abnormal temperature regulation, subjects may not complain of pain, fever, or other signs of infection or other illnesses. Other health issues seen in adults with PWS include scoliosis, hypoventilation, recurrent respiratory infections/aspiration, choking, sleep apnea, hypertension, osteoporosis, and leg ulceration [71].

Adults with PWS have early functional decline, making activities of daily living more difficult [149]. Psychiatric symptoms or psychosis may emerge, necessitating psychological evaluation and/or medical treatment. Tantrums and stubbornness may prevent adults with PWS from living in the community at large and retaining jobs. Group homes that operate with resources of a multidisciplinary team and emphasize control of diet and behavior management tend to be successful [17]. Additionally, most adults with PWS who are successfully employed are in sheltered workshops that provide a structured environment that is free from all sources of potentially edible food items. Many individuals with PWS have good fine motor skills. Thus, it is often beneficial for families to work with an attorney specializing in working with families of the disabled. Community resources for families are available through the Prader-Willi Syndrome Association in the United States.

Future studies and therapies

A lack of detailed understanding of the neuroendocrine control of appetite and obesity in PWS currently hampers progress into design of antiobesity drugs. However, some strides have been made. It is possible that specific ghrelin antagonists may assist in reducing PWS-related obesity. In addition, recent evidence suggests that central melanocortin agonists may block ghrelin-mediated feeding. Therefore, potential combinatorial therapy with a ghrelin antagonist and melanocortin agonist may ameliorate hyperghrelinemia effects in PWS.

These studies provide some hope, but many questions still remain unanswered. Future studies may aim at understanding genetic mechanisms of PWS obesity and relative insulin sensitivity, the regulation of ghrelin receptors and effect on appetite and weight, the cause for hyperghrelinemia, and the risks and benefits of therapies aimed at controlling appetite-regulating hormones.

SUMMARY

PWS has a unique phenotypic profile and remains the most common cause of syndromic obesity. Diagnostic advances have resulted in early detection of

PWS in infants and young children, allowing for early treatment and improved outcomes. GH therapy has been shown to have therapeutic benefits in PWS, and requires close monitoring for adverse events. Several top priority areas for GH research in PWS include determination of optimal timing and dosage of GH treatment initiation in early life, longer-term data on safety and efficacy of GH in PWS populations across international databases and registries, further evaluation of GH effects on behavior and cognition across development, longer-term data on appropriate monitoring for sleep-disordered breathing after-GH initiation, and randomized controlled trials to evaluate the effects of GH therapy in concert with other novel therapeutic strategies including bariatric surgery.

References

[1] Cassidy SB, Dykens E, Williams CA. Prader-Willi and Angelman syndromes: sister imprinted disorders. Am J Med Genet 2000;97(2):136–46.

[2] Bervini S, Herzog H. Mouse models of Prader–Willi syndrome: a systematic review. Front Neuroendocrinol 2013;34(2):107–19.

[3] Miller NLG, Wevrick R, Mellon PL. Necdin, a Prader–Willi syndrome candidate gene, regulates gonadotropin-releasing hormone neurons during development. Hum Mol Genet 2009;18(2):248–60.

[4] Bischof JM, Stewart CL, Wevrick R. Inactivation of the mouse Magel2 gene results in growth abnormalities similar to Prader-Willi syndrome. Hum Mol Genet 2007;16(22):2713–9.

[5] Ding F, Li HH, Zhang S, et al. SnoRNA Snord116 deletion causes growth deficiency and hyperphagia in mice. PLoS One 2008;3(3):e1709.

[6] Holm VA, Cassidy SB, Butler MG, et al. Prader-Willi syndrome: consensus diagnostic criteria. Pediatrics 1993;91(2):398–402.

[7] Gunay-Aygun M, Schwartz S, Heeger S, et al. The changing purpose of Prader-Willi syndrome clinical diagnostic criteria and proposed revised criteria. Pediatrics 2001;108(5):E92.

[8] Haqq AM, Grambow SC, Muehlbauer M, et al. Ghrelin concentrations in Prader-Willi syndrome (PWS) infants and children: changes during development. Clin Endocrinol (Oxf) 2008;69(6):911–20.

[9] Goldstone AP, Holland AJ, Butler JV, et al. Appetite hormones and the transition to hyperphagia in children with Prader-Willi syndrome. Int J Obes (Lond) 2012;36(12):1564–70.

[10] Erdie-Lalena CR, Holm VA, Kelly PC, et al. Ghrelin levels in young children with Prader-Willi syndrome. J Pediatr 2006;149(2):199–204.

[11] Cummings DE, Clement K, Purnell JQ, et al. Elevated plasma ghrelin levels in Prader Willi syndrome. Nat Med 2002;8(7):643–4.

[12] Irizarry KA, Bain J, Butler MG, et al. Metabolic profiling in Prader–Willi syndrome and non-syndromic obesity: sex differences and the role of growth hormone. Clin Endocrinol 2015;83(6):797–805.

[13] Haqq AM, Muehlbauer MJ, Newgard CB, et al. The metabolic phenotype of Prader-Willi syndrome (PWS) in childhood: heightened insulin sensitivity relative to body mass index. J Clin Endocrinol Metab 2011;96(1):E225–32.

[14] Gumus Balikcioglu P, Balikcioglu M, Muehlbauer MJ, et al. Macronutrient regulation of ghrelin and peptide YY in pediatric obesity and Prader-Willi syndrome. J Clin Endocrinol Metab 2015;100(10):3822–31.

[15] Butler MG, Meaney FJ. Standards for selected anthropometric measurements in Prader-Willi syndrome. Pediatrics 1991;88(4):853–60.

[16] Wollmann HA, Schultz U, Grauer ML, et al. Reference values for height and weight in Prader-Willi syndrome based on 315 patients. Eur J Pediatr 1998;157(8):634–42.

[17] Greenswag LR. Adults with Prader-Willi syndrome: a survey of 232 cases. Dev Med Child Neurol 1987;29(2):145–52.

[18] Costeff H, Holm VA, Ruvalcaba R, et al. Growth hormone secretion in Prader-Willi syndrome. Acta Paediatr Scand 1990;79(11):1059–62.

[19] Cappa M, Grossi A, Borrelli P, et al. Growth hormone (GH) response to combined pyridostigmine and GH-releasing hormone administration in patients with Prader-Labhard-Willi syndrome. Horm Res 1993;39(1–2):51–5.

[20] Angulo M, Castro-Magana M, Mazur B, et al. Growth hormone secretion and effects of growth hormone therapy on growth velocity and weight gain in children with Prader-Willi syndrome. J Pediatr Endocrinol Metab 1996;9(3):393–400.

[21] Grosso S, Cioni M, Buoni S, et al. Growth hormone secretion in Prader-Willi syndrome. J Endocrinol Invest 1998;21(7):418–22.

[22] Grugni G, Guzzaloni G, Moro D, et al. Reduced growth hormone (GH) responsiveness to combined GH-releasing hormone and pyridostigmine administration in the Prader-Willi syndrome. Clin Endocrinol (Oxf) 1998;48(6):769–75.

[23] Lindgren AC, Hagenas L, Muller J, et al. Growth hormone treatment of children with Prader-Willi syndrome affects linear growth and body composition favourably. Acta Paediatr 1998;87(1):28–31.

[24] Thacker MJ, Hainline B, St Dennis-Feezle L, et al. Growth failure in Prader-Willi syndrome is secondary to growth hormone deficiency. Horm Res 1998;49(5):216–20.

[25] Corrias A, Bellone J, Beccaria L, et al. GH/IGF-I axis in Prader-Willi syndrome: evaluation of IGF-I levels and of the somatotroph responsiveness to various provocative stimuli. Genetic Obesity Study Group of Italian Society of Pediatric Endocrinology and Diabetology. J Endocrinol Invest 2000;23(2):84–9.

[26] Eiholzer U, Stutz K, Weinmann C, et al. Low insulin, IGF-I and IGFBP-3 levels in children with Prader-Labhart-Willi syndrome. Eur J Pediatr 1998;157(11):890–3.

[27] Carrel AL, Myers SE, Whitman BY, et al. Growth hormone improves body composition, fat utilization, physical strength and agility, and growth in Prader-Willi syndrome: a controlled study. J Pediatr 1999;134(2):215–21.

[28] Burman P, Ritzen EM, Lindgren AC. Endocrine dysfunction in Prader-Willi syndrome: a review with special reference to GH. Endocr Rev 2001;22(6):787–99.

[29] Grugni G, Guzzaloni G, Morabito F. Impairment of GH responsiveness to GH-releasing hexapeptide (GHRP-6) in Prader-Willi syndrome. J Endocrinol Invest 2001;24(5):340–8.

[30] Brambilla P, Bosio L, Manzoni P, et al. Peculiar body composition in patients with Prader-Labhart-Willi syndrome. Am J Clin Nutr 1997;65(5):1369–74.

[31] Deal CL, Tony M, Höybye C, et al. Growth hormone research society workshop summary: consensus guidelines for recombinant human growth hormone therapy in Prader-Willi Syndrome. J Clin Endocrinol Metab 2013;98(6):E1072–87.

[32] Butler MG, Lee J, Manzardo AM, et al. Growth charts for non-growth hormone treated Prader-Willi syndrome. Pediatrics 2015;135(1):e126–135.

[33] Siemensma EP, Tummers-de Lind van Wijngaarden RF, Festen DA, et al. Beneficial effects of growth hormone treatment on cognition in children with Prader-Willi syndrome: a randomized controlled trial and longitudinal study. J Clin Endocrinol Metab 2012;97(7):2307–14.

[34] Aycan Z, Bas VN. Prader-Willi syndrome and growth hormone deficiency. J Clin Res Pediatr Endocrinol 2014;6(2):62–7.

[35] Eiholzer U, Blum WF, Molinari L. Body fat determined by skinfold measurements is elevated despite underweight in infants with Prader-Labhart-Willi syndrome. J Pediatr 1999;134(2):222–5.

[36] Bekx MT, Carrel AL, Shriver TC, et al. Decreased energy expenditure is caused by abnormal body composition in infants with Prader-Willi Syndrome. J Pediatr 2003;143(3):372–6.

[37] Festen DAM, De Lind van Wijngaarden R, Van Eekelen M, et al. Randomized controlled GH trial: effects on anthropometry, body composition and body proportions in a large group of children with Prader–Willi syndrome. Clin Endocrinol 2008;69(3):443–51.

[38] de Lind van Wijngaarden RF, Cianflone K, Gao Y, et al. Cardiovascular and metabolic risk profile and acylation-stimulating protein levels in children with Prader-Willi syndrome and effects of growth hormone treatment. J Clin Endocrinol Metab 2010;95(4):1758–66.

[39] de Lind van Wijngaarden RF, de Klerk LW, Festen DA, et al. Randomized controlled trial to investigate the effects of growth hormone treatment on scoliosis in children with Prader-Willi syndrome. J Clin Endocrinol Metab 2009;94(4):1274–80.

[40] Nagai T, Obata K, Tonoki H, et al. Cause of sudden, unexpected death of Prader-Willi syndrome patients with or without growth hormone treatment. Am J Med Genet A 2005;136(1):45–8.

[41] Sacco M, Di Giorgio G. Sudden death in Prader-Willi syndrome during growth hormone therapy. Horm Res 2005;63(1):29–32.

[42] Schrander-Stumpel CT, Curfs LM, Sastrowijoto P, et al. Prader-Willi syndrome: causes of death in an international series of 27 cases. Am J Med Genet A 2004;124A(4):333–8.

[43] Vogels A, Van Den Ende J, Keymolen K, et al. Minimum prevalence, birth incidence and cause of death for Prader-Willi syndrome in Flanders. Eur J Hum Genet 2004;12(3): 238–40.

[44] Van Vliet G, Deal CL, Crock PA, et al. Sudden death in growth hormone-treated children with Prader-Willi syndrome. J Pediatr 2004;144(1):129–31.

[45] Oiglane E, Ounap K, Bartsch O, et al. Sudden death of a girl with Prader-Willi syndrome. Genet Couns 2002;13(4):459–64.

[46] Eiholzer U, Nordmann Y, L'Allemand D. Fatal outcome of sleep apnoea in PWS during the initial phase of growth hormone treatment. A case report. Horm Res 2002;58(Suppl 3): 24–6.

[47] Nordmann Y, Eiholzer U, l'Allemand D, et al. Sudden death of an infant with Prader-Willi syndrome–not a unique case? Biol Neonate 2002;82(2):139–41.

[48] Schrander-Stumpel C, Sijstermans H, Curfs L, et al. Sudden death in children with Prader-Willy syndrome: a call for collaboration. Genet Couns 1998;9(3):231–2.

[49] Lindgren AC, Hellstrom LG, Ritzen EM, et al. Growth hormone treatment increases CO(2) response, ventilation and central inspiratory drive in children with Prader-Willi syndrome. Eur J Pediatr 1999;158(11):936–40.

[50] Haqq AM, Stadler DD, Jackson RH, et al. Effects of growth hormone on pulmonary function, sleep quality, behavior, cognition, growth velocity, body composition, and resting energy expenditure in Prader-Willi syndrome. J Clin Endocrinol Metab 2003;88(5): 2206–12.

[51] Carrel AL, Myers SE, Whitman BY, et al. Benefits of long-term GH therapy in Prader-Willi syndrome: a 4-year study. J Clin Endocrinol Metab 2002;87(4):1581–5.

[52] Lindgren AC, Ritzen EM. Five years of growth hormone treatment in children with Prader-Willi syndrome. Swedish National Growth Hormone Advisory Group. Acta Paediatr Suppl 1999;88(433):109–11.

[53] Eiholzer U, l'Allemand D. Growth hormone normalises height, prediction of final height and hand length in children with Prader-Willi syndrome after 4 years of therapy. Horm Res 2000;53(4):185–92.

[54] Myers SE, Carrel AL, Whitman BY, et al. Sustained benefit after 2 years of growth hormone on body composition, fat utilization, physical strength and agility, and growth in Prader-Willi syndrome. J Pediatr 2000;137(1):42–9.

[55] Carrel AL, Myers SE, Whitman BY, et al. Sustained benefits of growth hormone on body composition, fat utilization, physical strength and agility, and growth in Prader-Willi syndrome are dose-dependent. J Pediatr Endocrinol Metab 2001;14(8):1097–105.

[56] Lo S, Siemensma EC, Festen DM, et al. Behavior in children with Prader–Willi syndrome before and during growth hormone treatment: a randomized controlled trial and 8-year longitudinal study. Eur Child Adolesc Psychiatry 2015;24(9):1091–101.

[57] Whitman BY, Myers S, Carrel A, et al. The behavioral impact of growth hormone treatment for children and adolescents with Prader-Willi syndrome: a 2-year, controlled study. Pediatrics 2002;109(2):E35.

[58] Bakker NE, Kuppens RJ, Siemensma EP, et al. Eight years of growth hormone treatment in children with Prader-Willi syndrome: maintaining the positive effects. J Clin Endocrinol Metab 2013;98(10):4013–22.

[59] Sode-Carlsen R, Farholt S, Rabben KF, et al. Growth hormone treatment for two years is safe and effective in adults with Prader-Willi syndrome. Growth Horm IGF Res 2011;21(4):185–90.

[60] Höybye C. Growth hormone treatment of Prader–Willi syndrome has long-term, positive effects on body composition. Acta Paediatr 2015;104(4):422–7.

[61] Corrias A, Grugni G, Crino A, et al. Assessment of central adrenal insufficiency in children and adolescents with Prader-Willi syndrome. Clin Endocrinol (Oxf) 2012;76(6):843–50.

[62] Stevenson DA, Anaya TM, Clayton-Smith J, et al. Unexpected death and critical illness in Prader–Willi syndrome: report of ten individuals. Am J Med Genet A 2004;124A(2):158–64.

[63] Emerick J, Vogt K. Endocrine manifestations and management of Prader-Willi syndrome. Int J Pediatr Endocrinol 2013;2013(1):14.

[64] Barbara DW, Hannon JD, Hartman WR. Intraoperative adrenal insufficiency in a patient with Prader-Willi syndrome. J Clin Med Res 2012;4(5):346–8.

[65] McCandless SE. Clinical report-health supervision for children with Prader-Willi syndrome. Pediatrics 2011;127(1):195–204.

[66] Hirsch HJ, Eldar-Geva T, Bennaroch F, et al. Sexual dichotomy of gonadal function in Prader–Willi syndrome from early infancy through the fourth decade. Hum Reprod 2015;30(11):2587–96.

[67] Siemensma EPC, van Alfen-van der Velden AA, Otten BJ, et al. Ovarian function and reproductive hormone levels in girls with Prader-Willi syndrome: a longitudinal study. J Clin Endocrinol Metab 2012;97(9):E1766–73.

[68] Siemensma EPC, de Lind van Wijngaarden RFA, Otten BJ, et al. Pubarche and serum dehydroepiandrosterone sulphate levels in children with Prader–Willi syndrome. Clin Endocrinol 2011;75(1):83–9.

[69] Akefeldt A, Tornhage CJ, Gillberg C. A woman with Prader-Willi syndrome gives birth to a healthy baby girl. Dev Med Child Neurol 1999;41(11):789–90.

[70] Schulze A, Mogensen H, Hamborg-Petersen B, et al. Fertility in Prader-Willi syndrome: a case report with Angelman syndrome in the offspring. Acta Paediatr 2001;90(4):455–9.

[71] Butler JV, Whittington JE, Holland AJ, et al. Prevalence of, and risk factors for, physical ill-health in people with Prader-Willi syndrome: a population-based study. Dev Med Child Neurol 2002;44(4):248–55.

[72] Diene G, Mimoun E, Feigerlova E, et al. Endocrine disorders in children with Prader-Willi syndrome—data from 142 children of the French database. Horm Res Paediatr 2010;74(2):121–8.

[73] Talebizadeh Z, Butler MG. Insulin resistance and obesity-related factors in Prader-Willi syndrome: comparison with obese subjects. Clin Genet 2005;67(3):230–9.

[74] Lacroix D, Moutel S, Coupaye M, et al. Metabolic and adipose tissue signatures in adults with Prader-Willi syndrome: a model of extreme adiposity. J Clin Endocrinol Metab 2015;100(3):850–9.

[75] Purtell L, Viardot A, Sze L, et al. Postprandial metabolism in adults with Prader-Willi syndrome. Obesity (Silver Spring) 2015;23(6):1159–65.

[76] Schuster DP, Osei K, Zipf WB. Characterization of alterations in glucose and insulin metabolism in Prader-Willi subjects. Metabolism 1996;45(12):1514–20.

[77] Bray GA, Dahms WT, Swerdloff RS, et al. The Prader-Willi syndrome: a study of 40 patients and a review of the literature. Medicine (Baltimore) 1983;62(2):59–80.

[78] Sareen C, Ruvalcaba RH, Kelley VC. Some aspects of carbohydrate metabolism in Prader-Willi syndrome. J Ment Defic Res 1975;19(2):113–9.

[79] Senda M, Ogawa S, Nako K, et al. The glucagon-like peptide-1 analog liraglutide suppresses ghrelin and controls diabetes in a patient with Prader-Willi syndrome. Endocr J 2012;59(10):889–94.

[80] Sze L, Purtell L, Jenkins A, et al. Effects of a single dose of exenatide on appetite, gut hormones, and glucose homeostasis in adults with Prader-Willi syndrome. J Clin Endocrinol Metab 2011;96(8):E1314–9.

[81] Arens R, Gozal D, Omlin KJ, et al. Hypoxic and hypercapnic ventilatory responses in Prader-Willi syndrome. J Appl Physiol 1994;77(5):2224–30.

[82] Haqq AM, Muehlbauer M, Svetkey LP, et al. Altered distribution of adiponectin isoforms in children with Prader-Willi syndrome (PWS): association with insulin sensitivity and circulating satiety peptide hormones. Clin Endocrinol 2007;67(6):944–51.

[83] Berthoud HR, Powley TL. Morphology and distribution of efferent vagal innervation of rat pancreas as revealed with anterograde transport of DiI. Brain Res 1991;553(2):336–41.

[84] Cohen M, Hamilton J, Narang I. Clinically important age-related differences in sleep related disordered breathing in infants and children with Prader-Willi Syndrome. PLoS One 2014;9(6):e101012.

[85] De Cock VC, Diene G, Molinas C, et al. Efficacy of modafinil on excessive daytime sleepiness in Prader–Willi syndrome. Am J Med Genet Part A 2011;155(7):1552–7.

[86] Manni R, Politini L, Nobili L, et al. Hypersomnia in the Prader Willi syndrome: clinical-electrophysiological features and underlying factors. Clin Neurophysiol 2001;112(5):800–5.

[87] Fronczek R, Lammers GJ, Balesar R, et al. The number of hypothalamic hypocretin (orexin) neurons is not affected in Prader-Willi syndrome. J Clin Endocrinol Metab 2005;90(9):5466–70.

[88] Nevsimalova S, Vankova J, Stepanova I, et al. Hypocretin deficiency in Prader-Willi syndrome. Eur J Neurol 2005;12(1):70–2.

[89] Dykens E, Shah B. Psychiatric disorders in Prader-Willi syndrome: epidemiology and management. CNS Drugs 2003;17(3):167–78.

[90] Stein DJ, Keating J, Zar HJ, et al. A survey of the phenomenology and pharmacotherapy of compulsive and impulsive-aggressive symptoms in Prader-Willi syndrome. J Neuropsychiatry Clin Neurosci 1994;6(1):23–9.

[91] Reddy LA, Pfeiffer SI. Behavioral and emotional symptoms of children and adolescents with Prader-Willi Syndrome. J Autism Dev Disord 2007;37(5):830–9.

[92] Johnson L, Manzardo AM, Miller JL, et al. Elevated plasma oxytocin levels in children with Prader-Willi syndrome compared with healthy unrelated siblings. Am J Med Genet A 2016;170(3):594–601.

[93] Nelson R, Huse D, Holman R, et al. Nutrition, metabolism, body composition and response to the ketogenic diet in Prader-Willi syndrome. In: Holm VA, editor. Prader-Willi syndrome. Baltimore (MD): University Park Press; 1981. p. 105–20.

[94] Schoeller DA, Levitsky LL, Bandini LG, et al. Energy expenditure and body composition in Prader-Willi syndrome. Metabolism 1988;37(2):115–20.

[95] Butler MG. Management of obesity in Prader-Willi syndrome. Nat Clin Pract Endocrinol Metab 2006;2(11):592–3.

[96] Abbott WG, Howard BV, Ruotolo G, et al. Energy expenditure in humans: effects of dietary fat and carbohydrate. Am J Physiol 1990;258(2 Pt 1):E347–51.

[97] Scheimann AO, Butler MG, Gourash L, et al. Critical analysis of bariatric procedures in Prader-Willi syndrome. J Pediatr Gastroenterol Nutr 2008;46(1):80–3.

[98] Chen KY, Sun M, Butler MG, et al. Development and validation of a measurement system for assessment of energy expenditure and physical activity in Prader-Willi syndrome. Obes Res 1999;7(4):387–94.

[99] Lloret-Linares C, Faucher P, Coupaye M, et al. Comparison of body composition, basal metabolic rate and metabolic outcomes of adults with Prader Willi syndrome or lesional hypothalamic disease, with primary obesity. Int J Obes (Lond) 2013;37(9):1198–203.

[100] Goldstone AP, Brynes AE, Thomas EL, et al. Resting metabolic rate, plasma leptin concentrations, leptin receptor expression, and adipose tissue measured by whole-body magnetic resonance imaging in women with Prader-Willi syndrome. Am J Clin Nutr 2002;75(3): 468–75.

[101] van Mil EA, Westerterp KR, Gerver WJ, et al. Energy expenditure at rest and during sleep in children with Prader-Willi syndrome is explained by body composition. Am J Clin Nutr 2000;71(3):752–6.

[102] Schutz Y, Bessard T, Jequier E. Diet-induced thermogenesis measured over a whole day in obese and nonobese women. Am J Clin Nutr 1984;40(3):542–52.

[103] Segal KR, Edano A, Tomas MB. Thermic effect of a meal over 3 and 6 hours in lean and obese men. Metabolism 1990;39(9):985–92.

[104] Steiniger J, Karst H, Noack R, et al. Diet-induced thermogenesis in man: thermic effects of single protein and carbohydrate test meals in lean and obese subjects. Ann Nutr Metab 1987;31(2):117–25.

[105] Jequier E, Schutz Y. New evidence for a thermogenic defect in human obesity. Int J Obes 1985;9(Suppl 2):1–7.

[106] Maffeis C, Schutz Y, Grezzani A, et al. Meal-induced thermogenesis and obesity: is a fat meal a risk factor for fat gain in children? J Clin Endocrinol Metab 2001;86(1):214–9.

[107] Tentolouris N, Alexiadou K, Kokkinos A, et al. Meal-induced thermogenesis and macronutrient oxidation in lean and obese women after consumption of carbohydrate-rich and fat-rich meals. Nutrition 2011;27(3):310–5.

[108] D'Alessio DA, Kavle EC, Mozzoli MA, et al. Thermic effect of food in lean and obese men. J Clin Invest 1988;81(6):1781–9.

[109] Nardella MT, Sulzbacher SI, Worthington-Roberts BS. Activity levels of persons with Prader-Willi syndrome. Am J Ment Defic 1983;87(5):498–505.

[110] Davies PS, Joughin C. Using stable isotopes to assess reduced physical activity of individuals with Prader-Willi syndrome. Am J Ment Retard 1993;98(3):349–53.

[111] Rubin DA, Clark SJ, Ng J, et al. Hormonal and metabolic responses to endurance exercise in children with Prader-Willi syndrome and non-syndromic obesity. Metabolism 2015;64(3):391–5.

[112] Castner DM, Tucker JM, Wilson KS, et al. Patterns of habitual physical activity in youth with and without Prader-Willi Syndrome. Res Dev Disabil 2014;35(11):3081–8.

[113] Miller JL, Lynn CH, Driscoll DC, et al. Nutritional phases in Prader–Willi syndrome. Am J Med Genet Part A 2011;155(5):1040–9.

[114] Holm VA, Pipes PL. Food and children with Prader-Willi syndrome. Am J Dis Child 1976;130(10):1063–7.

[115] Stadler DD. Nutritional management. In: Greenswag LR, editor. Management of Prader-Willi syndrome. 2nd edition. New York: Springer-Verlag; 1995. p. 88–114.

[116] Hoffman CJ, Aultman D, Pipes P. A nutrition survey of and recommendations for individuals with Prader-Willi syndrome who live in group homes. J Am Diet Assoc 1992;92(7): 823–30, 833.

[117] Nelson R, Hayles A, Novak L, et al. Ketogenic diet and Prader-Willi syndrome. Am J Clin Nutr 1970;23:667.

[118] Heiman MF. The management of obesity in the post-adolescent developmentally disabled client with Prader-Willi syndrome. Adolescence 1978;13(50):291–6.

[119] Altman K, Bondy A, Hirsch G. Behavioral treatment of obesity in patients with Prader-Willi syndrome. J Behav Med 1978;1(4):403–12.

[120] Kriz JS, Cloninger BJ. Management of a patient with Prader-Willi syndrome by a dental-dietary team. Spec Care Dentist 1981;1(4):179–82.

[121] Evans PR. Hypogenital dystrophy with diabetic tendency. Guys Hosp Rep 1964;113:207–22.

[122] Jancar J. Prader-Willi syndrome. (Hypotonia, obesity, hypogonadism, growth and mental retardation). J Ment Defic Res 1971;15(1):20–9.

[123] Juul J, Dupont A. Prader-Willi syndrome. J Ment Defic Res 1967;11(1):12–22.

[124] Bistrian BR, Blackburn GL, Stanbury JB. Metabolic aspects of a protein-sparing modified fast in the dietary management of Prader-Willi obesity. N Engl J Med 1977;296(14):774–9.

[125] Collier SB, Walker WA. Parenteral protein-sparing modified fast in an obese adolescent with Prader-Willi syndrome. Nutr Rev 1991;49(8):235–8.

[126] Coplin SS, Hine J, Gormican A. Out-patient dietary management in the Prader-Willi syndrome. J Am Diet Assoc 1976;68(4):330–4.

[127] Pipes PL, Holm VA. Weight control of children with Prader-Willi syndrome. J Am Diet Assoc 1973;62(5):520–4.

[128] Caldwell ML, Taylor RL. A clinical note on food preference of individuals with Prader-Willi syndrome: the need for empirical research. J Ment Defic Res 1983;27(Pt 1):45–9.

[129] Silverthorn KH, Hornak JE. Beneficial effects of exercise on aerobic capacity and body composition in adults with Prader-Willi syndrome. Am J Ment Retard 1993;97(6):654–8.

[130] Bakker NE, Kuppens RJ, Siemensma EP, et al. Bone mineral density in children and adolescents with Prader-Willi syndrome: a longitudinal study during puberty and 9 years of growth hormone treatment. J Clin Endocrinol Metab 2015;100(4):1609–18.

[131] Longhi S, Grugni G, Gatti D, et al. Adults with Prader–Willi syndrome have weaker bones: effect of treatment with GH and sex steroids. Calcif Tissue Int 2015;96(2):160–6.

[132] Goldstone AP, Holland AJ, Hauffa BP, et al. Recommendations for the diagnosis and management of Prader-Willi syndrome. J Clin Endocrinol Metab 2008;93(11):4183–97.

[133] Eldar-Geva T, Hirsch HJ, Pollak Y, et al. Management of hypogonadism in adolescent girls and adult women with Prader–Willi syndrome. Am J Med Genet Part A 2013;161(12):3030–4.

[134] Einfeld SL, Smith E, McGregor IS, et al. A double-blind randomized controlled trial of oxytocin nasal spray in Prader Willi syndrome. Am J Med Genet Part A 2014;164(9):2232–9.

[135] Tauber M, Mantoulan C, Copet P, et al. Oxytocin may be useful to increase trust in others and decrease disruptive behaviours in patients with Prader-Willi syndrome: a randomised placebo-controlled trial in 24 patients. Orphanet J Rare Dis 2011;6:47.

[136] Artuch R, Salviati L, Jackson S, et al. Coenzyme Q(10) deficiencies in neuromuscular diseases. Adv Exp Med Biol 2009;652:117–28.

[137] Butler MG, Dasouki M, Bittel D, et al. Coenzyme Q10 levels in Prader-Willi syndrome: comparison with obese and non-obese subjects. Am J Med Genet Part A 2003;119A(2):168–71.

[138] Eiholzer U, Meinhardt U, Rousson V, et al. Developmental profiles in young children with Prader-Labhart-Willi syndrome: effects of weight and therapy with growth hormone or co-enzyme Q10. Am J Med Genet A 2008;146a(7):873–80.

[139] Miller JL, Lynn CH, Shuster J, et al. Carnitine and coenzyme Q10 levels in individuals with Prader-Willi syndrome. Am J Med Genet A 2011;155a(3):569–73.

[140] Hoffman KL. Animal models of obsessive compulsive disorder: recent findings and future directions. Expert Opin Drug Discov 2011;6(7):725–37.

[141] Ramirez-Nino AM, D'Souza MS, Markou A. N-acetylcysteine decreased nicotine self-administration and cue-induced reinstatement of nicotine seeking in rats: comparison with the effects of N-acetylcysteine on food responding and food seeking. Psychopharmacology (Berl) 2013;225(2):473–82.

[142] Miller JL, Angulo M. An open-label pilot study of N-acetylcysteine for skin-picking in Prader-Willi syndrome. Am J Med Genet A 2014;164a(2):421–4.

[143] Joharapurkar AA, Dhanesha NA, Jain MR. Inhibition of the methionine aminopeptidase 2 enzyme for the treatment of obesity. Diabetes Metab Syndr Obes 2014;7:73–84.

[144] Miller J, Drisoll D, Chen A, et al. Randomized, double-blind, placebo controlled 4 week proof of concept trial of beloranib, a novel treatment for Prader-Willi syndrome. Boston: The Obesity Society; 2014.

[145] Shoemaker AH, Proietto J, Abuzzahab J, et al. Randomized, double-blind, placebo-controlled 4 week proof of concept trial of beloranib resulted in rapid and significant weight loss in patients with hypothalamic injury associated obesity. San Diego (CA): Endocrine Society; 2015.

[146] Alqahtani AR, Elahmedi MO, Al Qahtani AR, et al. Laparoscopic sleeve gastrectomy in children and adolescents with Prader-Willi syndrome: a matched-control study. Surg Obes Relat Dis 2016;12(1):213–4.

[147] Fong AW, Wong SH, Lam CH, et al. Ghrelin level and weight loss after laparoscopic sleeve gastrectomy and gastric mini-bypass for Prader–Willi syndrome in Chinese. Obes Surg 2012;22(11):1742–5.

[148] Whittington JE, Holland AJ, Webb T. Ageing in people with Prader-Willi syndrome: mortality in the UK population cohort and morbidity in an older sample of adults. Psychol Med 2015;45(3):615–21.

[149] Sinnema M, Schrander-Stumpel CT, Maaskant MA, et al. Aging in Prader-Willi syndrome: twelve persons over the age of 50 years. Am J Med Genet A 2012;158a(6):1326–36.

Advances in Pediatrics 63 (2016) 79–102

ADVANCES IN PEDIATRICS

ELSEVIER
MOSBY

Advances in the Care of Transgender Children and Adolescents

Daniel E. Shumer, MD, MPH[a],*, Natalie J. Nokoff, MD[b], Norman P. Spack, MD[c]

[a]Division of Pediatric Endocrinology, Department of Pediatrics and Communicable Diseases, University of Michigan Health Systems, University of Michigan, 1500 East Medical Center Drive, Ann Arbor, MI 48109-5175, USA; [b]Division of Pediatric Endocrinology, Department of Pediatrics, University of Colorado School of Medicine, 13123 East 16th Avenue, Aurora, CO 80045, USA; [c]Endocrine Division, Boston Children's Hospital, Harvard Medical School, 300 Longwood Avenue, Boston, MA 02115, USA

Keywords
- Gender dysphoria • Transgender • Gender identity • Adolescent • Child

Key points
- Children and adolescents with gender dysphoria are presenting for medical attention at increasing rates.
- Standards of care have been developed that outline appropriate mental health support and hormonal interventions for transgender youth.
- Transgender issues have emerged from the periphery of the general conscious to a center stage cultural, human rights, and medical topic.

INTRODUCTION

The World Professional Association for Transgender Health (WPATH) first published Standards of Care for the heath of transsexual, transgender, and gender-nonconforming people in 1980, with the seventh edition released in 2012 [1]. In 2009, The Endocrine Society issued a clinical practice guideline for the treatment of transsexual persons, including support for pubertal suppression and cross-sex hormones in carefully screened and supported transgender adolescents [2]. In the 35 years since the publication of the first edition of the WPATH standards, transgender issues have emerged from the periphery of the general conscious to a center stage cultural, human rights, and medical topic

*Corresponding author. E-mail address: dshumer@med.umich.edu

0065-3101/16/$ – see front matter
http://dx.doi.org/10.1016/j.yapd.2016.04.018

in both lay media and scientific inquiry [3,4]. Gender management clinics have emerged to assess, support, and provide medical treatment for transgender adolescents across Europe and North America [5–9]. As transgender issues continue to emerge to the forefront of the public consciousness, the public is expecting knowledgeable, competent, and comprehensive mental health and medical care. Yet, only a minority of medical schools offer curriculum related to transgender-specific care [10]. This mismatch between provider education and patient expectation has left providers and health systems struggling to develop appropriate clinical care systems. This article defines critical terminology in the field, describes what is known about gender identity development, outlines the current mental health disparities faced by transgender persons in general and youth specifically, addresses current guidelines regarding medical treatment of the pediatric transgender patient, highlights persisting challenges and barriers to care, and concludes with case examples.

DEFINITIONS AND EPIDEMIOLOGY

Gender identity describes one's internal feeling of gender, for example, boy or girl, man or woman; agender (identifying as having no gender); or a nonbinary understanding of one's gender. This is in contrast to *biologic sex*, which describes the chromosomal, hormonal, and anatomic determinants that result in characterizing people as male or female. A *transgender* person feels a discrepancy between their sex assigned at birth and their gender identity [11]. The term *cisgender* has subsequently been introduced to describe individuals who have a gender identity congruent with or the same as their sex assigned at birth. *Gender role* or *gender expression* describes how a person presents themselves as masculine or feminine in the context of societal expectations. *Gender attribution* describes the process whereby other observers view a person as masculine or feminine. For example, a transgender woman who appears masculine owing to the development of male secondary sex characteristics may have a male *gender attribution* and struggle with "passing" as an affirmed woman. Finally, *sexual orientation* describes the persons one finds sexually desirable, for example, homosexual, heterosexual, bisexual, pansexual, or asexual [12].

   Gender dysphoria in childhood and *gender dysphoria in adolescents and adults* are defined in the *Diagnostic and Statistical Manual of Mental Health Disorders*, Fifth Edition (referred to *gender identity disorder* in previous editions) [13,14]. Both children and adolescents meet diagnostic criteria for gender dysphoria if they experience a marked difference between their experienced and assigned gender that persists for at least 6 months and causes significant distress or impaired functioning [14]. A *transsexual* person, as defined by the WPATH Standards of Care, describes "individuals who seek to change or have changed their primary and/or secondary sex characteristics through feminizing or masculinizing medical interventions (hormones and/or surgery), typically accompanied by a permanent change in gender role" [1].

   As evidenced by the American Psychiatric Association's decision to remove the stigmatizing word "disorder" from the lexicon, replacing *gender identity disorder* with *gender dysphoria*, there has been evolving depathologization for those whose gender identity differs from their sex assigned at birth. The idea that *gender identity* exists on a continuum and that *gender diversity* should be celebrated has gained cultural traction and has resulted in greater acceptance of gender nonconforming people in certain communities. See Table 1 for a list of commonly used terms.

The prevalence of gender dysphoria has been difficult to estimate. A calculated prevalence from the Netherlands in 1996 suggested 1 in 11,900 natal Dutch males and 1 in 30,400 natal Dutch females were transsexual [15]. However, the frequency of new referrals to pediatric gender programs suggests that these numbers understate the current prevalence in the United States. In addition, the proportion of natal male and natal female referrals seems to be closer to 1:1, conflicting with Dutch epidemiologic data [5]. In dramatic contrast with the Dutch data, a recent survey of 28,662 adults in Massachusetts found 0.5% self-identifying as transgender [16]. We suggest that as societal acceptance of gender diversity continues to advance and as barriers to care are removed, the transgender population will grow dramatically.

HISTORICAL PERSPECTIVES

Before the isolation of sex hormones, their development into an injectable or oral compound to be administered, and development of surgical techniques, there were no options to change one's secondary sex characteristics.

Table 1	
Terminology related to gender identity	
Gender identity	An internal feeling of one's gender as a boy or man, girl or woman, no gender, or a nonbinary understanding of one's gender
Biologic sex	The genetic, anatomic, and hormonal determinants of sex classified as male or female, or indeterminate owing to a disorder of sex development
Transgender	Having a gender identity that is not congruent with one's biologic sex
Cisgender	Having a gender identity that is congruent with one's biologic sex
Transsexual	A term most often used to describe a transgender person who is or has transitioned using hormones and/or surgical procedures
Gender nonconforming	Describes a person who behaviors, actions, or interests do not conform to the societal expectations based on their biologic sex
Gender role	The stereotypical role that members of each biologic sex are expected to play based on societal norms or expectations
Gender dysphoria	A diagnosis defined by the *Diagnostic and Statistical Manual of Mental Disorders* describing distress caused by an incongruence between gender identity and biologic sex
Agender	A gender identity characterized by feeling no identification with being a boy or man, girl or woman, or any other gender identity
Gender fluid	Gender identity that varies over time
Genderqueer	A term used by people who do not classify themselves using conventional gender distinctions, but may instead identify as neither gender, both genders, or a combination of male and female genders
Gender attribution	How an observer decides which sex or gender they believe another person to be

Charles-Édouard Brown-Séquard was among the first to conceptualize that hormones, or substances, may be secreted by a gland and enter the bloodstream to affect distant organs. He claimed to have injected himself with an extract derived from dog and guinea pig testes [17].

Testosterone was discovered in 1935 [18] and was synthesized from cholesterol soon after [19]. Estrone was isolated in 1929 to 1930 from the urine of pregnant women in the United States [20] and Germany [21] with the discovery of estriol shortly afterward [22]. Progesterone was discovered in 1934 by multiple groups [23,24]. The first orally active progestin was synthesized in 1938 and named "ethisterone" and was significantly androgenic [25]. The same group later synthesized estradiol, termed "ethynylestradiol" [26], which was widely used for decades including in the care of transgender women [27].

Magnus Hirschfeld was a Jewish German physician and sexologist who is known for advocating for the rights of homosexuals in turn-of-the century Germany. He coined the term "transvestite" and opened the Institute for Sexual Research in 1919 [28].

The first "modern" orchiectomy was performed in 1930 for a Danish natal male who sought a sex change. She then underwent a penectomy, implantation of ovarian tissue, and vaginoplasty [29]. There are older examples from history, for example, the Hijiras, an Indian Caste of men who lived as women and underwent ritual castration or a surgery performed in Australian aboriginal men to create a rudimentary vagina [30]. There were additional published cases of penectomy for gender dysphoria in the 1940s and 1950s in Germany [30].

The first widely published case in of a transgender female in the United States was Christine Jorgensen, who appeared on the front page of the *New York Daily News* on December 1, 1952 [31]. Christine, formerly George, served in World War II and after returning from war, started taking feminizing hormones. She underwent orchiectomy and sex reassignment surgery in Denmark, and later had a vaginoplasty in the United States [32].

The earliest case reports in the medical literature of surgical treatment of a transgender individual were in Germany in 1940s [33] and in *JAMA* in 1953 by Danish physicians [34]. A 24-year-old natal male presented with a desire to more fully live as a woman and was treated with estradiol monobenzoate injections and oral ethinyl estradiol. Per the patient's wishes, she underwent orchiectomy after permission was granted by the Danish Ministry of Justice [34]. After the initial operation, the patient had a penectomy and plastic surgery of the scrotum to construct "labia-like formations." A vaginoplasty was not performed and not desired by the patient. The authors were ahead of their time, calling on the "medical profession and authorities" to show a "more positive attitude toward the efforts at easing and facilitating the daily life of the victims of genuine transvestism" with an outline of suggestions to make this possible [34], which resonate with current recommendations.

Harry Benjamin was a German-born sexologist and endocrinologist who knew Magnus Hirschfeld and became widely known for his 1966 book,

The Transsexual Phenomenon [35]. He treated Christine Jorgensen. In 1979, the Harry Benjamin International Gender Dysphoria Association was formed, now renamed the WPATH. The first "standards of care" were published in 1979, now in their seventh version [1].

The first female-to-male (FTM) sex reassignment surgeries were performed at Johns Hopkins in 1966 after the Gender Identity Clinic was formed. The psychologist and sexologist John Money helped found the clinic and was later widely criticized for the John/Joan case [36]. Thousands of gender affirmation surgeries were later performed by Dr Stanley Biber in Trinidad, Colorado, which was later coined, the "sex change capital of the world." He performed his first sex reversal surgery in 1969 at his patient's request and after learning from sketches of surgical procedures.

In the 1980s, gonadotropin-releasing hormone (GnRH) agonists were first used for the treatment of central precocious puberty [37], and would prove to be a key treatment option for younger transgender patients. Before the late 1990s, treatment of children or adolescents with gender dysphoria was not considered. In 1998, Drs Cohen-Kettenis and van Goozen in the Netherlands published a report of an FTM transgender patient treated with triptorelin, a GnRH agonist, starting at the age of 13 years [38]. The Dutch practice methods of using pubertal suppression followed by cross-sex hormones for transgender adolescents subsequently became incorporated into the WPATH and The Endocrine Society Standards of Care [1,2].

THE DEVELOPMENT OF GENDER IDENTITY
Expectant parents can now learn the chromosomal sex of their fetus with first trimester cell-free fetal DNA and the anatomic sex on the second trimester ultrasound examination [39]. Many parents then spend the next few months preparing a nursery adorned in pink or blue, excited to welcome their new son or daughter into the world. The baby is born into a gendered world, where boys and girls dress differently and are often encouraged to pursue gender-specific games or styles of play. Although these stereotypical gender roles vary by culture and change over time, the different expectations of boys and girls are thought to impact the development of gender identity. Children as young as 2 years learn to label themselves as a boy or a girl, and by age 4 to 5, are able to understand that gender is a stable and lasting aspect of their identity [40]. Boys and girls have group differences in toy preference by as early as 12 months and can label other children as boys or girls by age 2 [41].

Development of gender identity development is complex, and likely a multifactorial process involving genetic, hormonal, and environmental factors. John Money and Anke Ehrhardt proposed the idea of brain sex [42], which has drawn controversy [43]. Several brain structures seem to be sexually dimorphic [44], which has led researchers to study whether transgender individuals have brain structures that more closely align with their affirmed gender. In 1 study, the volume of the bed nucleus of the stria terminalis in male-to-female (MTF) transgender persons was equivalent to the volume found in cisgender women

[45]. However, others argue that such "dimorphisms" are better thought of as small differences with significant overlap [43].

Studies of heritability of transgender identity have suggested that genetic factors may contribute to gender development. For example, in a recent review of twin studies, of 23 monozygotic male and female twin pairs where at least 1 twin met the criteria for gender identity disorder, 9 twin pairs (39.1%) were concordant for gender identity disorder [46]. Studies have failed to firmly establish causative genes [6].

The hormonal milieu of the developing fetal brain and its role on later gender identity has been another area of active research. Much of this research has been driven by the study of persons with disorders of sex development. Sex hormones, primarily androgens and estrogens, affect sex-specific changes in the developing fetus. During fetal life and infancy, there are significant sex-specific differences in the normal concentrations of these hormones. It has been posited that these differences may contribute to group differences in behaviors observed between males and females later in life [47,48]. Populations of patients with various disorders of sex development have served as natural experiments for this hypothesis. For example, infants with a 46,XX karyotype and congenital adrenal hyperplasia are most often raised as girls but have had fetal exposure to higher than normal concentrations of circulating androgens. In a metaanalysis, 5% of those assigned and raised female had gender dysphoria or a male gender identity, suggesting that prenatal androgen exposure may influence the development of a male-typical gender identity [49]. In another example, of 14 patients with 46,XY karyotype and cloacal extrophy raised female, 8 (57%) subsequently affirmed a male gender identity [50]. These and other studies (see Rosenthal [6] for a more complete review) suggest that the prenatal hormonal milieu, especially fetal androgen exposure, may play a role in gender identity development. Yet, the vast majority of transgender persons do not have an identified disorders of sex development or endocrinopathy.

Finally, individual environmental factors may influence the development of gender dysphoria. It has been suggested that the social relationship between the parent and infant [41] and cognitive learning about parental expectations and societal norms [51] contribute to gender development in all children. The observation that children with autism spectrum disorder are disproportionately affected by gender dysphoria has contributed to the discussion of environmental factors and gender identity. Children with autism spectrum disorder may, as a result of social cognitive impairment, feel less societal pressure to conform to their assigned sex at birth, which may manifest as persistence of gender dysphoria [52].

Children referred for assessment owing to gender nonconformity may demonstrate gender nonconforming behaviors at a very young age, sometimes as early as 3 years [53]. Others persons may disclose a transgender identity later in adolescence or adulthood, without a history of gender nonconformity in early childhood [6,54]. Young children who are gender nonconforming or who identify as transgender may or may not continue to identify as transgender as adolescents and adults. In fact, there is evidence to suggest that, for a majority of young children with cross-gender identity, this identity does not persist into adolescence; at the time of puberty, their transgender identity may desist and perhaps evolve into a gay or lesbian sexual orientation [55,56]. However, those who have persistence of transgender identity and/or worsening of gender dysphoria in puberty are thought to be much less likely to identify as cisgender as adolescence continues. Clinicians can use worsening gender dysphoria at the onset of puberty as a diagnostic tool of persistent transgender identity and as a criterion for eligibility for medical intervention [38,57].

There have been efforts to identify factors to differentiate prepubertal children who will persist in their transgender identity during adolescence and adulthood versus those who will desist. In a study of 53 adolescents in the Netherlands, those who persisted versus desisted in their gender identity had similar gender variant expression in childhood. Yet, those who experienced increased dysphoria in adolescence, starting between 10 and 13 years, were more likely to have a stable transgender identity. Important factors in early adolescence included the social environment, feelings toward pubertal changes, and the emergence of sexual attraction [58]. Additional study of desistance versus persistence suggested that children who persist may have more severe symptoms of gender dysphoria in childhood and are more likely to undergo a social transition in childhood (live as the affirmed gender) [59]. The uncertainty of future persistence, coupled with the idea that acceptance of a transgender identity in early childhood may be associated with persistence of transgender identity in adolescence and adulthood, has led to controversy regarding the appropriate counseling and mental health treatment strategies for prepubertal children with gender dysphoria.

MENTAL HEALTH

Transgender persons continue to be disproportionately affected by bias, persecution, and harassment [60], and have alarmingly high rates of depression, anxiety, self-harm behaviors, and suicidality. A staggering 41% of transgender adults have attempted suicide. Rates of suicide attempt are higher among nonwhite transgender adults, those who are unemployed or underemployed, poor, less educated, and young [61]. Transgender youth who experience verbal and physical abuse are more likely to attempt suicide [62], and transgender individuals are disproportionately victimized by physical abuse [63]. Transgender youth also have higher rates of alcohol, tobacco, cannabis, and other drug use [64], and MTF persons, in particular, have higher rates of sex work and human immunodeficiency virus infection [65]. In a recent study of mental health disparity, transgender youth had a 2- to 3-fold increased risk of depression, anxiety disorder, suicidal ideation, suicide attempt, self-harm behaviors, and use of both inpatient and outpatient mental health services compared with cisgender youth [66].

The 2011 National School Climate Survey of LGBT youth surveyed more than 8500 students ages 13 to 20 years in the United States, 700 of whom identified as transgender. Eighty percent of the transgender students reported feeling unsafe at school because of their gender expression and more than one-half of gender nonconforming students had experienced verbal harassment. School policies that affect transgender students include school dress codes, gender segregated sports and physical education, gender segregated bathrooms and locker rooms, gendered pronouns, and binary-only options on school forms [67].

It is, therefore, not surprising that youth presenting to gender management clinics are disproportionately affected by mental health comorbidities. At Boston Children's Hospital's Gender Management Services program, patients had a high prevalence of diagnosed psychiatric comorbidities (44%), history of self-mutilation (21%), history of psychiatric hospitalization (9%), and history of suicide attempt (9%) [5]. Among 101 transgender youth ages 12 to 24 followed at the Center for Transyouth Health and Development at Children's Hospital Los Angeles, 15% had mild depression, 9% had moderate depression, and 11% had severe depression as rated on the Beck Depression Inventory. One-half reported having thoughts about suicide, and 30% had attempted suicide [64]. As noted, rates of autism spectrum disorder may also be increased among children and adolescents presenting with gender dysphoria, with a rate of 7.8% reported from the gender program in the Netherlands, a rate exceeding that in the general population [68].

There is a lack of consensus among mental health providers regarding the goals of mental health treatment in prepubertal children [12]. Some argue that therapeutic goals should focus on reduction in dysphoria and acceptance of the biologic sex [69]. Affirmative approaches help families to support a child's transgender identity and assist children and families with the logistics of making a social transition [70]. There is less controversy about treatment goals for pubertal adolescents. Pubertal adolescents are less likely to desist, and supportive trans-affirmative mental health support is encouraged. The American Psychological Association recently published "Guidelines for Psychological Practice with Transgender and Gender Nonconforming People" containing 16 guidelines recommended for psychologists to assist with "culturally competent, developmentally appropriate, and trans-affirmative psychological practice" [71].

The WPATH Standards of Care and The Endocrine Society clinical practice guidelines describe comprehensive approaches aimed to mitigate mental health disparities and improve outcomes. Data from a pioneering Dutch group suggests that adolescents followed by a multidisciplinary gender team and treated with pubertal suppression followed by cross-sex hormones had improvement in psychological function with mental health outcomes in young adulthood similar to the general Dutch population [72,73]. The Endocrine Society guidelines recommend that children and adolescents with gender concerns be seen by a mental health professional with training in child and adolescent developmental psychology. The mental health professional should (1) determine whether the individual fulfills *Diagnostic and Statistical Manual of Mental Disorders* criteria for gender dysphoria, (2) inform the individual with respect to possibilities and limitations of sex reassignment and other treatments, and (3) assess for potential psychological comorbidities [2]. The WPATH Standards of Care requires that adolescents meet eligibility and readiness criteria before proceeding with hormone treatments; medical interventions can be initiated only after a referral from a qualified mental health professional [1]. Many multidisciplinary clinics require such documentation before hormones are prescribed. However, mental health providers with expertise in this area are limited, and many transgender youth may not have access to such providers given location, insurance coverage, and cost.

SEX DIFFERENTIATION AND NORMAL PUBERTY

Testosterone and estrogen are produced in the testes and ovaries beginning in early fetal life. Testosterone production in the fetus, and its subsequent conversion to dihydrotestosterone, leads to virilization of genital tissues and development of male genitalia. Absence of testosterone results in female external genitalia [74].

After the "minipuberty" of infancy, sex hormone production within the gonads enters a quiescent stage [75]. There is little difference in the hormonal milieu between prepubertal males and females; therefore, hormonal interventions are not indicated in prepubertal transgender children. The transgender prepubertal child can instead focus on better understanding their gender identity with the aid of a mental health professional and their family. When a prepubertal child makes a social transition, presenting themselves as their affirmed gender, their ability to "pass" as their affirmed gender is aided by the fact that they have not yet developed secondary sex characteristics.

Puberty, the life stage characterized by the development of secondary sex characteristics, begins with the activation of the GnRH pulse generator within the hypothalamus. Pulsatile GnRH leads, in turn, to pulsatile production luteinizing hormone (LH) and follicle-stimulating hormone (FSH) within the anterior pituitary gland. LH inspires production of testosterone in testicular Leydig cells. It also leads to production of androgens in ovarian theca cells, which are then converted to estrogen. FSH causes germ cell maturation and testicular enlargement in males and the growth and recruitment of ovarian follicles in females [76,77]. Male puberty, driven by testosterone and dihydrotestosterone, is characterized by enlargement of the testes and phallus, development of facial and body hair, enlargement of the larynx and deepening of the voice, increase of lean muscle to fat ratio, and skeletal changes such as masculinization of the facial bones and jaw and widening of the shoulders. In female puberty, estrogen production results in development of glandular breast tissue and redistribution of fat to the buttock and hips. Ovarian and endometrial development leads to menarche [78].

The onset of central puberty can be assessed clinically by the development of testicular enlargement and breast budding in biologic males and females, respectively. The beginnings of testicular enlargement and thinning of the scrotal skin in biologic males, and the development of breast budding in biologic females, are hallmarks of sexual maturity rating (SMR; Tanner stage) 2. Pubic hair development and the development of apocrine body odor may develop before central puberty as a result of adrenal androgen production. These changes by themselves should not be considered evidence of central puberty [79,80]. The average age of onset of puberty is 10 to 11 years in females and 11 to 12 years in males. Height velocity increases during puberty and peaks about 2.5 years after the start of the pubertal growth acceleration [81]. In biologic males, characteristics significantly affecting gender attribution, such as facial hair development, completion of voice change, and masculinization of facial bones, occur later in puberty compared with genital development. The lateness of these changes within normal male puberty provides incentive for pubertal suppression in MTF individuals presenting in late puberty. In FTM individuals, breast development typically progresses from SMR 2 to 5 (fully developed) within 4 to 5 years and menses typically begin 2 to 2.5 years after breast budding [78].

OVERVIEW OF MEDICAL MANAGEMENT
The WPATH standards of care and The Endocrine Society clinical practice guidelines both recommend the diagnosis of gender dysphoria be made by a mental health professional with expertise in gender identity before considering a hormonal intervention [1,2]. Some multidisciplinary gender programs employ mental health professionals to perform assessments for referred patients; other programs rely on community-based mental health providers to make the diagnosis of gender dysphoria [82]. Primary goals of medical interventions include (1) prevention of the development of unwanted secondary sex characteristics of the biologic sex and (2) promotion of the development of desired secondary sex characteristics of the affirmed gender. Broader objectives include reduction in dysphoric feelings; reduction in comorbid depression, anxiety, and suicidality; and enhanced ability to "pass" as the affirmed gender with subsequent improvement in quality of life and general functioning.

PREVENTION OF THE DEVELOPMENT OF UNWANTED SECONDARY SEX CHARACTERISTICS
Medical interventions that suppress sex hormone production or that block sex hormone action work to prevent the development of undesired secondary sex characteristics of the biologic sex (Table 2). These interventions include pubertal suppression using GnRH agonists, reduction in biologic hormone production using progestins, and use of androgen receptor antagonists such as spironolactone [6].

Use of a GnRH agonist to suppress puberty completely starting at SMR 2 followed by introduction of cross-sex hormones in later adolescence was first described by a pioneering gender center in Amsterdam, the Netherlands [38,57]. The rationale for using GnRH agonist medications to suppress puberty

Table 2
Medications used in the treatment of transgender adolescents

Class of medication	Medication names	Mechanism of delivery	Mechanism of action
Prevention of the development of unwanted secondary sex characteristics			
GnRH agonists	Leuprolide acetate	IM injection	Inhibition of the HPG axis
	Histrelin acetate	SC implant	
Progestins	Medroxyprogesterone acetate	Oral or intramuscular injection	Inhibition of the HPG axis
	Norethindrone	Oral	"
Androgen receptor inhibitors	Spironolactone	Oral	Inhibition of testosterone action
	Cyproterone acetate	Oral or intramuscular injection	"
Promotion of the development of desired secondary sex characteristics			
Testosterone	Testosterone enanthate	IM injection	Activation of androgen receptors
	Testosterone cypionate	IM injection	
	Other testosterone	Transdermal gels and patches	"
17ß-estradiol	17ß-estradiol	Oral or transdermal patch most common; also available as IM injection and sublingual	Activation of estrogen receptors

Abbreviations: HPG, hypothalamic–pituitary–gonadal; IM, intramuscular; SC, subcutaneous.

include that (1) it allows a transgender adolescent protected time to explore their gender identity with their mental health professional and family without continued progression into their biologic puberty, (2) halting the progression of puberty seems to improve behavioral and emotional problems, and reduces depressive symptoms [72], and (3) preventing the development of secondary sex characteristics of the biologic puberty can improve the ability to pass as the affirmed gender and obviate the need for procedures such as masculinizing chest surgery in biologic females, and electrolysis of facial and body hair, feminizing facial surgeries, and voice therapy in biologic males.

For example, an FTM patient who starts on GnRH agonist medication at SMR 2, and then starts on testosterone in later adolescence, may not require masculinizing chest surgery and will also forgo menstruation. If suppression occurs at SMR 3 or 4, before full breast development, a less invasive chest surgery (eg, through an areolar incision rather than an inframammary incision) may be considered. An FTM patient presenting after full breast development has occurred would get less benefit from GnRH agonist treatment. Although a GnRH agonist would suppress dysphoric menses, other more cost-effective interventions, such as treatment with a progestin, may accomplish a similar result.

For MTF, use of GnRH agonist medication before the development of male secondary sex characteristics can dramatically improve gender attribution and the ability to pass as the affirmed female gender. For example, an MTF who starts on GnRH agonist medication at SMR 2, who continues on it as estrogen therapy is initiated in later adolescence, and then proceeds with gonadectomy and vaginoplasty after age 18, will never develop masculine facial and body hair, will not have a deep voice, and will not have masculinization of the facial bones and skeletal frame [12].

Both WPATH and The Endocrine Society Guidelines recommend consideration of GnRH agonist therapy only after the start of puberty (SMR 2) [1,2]. Use of pubertal suppression to prevent puberty from starting, starting at SMR 1, is not recommended. This is because persistence of gender dysphoria during early puberty can be used as an important diagnostic tool, predicting continued transgender identity in older adolescence and adulthood. Additionally, starting at SMR 1 would add unnecessary treatment and cost for a prepubertal patient not requiring pubertal suppression.

GnRH agonist medications have been used extensively in the pediatric age group for treatment of precocious puberty for more than 25 years. They are considered safe and reversible medications [83]. In the transgender population, theoretic risks include reduction in bone mineral density z-score while on treatment. However, new evidence suggests that bone density accrual improves after starting treatment with cross-sex hormones [57]. Although the effects of GnRH agonists are reversible, they are often started with the intent of initiating cross-sex hormones later on, and the combination of the two results in permanent and semipermanent effects. It is important that families receive counseling regarding the fertility effects of GnRH agonists and cross-sex hormones. A child who starts on GnRH agonist therapy at SMR stage 2 and continues on the mediation as cross-sex hormones are introduced later in adolescence will never have spermatogenesis or menarche, and will not have the opportunity to bank gametes using cryopreservation. Yet for many patients and families, after appropriate informed consent, the benefits of pubertal suppression still outweigh the risks [1,2]. GnRH agonists can be continued during treatment with cross-sex hormones. For example, an MTF individual may be treated concurrently with a GnRH agonist and estrogen until gonadectomy is performed, at which point GnRH agonist therapy would no longer be needed. An FTM individual may use a GnRH agonist and testosterone until masculinizing chest surgery, at which point monotherapy with testosterone should suffice to prevent continued menstruation.

GnRH agonists provide a constant level of stimulation to the GnRH receptor and, as a result, inhibit the pulsatile secretion of LH and FSH from the anterior pituitary. Common forms of administration include an intramuscular injection administered every 30 or 90 days (leuprolide acetate) or a subcutaneous implant, replaced annually (histrelin acetate). In our experience, histrelin acetate implants in either the pediatric preparation (distributed in the United States as Supprelin, designed to deliver 65 µg/d of active medication) or adult preparation (distributed in the United States as Vantas, designed to deliver 50 µg/d of active medication) are both effective at suppressing puberty in transgender adolescents for longer than 1 year. GnRH agonists can also be given as intranasal preparations; however, there are no reports of use of this preparation in transgender individuals. Choice of GnRH agonist preparation in the United States is often based on availability, insurance coverage, patient age, and patient and family preference. We have often used Vantas in situations where insurance coverage is denied because it is more affordable for out-of-pocket payment compared with other preparations. The use of any GnRH agonist preparation for pubertal suppression in transgender adolescents is considered "off-label" in the United States. The Food and Drug Administration has not listed gender dysphoria as a clinical indication for their use, although this is current standard of care.

In addition to GnRH agonists, other medications that reduce the production of sex hormones or inhibit their actions can be useful in the transgender adolescent. Even before the development of GnRH agonist medications, progestins, more specifically medroxyprogesterone acetate, had been used in the treatment of precocious puberty to suppress sex hormone production [84]. Progestins, including medroxyprogesterone acetate and norethindrone, reduce the pulsatile release of LH and also directly inhibit sex hormone production at the level of the gonad [6]. Medroxyprogesterone acetate can be given as an intramuscular injection every 3 months (Depo-Provera) or as a daily oral medication (Provera), and norethindrone as a daily oral medication (as Micronor or Aygestin). In our experience, treatment with progestins have been especially helpful in a few specific situations. (1) In an FTM individual who has already completed breast development and started menstruating, but who is either too young or still in the process of considering treatment with testosterone; in this situation, treatment with a progestin can aid in reducing dysphoria by suppressing menses. (2) In an MTF individual who has started on cross-sex hormone therapy with estradiol and who cannot receive GnRH agonist therapy owing to lack of insurance coverage; in this situation, if the estrogen monotherapy is insufficient to bring testosterone down to a level that would support normal breast development, use of estrogen therapy with concurrent use of a progestin can help to promote normal breast development and minimize further masculinization from testicular production of testosterone. Note that, conversely, an FTM individual on monotherapy with testosterone will most often have adequate suppression of menses and should not require pubertal suppression with GnRH or treatment with a progestin.

Finally, spironolactone is an oral medication most commonly used as a weak diuretic, which also acts as a weak androgen receptor antagonist. This medication can be used by MTF individuals to reduce the effects of testicular androgen production [6]. We most commonly use spironolactone when the patient is troubled by the development of facial and body hair. Although spironolactone will not cause regression of the terminal hair follicles, patients on spironolactone therapy may require less frequent shaving or electrolysis treatments. Cyproterone acetate is another antiandrogen medication not approved for use in the United States, but is used in MTF patients in other countries [6].

PROMOTION OF THE DEVELOPMENT OF DESIRED
SECONDARY SEX CHARACTERISTICS

The use of hormonal interventions, often referred to as *cross-sex or gender affirming hormones*, to promote the development of desired secondary sex characteristics in transgender persons can be considered in carefully screened and counseled adolescents with gender dysphoria (see Table 2). Specifically, the use of 17β-estradiol in MTF individuals, and testosterone in FTM individuals, are used to induce the development of the secondary sex characteristics of the affirmed gender. Broad goals of treatment are to improve psychological functioning and general well-being, and enhance the patient's ability to present as their affirmed gender in social life. The WPATH standards of care do not specify an age at which cross-sex hormones can be administered, but suggest obtaining parental consent [1]. The Endocrine Society suggests that cross-sex hormones can be considered "around age 16" [2]. In our practice, we have found that for many patients there is significant psychosocial risk in waiting until age 16 years to start cross-sex hormones if the patient is otherwise stable in their transgender identity. It is therefore our practice, and the practice of similar institutions, to consider cross-sex hormone treatment initiation as young as age 14 years [5,6].

MTF individuals are treated with 17β-estradiol to induce female secondary sex characteristics. Treatment with 17β-estradiol will promote the development of breast tissue and development of a more feminine body habitus. These changes are more effective when testosterone production is reduced, either by using GnRH agonist medication or a progestin concurrently. Higher doses of 17β-estradiol would be required to produce feminizing changes if the testosterone concentration is in the normal male range.

17β-Estradiol is available in oral, sublingual, transdermal, and intramuscular preparations [6]. We prefer to use oral or transdermal 17β-estradiol. In a patient who is concurrently being treated with a GnRH agonist, we would use oral 17β-estradiol (Estrace) 0.5 mg/d and increase gradually to 2 mg/d, with dose increases every 4 to 6 months, or transdermal 17β-estradiol (such as Climara or Vivelle-Dot) starting at 12.5 or 25 µg weekly. In our practice, adolescent patients on GnRH agonist therapy concurrent with 17β-estradiol are able to achieve normal breast development without need or desire for later breast modification surgery. Similar results may be possible using a combination of medroxyprogesterone and 17β-estradiol or norethindrone and 17β-estradiol. Without any concurrent suppression using GnRH agonist or progestin, patients require higher doses of estrogen to suppress testosterone production and overcome its androgenic effect on the breast tissue. Cosmetic results may be less favorable and higher dose estrogen therapy carries thrombogenic risk. Once a patient undergoes gonadectomy as part of gender confirmation surgery, monotherapy with 17β-estradiol is sufficient. Additionally, some centers use progesterone concurrently with estradiol to improve breast development, although the effects have not been adequately studied.

FTM individuals are prescribed testosterone to promote the development of male secondary sex characteristics. Testosterone is available via many different preparations, including intramuscular, gels, creams, and patches. Testosterone for pubertal induction has classically been given as an intramuscular preparation (as testosterone cypionate or testosterone enanthate). Intramuscular testosterone, when used for male pubertal induction, is often used starting at 25 mg every 2 weeks with gradual dose increases to 100 to 200 mg every 2 weeks. Many centers use testosterone cypionate or testosterone enanthate administered as a subcutaneous injection administered by the patient or his parent weekly. It can be started at 12.5 to 25 mg weekly increasing to 50 to 100 mg weekly [6]. Doses are adjusted to keep the testosterone concentration in the normal male range for age, and based on clinical response. The subcutaneous method allows for in-home administration after a brief in-office education on the subcutaneous administration technique. Because testosterone for injection is suspended in oil, it does not draw readily through a standard insulin syringe. Instead, a thicker gauge needle, such as a 21-gauge needle for drawing, and a 25-gauge needle for injecting, must be prescribed for administration.

LONGITUDINAL SCREENING AND ANTICIPATORY GUIDANCE

Patients being treated with pubertal suppression, spironolactone, 17β-estradiol, and/or testosterone require continued support from a mental health professional, longitudinal follow-up to assess clinical response and development of untoward side effects of treatment, and laboratory monitoring. Rosenthal [6] suggests that patients undergoing pubertal suppression using GnRH agonist medication should have a physical examination, including monitoring of height, weight, and pubertal staging, as well as biochemical assessment of puberty using LH, FSH, and estradiol or testosterone measurement every 3 months and a bone age evaluation annually. Additionally, owing to the delay in bone density accrual in patients undergoing pubertal suppression, it is advised to follow bone health using measurement of calcium, phosphorus, alkaline phosphatase, and 25-hydroxyvitamin D annually, as well as consideration for dual-energy x-ray absorptiometry annually [6]. Spironolactone can cause hyperkalemia; therefore, we obtain a baseline electrolyte panel and repeat with each dose adjustment and when obtaining other laboratory evaluations. In patients prescribed 17β-estradiol or testosterone, Rosenthal [6] suggests clinical follow-up every 3 months to assess height, weight, blood pressure, and pubertal progression. At these visits, LH, FSH, and estradiol and/or testosterone can be assessed. In addition, he suggests following calcium, phosphorus, alkaline phosphatase, 25-hydroxyvitamin D, complete blood count, renal function, liver function, fasting lipids, glucose, insulin, and hemoglobin A1C, plus prolactin in MTF patients [6]. Patients who had puberty suppressed and who are subsequently being treated with cross-sex hormones can also be monitored for gains in bone density using dual-energy x-ray absorptiometry [6].

Although long-term health data are sparse with regard to adolescents, some data exist in the adult transgender literature. In longitudinal studies of FTM adults, testosterone administration (250 mg IM every 2 weeks) is associated with lower high-density lipoprotein cholesterol and higher triglycerides after 6 to 12 months of treatment compared with baseline [85–87]. However, long-term testosterone administration does not seem to alter fasting insulin or glucose use in FTM adults compared with a pretestosterone baseline assessment [86]. A Dutch study of FTM adults on testosterone did not suggest an increased incidence of cardiovascular events or increased mortality compared with the general population [88].

Elevated blood pressure, fasting insulin, and decreased insulin sensitivity have been reported in MTF adults treated with ethinyl estradiol [86,87]. Treatment of MTF adults with ethinyl estradiol has also been associated with increased risk of cardiovascular death [88]. After 1990, 17ß-estradiol was used in the Netherlands in favor of ethinyl estradiol owing to its more favorable cardiovascular risk profile.

We advise discussing potential impairment to fertility, not only before starting cross-sex hormones, but also before starting pubertal suppression. Even though pubertal suppression using GnRH agonist medications by themselves do not impair future fertility, their use combined with cross-sex hormones does impair fertility. In our experience, many adolescent patients, even those who are not transgender, are often reticent to discuss their future fertility. The conversation can be more complex in transgender adolescents, who may have some desire to have biologic children, but who bristle at the idea of using their own anatomy to accomplish this. If a patient has progressed far enough into natal puberty such that cryopreservation of sperm or oocytes is possible, this option should be discussed. Providers treating transgender adolescents should familiarize themselves with cryopreservation options in their community. The cost of preservation methods, especially the preservation of oocytes, is often a significant barrier.

GENDER AFFIRMATIVE SURGERY

Mental health and medical providers caring for transgender adolescents should become familiar with common surgical interventions used in the transgender patient population, and should be knowledgeable about what surgical resources are available in the community. Surgical interventions used in transgender persons for the purposes of transition are often referred to as *gender affirmation* surgeries. Procedures may include genital surgeries, chest surgeries, and a variety of other gender affirming procedures. The most common surgical procedures performed in MTF individuals include breast augmentation surgery; genital surgery including penectomy, orchiectomy, and vaginoplasty; facial feminization surgeries; voice surgery; thyroid cartilage reduction; and hair reconstruction. Electrolysis or laser hair removal is also commonly performed. In FTM individuals, surgical procedures include mastectomy and genital surgeries including hysterectomy/salpingoophorectomy, metoidioplasty with phalloplasty, vaginectomy, scrotoplasty, and implantation of erectile and testicular prostheses. Genital surgeries are typically not recommended until the patient has reached the legal age of majority. Chest surgery in FTM patients can be considered earlier [1].

OUTCOMES

Treatment with pubertal suppression in transgender adolescents improves psychological functioning and decreases depressive symptoms; however, it does not seem to eliminate gender dysphoria [72]. Long-term outcomes data from the Netherlands suggests that transgender persons treated with pubertal suppression, followed by cross-sex hormones and finally gender affirmation surgery in young adulthood, yields positive outcomes with none regretting starting gender affirming medical treatments [73]. In a study primarily sampling participants from the United States, FTM individuals reported diminished quality of life compared with cisgender males and females; however, those who have received testosterone report significantly higher quality of life compared with those who have not [89].

More robust long-term outcomes data may be necessary for the WPATH and The Endocrine Society recommendations to be more fully adopted, embraced, and refined. In addition, these interventions will remain "off-label" in the United States until approved by the US Food and Drug Administration. That said, it is evident by the growing demand for these interventions and the increase in pediatric gender programs in the United States, that gender affirming medical interventions for appropriately assessed patients has become the standard of care.

CHALLENGES AND BARRIERS TO CARE

The National Transgender Discrimination Survey Report on Health and Health Care in 2010 surveyed more than 6000 transgender adults in the United States and US territories, and found that transgender adults experience discrimination by medical providers, with 19% of respondents reporting that they have been refused care owing to their gender identity. More than one-quarter responded that they have been harassed verbally in a medical setting and more than one-half had to teach their provider about transgender health care. More than one-quarter reported postponing or delaying needed either preventive care or care when they were sick or injured [61]. Transgender individuals who belong to racial and ethnic minorities experience more discrimination [90]. Finally, insurance company denial of transgender-related interventions remains a significant barrier to care [12]. There have been efforts to improve resident and medical student education and comfort with taking care of transgender patients [10,91], including a recent report by the Association of American Medical Colleges on implementation of curricular changes [92].

CURRENT GENDER MANAGEMENT PROGRAMS IN THE UNITED STATES AND CANADA

A recent report provides descriptions and contact information for 35 gender programs in the United States and Canada [93]. In addition to these programs, several other programs are known to exist by the authors. The descriptions of the various programs in this report makes clear that different centers have approached providing gender services to children and adolescents in diverse ways. For example, providers from the fields of pediatric endocrinology, adolescent medicine, gynecology, primary care, and nurse clinicians are working in these programs to provide hormonal interventions. Programs often employ mental health providers from the fields of social work, psychology, and psychiatry to provide individual counseling, assessments, family therapy, and/or group therapy. Some programs serve as a primary care medical home for patients, whereas others function as a consultative program [93].

We suggest that other roles of multidisciplinary programs could include providing training programs for hospital staff and other members of the health care system, advocating for changes to paper forms and the electronic medical record to make them more gender inclusive, providing education for medical students and trainees, promoting community partnerships, collaborating with and/or providing education to school systems, promoting research, and assisting with transition to adult care.

CASE EXAMPLES
Patient 1
An 11-year-old biologic male presented to the pediatrician with concerns regarding gender identity. The child had been interested in stereotypically feminine toys and play from a very young age, and the parents had assumed that the child would grow up to be a gay man. However, more recently the child has clearly expressed a female gender identity to the parents. The child has declared herself to be transgender and insisted on use of female pronouns at home. The parents noted that school performance had suffered and the child has become withdrawn and depressed over the past year. The pediatrician referred the family to a mental health professional with experience in gender identity in children. After several sessions, the mental health professional confirmed a diagnosis of gender dysphoria and recommended referral to a medical clinic with experience in gender dysphoria. At the clinic, the child was found to be at SMR 2. After discussion of risks and benefits of intervention, the child and family elected to proceed with pubertal suppression. A bone age and dual-energy x-ray absorptiometry test were found to be normal for age, and 25-hydroxyvitamin D was slightly low. A histrelin acetate implant was placed and vitamin D supplementation was initiated. Pubertal suppression continued until age 14. By that time, the child had made a complete social transition, using a female name and pronouns at home and at school, and had been supported by ongoing therapy from her mental health professional. Oral 17ß-estradiol was started and pubertal suppression with histrelin acetate was continued. The child proceeded through a normal female puberty on 17ß-estradiol treatment. At age 18, she elected to have gender affirmation surgery, including orchiectomy and vaginoplasty, at which point histrelin acetate was discontinued.

Patient 2

A 10-year-old biologic female with characteristically male interests and behaviors became distressed with the development of breast budding. The patient also disclosed a male gender identity to friends, and then to parents. After a diagnosis of gender dysphoria was made by a mental health professional, the child was referred to a gender program. The clinic physician confirmed breast maturity rating 2, and after discussion with the patient and family, suppression of puberty was initiated using leuprolide acetate, administered every 90 days. The treatment halted progression of breast development. At age 15, after the child had made a complete social transition, testosterone enanthate was initiated, administered subcutaneously weekly at home. At age 19, the patient elected to undergo hysterectomy/salpingoophorectomy and leuprolide acetate was discontinued.

Patient 3

A 15-year-old biologic male with female affirmed gender identity presented to a gender clinic after being referred by their primary care physician and mental health professional for treatment of gender dysphoria. The adolescent was found to be at SMR 4. Goals of treatment were determined to be suppression of continued masculinization and promotion of feminization, including breast development. The provider attempted to prescribe a GnRH agonist, but it was rejected by the patient's insurance. The provider instead prescribed norethindrone to suppress androgen production, spironolactone to inhibit androgen action, and 17ß-estradiol to promote breast development and feminization.

Patient 4

A 16-year-old biologic female presented to a gender clinic after receiving a diagnosis of gender dysphoria by a mental health professional. The teen was especially dysphoric with monthly menses, but the family was uneasy about committing to irreversible therapy with testosterone. Treatment with norethindrone 5 mg oral daily was initiated, and the monthly menses were suppressed, with resulting improvement in well-being. At age 18, the patient had made a complete social transition and elected to start testosterone, prescribed at 50 mg subcutaneous weekly, at which point norethindrone was discontinued without subsequent return of menses on testosterone monotherapy.

Patient 5

A 12-year-old biologic male presented to the gender clinic after referral by a mental health professional. The child had been having dysphoric feelings about his male pubertal development, and was found to be at SMR rating 3. Treatment with a GnRH agonist was initiated. The child continued in therapy and by age 14 had developed a better understanding of their gender identity. The child accepts that they do not identity completely with a male or female gender identity, and begins to refer to themself as genderqueer. They prefer to be referred to using the them/they/their pronouns. After discussion with the family and mental health professional, the decision is made to withdraw the GnRH agonist medication and allow male puberty to progress with continued supportive counseling in place.

Acknowledgments

Thank you to the wonderful children, teenagers, and families who come to our clinics. Also thank you to the clinicians and staff at The Center for Transyouth Health and Development at Children's Hospital Los Angeles for allowing Dr N.J. Nokoff to visit and gain insight into the wonderful care they provide for transgender and gender nonconforming youth.

References

[1] Coleman E, Bockting W, Botzer M, et al. Standards of care for the health of transsexual, transgender, and gender-nonconforming people, version 7. Int J Transgend 2012;13(4): 165–232.

[2] Hembree WC, Cohen-Kettenis P, Delemarre-van de Waal HA, et al. Endocrine treatment of transsexual persons: an Endocrine Society clinical practice guideline. J Clin Endocrinol Metab 2009;94(9):3132–54.

[3] Mcinroy LB, Craig SL. Transgender representation in offline and online media: LGBTQ youth perspectives. J Hum Behav Soc Environ 2015;25(6):606–17.

[4] Glicksman E. Transgender today. Monitor on Psychology 2013;44(4):36.

[5] Spack NP, Edwards-Leeper L, Feldman HA, et al. Children and adolescents with gender identity disorder referred to a pediatric medical center. Pediatrics 2012;129(3):418–25.

[6] Rosenthal SM. Approach to the patient: transgender youth: endocrine considerations. J Clin Endocrinol Metab 2014;99(12):4379–89.

[7] Sherer I, Rosenthal S, Ehrensaft D, et al. Child and Adolescent Gender Center: a multidisciplinary collaboration to improve the lives of gender nonconforming children and teens. Pediatr Rev 2012;33:273–5.

[8] De Vreis A, Cohen-Kettenis PT. Clinical management of gender dysphoria in children and adolescents: the Dutch approach. J Homosex 2012;59:301–20.

[9] Zucker K, Bradley S, Owen-Anderson A, et al. Is gender identity disorder in adolescents coming out of the closet? J Sex Marital Ther 2008;34:287–90.

[10] Obedin-Maliver J, Goldsmith E, Stewart L, et al. Lesbian, gay, bisexual, and transgender-related content in undergraduate medical education. JAMA 2011;306(9):971–7.

[11] Institute of Medicine. The health of lesbian, gay, bisexual, and transgender people: building a foundation for better understanding. Washington, DC: The National Academies Press; 2011.

[12] Shumer DE, Spack NP. Current management of gender identity disorder in childhood and adolescence: guidelines, barriers and areas of controversy. Curr Opin Endocrinol Diabetes Obes 2013;20(1):69–73.

[13] American Psychiatric Association. Diagnostic and statistical manual of mental disorders. 4th edition. Arlington (VA): American Psychiatric Publishing; 2000.

[14] American Psychiatric Association. Diagnostic and statistical manual of mental disorders. 5th edition. Arlington (VA): American Psychiatric Publishing; 2013.

[15] Van Kesteren PJ, Gooren LJ, Megens JA. An epidemiological and demographic study of transsexuals in The Netherlands. Arch Sex Behav 1996;25:589–600.

[16] Conron K, Scott G, Stowell G, et al. Transgender health in Massachusetts: results from a household probability sample of adults. Am J Public Health 2012;102:118–22.

[17] Brown-Sequard CE. Note on the effects produced on man by subcutaneous injections of a liquid obtained from the testicles of animals. Lancet 1889;134:105–7.

[18] David KG, Dingemanse E, Freud J, et al. On crystalline male hormone from testicles (testosterone) effective as from urine or from cholesterol. Hoppe Seylers Z Physiol Chem 1935;233:281.

[19] Ruzicka L, Wettstein A. Sexualhormone VII. Über die künstliche Herstellung des Testikelhormons Testosteron (Androsten-3-on-17-ol). Helv Chim Acta 1935;18(1):1264–75.

[20] Veler CD, Thayer S, Doisy EA. The preparation of the crystalline follicular ovarian hormone: Theelin. J Biol Chem 1930;87(2):357–71.

[21] Butenandt A. Über 'Progynon' ein krystallisiertes weibliches Sexualhormon. Naturwissenschaften 1929;17(45):879.

[22] Marrian GF. The chemistry of oestrin. Biochem J 1930;24:435–45.

[23] Slotta KH, Ruschig H, Fels E. Reindarstellung der Hormone aus dem Corpus luteum (II. Mitteil.). Ber Dtsch Chem Ges 1934;67(9):1624–6.

[24] Wintersteiner O, Allen WM. Crystalline progestin. J Biol Chem 1934;107(1):321–36.

[25] Inhoffen HH, Logemann W, Hohlweg W, et al. Sex hormone series. Ber Dtsch Chem Ges 1938;71:1024–32.

[26] Inhoffen HH, Hohlweg W. Neue per os-wirksame weibliche Keimdrüsenhormon-Derivate: 17-Aethinyl-oestradiol und Pregnen-in-on-3-ol-17. Naturwissenschaften 1938;26(6):96.

[27] Gooren LJ, Giltay EJ, Bunck MC. Long-term treatment of transsexuals with cross-sex hormones: extensive personal experience. J Clin Endocrinol Metab 2008;93:19–25.

[28] Hirschfeld M. Sexualpathologie: T. Sexuelle Zwischenstufen; Das Männliche Weib Und der Weibliche Mann, vol. 2. Bonn (Germany): A. Marcus & E. Webers; 1918.

[29] Elbe L. Man into woman: an authentic record of a change of sex. Norwich (England): Jarrold Publishers; 1933.

[30] Goddard JC, Vickery RM, Terry TR. Development of feminizing genitoplasty for gender dysphoria. J Sex Med 2007;4(4 Pt 1):981–9.

[31] Christine J. Available at: www.christinejorgensen.org. Accessed December 16, 2015.

[32] Dec. 1, 1952: Ex-GI becomes blonde beauty. Wired. 2010. Available at: www.wired.com/2010/12/1201first-sex-change-surgery, Accessed December 16, 2015.

[33] Huelke H. Ein Transvestit. Z Kriminalistische Wissen 1949;3:91–2.

[34] Hamburger C, Stürup GK, Dahl-Iversen E. Transvestism: hormonal, psychiatric, and surgical treatment. JAMA 1953;152(5):391–6.

[35] Benjamin H. The transsexual phenomenon: a scientific report on transsexualism and sex conversion in the human male and female. New York: The Julian Press, Inc. Publishers; 1966.

[36] Colapinto J. As nature made him: the boy who was raised as a girl. 2nd edition. New York: Harper Perennial; 2006.

[37] Mansfield MJ, Beardsworth DE, Loughlin JS, et al. Long-Term treatment of central precocious puberty with a long-acting analogue of luteinizing hormone-releasing hormone. N Engl J Med 1983;309(21):1286–90.

[38] Cohen-Kettenis PT, van Goozen S. Pubertal delay as an aid in diagnosis and treatment of a transsexual adolescent. Eur Child Adolesc Psychiatry 1998;7(4):246–8.

[39] Devaney SA, Palomaki GE, Scott JA, et al. Non invasive fetal sex determination using cell-free DNA: a systematic review and meta-analysis. JAMA 2011;306(6):627–36.

[40] Kohlberg LA. A cognitive-developmental analysis of children's sex role concepts and attitudes. In: Maccoby E, editor. The development of sex differences. Stanford (CA): Stanford University; 1966. p. 82–173.

[41] Fausto-Sterling A. The dynamic development of gender variability. J Homosex 2012;59(3): 398–421.

[42] Money J, Ehrhardt A. Fetal hormones and the brain: effect on sexual dimorphism of behavior - a review. Arch Sex Behav 1971;1(3):241–62.

[43] Fausto-Sterling A. Sex/gender: biology in a social world. New York: Routledge; 2012.

[44] Goldstein J, Seidman L, Horton N, et al. Normal sexual dimorphism of the adult human brain assessed by in vivo magnetic resonance imaging. Cereb Cortex 2001;11(6):490–7.

[45] Zhou J-N, Hofman MA, Gooren LJG, et al. A sex difference in the human brain and its relation to transsexuality. Nature 1995;378:68–70.

[46] Heylens G, De Cuypere G, Zucker KJ, et al. Gender identity disorder in twins: a review of the case report literature. J Sex Med 2012;9(3):751–7.

[47] Berenbaum SA, Beltz AM. Sexual differentiation of human behavior: effects of prenatal and pubertal organizational hormones. Front neuroendocrinology 2011;32(2):183–200.

[48] Jordan-Young RM. Hormones, context, and "brain gender": a review of evidence from congenital adrenal hyperplasia. Soc Sci Med 2012;74(11):1738–44.

[49] Dessens A, Slijper F, Drop S. Gender dysphoria and gender change in chromosomal females with congenital adrenal hyperplasia. Arch Sex Behav 2005;34:389–97.

[50] Reiner W, Gearhart J. Discordant sexual identity in some genetic males with cloacal exstrophy assigned to female sex at birth. N Engl J Med 2004;350:333–41.

[51] Martin CL, Ruble DN, Szkrybalo J. Cognitive theories of early gender development. Psychol Bull 2002;128(6):903–33.

[52] Strang JF, Kenworthy L, Dominska A, et al. Increased gender variance in autism spectrum disorders and attention deficit hyperactivity disorder. Arch Sex Behav 2014;43(8):1525–33.

[53] Shechner T. Gender Identity disorder: a literature review from a developmental perspective. Isr J Psychiatry Relat Sci 2010;47(2):132–8.

[54] Gooren LJ. Clinical practice. Care of transsexual persons. N Engl J Med 2011;364(13):1251–7.

[55] Drummond K, Bradley S, Peterson-Badali M, et al. A follow-up study of girls with gender identity disorder. Dev Psychol 2008;44:34–45.

[56] Wallien MSC, Cohen-Kettenis PT. Psychosexual outcome of gender dysphoric children. J Pers Assess 2009;91:545–52.

[57] Delemarre-van de Wall HA, Cohen-Kettenis PT. Clinical management of gender identity disorder in adolescents: a protocol on psychological and paediatric endocrinology aspects. Eur J Endocrinol 2006;155(Suppl 1):S131–7.

[58] Steensma TD, Biemond R, de Boer F, et al. Desisting and persisting gender dysphoria after childhood: a qualitative follow-up study. Clin Child Psychol Psychiatry 2011;16(4):499–516.

[59] Steensma TD, McGuire JK, Kreukels B, et al. Factors associated with desistence and persistence of childhood gender dysphoria: a quantitative follow-up study. J Am Acad Child Adolesc Psychiatry 2013;52:582–90.

[60] Bradford J, Reisner SL, Honnold JA, et al. Experiences of transgender-related discrimination and implications for health: results from the Virginia Transgender Health Initiative Study. Am J Public Health 2013;103(10):1820–9.

[61] Grant JM, Mottet LA, Tanis JD, et al. National transgender discrimination survey report on health and health care. Washington, DC: National Center for Transgender Equality; National Gay and Lesbian Task Force; 2010.

[62] Grossman A, D'Augelli A. Transgender youth and life-threatening behaviors. Suicide Life Threat Behav 2007;37(5):527–37.

[63] Nuttbrock L, Hwahng S, Bockting W, et al. Psychiatric impact of gender-related abuse across the life course of male-to-female transgender persons. J Sex Res 2010;47(1):12–23.

[64] Olson J, Schrager S, Belzer M, et al. Baseline physiologic and psychosocial characteristics of transgender youth seeking care for gender dysphoria. J Adolesc Health 2015;57(4):374–80.

[65] Wilson E, Garafalo R, Harris R, et al. Transgender female youth and sex work: HIV risk and a comparison of life factors related to engagement in sex work. AIDS Behav 2009;13(5):902–13.

[66] Reisner SL, Vetters R, Leclerc M, et al. Mental health of transgender youth in care at an adolescent urban community health center: a matched retrospective cohort study. J Adolesc Health 2015;56(3):274–9.

[67] Kosciw J, Greytak E, Bartkiewicz M, et al. The 2011 National School Climate Survey: the experiences of lesbian, gay, bisexual and transgender youth in our Nation's schools. New York: Gay, Lesbian & Straight Education Network; 2012.

[68] De Vries ALC, Noens ILJ, Cohen-Kettenis PT, et al. Autism spectrum disorders in gender dysphoric children and adolescents. J Autism Dev Disord 2010;40(8):930–6.

[69] Zucker KJ, Wood H, Singh D, et al. A developmental, biopsychosocial model for the treatment of children with gender identity disorder. J Homosex 2012;59:369–97.

[70] Hill DB, Menvielle E, Sica KM, et al. An affirmative intervention for families with gender variant children: parental ratings of child mental health and gender. J Sex Marital Ther 2010;36(1):6–23.

[71] American Psychological Association. Guidelines for psychological practice with transgender and gender nonconforming people. Am Psychol 2015;70(9):832–64.

[72] De Vries ALC, Steensma TD, Doreleijers TA, et al. Puberty suppression in adolescents with gender identity disorder: a prospective follow-up study. J Sex Med 2011;8: 2276–83.

[73] De Vries ALC, McGuire JK, Steensma TD, et al. Young adult psychological outcome after puberty suppression and gender reassignment. Pediatrics 2014;134(4):1–9.

[74] Witchel SF, Lee PA. Differentiation of external genital structures. In: Sperling MA, editor. Pediatric endocrinology. 3rd edition. Philadelphia: Saunders Elsevier; 2008. p. 132.

[75] Kuiri-Hänninen T, Sankilampi U, Dunkel L. Activation of the hypothalamic-pituitary-gonadal axis in infancy: minipuberty. Horm Res Paediatr 2014;82(2):73–80.

[76] Hughes IA. Puberty and the testis. In: Sperling MA, editor. Pediatric endocrinology. 3rd edition. Philadelphia: Saunders Elsevier; 2008. p. 676–9.

[77] Rosenfield RL, Cooke DW, Radovick S. Development of the female reproductive system. In: Sperling MA, editor. Pediatric endocrinology. 3rd edition. Philadelphia: Saunders Elsevier; 2008. p. 532–59.

[78] Marcell AV. Adolescence. In: Kligman RM, Behrman RE, Jenson HB, et al, editors. Nelson textbook of pediatrics. 18th edition. Philadelphia: Saunders Elsevier; 2007. p. 60–5.

[79] Marshall WA, Tanner JM. Variations in pattern of pubertal changes in girls. Arch Dis Child 1969;44(235):291–303.

[80] Marshal WA, Tanner JM. Variations in the pattern of pubertal changes in boys. Arch Dis Child 1970;45(239):13–23.

[81] Abbassi V. Growth and normal puberty. Pediatrics 1998;101(Suppl 3):507–11.

[82] Tishelman AC, Kaufman R, Edwards-Leeper L, et al. Serving transgender youth: challenges, dilemmas, and clinical examples. Prof Psychol Res Pr 2015;46(1):37–45.

[83] Boepple PA, Mansfield MJ, Wierman ME, et al. Use of a potent, long acting agonist of gonadotropin-releasing hormone in the treatment of precocious puberty. Endocr Rev 1986;7(1):24–33.

[84] Warren M, Mathews J, Morishima A, et al. The effect of medroxyprogesterone acetate on gonadotropin secretion in girls with precocious puberty. Am J Med Sci 1975;269(3): 375–81.

[85] Elamin M, Garcia M, Murad M, et al. Effect of sex steroid use on cardiovascular risk in transsexual individuals: a systematic review and meta-analyses. Clin Endocrinol (Oxf) 2010;72(1):1–10.

[86] Elbers J, Giltay E, Teerlink T, et al. Effects of sex steroids on components of the insulin resistance syndrome in transsexual subjects. Clin Endocrinol (Oxf) 2003;58(5):562–71.

[87] Giltay E, Lambert J, Gooren L, et al. Sex steroids, insulin, and arterial stiffness in women and men. Hypertension 1999;34(4 Pt 1):590–7.

[88] Asscheman H, Giltay E, Megens J, et al. A long-term follow-up study of mortality in transsexuals receiving treatment with cross-sex hormones. Eur J Endocrinol 2011;164(4): 635–42.

[89] Newfield E, Hart S, Dibble S, et al. Female-to-male transgender quality of life. Qual Life Res 2006;15(9):1447–57.

[90] Miller L, Grollman E. The social costs of gender nonconformity for transgender adults: implications for discrimination and health. Socio Forum 2005;30(3):809–31.

[91] Thomas D, Safer J. A simple intervention raised resident-physician willingness to assist transgender patients seeking hormone therapy. Endocr Pract 2015;21(10): 1134–42.

[92] Hollenback A, Eckstrand K, Dreger A. Implementing curricular and institutional climate changes to improve health care for individuals who are LGBT, gender nonconforming, or born with DSD. Washington, DC: Association of American Medical Colleges; 2014.

[93] Hsieh S, Leininger J. Resource list: clinical care programs for gender-nonconforming children and adolescents. Pediatr Ann 2014;43(6):238–44.

Advances in Pediatrics 63 (2016) 103–126

ADVANCES IN PEDIATRICS

ELSEVIER
MOSBY

Asthma Management for Children
Risk Identification and Prevention

Monica J. Federico, MD[a], Heather E. Hoch, MD[a],
William C. Anderson III, MD[b], Joseph D. Spahn, MD[b],
Stanley J. Szefler, MD[a],*

[a]Department of Pediatrics, University of Colorado School of Medicine, Children's Hospital
Colorado, 13123 East 16th Avenue, Aurora, CO 80045, USA; [b]Pediatric Allergy & Immunology,
University of Colorado School of Medicine, Children's Hospital Colorado, 13123 East 16th
Avenue, Aurora, CO 80045, USA

Keywords
• Asthma • Early asthma • Inhaled corticosteroids • Lebrikizumab • Mepolizumab
• Omalizumab • Severe asthma • Tiotropium

Key points

- Children with frequent wheeze, allergies, parental history of asthma, early illness, and environmental exposures to tobacco smoke and violence or stress may be at higher risk to progress to persistent wheeze or asthma.

- Although strides have been made in terms of developing predictors of asthma exacerbations in children, continued research is needed to further refine these predictors.

- Children with severe asthma are less likely to require chronically administered oral glucocorticoids, have improved lung function, and require less rescue short-acting beta-agonist therapy compared with children in the recent past.

Continued

Disclosure Information: S.J. Szefler has consulted for Aerocrine, Astra Zeneca, Boehringer-Ingelheim, Daiischi
Sankyo, Glaxo Smith Kline, Genentech, Merck, Novartis, and Roche and has received research support from
the National Institutes of Health, the National Heart, Lung, and Blood Institute (HL098075), the National
Institute for Allergy and Infectious Diseases (AI90052), the National Institute for Environmental and Health
Sciences (ES018181) and the Environmental Protection Agency, the Colorado Cancer, Cardiovascular, and
Pulmonary Disease Program (13-FLA76546), and Glaxo Smith Kline.
No conflict of interest (W.C. Anderson; M.J. Federico; H.E. Hoch; J.D. Spahn).

*Corresponding author. E-mail address: stanley.szefler@childrenscolorado.org

Continued

- New electronic monitoring devices have the potential to significantly improve adherence and significantly reduce the disproportionate morbidity and mortality in children with severe persistent asthma.
- Emerging therapies are adding to the options of therapeutics for preventing and managing acute asthma exacerbations.

INTRODUCTION

Almost every 10 years there is a paradigm shift in the way that we look at and manage asthma. For the last 10 years, we have been focused on asthma control. The asthma guidelines and strategies, nationally and worldwide, have focused on achieving control through careful assessment, education, environmental control, and therapeutic intervention. It is now time to look at the disease in terms of risk factors for breakthrough symptoms, including exacerbations, as well as progression of disease that may result in chronic obstructive lung disease persisting into adulthood. This article reviews recent publications regarding early asthma, asthma exacerbations, severe asthma, and new medications. These 4 sections summarize new information on early asthma, asthma exacerbations, severe asthma, and new medications.

EARLY ASTHMA

The diagnosis of asthma at less than 5 years of age is a subject of debate in scientific literature and among providers who care for children who have symptoms of airway obstruction (eg, cough, wheeze) and albuterol response before 5 years of age. The urgency for diagnosing and treating those children is due not only to the increasing prevalence of asthma and cost of asthma care in young children but also to recent data indicating that children who are diagnosed with asthma may have lower lung functions as adults and be at higher risk for chronic obstructive lung disease [1].

Epidemiology of preschool and early wheeze

The prevalence of asthma in children younger than 5 years is increasing. The Centers for Disease Control and Prevention (CDC) in the United States reported in 2013 that children aged 0 to 4 years are more likely to have an asthma attack with a prevalence ratio of 1.9 (95% confidence interval 1.5–2.4). The demographics of early asthma are not as clear because children aged 0 to 4 years are often included as part of the demographic of children aged 0 to 17 years. The CDC data published in 2011 show that 14.6% of black children aged 0 to 17 years, 8.2% of white children, and 18.4% of children of Puerto Rican descent report asthma. The prevalence of asthma for children who live at or at less than the Federal Poverty Level (FPL) is 11.7% versus 8.2% of children living at 2 or more times the FPL [2].

Risk factors for preschool and early wheeze

The risk of wheeze in early childhood correlates with patient- and family specific factors and environmental exposures. The risk factors for asthma and for early wheeze are different. Early wheeze is discussed in this section. The Tucson Birth Cohort Study and the Prevention and Incidence of Asthma and Mite Allergy along with other birth cohort studies show that early wheeze in infants that resolves in the first 3 to 5 years (transient early wheeze) is associated with viral, lower respiratory tract infections. Later-onset wheeze and persistent wheeze is associated with parental history of allergy and aeroallergen sensitization [3,4]. Preterm birth is also associated with early wheeze and, in the setting of rapid weight gain in infancy, asthma [5,6]. Several studies, including the Tucson Birth Cohort Study, have evaluated the effect of a child's genetic risk factors. No one has reported definitive data showing that variation of specific genetic loci or mutation are predictable risk factors for wheeze or asthma. However, there is strong evidence that methylation of the DNA (epigenetic change) at specific loci may increase the risk of wheeze and asthma [7]. Epigenetic changes may be due to maternal- or child-specific factors, such as early infection or exposure to tobacco smoke or prenatal stress.

Environmental factors, including pollution and tobacco smoke, psychological stress, aeroallergens, and viral illness, affect risk for wheeze in early childhood. Tobacco smoke both prenatally and after birth is associated with increased risk for wheeze and more severe illness [8]. Brunst and colleagues [9] demonstrated that high traffic-related air pollution is associated with transient and persistent wheeze. Psychological stress and prenatal community violence during pregnancy and after birth is also associated with increased risk for wheezing illness [10]. Chiu and colleagues [11] found that prenatal stress may even modify the effect of traffic-related pollution such that there may be increased impact even at lower levels of pollution.

Human rhinovirus and respiratory syncytial virus have been associated with recurrent wheeze in early childhood. Children with a first-degree relative with allergy or asthma followed in the Melbourne Atopy Cohort study were more likely to have early onset recurrent wheeze if they had a documented lower respiratory tract infection [4]. In children who are atopic, early infection may be associated with persistent wheeze in school-aged children [12].

The impact of aeroallergens is unclear. Children who are positive for aeroallergen sensitivity are more likely to have persistent wheeze and recurrent wheeze starting later in early childhood (3 years) [3,13]. However, the impact of exposure to aeroallergens is variable depending on the timing of the exposure and the sensitivity of the child.

Phenotypes of preschool wheeze

Over the past 30 years, birth cohort studies have been conducted to evaluate and describe the clinical and physiologic phenotypes of wheeze seen in children younger than 5 years. One of the challenges to creating those categories is that there is not a gold standard for the diagnosis of asthma in young wheezing children.

Several birth cohort studies created similar phenotypes based on the age symptoms start in the child's life, the presence or absence of atopy, and the frequency of symptoms. The clinical application of those early wheeze phenotypes is complicated by the variability of symptoms and wheezing patterns in individual patients over time [14]. The addition of other biomarkers of disease may lead to an improved ability to predict long-term outcomes using early wheezing phenotypes [15].

Pathophysiology of preschool wheeze

The pathophysiology of inflammation and wheeze in children who wheeze before 5 years of age is unclear [16]. Two recent studies suggest that early inflammation does not correlate with long-term clinical outcomes [17,18]. Another study of children with episodic wheeze and control shows no difference in airway inflammation between the groups [19].

Airway obstruction as measured by infant lung function studies of children with preschool wheeze may explain wheeze in children less than 3 years of age [20]. Children with low infant lung function are more likely to have wheeze with viral illness [21]. Conversely, infant lung function has not been shown to correlate with a diagnosis of persistent wheeze in school-aged children [15,22].

Treatment of preschool wheeze

Limited understanding of the pathophysiology of preschool wheeze leads to difficulties in predicting the response to treatment. The natural history of preschool wheeze is waxing and waning symptoms, suggesting that treatment needs may also vary. Inhaled corticosteroids (ICS) are the cornerstone of asthma treatment in school-aged children through adulthood. Studies and meta-analyses evaluating the response to chronic therapy options including intermittent ICS versus daily ICS are variable. The inconsistent results could be due to study populations, design, the timing of the initiation of inhaled therapy, the dose, and the length of therapy [22].

The final recommendation of the most recent review by Ducharme and colleagues [21] is that daily ICS are more effective than intermittent ICS in controlling exacerbations. Daily inhaled therapy has not been shown to prevent future wheeze or the progression to persistent asthma [22]. There are also no data indicating that daily therapy affects lung function in preschool children [21].

The benefits of daily and intermittent ICS therapy in children must be weighed against the risks of side effects. Guilbert and colleagues [23] demonstrated the significant impact on linear growth, especially in 2-year-old children less than 15 kg who were on daily inhaled fluticasone compared with placebo. The Childhood Asthma Management Program (CAMP) Study demonstrated a decrease in final height in children, aged 5 to 13 years, who were started on budesonide for asthma. The impact was greatest in prepubertal children [24].

The impact on height of high-dose intermittent inhaled therapy is less than daily, although further studies are needed to confirm [25,26].

Several national and international guidelines for the diagnosis and management of children less than 5 years old with wheeze and asthma make treatment recommendations based on the evidence available and expert opinion. These guidelines not only summarize the evidence but also discuss the implementation of the evidence into practice. Australia and Canada published updated guidelines in 2015 [27,28]. The Global Initiative for Asthma (GINA) update was released in 2014 [28,29]. All of these guidelines and proposed strategies recommend daily controller therapy for children who meet specific criteria, such as frequent and poorly controlled symptoms suggesting asthma and the frequency and severity of wheezing episodes (Table 1). They do not recommend intermittent controller medications for these children. The type of daily medication recommendation varies by age in the Australian guidelines. All of these guidelines also recommend frequent reassessment of symptoms and evaluation of side effects of therapy for any child less than 5 years of age on controller therapy. None of the guidelines recommend oral corticosteroids for initiation at home for an exacerbation of wheeze.

Progression to persistent wheeze and asthma

It is difficult to predict whether children who wheeze as toddlers will develop asthma. Many of the children who wheeze before 5 years of age will stop wheezing by 6 years of age [21]. Predictors of persistent wheeze in cohort studies include patient characteristics, such as history of wheeze, atopy, and parental history of asthma, male sex, and tobacco smoke exposure [4,30–32]. Several cohorts developed prediction scores based on the phenotypes identified early in childhood. The Asthma Predictive Index (API) developed as part of the Tucson birth cohort study and modified for the Prevention of Early Asthma in Kids study is the most widely tested and used [33,34]. This index, like others, has a low sensitivity and positive predictive value for asthma.

Table 1
Long-term controller therapy for young children

Guideline	Publication date	Controller medication if needed	Oral corticosteroids	Link
GINA	2014	Daily	Severe exacerbations only	http://www.ginasthma.org/
Canada	2015	Daily	Severe exacerbations only	http://www.respiratoryguidelines.ca/
Australia	2015	Daily	Severe exacerbations only	http://www.nationalasthma.org.au/ handbook

However, the specificity of the index, which has been tested in several large cohorts, is more than 92%. Unfortunately, because of the low sensitivity, a negative API or modified API is not an absolute test of the likelihood of developing asthma; these children should be followed closely [35].

Bacharier and colleagues [36] recommend that the API can be used in conjunction with other factors, such as aeroallergen sensitivity, recent severe exacerbation, and sex, to predict response to ICS. A recent study by Klaassen and colleagues [37] reports that the ability of the API to predict asthma at 8 years old is significantly improved when combined with exhaled biomarkers of asthma. Further work will be needed to develop an objective, widely available, predictive score with a high positive predictive value [23,38].

Long-term sequelae preschool wheeze

The long-term clinical outcome of children with early childhood wheeze varies by the severity and persistence of disease. Infant lung function before 12 months of age is decreased in children with early onset transient wheeze (wheeze that resolves by 3 years old). However, neither low infant lung function nor transient wheeze seem to predict asthma [15,39]. Cohort studies suggest that children who have persistent wheeze early in life seem to have lower lung function, increased airway hyperresponsiveness (AHR), and diminished growth in forced expiratory volume in the first second of expiration (FEV_1) until at least 18 years of age [21,40]. Children with an early rhinovirus and persistent wheeze may be specifically more likely to have low lung function until age 8 years of age [23]. The evidence of early changes in lung function suggests that the decrease in lung function seen in children begins early in life and there may be an opportunity to alter that trajectory if treatment is initiated early. Further studies are needed to evaluate whether preventative treatment should be focused on prevention of early epigenetic change by decreasing exposures, such as smoke and stress; altering the early microbiome; or preventing early allergy and inflammation. A combination of strategies may be needed, and treatment will most likely need to be tailored to each family and child to improve the short- and long-term clinical outcomes in these children.

ASTHMA EXACERBATIONS

Asthma exacerbations remain a target of both asthma therapy and research for many reasons, perhaps the most important being that exacerbations account for a significant proportion of the cost of asthma-related care [41] as well as contribute to significant asthma morbidity. Therefore, predicting and treating asthma exacerbations is highly important and a focus of recent research.

Predicting asthma exacerbations

Forno and Celedon [42] summarized several risk factors identified in the asthma literature for asthma exacerbations, including poor control, recent history of severe exacerbations, viral infections, allergen exposure, winter season, younger age, nonwhite race, tobacco smoke exposure, and outdoor air pollution. Among these, the investigators concluded that a history of recent exacerbation was the single best predictor of future exacerbation. An analysis of The Epidemiology and Natural History of Asthma (TENOR) cohort of more than 4000 children with severe or difficult-to-treat asthma found that prior asthma exacerbations, short-acting beta-agonist use, and lung function as well as the Asthma Therapy Assessment Questionnaire were independent predictors of asthma exacerbations [43]. The National Institute of Allergy and Infectious Diseases (NIAID) Inner City Asthma Consortium evaluated 400 inner-city children with asthma to determine season-specific risk factors, due to the seasonal nature of asthma exacerbations [44]. They found that significant risk factors for exacerbations exist (including age, total immunoglobulin E [IgE], allergen skin test positivity, blood eosinophils, exacerbation in the prior season, treatment step, FEV_1/forced vital capacity [FVC] ratio, and exhaled nitric oxide); for each season, different risk factors were proportionally responsible for most of the risk. Furthermore, they were able to develop a predictive index to score individual patients' risk of exacerbations. To predict imminent asthma exacerbations, a combination of change in symptoms and decrease to less than 70% of personal best in peak flow has good predictive value in the 1-week window before an asthma exacerbation in one evaluation [45].

Environmental factors
Increasing numbers of recent studies have focused on the impact of environmental factors on asthma exacerbations. Ecological studies have compared climatic factors and air pollution with school health records and found that upper atmosphere temperature, dew point, mixing ratio, and air pollutants predicted the probability of asthma exacerbations in elementary school-aged children [46,47]. Another ecological study found that high levels of particulate matter and other air pollutants predicted asthma exacerbations in elementary school-aged children in the United States. [48]. These investigators postulate that monitoring of air pollutants over time could allow for mathematical modeling to predict asthma exacerbations over large groups of children. Ultrafine pollution particles and carbon monoxide were found to be particularly associated with increased odds of a pediatric asthma visit in another study [49]. As national and international focus continues to be directed toward environmental changes and triggers of human disease, the effect of the environment on asthma health will continue to be evaluated.

Biomarkers
Forno and Celedon [42] also summarized biomarkers that had been studied for exacerbation prediction, including exhaled nitric oxide, sputum eosinophilia, urine bromotyrosine, urine metabolome studies, and serum vitamin D. Interestingly, urinary bromotyrosine has been shown to track with asthma control as well as predict the risk of future exacerbations [50]. Exhaled nitric oxide has even been tested in infants and toddlers and was shown to be predictive of future acute exacerbations and prediction of wheezing at 3 years of age [51], though its utility in predicting exacerbations in other ages has not been

consistent [52]. Children with asthma exposed to secondhand smoke are at a particularly high risk for exacerbations, and urinary leukotriene E_4 has been identified as a predictor of asthma exacerbations in those exposed to second-hand smoke [53]. Although these biomarkers have shown promise, no one definable biomarker has shown itself to be an adequate predictive marker on its own. Additionally, the biomarkers discussed earlier are only a small portion of those currently being assessed for clinical use.

Preventing and managing asthma exacerbations

As the science of predicting asthma exacerbations advances, clinicians are left with the question of how to treat those who do exacerbate. Acute asthma exacerbations result in more than 2 million emergency department (ED) visits per year [54]; in 2013, 57.9% of children with a current diagnosis of asthma experienced an exacerbation [55]. Currently available therapies include oxygen; fluids; steroids; beta-agonists, including albuterol and terbutaline; and anticholinergics, including ipratropium, magnesium sulfate, methylxanthines, heliox, and ketamine [56]. Although therapies, such as beta-agonist and systemic corticosteroid therapy, have been a mainstay for many years, treatment of acute asthma exacerbations continues to evolve.

Corticosteroids

Corticosteroids are effective against both acute and chronic inflammation and have been a mainstay of acute asthma therapy for some time [56]. One current area of active investigation is the effectiveness of dexamethasone versus prednisone in the treatment of acute asthma exacerbations. Dexamethasone has been considered as an alternative to prednisone/prednisolone because of its increased tolerability. Studies have evaluated the use of dexamethasone in the ED setting and found that dexamethasone is a viable alternative to prednisone, with equivalent effectiveness and improved compliance, palatability (decreased vomiting), and cost profile [57–59].

Although ICSs have been largely used chronically rather than in acute exacerbations, recent studies have sought to evaluate their use in the acute setting. Chen and colleagues [60] found that the addition of inhaled high-dose budesonide to nebulized beta-agonists and ipratropium led to clinical improvement and reduced need for oral corticosteroids. In fact, one systematic review of 8 pediatric studies found that there was no difference between ICS and systemic corticosteroids in terms of hospital admission rates, unscheduled visits for asthma symptoms, and the need for an additional course of systemic corticosteroids [61].

Anticholinergics

Inhaled anticholinergics are another option to consider. Inhaled anticholinergics are frequently combined with short-acting beta-agonists in the ED setting and have been shown to decrease the risk of hospital admission when used in this way [62], though they have not been shown to be efficacious when used on their own [63]. However, studies have not supported the use of inhaled anticholinergics in hospitalized patients because of the lack of significant benefits in terms of hospital length of stay and other markers of response to therapy [64].

Other emerging therapies
Other medications are emerging as potential therapies for acute asthma exacerbations. Magnesium sulfate is under study because of its properties as a smooth muscle relaxant [64]. One retrospective study evaluated the use of intravenous magnesium sulfate in pediatric patients in the ED and found that it was largely well tolerated, with only one patient experiencing hypotension, but also found that dosage as well as time of administration varied widely across the centers studied [65]. A randomized controlled trial of intravenous magnesium sulfate found that infusion within the first hour of hospitalization significantly reduced the percentage of children who required mechanical ventilation [66]. Magnesium sulfate is also available in an inhaled formulation. One systematic Cochrane review found no good evidence that inhaled magnesium sulfate should be used as a substitute for beta-agonist therapy as well as no clear evidence of improved pulmonary function or reduced hospital admissions, though individual studies suggested possible improvement in severe asthmatic patients with low lung function (FEV_1 <50% predicted) [67]. Additionally, it may be efficacious in asthmatic patients with more severe exacerbations [68]. Another therapeutic target includes inhaled furosemide, which shows promise as an adjunct to currently available asthma therapies [69].

Preventing asthma exacerbations
Another recent study from the NIAID Inner City Asthma Consortium indicated that a preseasonal approach using omalizumab therapy (anti-IgE) was effective in preventing a fall exacerbation in those participants with a history of an asthma exacerbation in the prior year. This strategy was particularly effective in those children who had an asthma exacerbation in the 6-month observation period before starting omalizumab therapy and those who required high levels of treatment of asthma control, namely, high-dose ICS with supplemental controller therapy [70].

SEVERE ASTHMA
With the development of very effective asthma control medications, most children with asthma can attain and maintain good asthma control. Unfortunately, a small group of severe asthmatic children will continue to have difficult-to-control asthma despite maximal medical therapy. These children are often described as having difficult-to-control, refractory, treatment refractory, steroid-resistant, or steroid-insensitive asthma. Most definitions of severe asthma have included frequent day and nighttime symptoms, need for rescue bronchodilator therapy several times a day, and an FEV_1 less than 60% of predicted. The European Respiratory Society/American Thoracic Society Task Force Report on severe asthma recently simplified the definition of severe asthma by stating that severe asthma requires treatment with high-dose ICS

plus a second controller and/or systemic corticosteroids to prevent it from becoming uncontrolled or that remains uncontrolled despite this therapy [71]. In addition, severe asthma must be distinguished from uncontrolled asthma.

Although severe asthma has been estimated to affect 5% to 10% of all asthmatic patients, the exact prevalence has been difficult to determine because of the lack of a consistent definition. In a recently published study, Hekking and colleagues [72] sought to determine the prevalence of difficult-to-treat versus severe refractory asthma. Patients with difficult-to-treat asthma were those with uncontrolled symptoms despite high-intensity treatment, whereas patients with severe refractory asthma were the fraction of difficult-to-treat asthmatic patients who had both good adherence and inhalation technique. Approximately 17% of asthmatic patients had difficult-to-treat asthma. Because 50% were nonadherent and 58% had poor inhaler technique, only 20% of the difficult-to-control asthmatic patients had severe refractory asthma. Thus, severe asthma comprised only 3.6% of the adult asthmatic population, a value less than the estimated prevalence of 5% to 10%. Although difficult-to-control asthma is relatively common, only a fraction of these patients will have severe refractory asthma. To determine the true prevalence of severe refractory childhood asthma, future studies must take into account both inhaler technique and adherence.

Natural history of severe asthma

Reddy and colleagues [73] sought to determine whether the recent introduction of highly effective asthma therapies have altered the natural history of severe childhood asthma. The investigators compared 2 cohorts of children with severe asthma referred to a national asthma referral center before (Historic Cohort 1993–1997) and following the widespread use of second-generation ICS alone or in combination with long-acting beta-agonists (LABAs) and leukotriene receptor antagonists (Current Cohort 2003–2007). Children from the Current Cohort were much less likely to require chronically administered oral corticosteroid therapy; in those that did, their oral corticosteroid dose was much lower and they required it for a much shorter period of time compared with children from the Historic Cohort. Children in the Current Cohort also had better lung function, required significantly less rescue albuterol, and were less likely to have required intubation/mechanical ventilation in the past but had more asthma exacerbations per year. They were also less growth suppressed and had fewer Cushingoid stigmata, but they were as likely to have osteopenia as the Historic Cohort.

The data presented suggest that, with the development of highly effective medications, children with severe asthma are less likely to be steroid dependent, have better baseline lung function, require far less rescue albuterol, and are less growth suppressed. Despite these gains, children with severe asthma continue to have frequent exacerbations and osteopenia continues to be a common steroid-induced adverse effect.

Whether frequent asthma exacerbations result in a more rapid decline in lung function over time was addressed by the TENOR study, whereby the effect of asthma exacerbations on annual lung function decline was studied in more than 2000 subjects with severe asthma over a 3-year period [74]. This large prospective study found that asthma exacerbations contribute to progressive loss of lung function, especially in children. In addition, ICS therapy did not seem to ameliorate this effect, as nearly all subjects were on this therapy.

Matsunaga and colleagues [75] made similar observations; they prospectively evaluated the effect of asthma exacerbations on lung function in adults with stable asthma on ICS therapy over a 3-year period. At least 25% of the patients had 1 or more asthma exacerbations requiring prednisone or hospitalization during the study. Not only were exacerbations related to loss of lung function but also those with the most exacerbations had the greatest decline in lung function.

Of the 25% of participants enrolled in the NHLBI CAMP study who displayed an annual decline in lung function, ICS therapy failed to protect against this loss, as there was no difference in the percentage of or rate of decline between those who received budesonide versus those who received a matching placebo over a 5-year period [76].

The annual declines in lung function in the studies mentioned earlier were small, but the cumulative effect over time is likely to result in a significant reduction in lung function and may explain why adults with severe asthma have FEV_1 values that are much lower than children with severe asthma [77]. In addition, these studies suggest that ICS therapy does not seem to ameliorate loss of lung function and that asthma exacerbations contribute to asthma progression.

Severe asthma phenotypes

Cluster analysis is an analytical technique that has recently been used to identify asthma phenotypes. Its advantage comes from its ability to distinguish complex phenotypes without a priori (ie, biased) definitions of disease severity. The NHLBI Severe Asthma Research Program (SARP) study team, using a cluster approach, found children with severe asthma to be distributed across 4 distinct clusters [78]. Children in cluster 4 (early onset atopic asthma with advanced airflow limitation) had the lowest lung function, required several asthma control medications, and had the most asthma symptoms. The mean prebronchodilator FEV_1 of these children was 75% of predicted with a postbronchodilator FEV_1 of 90% of predicted. That children with severe asthma were likely to have FEV_1 values of greater than 60% of predicted was first described a decade ago [79,80].

Of interest, all 4 childhood clusters had varying degrees of atopy. The childhood clusters differed substantially from those identified among the adults with severe asthma, which were based on age of onset, allergen sensitization, baseline lung function, beta-agonist reversibility, and medication use/health care utilization [81]. When comparing the two cohorts, children had less airway limitation but required rescue albuterol more frequently. The children were also found to have frequent exacerbations, yet had little impairment and normal lung function between exacerbations. This observation has been replicated in several NHLBI-sponsored studies in children with mild and moderate persistent asthma [82,83].

A second cluster analysis from France identified 2 distinct severe asthma clusters [84]. Children in cluster 1 were the most atopic, had the highest circulating IgE levels and circulating eosinophils, had long-standing and uncontrolled asthma despite high-dose ICS, and were most likely to have been hospitalized. Children in cluster 2 were older, had a higher body mass index, had increased circulating neutrophils, had elevated IgG, IgA, and IgM levels, and had the lowest lung function. There was no predominance of severe asthma in any one cluster, and atopic features were present in both groups. Unlike the SARP study, the nature of inflammation varied among the clusters, with cluster 1 patients having a T_H2-mediated and cluster 2 patients having more of a T_H1-mediated inflammatory process.

Mechanisms of severe asthma

In adults with severe asthma, YKL-40 expression is upregulated in CD8+ cells and serum YKL-40 levels are elevated, correlate positively with airway remodeling, and inversely correlate with lung function [85,86]. Whether YKL-40 levels are also elevated in children with severe asthma was studied by Santos and colleagues [87], who compared lung function, YKL-40, IgE, and exhaled nitric oxide (eNO) levels in children with mild, moderate, and severe persistent asthma to adults with severe asthma. Children with severe asthma did not have elevated YKL-40 (26 ng/mL) levels compared with the adults with severe asthma (62 ng/mL). Children with severe asthma also had better lung function and higher IgE and eNO levels compared with the adults with severe asthma who had significant airflow limitation and low serum IgE and eNO levels. Lastly, no relationship between YKL-40 levels and asthma severity was found among the children studied. These data support the contention that there are distinct pathophysiologic differences in severe asthma that depend on one's age.

Airway remodeling, which involves thickening of the reticular basement membrane (RBM), goblet cell, and submucous gland hyperplasia, airway smooth muscle (ASM) hyperplasia, and hypertrophy and angiogenesis, is a characteristic histologic finding in grade school–aged children and adults with asthma [15,88]. At present, it remains to be determined when airway remodeling begins, although remodeling was not seen in infants with frequent wheeze [88].

Lezmi and colleagues [15] evaluated airway remodeling and inflammation in preschool-aged children with severe recurrent wheeze. Children 36 months of age or younger comprised group 1, whereas children aged 37 to 59 months comprised group 2. Group 3 consisted of school-aged asthmatic children. RBM thickness increased with age, with ASM area being greatest in the school-aged children. ASM was found to be greater among the atopic versus nonatopic preschool-aged children. Airway inflammatory cells were similar in both groups 1 and 2 with an absence of eosinophils and a predominance of neutrophils noted, whereas eosinophils were the predominant airway inflammatory cell in the grade school–aged children. No relationships were noted between airway inflammation and airway wall structural changes, and there was no correlation between inhaled steroid dosage and degree of airway wall remodeling.

Thus, in preschool-aged children with severe wheezing, airway remodeling is present by 3 years of life and progresses over time. Remodeling and inflammation seem to occur in conjunction, yet the two processes seem to be unrelated. Neutrophilic inflammation is present in both wheezing infants and preschool-aged children with severe recurrent wheeze. As eosinophilic inflammation is a characteristic finding in older children and adults, a switch from a neutrophil- to an eosinophil-driven inflammatory process must occur in genetically predisposed children with recurrent wheeze who go on to have persistent asthma. The mechanisms involved in this switch have yet to be determined.

Tumor necrosis factor α (TNFα) plays an important role in T_H1-driven diseases, such as rheumatoid arthritis and inflammatory bowel disease. TNFα has also been noted in the bronchoalveolar lavage fluid of adults with severe asthma. At one time, TNFα was thought to be an important mediator in severe asthma as small studies using TNFα antagonists improved lung function, reduced bronchial hyperresponsiveness, and improved quality of life in adults with severe asthma [89]. When a large placebo-controlled trial evaluating golimumab, a TNFα antagonist, was discontinued prematurely because of its adverse effects and lack of efficacy, interest in TNFα and its antagonists waned [90].

Whether TNFα may play a role in children with severe asthma was the aim of Brown and colleagues [91] who measured plasma TNFα concentrations and TNFα mRNA expression in children with asthma. This study suggested that, as in adults with severe asthma, a phenotype of severe childhood asthma exists that is characterized by TNFα overexpression and poor asthma control despite high-dose ICS therapy. It is possible that targeted therapy with TNFα antagonists in this asthma phenotype may be an effective therapy.

Adherence

Suboptimal adherence to prescribed medication is an important contributor to severe asthma, as many patients who are thought to have severe asthma end up having poorly controlled asthma due to suboptimal adherence with prescribed asthma medications. The monitoring of refill rates of prescribed medications provides a simple and robust measure of adherence, as one cannot be adherent if one does not fill one's prescriptions. With that said, adherence may be overestimated, as filling a prescription does not provide proof that the patient actually took the medication. Murphy and colleagues [92] analyzed prescription refill rates in patients with difficult-to-control asthma residing in Leicester, United Kingdom. Prescription data were compared with the patients' prescribed medication regimen to determine each patient's level of adherence, with good adherence defined as 80% or greater. Patients with suboptimal adherence had lower FEV_1 values, higher sputum eosinophil counts, and were more likely to have required mechanical ventilation. For every 10% decrease in ICS adherence, the odds of having required mechanical ventilation increased 1.4 times. This finding is in line with that of an epidemiologic study that found the risk of death from asthma decreased 21% for every additional ICS canister filled [93].

Another study using prescription refill rates to measure adherence came from Ireland [94]. In this study, 35% of patients filled their prescribed combination inhaler 50% or less of the time. These poorly adherent patients were more likely to have been hospitalized 3 or more times in past year, had lower asthma-specific quality-of-life scores, were on a higher prescribed ICS dose, and required more frequent use of short-acting beta-2 agonists than patients with good adherence. Three variables were associated with nonadherence: female sex, quality of life, and hospital admissions in the preceding 12 months.

Thus, poor adherence is common among patients with severe asthma. Poorly adherent patients are more likely to have required frequent hospitalizations, have been mechanically ventilated, have greater airflow obstruction, higher sputum eosinophils counts, and a lower quality of life. Thus, poor adherence is a significant contributor to poor asthma control. As patient self-reporting is a poor identifier of adherence, objective assessment of adherence must be part of any systematic evaluation protocol for severe asthma.

NEW MEDICATIONS

Children who are more adherent to controller medications are 21% to 68% less likely to have asthma exacerbations than those who are not [95]. Unfortunately, adherence to asthma controller therapies only ranges from 30% to 70% [96]. Patients are poor self-reporters of their own adherence, with a large discrepancy existing between their reported medication use, including on diary cards, and their actual use [97–100].

Electronic monitoring devices (EMDs) are a new approach to achieving asthma control, increasing adherence, and preventing exacerbations. EMDs provide accurate, objective, and detailed information on patient adherence without significantly disrupting their natural medication taking behavior [100]. EMDs may record the date, time, and even location of each actuation through Global Positioning System monitoring as well as provide reminder prompts to take the medication [100]. EMDs with audiovisual reminders have been proven to increase adherence rates in both adults and adolescents as well as children [101–103]. A consistent benefit in asthma outcomes with EMDs has not been demonstrated, including improvement in exacerbations over time, school absenteeism, caregiver work absenteeism, FEV_1, or ED visits [103]. Possible reasons for this lack of benefit include the sample sizes involved, limited duration of intervention, patient awareness of adherence monitoring, or multiple asthma phenotypes requiring different treatment modalities [104].

Current treatment modalities, including second-generation ICSs and combination ICS/LABAs, are likely responsible for the change in the course of asthma over the last 20 years, including less use of chronic oral corticosteroids and improved asthma control [73]. ICSs and ICS/LABAs may not be sufficient alone for the management of patients with severe asthma, whose persistent symptoms place them at an increased risk of exacerbations, hospitalizations, ED visits, and oral corticosteroid use [105]. In patients whose symptoms remain poorly controlled despite close adherence with optimal current therapy, new therapeutics, including tiotropium and T_H2-directed biologics, may be key to improving control and preventing exacerbations [106].

When considering the use of new pharmaceutical agents in children with asthma, attention must be paid to the specific pediatric evidence for their use. Most recently approved therapies, including omalizumab, mepolizumab, and tiotropium, are only approved by the Food and Drug Administration (FDA) for use in patients as young as 12 years old [107–109]. Age-limited studies often lead to the off-label use of asthma drugs in the pediatric population [110]. Such extrapolation of pharmacologic results from adults to children cannot be readily made secondary to differences in pediatric respiratory function, immunology, and disease pathogenesis [111].

Tiotropium

Tiotropium is a long-acting once-daily anticholinergic initially approved for the treatment of persistent asthma in 2015 [109]. Tiotropium studies were first conducted with the HandiHaler and then the Respimat device (Boehinger Ingelheim, Ingelheim am Rhein, Germany), which is the currently approved device for the treatment of persistent asthma [109]. Tiotropium has been studied as an add-on therapy to ICSs in adolescents and children [112–114]. An improvement in lung function has been demonstrated in symptomatic pediatric and adolescent patients with asthma with the addition of tiotropium to ICS, improving peak and trough FEV_1 and morning and evening peak expiratory flow (PEF) [112–114]. However, these pediatric and adolescent studies did not show a statistically significant improvement in asthma control or quality of life [112,114], and an effect on asthma exacerbations was not investigated.

Clinical characteristics predicting a response to tiotropium have only been derived from adult studies. An improvement in FEV_1 and PEF with the addition of tiotropium to low-dose ICS was predicated by a response to albuterol, a decreased FEV_1/FVC ratio, and a higher cholinergic tone, reflected by a lower resting heart rate [115]. Tiotropium has not demonstrated a response association with allergic markers, including atopy, IgE level, sputum eosinophil count, or exhaled nitric oxide (F_{ENO}) [115,116].

Omalizumab

Omalizumab is indicated as an add-on therapy in steps 5 and 6 of the NHLBI Expert Panel Report-3 guidelines for patients 12 years of age and older with moderate to severe persistent asthma [117]. In this adolescent and adult population, omalizumab decreases rates of asthma exacerbations, annualized rate of hospital admissions, total emergency visits, unscheduled doctor visits, rescue therapy use, and ICS dose [118–121]. It also improves asthma symptom scores, quality of life, and time to first asthma exacerbations [119].

Omalizumab has shown a similar benefit in pediatric patients, aged 6 years and older, with moderate to severe persistent or uncontrolled asthma with reductions in asthma exacerbation rates, symptom days, hospitalizations, urgent physician office visits, missed school days, and daily rescue medication use [122–124]. The impact of omalizumab on pediatric exacerbations was highlighted in the NIAID Inner-City Anti-IgE Therapy for Asthma (ICATA) trial, which demonstrated near-complete elimination of the seasonal variability of asthma exacerbations in the fall and spring with its use [122]. Especially important in the pediatric population is the ability of omalizumab to improve exacerbation rates while reducing ICS [70,122–124].

Although omalizumab dosing is based on IgE, weight, and aeroallergen sensitization, its use may be most beneficial in those patients with elevated eosinophilic biomarkers [107]. In adolescents and adults, a greater reduction in asthma exacerbations was observed in patients with high compared with low baseline F_{ENO}, peripheral eosinophil count, and periostin, based on median split [119,125,126]. Similarly, in the ICATA trial, pediatric patients with a F_{ENO} 20 ppb or greater, a peripheral eosinophil count of 2% or greater, and a body mass index of 25 or greater had significantly fewer exacerbations with omalizumab treatment compared with those with lower values of these parameters [127].

Mepolizumab

Mepolizumab is a humanized monoclonal antibody directed against interleukin 5 (IL-5) that was FDA approved in 2015 as an add-on therapy for the treatment of severe eosinophilic asthma in patients 12 years of age and older [108]. Mepolizumab studies defined eosinophilic asthma as sputum eosinophil count of 3% or greater, F_{ENO} of 50 ppb or greater, or a peripheral eosinophil count of 0.3 or greater $\times 10^9$/L [128,129]. Several studies demonstrate a decrease in eosinophil counts in asthmatic patients with its use [128–132]. In adolescents and adults, mepolizumab has been proven to reduce the rates of asthma exacerbations, to decrease exacerbations requiring admission or ED visits, and to delay the time to first exacerbation [128,129,133]. Later studies demonstrated an improvement in FEV_1 and asthma control questionnaire (ACQ) scores [129,133]. Mepolizumab has also been proven to reduce the daily maintenance oral corticosteroid dose while still improving rates of asthma exacerbations [133]. The rate of clinically significant exacerbations with mepolizumab correlated with blood eosinophil count and number of exacerbations in the year before baseline but not atopic status, IgE concentrations, FEV_1, or bronchodilator response [128].

Reslizumab

Reslizumab is an IgG4κ humanized monoclonal antibody that also binds IL-5 and reduces serum eosinophilia in patients with asthma similar to mepolizumab [134,135]. Also like mepolizumab, reslizumab has only been studied in patients greater than 12 years old [134,135]. However, the definition of eosinophilic asthma differs between these two therapies with reslizumab using a peripheral eosinophil count of 400/μL or greater [135]. When used as an add-on therapy to adult and adolescent patients on ICS or ICS/LABA, reslizumab reduced asthma exacerbation rates comparable with that seen with mepolizumab, increased time to first exacerbation, increased FEV_1, and improved ACQ and quality of life scores [134,135].

Lebrikizumab

Lebrikizumab is an IgG4 humanized monoclonal against IL-13, with published studies to date only in adults. The addition of lebrikizumab to ICS in patients with high periostin and F_{ENO} levels, based on median splits, each correlated with an improvement in prebronchodilator FEV_1 [136]. Furthermore, those patients with a high periostin level had a greater decline in F_{ENO} with lebrikizumab [136]. Those patients with an IgE level greater than 100 IU/mL and a peripheral eosinophil count greater than 0.14×10^9 cells per liter had a decrease in their asthma exacerbation rates with lebrikizumab [136].

Questions exist about the utility of periostin as a biomarker in the pediatric population as it is a product of bone turnover, leading to higher levels in growing children compared with adults [137]. However, within the pediatric population, higher levels of periostin have been identified in children who developed asthma by 6 years of age compared with those who did not and in healthy children 6 to 15 years of age compared with asthmatic patients [137,138]. Additional studies examining periostin in relation to IL-13 and lebrikizumab in the pediatric population are needed.

SUMMARY

Based on the summary provided here on the current literature, it seems that the management of children will be continually changing in the coming years. With new insights into the development of asthma, we can begin to identify those children at risk for asthma onset, exacerbations, and progression. We can also begin to develop interventions for those who are at risk using risk profiles. That will lead to new intervention strategies. Because the new immunomodulators have been effective in reducing exacerbations, it is possible that they may also be helpful in preventing the progression of disease and reversing the natural history of asthma, including progression to chronic obstructive airway disease in adults. The future is bright for developing new strategies for managing asthma in children and reducing the burden of disease not only in children but also in adults. This development will take a concerted collaborative effort among patients, families, clinicians, and the pharmaceutical industry to keep moving forward and the health care system in reviewing available data and continuing to help those children who are not receiving adequate management.

Acknowledgments

The authors would like to thank Dr Michael Kappy for the invitation to contribute to *Advances in Pediatrics* and to Gretchen Hugen for assistance with preparation of this review.

References

[1] Yagiyeva N, Devereux G, Fielding S, et al. Outcomes of childhood asthma and wheezy bronchitis- a 50-year cohort study. Am J Respir Crit Care Med 2016;193:23–30.

[2] Akinbami LJ, Moorman JE, Simon AE, et al. Trends in racial disparities for asthma outcomes among children 0 to 17 years, 2001-2010. J Allergy Clin Immunol 2014;134:547–53.

[3] Savenije OE, Granell R, Caudri D, et al. Comparison of childhood wheezing phenotypes in 2 birth cohorts: ALSPAC and PIAMA. J Allergy Clin Immunol 2011;127:1505–12.

[4] Lodge CJ, Zaloumis S, Lowe AJ, et al. Early-life risk factors for childhood wheeze phenotypes in a high-risk birth cohort. J Pediatr 2014;164:289–94.

[5] Harju M, Kreski-Nisula L, Georgiadis L, et al. The burden of childhood asthma and late preterm and early term births. J Pediatr 2014;164:295–9.

[6] Sonnenschein-van der Voort AM, Arends LR, de Jongste JC, et al. Preterm birth, infant weight gain and childhood asthma risk: a meta-analysis of 147,000 European children. J Allergy Clin Immunol 2014;133:1317–29.

[7] Sharma S, Zhou X, Thibault DM, et al. A genome-wide survey of CD4(+) lymphocyte regulatory genetic variants identifies novel asthma genes. J Allergy Clin Immunol 2014;134: 1153–62.

[8] Burke H, Leonardi-Bee J, Hashim A, et al. Prenatal and passive smoke exposure and incidence of asthma and wheeze: systematic review and meta-analysis. Pediatrics 2012;129:735–44.

[9] Brunst KJ, Ryan PH, Brokamp C, et al. Timing and duration of traffic-related air pollution exposure and the risk for childhood wheeze and asthma. Am J Respir Crit Care Med 2015;192:421–7.

[10] Guxens M, Sonnenschein-van der Voort AM, Timeier H, et al. Parental psychological distress during pregnancy and wheezing in preschool children: the Generation R Study. J Allergy Clin Immunol 2014;133:59–67.

[11] Chiu YH, Coull BA, Sternthal MJ, et al. Effects of prenatal community violence and ambient air pollution on childhood wheeze in an urban population. J Allergy Clin Immunol 2014;133:713–22.

[12] Jackson DJ, Gangnon RE, Evans MD, et al. Wheezing rhinovirus illnesses in early life predict asthma development in high-risk children. Am J Respir Crit Care Med 2008;178: 667–72.

[13] Taussig LM, Wright AL, Holberg CJ, et al. Tucson Children's Respiratory Study: 1980 to present. J Allergy Clin Immunol 2003;111:661–75.

[14] Ducharme FM, Noya FJ, Allen-Ramey FC, et al. Clinical effectiveness of inhaled corticosteroids versus montelukast in children with asthma: prescription patterns and patient adherence as key factors. Curr Med Res Opin 2012;28:111–9.

[15] Lezmi G, Gosset P, Deschildre A, et al. Airway remodeling in preschool children with severe recurrent wheeze. Am J Respir Crit Care Med 2015;192:164–71.

[16] Sonnappa S, Bastardo CM, Saglani S, et al. Relationship between past airway pathology and current lung function in preschool wheezers. Eur Respir J 2011;38:1431–6.

[17] Malmstrom K, Malmberg LP, O'Reilly R, et al. Lung function, airway remodeling and inflammation in infants: outcome at 8 years. Ann Allergy Asthma Immunol 2015;114:90–6.

[18] Murray CS, Pipis SD, McArdle EC, et al, National Asthma Campaign-Manchester Asthma and Allergy Study Group. Lung function at one month of age as a risk factor for infant respiratory symptoms in a high risk population. Thorax 2002;57:388–92.

[19] Borrego LM, Stocks J, Leiria-Pinto P, et al. Lung function and clinical risk factors for asthma in infants and young children with recurrent wheeze. Thorax 2009;64:203–9.

[20] Turner SW, Palmer LJ, Rye PJ, et al. Infants with flow limitation at 4 weeks: outcome at 6 and 11 years. Am J Respir Crit Care Med 2002;165:1294–8.

[21] Ducharme FM, Tse SM, Chauhan B. Diagnosis, management and prognosis of preschool wheeze. Lancet 2014;383:1593–604.

[22] Guilbert TW, Morgan WJ, Zeiger RS, et al. Long term inhaled corticosteroids in preschool children at high risk for asthma. N Engl J Med 2006;354:1985–97.

[23] Guilbert TW, Mauger DT, Allen DB, et al. Growth of preschool children at high risk for asthma 2 years after discontinuation of fluticasone. J Allergy Clin Immunol 2011;128: 956–63.

[24] Kelly HW, Sternberg AL, Lescher R, et al. Effect of inhaled glucocorticoids in childhood on adult height. N Engl J Med 2012;367:904–12.

[25] Bacharier LB, Guilbert TW, Zeiger RS, et al, for the Childhood Asthma Research and Education Network of the National Heart, Lung and Blood Institute. Patient characteristics associated with improved outcomes with use of an inhaled corticosteroid in preschool children at risk for asthma. J Allergy Clin Immunol 2009;123:1077–82.

[26] Ducharme FM, Zemek RL, Schuh S. Oral corticosteroids in children with wheezing. N Engl J Med 2009;360:1674.

[27] National Asthma Council Australia. Australian Asthma Handbook. Available at: http://www.nationalasthma.org.au/handbook. Accessed January 21, 2016.

[28] Canadian Thoracic Society. Canadian respiratory guidelines. Available at: http://www.respiratoryguidelines.ca/. Accessed January 21, 2016.

[29] Boulet LP, FitzGerald JM, Reddel HK. The revised 2014 GINA strategy report: opportunities for change. Curr Opin Pulm Med 2015;21:1–7.

[30] Caudri D, Savenije OE, Smit HA, et al. Perinatal risk factors for wheezing phenotypes in the first 8 years of life. Clin Exp Allergy 2013;43:1395–405.

[31] Matricardi PM, Illi S, Gruber C, et al. Wheezing in childhood: incidence, longitudinal patterns and factors predicting persistence. Eur Respir J 2008;32:585–92.

[32] Guilbert TW, Mauger DT, Lemanske RF. Childhood asthma-predictive phenotype. J Allergy Clin Immunol Pract 2014;2:664–70.

[33] Castro-Rodriguez JA, Holberg CJ, Wright AL, et al. A clinical index to define risk of asthma in young children with recurrent wheezing. Am J Respir Crit Care Med 2000;162: 1403–6.

[34] Guilbert TW, Morgan WJ, Krawiec M, et al, for the Childhood Asthma Research and Education Network. Prevention of early asthma in kids study: design, rationale and methods for the Childhood Asthma Research and Education network. Control Clin Trials 2004;25: 286–310.

[35] Huffaker MF, Phipatanakul W. Utility of the Asthma Predictive Index in predicting childhood asthma and identifying disease-modifying interventions. Ann Allergy Asthma Immunol 2014;112:188–90.

[36] Bacharier LB, Phillips BR, Zeiger RS, et al. Episodic use of an inhaled corticosteroid or leukotriene receptor antagonist in preschool children with moderate-to-severe intermittent wheezing. J Allergy Clin Immunol 2008;122:1127–35.

[37] Klaassen EM, van de Kant KD, Jobsis Q, et al. Exhaled biomarkers and gene expression at preschool age improve asthma prediction at 6 years of age. Am J Respir Crit Care Med 2015;191:201–7.

[38] Savenije OE, Kerkhof M, Koppelman GH, et al. Predicting who will have asthma at school age among preschool children. J Allergy Clin Immunol 2012;130:325–31.

[39] Lodge CJ, Lowe AJ, Allen KJ, et al. Childhood wheeze phenotypes show less than expected growth in FEB1 across adolescence. Am J Respir Crit Care Med 2014;189:1351–8.

[40] Grad R, Morgan WJ. Long-term outcomes of early-onset wheeze and asthma. J Allergy Clin Immunol 2012;130:299–307.

[41] Ivanova JI, Bergman R, Birnbaum HG, et al. Effect of asthma exacerbations on health care costs among asthmatic patients with moderate and severe persistent asthma. J Allergy Clin Immunol 2012;129(5):1229–35.

[42] Forno E, Celedon JC. Predicting asthma exacerbations in children. Curr Opin Pulm Med 2012;18(1):63–9.

[43] Zeiger RS, Yegin A, Simons FE, et al. Evaluation of the National Heart, Lung, and Blood Institute guidelines impairment domain for classifying asthma control and predicting asthma exacerbations. Ann Allergy Asthma Immunol 2012;108(2):81–7.

[44] Teach SJ, Gergen PJ, Szefler SJ, et al. Seasonal risk factors for asthma exacerbations among inner-city children. J Allergy Clin Immunol 2015;135(6):1465–73.e5.

[45] Honkoop PJ, Taylor DR, Smith AD, et al. Early detection of asthma exacerbations by using action points in self-management plans. Eur Respir J 2013;41(1):53–9.

[46] Jayawardene WP, Youssefagha AH, Lohrmann DK, et al. Prediction of asthma exacerbations among children through integrating air pollution, upper atmosphere, and school health surveillances. Allergy Asthma Proc 2013;34(1):e1–8.

[47] Youssefagha AH, Lohrmann DK, Jayawardene WP, et al. Upper-air observation indicators predict outbreaks of asthma exacerbations among elementary school children: integration of daily environmental and school health surveillance systems in Pennsylvania. J Asthma 2012;49(5):464–73.

[48] Youssefagha AH, Jayawardene WP, Lohrmann DK, et al. Air pollution indicators predict outbreaks of asthma exacerbations among elementary school children: integration of daily environmental and school health surveillance systems in Pennsylvania. J Environ Monit 2012;14(12):3202–10.

[49] Evans KA, Halterman JS, Hopke PK, et al. Increased ultrafine particles and carbon monoxide concentrations are associated with asthma exacerbation among urban children. Environ Res 2014;129:11–9.

[50] Wedes SH, Wu W, Comhair SA, et al. Urinary bromotyrosine measures asthma control and predicts asthma exacerbations in children. J Pediatr 2011;159(2):248–55.e1.

[51] Elliott M, Heltshe SL, Stamey DC, et al. Exhaled nitric oxide predicts persistence of wheezing, exacerbations, and decline in lung function in wheezy infants and toddlers. Clin Exp Allergy 2013;43(12):1351–61.

[52] Gruchalla RS, Sampson HA, Matsui E, et al. Asthma morbidity among inner-city adolescents receiving guidelines-based therapy: role of predictors in the setting of high adherence. J Allergy Clin Immunol 2009;124(2):213–21, 221.e1.

[53] Rabinovitch N, Reisdorph N, Silveira L, et al. Urinary leukotriene E(4) levels identify children with tobacco smoke exposure at risk for asthma exacerbation. J Allergy Clin Immunol 2011;128(2):323–7.

[54] Jones BP, Paul A. Management of acute asthma in the pediatric patient: an evidence-based review. Pediatr Emerg Med Pract 2013;10(5):1–23 [quiz: 23–4].

[55] CDC-most recent asthma data. 2013. Available at: http://www.cdc.gov/asthma/most_recent_data.htm. Accessed December 22, 2015.

[56] Nievas IF, Anand KJ. Severe acute asthma exacerbation in children: a stepwise approach for escalating therapy in a pediatric intensive care unit. J Pediatr Pharmacol Ther 2013;18(2):88–104.

[57] Meyer JS, Riese J, Biondi E. Is dexamethasone an effective alternative to oral prednisone in the treatment of pediatric asthma exacerbations? Hosp Pediatr 2014;4(3):172–80.

[58] Keeney GE, Gray MP, Morrison AK, et al. Dexamethasone for acute asthma exacerbations in children: a meta-analysis. Pediatrics 2014;133(3):493–9.

[59] Andrews AL, Wong KA, Heine D, et al. A cost-effectiveness analysis of dexamethasone versus prednisone in pediatric acute asthma exacerbations. Acad Emerg Med 2012;19(8):943–8.

[60] Chen AH, Zeng GQ, Chen RC, et al. Effects of nebulized high-dose budesonide on moderate-to-severe acute exacerbation of asthma in children: a randomized, double-blind, placebo-controlled study. Respirology 2013;18(Suppl 3):47–52.

[61] Beckhaus AA, Riutort MC, Castro-Rodriguez JA. Inhaled versus systemic corticosteroids for acute asthma in children. A systematic review. Pediatr Pulmonol 2014;49(4):326–34.

[62] Griffiths B, Ducharme FM. Combined inhaled anticholinergics and short-acting beta2-agonists for initial treatment of acute asthma in children. Cochrane Database Syst Rev 2013;(8):CD000060.

[63] Teoh L, Cates CJ, Hurwitz M, et al. Anticholinergic therapy for acute asthma in children. Cochrane Database Syst Rev 2012;(4):CD003797.

[64] Vezina K, Chauhan BF, Ducharme FM. Inhaled anticholinergics and short-acting beta(2)-agonists versus short-acting beta2-agonists alone for children with acute asthma in hospital. Cochrane Database Syst Rev 2014;7:CD010283.

[65] Kokotajlo S, Degnan L, Meyers R, et al. Use of intravenous magnesium sulfate for the treatment of an acute asthma exacerbation in pediatric patients. J Pediatr Pharmacol Ther 2014;19(2):91–7.

[66] Torres S, Sticco N, Bosch JJ, et al. Effectiveness of magnesium sulfate as initial treatment of acute severe asthma in children, conducted in a tertiary-level university hospital: a randomized, controlled trial. Arch Argent Pediatr 2012;110(4):291–6.

[67] Powell C, Dwan K, Milan SJ, et al. Inhaled magnesium sulfate in the treatment of acute asthma. Cochrane Database Syst Rev 2012;12:CD003898.

[68] Powell CV, Kolamunnage-Dona R, Lowe J, et al. MAGNEsium Trial In Children (MAGNETIC): a randomised, placebo-controlled trial and economic evaluation of nebulised magnesium sulphate in acute severe asthma in children. Health Technol 2013;17(45): v–vi, Assess. 1–216.

[69] Inokuchi R, Aoki A, Aoki Y, et al. Effectiveness of inhaled furosemide for acute asthma exacerbation: a meta-analysis. Crit Care 2014;18(6):621.

[70] Teach SJ, Gill MA, Togias A, et al. Preseasonal treatment with either omalizumab inhaled corticosteroid boost to prevent fall asthma. J Allergy Clin Immunol 2015;136:1476–85.

[71] Chung KF, Wenzel SE, Brozek JL, et al. International ERS/ATS guidelines on definition, evaluation and treatment of severe asthma. Eur Respir J 2014;43:343–73.

[72] Hekking P-PW, Wener RR, Amelink M, et al. The prevalence of severe refractory asthma. J Allergy Clin Immunol 2015;135:896–902.

[73] Reddy MB, Doshi J, Covar R, et al. The changing face of severe childhood asthma: a comparison of two cohorts of children evaluated at National Jewish Health over the past two decades. Allergy Asthma Proc 2014;35:119–25.

[74] Calhoun WJ, Haselkorn T, Miller DP, et al. Asthma exacerbations and lung function in patients with severe or difficult-to-treat asthma. J Allergy Clin Immunol 2015;136:1125–7.

[75] Matsunaga K, Hirano T, Oka A, et al. Progression of irreversible airflow limitation in asthma: correlation with severe exacerbations. J Allergy Clin Immunol Pract 2015;3: 759–64.

[76] Covar RA, Spahn JD, Murphy JR, et al. Progression of asthma measured by lung function in the Childhood Asthma Management Program. Am J Respir Crit Care Med 2004;170: 234–41.

[77] Jenkins HA, Szefler SJ, Covar R, et al. A comparison of the clinical characteristics of children and adults with severe asthma. Chest 2003;124:1318–24.

[78] Fitzpatrick AM, Teague G, Meyers DA, et al. Heterogeneity of severe asthma in childhood: confirmation by cluster analysis of children in the National Institutes of Health/National Heart, Lung, and Blood Institute Severe Asthma Research Program. J Allergy Clin Immunol 2011;127:382–9.

[79] Spahn JD, Cherniack R, Paull K, et al. Is the forced expiratory volume in one second the best measure of severity in childhood asthma? Am J Respir Crit Care Med 2004;169:784–6.

[80] Paull K, Covar R, Jain N, et al. Do the NHLBI lung function criteria apply to children? A cross-sectional evaluation of childhood asthma at National Jewish Medical Center 1999-2002. Pediatr Pulmonol 2005;39:311–7.

[81] Moore WC, Meyers DA, Wenzel SE, et al. Identification of asthma phenotypes using cluster analysis in the Severe Asthma Research Program. Am J Respir Crit Care Med 2010;181:315–23.

[82] Martinez FD, Chinchilli VM, Morgan WJ, et al. Use of beclomethasone dipropionate as rescue treatment for children with mild persistent asthma (TREXA): a randomized, double-blind, placebo-controlled trial. Lancet 2011;377:650–7.

[83] Lemanske RF, Mauger DT, Sorkness CA, et al. Step-up therapy for children uncontrolled asthma while receiving inhaled corticosteroids. N Engl J Med 2010;362:975–85.

[84] Just J, Gouvis-Echraghi R, Rouve S, et al. Two novel, severe asthma phenotypes identified during childhood using a clustering approach. Eur Respir J 2012;40:55–60.

[85] Tsitsiou E, Williams AE, Moschos SA, et al. Transcriptome analysis shows activation of circulating CD8+ T cells in patients with severe asthma. J Allergy Clin Immunol 2012;129:95–103.

[86] Chupp GL, Lee CG, Jarjour N, et al. A chitinase-like protein in the lung and circulation of patients with severe asthma. N Engl J Med 2007;357:2016–27.

[87] Santos CB, Davidson J, Covar R, et al. The chitinase-like protein YKL-40 is not a useful biomarker for severe asthma in children. Ann Allergy Asthma Immunol 2014;113:263–6.

[88] Saglani S, Malmstrom K, Pelkonen AS, et al. Airway remodeling and inflammation in symptomatic infants with reversible airflow obstruction. Am J Respir Crit Care Med 2005;171:722–7.

[89] Berry MA, Hargadon B, Shelley M, et al. Evidence for a role of tumor necrosis factor α in refractory asthma. N Engl J Med 2006;354:697–708.

[90] Wenzel SE, Barnes PJ, Bleecker ER, et al. A randomized, double-blind, placebo-controlled study of tumor necrosis factor-α blockade in severe persistent asthma. Am J Respir Crit Care Med 2009;179:549–58.

[91] Brown SD, Brown LA, Stephenson S, et al. Characterization of a high TNF-α phenotype in children with moderate-to-severe asthma. J Allergy Clin Immunol 2015;135:1651–4.

[92] Murphy AC, Proeschal A, Brightling CE, et al. The relationship between clinical outcomes and medication adherence in difficult-to-control asthma. Thorax 2012;67:751–3.

[93] Suissa S, Ernst P, Benayoun S, et al. Low-dose inhaled corticosteroids and the prevention of death from asthma. N Engl J Med 2000;343:332–6.

[94] Gamble J, Stevenson M, McClean E, et al. The prevalence of non-adherence in difficult asthma. AM J Respir Crit Care Med 2009;180:817–22.

[95] Engelkes M, Janssens HM, de Jongste JC, et al. Medication adherence and the risk of severe asthma exacerbations: a systematic review. Eur Respir J 2015;45(2):396–407.

[96] Eakin MN, Rand CS. Improving patient adherence with asthma self-management practices: what works? Ann Allergy Asthma Immunol 2012;109(2):90–2.

[97] Weinstein AG. Asthma adherence management for the clinician. J Allergy Clin Immunol Pract 2013;1(2):123–8.

[98] Bender B, Wamboldt FS, O'Connor SL, et al. Measurement of children's asthma medication adherence by self report, mother report, canister weight, and Doser CT. Ann Allergy Asthma Immunol 2000;85(5):416–21.

[99] Patel M, Perrin K, Pritchard A, et al. Accuracy of patient self-report as a measure of inhaled asthma medication use. Respirology 2013;18(3):546–52.

[100] Chan AH, Harrison J, Black PN, et al. Using electronic monitoring devices to measure inhaler adherence: a practical guide for clinicians. J Allergy Clin Immunol Pract 2015;3(3):335–49.e5.

[101] Charles T, Quinn D, Weatherall M, et al. An audiovisual reminder function improves adherence with inhaled corticosteroid therapy in asthma. J Allergy Clin Immunol 2007;119(4): 811–6.

[102] Foster JM, Usherwood T, Smith L, et al. Inhaler reminders improve adherence with controller treatment in primary care patients with asthma. J Allergy Clin Immunol 2014;134(6):1260–8.e3.

[103] Chan AH, Stewart AW, Harrison J, et al. The effect of an electronic monitoring device with audiovisual reminder function on adherence to inhaled corticosteroids and school

attendance in children with asthma: a randomised controlled trial. Lancet Respir Med 2015;3(3):210–9.

[104] Chan AH, Reddel HK, Apter A, et al. Adherence monitoring and e-health: how clinicians and researchers can use technology to promote inhaler adherence for asthma. J Allergy Clin Immunol Pract 2013;1(5):446–54.

[105] Haselkorn T, Fish JE, Zeiger RS, et al. Consistently very poorly controlled asthma, as defined by the impairment domain of the Expert Panel Report 3 guidelines, increases risk for future severe asthma exacerbations in The Epidemiology and Natural History of Asthma: Outcomes and Treatment Regimens (TENOR) study. J Allergy Clin Immunol 2009;124(5):895–902.e1–4.

[106] Anderson WC III, Szefler SJ. New and future strategies to improve asthma control in children. J Allergy Clin Immunol 2015;136(4):848–59.

[107] Genentech I. Xolair: FDA prescribing information. 2015. Available at: http://www.gene.com/download/pdf/xolair_prescribing.pdf. Accessed December 8, 2015.

[108] GlaxoSmithKline. Nucala: FDA prescribing information. 2015. Available at: https://www.gsksource.com/pharma/content/dam/GlaxoSmithKline/US/en/Prescribing_Information/Nucala/pdf/NUCALA-PI-PIL.PDF. Accessed December 8, 2015.

[109] Boehringer Ingelheim. Spiriva Respimat: FDA prescribing information. 2015. Available at: http://docs.boehringer-ingelheim.com/Prescribing%20Information/PIs/Spiriva%20Respimat/spirivarespimat.pdf. Accessed December 4, 2015.

[110] Silva D, Ansotegui I, Morais-Almeida M. Off-label prescribing for allergic diseases in children. World Allergy Organ J 2014;7(1):4.

[111] Szefler SJ, Chmiel JF, Fitzpatrick AM, et al. Asthma across the ages: knowledge gaps in childhood asthma. J Allergy Clin Immunol 2014;133(1):3–13 [quiz: 4].

[112] Vogelberg C, Engel M, Moroni-Zentgraf P, et al. Tiotropium in asthmatic adolescents symptomatic despite inhaled corticosteroids: a randomised dose-ranging study. Respir Med 2014;108(9):1268–76.

[113] Hammelmann E, Boner A, Bernstein J, et al. 1-year efficacy and safety study of tiotropium Respimat add-on to ICS in adolescent patients with symptomatic asthma. Eur Respir J 2014;44:1889.

[114] Vogelberg C, Moroni-Zentgraf P, Leonaviciute-Klimantaviciene M, et al. A randomised dose-ranging study of tiotropium Respimat(R) in children with symptomatic asthma despite inhaled corticosteroids. Respir Res 2015;16:20.

[115] Peters SP, Bleecker ER, Kunselman SJ, et al. Predictors of response to tiotropium versus salmeterol in asthmatic adults. J Allergy Clin Immunol 2013;132(5):1068–74.e1.

[116] Kerstjens HA, Engel M, Dahl R, et al. Tiotropium in asthma poorly controlled with standard combination therapy. N Engl J Med 2012;367(13):1198–207.

[117] (EPR-3) EPR. Guidelines for the diagnosis and management of asthma - summary report 2007. J Allergy Clin Immunol 2007;120:S94–138.

[118] Bousquet J, Cabrera P, Berkman N, et al. The effect of treatment with omalizumab, an anti-IgE antibody, on asthma exacerbations and emergency medical visits in patients with severe persistent asthma. Allergy 2005;60(3):302–8.

[119] Hanania NA, Alpan O, Hamilos DL, et al. Omalizumab in severe allergic asthma inadequately controlled with standard therapy: a randomized trial. Ann Intern Med 2011;154(9):573–82.

[120] Humbert M, Beasley R, Ayres J, et al. Benefits of omalizumab as add-on therapy in patients with severe persistent asthma who are inadequately controlled despite best available therapy (GINA 2002 step 4 treatment): INNOVATE. Allergy 2005;60(3):309–16.

[121] Holgate ST, Chuchalin AG, Hebert J, et al. Efficacy and safety of a recombinant anti-immunoglobulin E antibody (omalizumab) in severe allergic asthma. Clin Exp Allergy 2004;34(4):632–8.

[122] Busse WW, Morgan WJ, Gergen PJ, et al. Randomized trial of omalizumab (anti-IgE) for asthma in inner-city children. N Engl J Med 2011;364(11):1005–15.

[123] Milgrom H, Berger W, Nayak A, et al. Treatment of childhood asthma with anti-immunoglobulin E antibody (omalizumab). Pediatrics 2001;108(2):E36.

[124] Lanier B, Bridges T, Kulus M, et al. Omalizumab for the treatment of exacerbations in children with inadequately controlled allergic (IgE-mediated) asthma. J Allergy Clin Immunol 2009;124(6):1210–6.

[125] Hanania NA, Wenzel S, Rosen K, et al. Exploring the effects of omalizumab in allergic asthma: an analysis of biomarkers in the EXTRA study. Am J Respir Crit Care Med 2013;187(8):804–11.

[126] Fajt ML, Wenzel SE. Asthma phenotypes and the use of biologic medications in asthma and allergic disease: the next steps toward personalized care. J Allergy Clin Immunol 2015;135(2):299–310 [quiz: 1].

[127] Sorkness CA, Wildfire JJ, Calatroni A, et al. Reassessment of omalizumab-dosing strategies and pharmacodynamics in inner-city children and adolescents. J Allergy Clin Immunol Pract 2013;1(2):163–71.

[128] Pavord ID, Korn S, Howarth P, et al. Mepolizumab for severe eosinophilic asthma (DREAM): a multicentre, double-blind, placebo-controlled trial. Lancet 2012;380(9842):651–9.

[129] Ortega HG, Liu MC, Pavord ID, et al. Mepolizumab treatment in patients with severe eosinophilic asthma. N Engl J Med 2014;371(13):1198–207.

[130] Haldar P, Brightling CE, Hargadon B, et al. Mepolizumab and exacerbations of refractory eosinophilic asthma. N Engl J Med 2009;360(10):973–84.

[131] Nair P, Pizzichini MM, Kjarsgaard M, et al. Mepolizumab for prednisone-dependent asthma with sputum eosinophilia. N Engl J Med 2009;360(10):985–93.

[132] Flood-Page P, Swenson C, Faiferman I, et al. A study to evaluate safety and efficacy of mepolizumab in patients with moderate persistent asthma. Am J Respir Crit Care Med 2007;176(11):1062–71.

[133] Bel EH, Wenzel SE, Thompson PJ, et al. Oral glucocorticoid-sparing effect of mepolizumab in eosinophilic asthma. N Engl J Med 2014;371(13):1189–97.

[134] Castro M, Mathur S, Hargreave F, et al. Reslizumab for poorly controlled, eosinophilic asthma: a randomized, placebo-controlled study. Am J Respir Crit Care Med 2011;184(10):1125–32.

[135] Castro M, Zangrilli J, Wechsler ME, et al. Reslizumab for inadequately controlled asthma with elevated blood eosinophil counts: results from two multicentre, parallel, double-blind, randomised, placebo-controlled, phase 3 trials. Lancet Respir Med 2015;3(5):355–66.

[136] Corren J, Lemanske RF, Hanania NA, et al. Lebrikizumab treatment in adults with asthma. N Engl J Med 2011;365(12):1088–98.

[137] Anderson HM, Lemanske RJ Jr, Arron JR, et al. Developmental assessment of serum periostin as an asthma biomarker in children. J Allergy Clin Immunol 2014;133(Suppl 2):AB85.

[138] Song JS, You JS, Jeong SI, et al. Serum periostin levels correlate with airway hyper-responsiveness to methacholine and mannitol in children with asthma. Allergy 2015;70(6):674–81.

Advances in Pediatrics 63 (2016) 127–146

ADVANCES IN PEDIATRICS

The Optic Nerve Hypoplasia Spectrum
Review of the Literature and Clinical Guidelines

Anna Ryabets-Lienhard, DO[a],*, Carly Stewart, MHA[b],
Mark Borchert, MD[b,c], Mitchell E. Geffner, MD[a,c]

[a]Center for Endocrinology, Diabetes, and Metabolism, Children's Hospital Los Angeles, 4650
Sunset Boulevard, Los Angeles, CA 90027, USA; [b]The Vision Center, Children's Hospital Los
Angeles, 4650 Sunset Boulevard, Los Angeles, CA 90027, USA; [c]The Saban Research Institute,
Children's Hospital Los Angeles, 4661 Sunset Boulevard, Los Angeles, CA 90027, USA

Keywords

- Optic nerve hypoplasia • Septo-optic dysplasia • Epidemiology • Hypopituitarism
- Hypothalamic-pituitary dysfunction • Clinical presentation • Diagnosis
- Management

Key points

- Optic nerve hypoplasia (ONH) is a complex congenital disorder of unknown etiology and is the leading cause of permanent, congenital visual impairment in children in the western world.
- The causes of ONH are complex and multifactorial, with most cases being sporadic. Further studies are necessary to elucidate the causes of ONH.
- ONH is frequently associated with congenital brain malformations, hypothalamic-pituitary dysfunction, neurocognitive disability, obesity, and autism spectrum disorders.
- Hypothalamic-pituitary dysfunction in ONH occurs independently of brain malformations and may evolve over time, necessitating long-term evaluation and follow-up.

Financial Disclosures: M.E. Geffner is a clinical trial consultant for Daiichi-Sankyo; is on the data safety monitoring board for Tolmar; has research contracts from Novo Nordisk and Versartis; serves on advisory boards for Ipsen, Pfizer, Inc, and Sandoz; is a lecturer for Sandoz; and receives royalties from McGraw-Hill and UpToDate. The other authors have no disclosures to report.

*Corresponding author. Children's Hospital Los Angeles, 4650 Sunset Boulevard, MS #61, Los Angeles, CA 90027. *E-mail address:* aryabets@chla.usc.edu

0065-3101/16/$ – see front matter
http://dx.doi.org/10.1016/j.yapd.2016.04.009

INTRODUCTION

Optic nerve hypoplasia (ONH) is a common complex congenital disorder of unknown cause, involving a spectrum of anatomic malformations and clinical manifestations ranging from isolated hypoplasia of 1 or both optic nerves, with a variable degree of visual impairment, to extensive brain malformations, hypothalamic-pituitary dysfunction, neurocognitive disability, and/or autism spectrum disorders (ASDs) [1,2]. ONH is the second leading cause of congenital visual impairment, superseded only by cortical visual impairment [3,4]. According to the United States (US) Babies Count registry for children with visual impairment from birth to age 3 years, ONH carries a worse visual prognosis compared with cortical visual impairment, retinopathy of prematurity, and albinism [5]. It is the single leading cause of permanent legal blindness in children in the western world [3].

Owing to early observations of co-occurrence with agenesis of the septum pellucidum and hypopituitarism [6,7], ONH has long been recognized as part of the septo-optic dysplasia (SOD) syndrome, a clinically inaccurate term that attributes prognostic importance of the hypothalamic-pituitary dysfunction development to the absent septum pellucidum and/or other midline brain malformations. More recent, larger studies have demonstrated ONH to be an independent risk factor for hypothalamic-pituitary dysfunction, with abnormalities of the septum pellucidum having no prognostic value [1,8–11].

Currently, there are no consensus or clinical practice guidelines available for evaluation and management of children with ONH. This article focuses on the current state of knowledge about the prevalence, causes, and associated clinical features of the ONH spectrum, including their presentation, diagnosis, and management. The authors recommend a family-centered, multidisciplinary approach to caring for all children with ONH. Herein, are presented comprehensive guidelines for clinical evaluation and management based on an extensive literature review and the authors' clinical experience.

EPIDEMIOLOGY

The prevalence of ONH has increased substantially since the 1980s. The Swedish Register of Visually Impaired Children reported a fourfold increase in prevalence between 1980 and 1999 [12]. In an epidemiologic study conducted between 1944 and 1974, the prevalence of ONH in British Columbia, Canada, was reported to be 1.8 per 100,000 [13]. In 1997, Blohme and Tornqvist [4] reported that 7.1 per 100,000 children younger than 20 years of age with visual impairment or blindness in Sweden had ONH. The most recent estimates from the United Kingdom reported a prevalence of 10.9 per 100,000 in children younger than 16 years of age [14] and, from Stockholm, Sweden, 17.3 per 100,000 children younger than 18 years of age [2]. In another 2014 report using data derived from a registry of children with severe visual impairment in New Zealand, ONH was found in 6.3% of cases of children younger than 16 years of age [9]. This finding most likely underestimates the true prevalence because mild and/or unilateral cases are not consistently enrolled in the registry.

In the US, the prevalence of ONH in visually impaired children is not exactly known. According to the 2007 US Babies Count, ONH was the cause of blindness in 9.7% of children with vision impairment [5]. Among 3070 students from schools for the blind in 2012, ONH was the cause of blindness in 15%, more than double that reported in 1999 (7%) [3]. This prevalence is most likely underestimated because schools for the blind may exclude children with functional vision, unilateral ONH, or severe developmental disabilities. In fact, in the US, only about 13% of visually impaired children attend schools for the blind; all others attend mainstream schools [3]. In 2013, the Mayo Clinic College of Medicine analyzed medical records of all known cases of ONH in Olmsted County, Minnesota, between 1984 and 2008, generating an annual incidence of 2.4 per 100,000 children younger than 19 years of age (1 in 2287 live births) [15].

CAUSES AND RISK FACTORS
Prenatal factors and maternal age
Although the causes of ONH are not known, retrospective and prospective studies have consistently reported young maternal age and primiparity as predominant, independent prenatal factors associated with ONH [9,16–22]. In a 2012 study of 88 subjects with SOD, first-trimester bleeding was more common compared with the general population [18]. The investigators supported a previously proposed hypothesis that ONH may be due to a vascular disruption sequence, perhaps involving the anterior cerebral artery during a critical period of neuroembryogenesis [18,23]. Early gestational vaginal bleeding was also noted and introduced as a potential etiologic factor by a large prospective study of more than 200 children [16].

Recent reports have pointed to factors of deprivation and geographic differences associated with higher rates of ONH, especially in areas of lower socioeconomic status [9,14,18]. Garcia-Filion and colleagues [16] found an association of poor prenatal maternal weight gain or weight loss, suggesting a contributory role for prenatal nutrition.

High-risk behaviors, such as smoking, alcohol use, and recreational and/or prescription drug use, have been associated with higher rates of ONH [14,19,24–26]. However, these findings, specifically alcohol and drug exposures, were not supported by larger, prospective studies [16,17,21]. At this time, young maternal age and primiparity remain the most consistent risk factors, although more studies are needed to elucidate the mechanisms by which these factors contribute to the pathogenesis of ONH.

Genetics
Genetic causes and familial cases of ONH are uncommon, with most cases being sporadic [27–29]. Current understanding of the basis for ONH points towards environmental effects contributing to the congenital development of ONH during a vulnerable period of neuroembryogenesis. However, familial cases of ONH exist, including 1 set of monozygotic twins [30–33]. *HESX1* mutations have been identified in patients with SOD and/or hypopituitarism with

and without midline malformations, though not necessarily with ONH [34]. In the cases with ONH, *HESX1* mutations were rarely found [28,33,35,36]. In 1 series of 850 subjects with SOD, with or without ONH, mutations of *HESX1* were found in less than 1% of cases, supporting the rarity of mutations of this gene in a heterogeneous cohort of subjects [28]. In the literature, there is 1 case of *OTX2* gene mutation and another in *PROKR2*; however, in both cases, ONH was diagnosed by MRI without direct ophthalmologic examination [37,38]. It is also unclear how these mutations may be involved in the pathogenesis of ONH, and there are no genotype-phenotype correlations or animal models to establish the causation.

In the prospective, clinical registry of children with ONH established in 1992 at Children's Hospital Los Angeles, there is 1 set of monozygotic twins and 1 pair of brothers, among more than 320 enrolled subjects. Although it remains possible that a genetic cause or predisposition underlies ONH, perhaps involving various genes that affect similar biological pathways, the disease most likely has a multifactorial etiology with predominantly environmental causes. Next-generation genomic sequencing studies of children and families with ONH are an important future step to gaining a better understanding of a possible genetic basis.

CLINICAL APPROACH TO CHILDREN WITH OPTIC NERVE HYPOPLASIA

The wide spectrum of anatomic malformations and clinical presentations in patients with ONH necessitates a comprehensive guide to optimize care for these medically complex individuals. Table 1 summarizes neuroanatomical, neuroendocrine, cognitive, and behavioral features of ONH, their known frequencies, and previously reported correlations [1,2,8–11,17,18,39–54]. To date, there are no well-established predictive factors that can guide clinicians in the care and counseling of patients with ONH and their families. The presence of ONH alone, independent of laterality or neuroanatomical abnormalities, poses an increased risk for hypothalamic-pituitary dysfunction, seen in approximately 60% to 80% of cases [8,10,18,40,43,48,51–53], which, if unrecognized, may lead to significant morbidity and mortality [55]. Growth hormone (GH) deficiency (GHD) is the most common hypothalamic-pituitary abnormality in children with ONH presenting alone or in combination with other hormone deficiencies (see Table 1). Early recognition, diagnosis, treatment, and diligent surveillance using a family-centered, multidisciplinary approach is imperative to maximize the well-being of these patients. Timely evaluation is contingent on recognition of age-dependent presenting features of ONH, and should involve hypothalamic-pituitary and ophthalmologic assessments along with brain and sella imaging (Fig. 1, Table 2).

Clinical presentations and associated features in optic nerve hypoplasia
Neonatal period to infancy
Table 2 describes presenting clinical signs and symptoms in patients with ONH by age. Visual problems usually do not become apparent until 1 to 3 months of age [1]. Presentation with hypothalamic-pituitary dysfunction is

Table 1
Clinical features of optic nerve hypoplasia by frequency and correlations

Major associated features	Frequencies (%)	Correlations
ONH		Young maternal age and primiparity
Bilateral	55–80	Higher risk of hypothalamic-pituitary dysfunction, developmental delay
Unilateral	20–45	—
Hypothalamic-pituitary dysfunction	60–80	Higher in bilateral ONH, pituitary gland abnormalities
GHRH or GHD	70	Hyperprolactinemia
TRH-TSH deficiency	35–43	Developmental delay, worse visual outcomes
CRH-ACTH deficiency	17–27	GH deficiency
ADH deficiency	4–5	Unknown
Hyperprolactinemia	49–72	GHRH-GH deficiency
Pubertal abnormalities[a]	Unknown	Unknown
Other hypothalamic dysfunction		
Overweight or obesity	20–44	Unknown
Autonomic dysfunction	Unknown	Unknown
Disordered sleep	30	Severe visual impairment, developmental delay, and multiple hormone deficiencies
Neuroanatomical malformations	46–82	—
Hypoplasia of corpus callosum	51	Developmental delay
Absent septum pellucidum	38	Unknown
Pituitary gland abnormality[b]	6–64	Hypothalamic-pituitary dysfunction
Other major malformations[c]	22	Developmental delay, focal deficits, or seizures
Behavioral or developmental abnormalities	71	Bilateral ONH, hypoplasia of corpus callosum, and other major malformations
ASDs	25	Severe visual impairment

Abbreviations: ACTH, adrenocorticotrophic hormone; ADH, antidiuretic hormone; GHD, growth hormone deficiency; TSH, thyroid-stimulating hormone; GHRH, growth hormone releasing hormone; TRH, thyrotropin releasing hormone, CRH, corticotropin releasing hormone.
[a]Central precocious puberty, rapid tempo puberty, delayed puberty, and arrested or absent development.
[b]Absent pituitary, ectopic neurohypophysis, absent neurohypophysis, and/or adenohypophysis abnormality.
[c]Cortical heterotopia, schizencephaly, polymicrogyria, pachygyria, cerebellar hypoplasia, white matter hypoplasia, hydrocephalus, and/or ventriculomegaly.

common in infants and children subsequently diagnosed with ONH [8,22,56,57]. This phenotype is characterized by the typical manifestations of congenital GHD or hypopituitarism, which include transient or permanent hypoglycemia (which may be attributed to GHD and/or adrenal insufficiency), micropenis, and/or cryptorchidism in boys, prolonged hyperbilirubinemia after birth due to cholestasis resulting in a usually reversible form of giant-cell

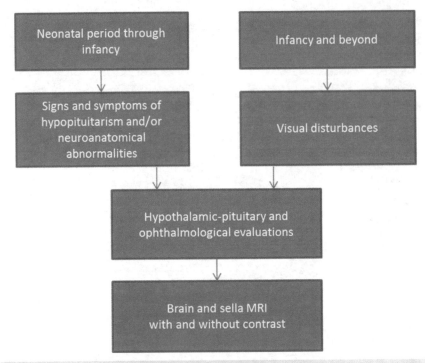

Fig. 1. Algorithm for initial evaluation of suspected ONH based on clinical presentation by age. Presenting clinical features detailed in Table 2.

Table 2
Clinical presentation by age

Neonatal period through infancy[a]	Infancy and beyond
Prolonged jaundice with or without giant-cell hepatitis	Unilateral or bilateral visual disturbances
Hypoglycemia	Nystagmus
Micropenis and/or cryptorchidism (boys)	Strabismus
Lethargy	Amblyopia
Poor feeding	Growth failure
Failure-to-thrive	Polyuria[b]
Polyuria	Polydipsia[b]
Irritability	
Neurologic deficits	
Seizures	
Vital sign instability	

[a]These features may occasionally be presenting signs during infancy and beyond.
[b]Polydipsia and polyuria may be psychogenic due to dysregulation of thirst to water balance in hypothalamus, or be a presenting feature of diabetes insipidus.

hepatitis, and/or poor linear growth that may begin at birth or, more likely, later in the first year of life [58–63]. The presence of any 1 or a combination of these findings should incite prompt investigation of the hypothalamic-pituitary axis and central nervous system, and referral to a pediatric endocrinologist and ophthalmologist, preferably a pediatric neuro-ophthalmologist (see Fig. 1). Timely hormonal replacement alleviates hypoglycemia and facilitates treatment of giant-cell hepatitis due to cholestasis [63]. In 62 cases of biopsy-confirmed neonatal giant-cell hepatitis, 16% were due to hypopituitarism [64]. Importantly, in 1 series of cases of neonatal hepatitis with significant delay in treatment until 5 years of age, cirrhosis and liver failure developed, necessitating liver transplant [62].

Central congenital hypothyroidism is often missed on newborn screening (NBS) in states that use initial thyroid-stimulating hormone (TSH) testing to detect the more commonly seen primary form of congenital hypothyroidism [65]. In a study of 135 subjects with ONH, approximately 50% who had low-normal TSH on NBS were diagnosed with central hypothyroidism on subsequent testing [66]. In this cohort, initial NBS TSH was significantly lower in those subsequently diagnosed with hypothyroidism compared with those who remained euthyroid (3.2 vs 4.5 μIU/mL; $P = .006$). In addition, subjects with hypothyroidism were found to have significantly worse vision outcomes compared with the euthyroid group [66]. Receiver-operating characteristic analysis suggested an optimal NBS TSH cut-off of 3.3 μIU/mL, over which there were relatively better vision outcomes. The study concluded that children with ONH and lower TSH levels on NBS are more likely to develop central hypothyroidism and poorer vision than those with higher TSH values.

Polyuria and polydipsia, as manifestations of diabetes insipidus (DI) due to a deficiency of antidiuretic hormone (ADH), also may occur, though posterior pituitary dysfunction in children with ONH is relatively uncommon [67]. The presence of DI in patients with ONH, similar to other forms of congenital DI, increases the risk for morbidity and mortality during the neonatal period because diagnosis and management in neonates are particularly challenging [67]. Patients with DI are also at increased risk for developing anterior pituitary hormone deficiencies during the neonatal period or later [67].

Infancy and beyond
Poor visual behavior in infants with ONH, presenting most commonly with wandering (searching) nystagmus, typically becomes evident at 1 to 3 months of life (see Table 2). In unilateral cases, strabismus (usually esotropia) is the main presenting feature, which typically develops in the first year of life. Unilateral cases are often diagnosed at later ages and have better visual function but possess significant risk for hypothalamic-pituitary dysfunction, though less than in bilateral cases [8,10,53]. Visual acuity in children with ONH ranges from functional vision to complete blindness. Vision impairment is nonprogressive and, in fact, improvement in vision, mainly in the first years of life, has been reported [1,66]. This is thought to be related to improvement in

superimposed cortical visual impairment, continuing optic nerve myelination, and/or thyroid status [1]. Approximately 80% of cases of ONH are bilateral, and most are legally blind [9,16,49].

Hypothalamic-pituitary dysfunction, most commonly presenting with growth failure due to GHD alone or in combination with other hormone deficiencies (see previous discussion), may present in infancy or evolve over time [9,10,40,68]. Normal linear growth velocity despite GHD is a documented phenomenon in children with ONH, though deceleration eventually occurs in most such cases, starting around age 3.5 years [48,69]. In the registry study, the authors examined the prevalence of endocrinopathies in 47 children at the time of enrollment (mean age 15.2 ± 10.6 months) and followed their subsequent growth patterns over time (until 59.0 ± 6.2 months of age) [8]. The overall prevalence of hypothalamic-pituitary dysfunction was 72%, with 64% of subjects having GHD, 49% hyperprolactinemia, 35% hypothyroidism, 17% adrenal insufficiency, and 4% DI. This hierarchy of hormonal dysfunction, with GHD being most common, is similar to that seen with other causes of congenital hypopituitarism, although the prevalence of TSH, adrenocorticotrophic hormone (ACTH), and ADH deficiencies may be greater in patients with ONH as suggested by 1 prior study [70]. An array of pubertal disturbances, including delayed, absent, precocious, and unduly rapid tempo variants, can occur, with the former 2 much more common than the latter 2, and typically only discernible after 10 years of age [45,71–76]. In addition, the authors' unpublished data show pubertal abnormalities may be present in children with no prior endocrinopathies; thus, long-term follow-up through adolescence is necessary. The prospective findings confirm or exceed the high prevalence of hypothalamic-pituitary dysfunction in children with ONH reported in previous retrospective studies [57,74].

Overweight or obesity is another manifestation of hypothalamic dysfunction and a major source of lifelong morbidity in patients with ONH. The prevalence of overweight (body mass index [BMI] > 85th percentile) in the registry was found to be 44% and was higher in children with co-existing GHD (52%) [8]. Mild hyperprolactinemia often occurs in subjects with disorders of the hypothalamus as a reflection of loss of normal inhibitory dopaminergic control of prolactin secretion. In a study of 125 children (age 13.2 ± 9.3 months) with ONH, 72% of subjects had elevated initial serum prolactin levels. By age 5 years, 60% of subjects with hyperprolactinemia had hypopituitarism, 31% were overweight, and 20% were obese. Though early hyperprolactinemia correlated with the presence of GHD, it did not predict future endocrinopathies or overweight or obesity [39].

Developmental delay and behavioral abnormalities are common but usually are not the main presenting features of ONH (see Table 1). In the registry, developmental delay was found in 71% of subjects and was associated with hypoplasia of the corpus callosum, hypothyroidism, and laterality of ONH (unilateral 39% vs bilateral 78%) [10]. In a recent population-based study of children younger than 18 years of age in Stockholm, Sweden, behavioral problems were also more common in cases of bilateral ONH compared with unilateral ones [2]. In addition, ASDs, which are over-represented in the visually impaired population [54,77], are prevalent in children with ONH [77,78]. In 1 study, 31% of children with ONH or SOD had a clinical diagnosis of ASDs, which was more common in patients with profound visual impairment [79]. However, given the overlapping behavioral characteristics of ONH and ASDs (including echolalia, pronoun reversal, stereotypic motor movements, and delays in developing imaginative play) [77], along with the inadequacy of current methods for diagnosing ASDs in visually-impaired children, the true prevalence in the ONH population is unknown.

Other common presenting features in ONH, including vital sign dysregulation (most notably temperature), hyperphagia or hypophagia with oral aversion, and disordered wake-sleep cycles, are thought to be due to hypothalamic dysfunction affecting critical regions or nuclei in the hypothalamus [1]. In a prospective study of 23 children with ONH, abnormal wake-sleep cycles were present in 30%, which correlated with severity of visual impairment, developmental delay, and hypothalamic-pituitary dysfunction [42].

Seizures and neurologic deficits have been described in patients with ONH with major neuroanatomical abnormalities on MRI, specifically, schizencephaly, polymicrogyria, and hydrocephalus [1]. Hypoplasia of the corpus callosum with or without an absent septum pellucidum has been associated with developmental delay and is the most common neuroanatomical malformation found in ONH (Fig. 2A) [10]. Similarly, in a recent evaluation of 94 children with ONH in New Zealand, neuroanatomical abnormalities were found in 60% of cases and were associated with a higher incidence of developmental delay [9].

There persists an assumption that the presence of various anatomic abnormalities of the brain in patients with ONH, most notably absence of the septum

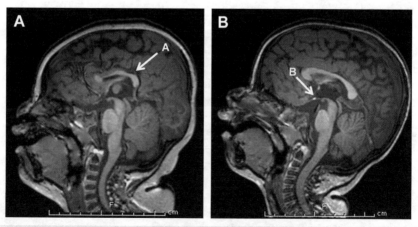

Fig. 2. ONH is commonly associated with neuroanatomical abnormalities (arrows), including (A) hypoplasia of (A) the corpus callosum and (B) an ectopic neurohypophysis.

pellucidum, is predictive of hypothalamic-pituitary dysfunction in ONH. This belief also seems to underlie the schedule of biochemical evaluations of pituitary function used by many clinicians.

In the registry study, Garcia-Filion and colleagues recently evaluated the spectrum of brain malformations by MRI and associations with hypopituitarism in children (personal communication, 2016). Subjects in the registry study undergo annual pituitary hormone testing until age 5 years and baseline neuroimaging. Noteworthy radiological findings in the cohort included abnormalities of the corpus callosum in 51%, the septum pellucidum in 38%, and the pituitary gland in 9% (see Fig. 2). Other major brain malformations affected 22% of the group and occurred independent of ONH laterality. In agreement with other reports [9,40,44], the study found that hypopituitarism was not associated with abnormalities of the corpus callosum, absent septum pellucidum, or other major brain malformations, except for malformations of the pituitary gland. Importantly, however, an intact pituitary gland and absence of neuroanatomical malformations do not preclude the development of hypothalamic-pituitary dysfunction [9,11,45,50,56] (personal communication, 2016). The authors' unpublished data show that, though all subjects with a pituitary gland malformation developed hypothalamic-pituitary dysfunction, 66% of patients with a normal pituitary gland on MRI also had hypothalamic-pituitary dysfunction (personal communication, 2016). The presence of ONH alone remains the main risk factor for the development of hypothalamic-pituitary dysfunction, independent of neuroradiographical findings.

An interesting but poorly explored observation is the occurrence of other systemic, non-neuroendocrine abnormalities occurring in as many as 47% of children with ONH as reported in a systematic retrospective review of 100 subjects [46]. The most commonly reported findings included facial dysmorphism, gastroesophageal reflux, cardiac or great vessel malformations, inguinal hernia, and hearing impairment. Several other case reports or series have described presence of gastroschisis, omphalocele, cleft lip or palate, and rare syndromes such as Williams and Donnai-Barrow syndromes [46,80–83]. The true prevalence and possible etiologic basis of these non-neuroendocrine abnormalities are not known. However, it is important to raise awareness that ONH may be found in patients with other systemic abnormalities or syndromes to avoid delayed diagnosis or treatment.

Evaluation and management of children with optic nerve hypoplasia
Vision
ONH is diagnosed by an ophthalmologist via direct ophthalmoscopy, confirming a small optic disc [1]. Fundus photographs are useful for confirming the diagnosis by measurement of the optic disc [1,2] (Fig. 3). A relative ratio of disc diameter to the distance between the macula and the temporal edge of the disc of less than 0.35 correlates with poor vision outcomes, though there is a gray zone of 0.30 to 0.35, in which normal vision has been reported [1,84]. Diagnosis in mild cases may be challenging but is improved by findings

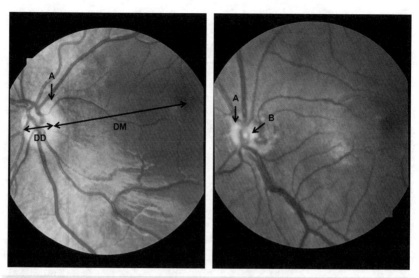

Fig. 3. Fundoscopic images of ONH. (*Left*) A mild case of ONH with disc diameter (DD) to disc to macula (DM) ratio of 0.22. (*Right*) A severely hypoplastic optic nerve (B). Both images display a hypopigmented double ring (A).

of tortuous retinal arterioles and/or venules, or abnormally straight retinal vessels with minimal branching [1]. Another common finding in ONH is a double-ring sign, which represents a hypopigmented or hyperpigmented area surrounding the disc, and is hypothesized to be due to a migrational defect of the sensory retina and/or pigment epithelium to the hypoplastic optic disc [53,85] (see Fig. 3). An MRI of the brain and orbits may be used as an adjunct to ophthalmoscopy in the diagnosis of ONH, though age needs to be taken into account when using MRI for this purpose [86].

ONH is an incurable congenital disorder. Though a growing number of international providers offer stem cell therapy for ONH, a small, case-controlled study showed no improvement in visual acuity in children who underwent stem cell therapy, the long-term risks of which are unknown [87]. Children with ONH should be monitored and treated by a neuro-ophthalmologist at least annually for refractive errors and amblyopia [1]. Children with unilateral or severely asymmetrical ONH should avoid patching. Strabismus surgery should be performed as early as possible in symmetric cases with good potential for binocular vision. Cosmetic surgery should be performed if psychosocial issues arise [1]. A referral to a teacher for the visually impaired may be beneficial to children with ONH at any age to help optimize residual vision.

Neuroanatomic malformations and neuropsychological abnormalities
An MRI of the brain and sella with and without contrast should be done on all patients with ONH. Severe major malformations, such as hydrocephalus and

schizencephaly and/or polymicrogyria, need to be evaluated and treated by a neurosurgeon and a neurologist, respectively, especially if seizures or neurologic deficits are present [53]. In addition to major brain malformations, the finding of a hypoplastic corpus callosum provides prognostic value for risk of delayed development (see Fig. 2).

All children with ONH should be referred to the local Early Head Start or Early Intervention program for early evaluation of deficits and, if needed, therapeutic services specific to visually impaired children. Physical therapy should focus on development of motor skills, especially ambulation. Oral aversions that make feeding a challenge may be remedied with occupational therapy focused on swallowing skills and tactile exposure. Speech therapy is often initiated to help with delays in communication development [1]. Orientation and mobility are critical for ambulatory patients to learn to safely navigate their environment. Behavioral therapy is frequently required in older children with emotional and behavioral problems related to ASDs, attention deficit disorders, or other neurologic dysfunction. A developmental pediatrician and/or neuropsychologist specializing in children with visual impairment should evaluate and treat children with ASDs and related developmental and learning challenges (Table 3).

Hypothalamic-pituitary axis

All children with a clinical presentation suggestive of hypothalamic-pituitary dysfunction or with a diagnosis of ONH should undergo hormonal testing and routine retesting to identify abnormalities in their earliest stages (see Fig. 1, Table 3). The authors suggest obtaining fasting blood tests, including cortisol, basic metabolic panel (for evaluation of fasting glucose and sodium), TSH, free T4, insulin-like growth factor (IGF)-I, IGF binding protein-3 (BP-3), and urine specific gravity at diagnosis. For young patients presenting with suspected hypoglycemia or DI, inpatient evaluation should be strongly considered. In children diagnosed between 3 weeks and 6 months of life, during the transient physiologic minipuberty period of infancy, initial blood testing should also include luteinizing hormone, follicle-stimulating hormone, and testosterone in boys or estradiol in girls. In addition, a prolactin level may be evaluated after 6 months of life (when the influence of normally higher physiologic levels in infancy is no longer an issue). Anthropometric measurements and morning screening blood tests should be obtained every 4 to 6 months in the first 3 years of life and annually thereafter for surveillance of evolving hypothalamic-pituitary dysfunction. Children with low levels of cortisol and/or IGF-I and IGFBP-3 on screening blood tests should undergo stimulation testing for corticotropin releasing hormone (CRH)-ACTH and growth hormone releasing hormone (GHRH)-GH deficiencies, respectively, which may be done simultaneously with a glucagon stimulation test [53].

Currently, there is no consensus on how long children with ONH and initially normal hypothalamic-pituitary function should be monitored. Some investigators have found that most children develop hypothalamic-pituitary hormone dysfunction in the first 2 years of life [57]. However, other studies have demonstrated endocrinopathies may evolve at a later age [40,68]. Ma and colleagues [68] found a clinically significant number of children with ONH developed central hypothyroidism after normal thyroid function tests at an earlier age. Eight subjects with ONH developed central hypothyroidism between the ages of 20 to 51 months. One child at age 28 months developed central hypothyroidism within 4 months of prior normal thyroid test results. The study concluded that evolving central hypothyroidism, along with other hormonal aberrations, is a common occurrence in ONH and that ongoing surveillance testing is necessary throughout early childhood. This recommendation has been made in at least 1 other study [88]. Borchert [53] recommends continued monitoring until at least 4 years of age. Others have suggested that lifelong monitoring and surveillance may be necessary [9]. Because pubertal dysfunction in children with ONH is common and may manifest as precocious, rapid tempo, delayed, arrested, or absent pubertal development, the authors recommend that children with ONH be screened and closely monitored at least through adolescence. More studies are needed to investigate the incidence and risk of development of hypothalamic-pituitary dysfunction over time in children and adolescents with ONH. Children with diagnosed hormone deficiencies should be treated with appropriate hormonal replacement. The efficacy of hormonal therapy mimics that seen in other forms of congenital hypopituitarism. Interestingly, in children with ONH, initial growth may be normal despite documented GHD [48,53,69,89]. Children with ONH should have IGF-I and IGFBP-3 levels measured even with a normal growth pattern. The long-term growth phenotype of children with ONH includes an increased propensity toward obesity with a reported prevalence of up to 44% [8,22].

All children and families should receive counseling on hormonal abnormalities, their signs and symptoms, monitoring, and treatment from an endocrinologist or specially trained advanced practice provider. For those with adrenal insufficiency, proper education on glucocorticoid replacement and stress-dosing during illness or injury, including availability of emergency intramuscular hydrocortisone administration and an emergency letter describing the patient's diagnosis and treatment, should be provided to all patients and families. In addition, written instructions and emergency hydrocortisone should be provided to the child's school and major caregivers outside the home. Skills and knowledge should be reassessed at subsequent visits.

Other hypothalamic abnormalities
Children with ONH have a high prevalence of overweight or obesity [8,39], which may be due to hyperphagia and disordered leptin sensitivity in the hypothalamus [1]. Although some research suggests a connection between GHD and obesity, simply treating with GH has not been proven to mitigate the excess weight. A recent study evaluated the effects of GH replacement on body composition in 17 children with ONH and GHD, and found a modest reduction in body fat percentage but no improvement in BMI or weight-for-stature standard

Table 3
Guidelines for evaluation and management of children with optic nerve hypoplasia

Problem	Screening and referral	Timing of evaluations
Vision	Dilated direct ophthalmoscopic examination and evaluation for other visual deficits Ophthalmology referral	At diagnosis and yearly, and as clinically indicated for treatment of refractive errors, strabismus, and amblyopia
Neuroanatomical problems	MRI of the brain and sella with and without contrast Neurology and/or neurosurgery referral as needed	At diagnosis and as clinically indicated
Hormone deficiencies[a]	8 AM[b] fasting blood tests: BMP (CMP at diagnosis), serum osmolality, cortisol, TSH, free T4, IGF-I, and IGFBP-3, prolactin (>6 mo of age), and urine osmolality LH, FSH, and estradiol or testosterone[c] Bone-age radiograph[d] Endocrinology referral	At diagnosis, every 4–6 mo in the first 3 y of life, and yearly thereafter 3 wk–6 mo of life and as clinically indicated[c] As clinically indicated for growth and puberty Hormone replacement monitoring every 3 mo
Failure-to-thrive[a]	Nutritional evaluation and swallow testing OT and/or gastroenterology referral	When present as clinically indicated
Overweight or obesity[a]	Nutritional evaluation or weight management programs	When present as clinically indicated

Condition	Intervention	Timing
Seizures[a]	EEG or MRI Neurology referral	At presentation of symptoms and signs
Sleep problems[a]	Counseling on bedtime routine and trial of melatonin Developmental pediatrician referral as needed	When present as clinically indicated
Developmental delay[a]	Developmental assessment tailored for visually impaired children Developmental pediatrician, psychologist, PT, OT, and/or speech therapy	Assessment at every visit by pediatrician
Behavioral problems or ASDs[a]	Behavioral or autism assessment Behavioral specialist or psychologist	As clinically indicated
School performance and quality-of-life	IFSP or IEP, counseling, and special needs assessment Early intervention, schools for blind children, and orientation and mobility referrals as needed	At diagnosis, when entering school and as needed

Abbreviations: BMP, basic metabolic panel; CMP, comprehensive metabolic panel; EEG, electroencephalogram; FSH, follicle stimulating hormone; IEP, individualized education program; IFSP, individual family service plan; IGFBP-3, insulin growth factor binding protein-3; IGF-I, insulin growth factor-I; GnRH, gonadotropin releasing hormone; LH, luteinizing hormone; OT, occupational therapy; PT, physical therapy; T4, thyroxine.

[a] At every visit, assess history, physical examination, vital signs, and growth with anthropometric data, including BMI and BSA.

[b] Before 6 months of age, screening tests may be done at any time of the day.

[c] Assessment of GnRH-LH-FSH function may be done during minipuberty, which is the physiologic, transient activation of hypothalamic-pituitary-gonadal axis of infancy. Subsequently, this assessment should be done when precocious puberty is suspected (signs of puberty <8 years in girls and <9 years of age in boys), or when delayed puberty is suspected (no signs of puberty in boys >14 years and girls >13 years), and/or with arrest of pubertal development.

[d] Delayed bone age is seen in GHD and/or delayed puberty, whereas advanced bone age is seen in precocious puberty. In children presenting concomitantly with GHD and precocious puberty, bone age as well as height velocity may be normal.

deviation scores [69]. Currently, as with other children who suffer from hypothalamic obesity, there is no effective treatment of this pernicious problem in children with ONH. Nutritional counseling for parents, early nutritional interventions, and weight management programs may be of some help.

Failure-to-thrive due to hypophagia and/or feeding challenges is seen in some children, and may necessitate nutritional and gastroenterological evaluations and management. DI should be evaluated in children presenting with failure-to-thrive and/or polydipsia because many young children with severe polydipsia may have poor growth and weight gain due to decreased caloric intake [90]. Additionally, water-seeking behavior is not uncommon and may be mistaken for DI. Conversely, some children with hypothalamic dysfunction may exhibit a diminished thirst mechanism, even in cases of DI.

Abnormal sleep-wake cycle and vital signs, including temperature dysregulation, may, in some instances, be managed through medical intervention. Disruption in these areas causes significant difficulties in daily life for the patients and families. Melatonin may be used to help with disordered sleeping, with low doses of 0.1 to 0.5 mg given daily before bedtime or higher doses of 3 to 5 mg for sporadic as-needed indications [91]. Vital sign dysregulation causing dysautonomia may pose a challenge for clinicians and families taking care of these children, especially in those with secondary adrenal insufficiency, frequently necessitating emergency room visits and glucocorticoid stress-dosing due to difficulty in objectively discerning true illness from dysautonomia.

SUMMARY

Overall, ONH is a complex condition of unknown causes with abnormalities of the septum pellucidum having no prognostic significance. The authors believe that the neuroendocrinologic manifestations of ONH require ongoing monitoring, even in those patients with normal brain imaging, and replacement of pituitary hormones when necessary (see Tables 1 and 3). Additionally, a long-term, family-centered multidisciplinary approach involving pediatric specialists in ophthalmology, endocrinology, neurology, and neuropsychology, as well as therapists and educators, is critical to optimize development and well-being of all children with ONH.

References

[1] Garcia-Filion P, Borchert M. Optic nerve hypoplasia syndrome: a review of the epidemiology and clinical associations. Curr Treat Options Neurol 2013;15(1):78–89.

[2] Tear Fahnehjelm K, Dahl S, Martin L, et al. Optic nerve hypoplasia in children and adolescents; prevalence, ocular characteristics and behavioural problems. Acta Ophthalmol 2014;92(6):563–70.

[3] Kong L, Fry M, Al-Samarraie M, et al. An update on progress and the changing epidemiology of causes of childhood blindness worldwide. J AAPOS 2012;16(6):501–7.

[4] Blohme J, Tornqvist K. Visual impairment in Swedish children. III. Diagnoses. Acta Ophthalmol Scand 1997;75(6):681–7.

[5] Hatton DD, Schwietz E, Boyer B, et al. Babies Count: the national registry for children with visual impairments, birth to 3 years. J AAPOS 2007;11(4):351–5.

[6] St John JR, Reeves DL. Congenital absence of the septum pellucidum: a review of the literature with case report. Am J Surg 1957;94(6):974–80.

[7] Hoyt WF, Kaplan SL, Grumbach MM, et al. Septo-optic dysplasia and pituitary dwarfism. Lancet 1970;1(7652):893–4.

[8] Ahmad T, Garcia-Filion P, Borchert M, et al. Endocrinological and auxological abnormalities in young children with optic nerve hypoplasia: a prospective study. J Pediatr 2006;148(1):78–84.

[9] Goh YW, Andrew D, McGhee C, et al. Clinical and demographic associations with optic nerve hypoplasia in New Zealand. Br J Ophthalmol 2014;98(10):1364–7.

[10] Garcia-Filion P, Epport K, Nelson M, et al. Neuroradiographic, endocrinologic, and ophthalmic correlates of adverse developmental outcomes in children with optic nerve hypoplasia: a prospective study. Pediatrics 2008;121(3):e653–9.

[11] Brodsky MC, Glasier CM. Optic nerve hypoplasia. Clinical significance of associated central nervous system abnormalities on magnetic resonance imaging. Arch Ophthalmol 1993;111(1):66–74.

[12] Blohme J, Bengtsson-Stigmar E, Tornqvist K. Visually impaired Swedish children. Longitudinal comparisons 1980-1999. Acta Ophthalmol Scand 2000;78(4):416–20.

[13] Jan JE, Robinson GC, Kinnis C, et al. Blindness due to optic-nerve atrophy and hypoplasia in children: an epidemiological study (1944-1974). Dev Med Child Neurol 1977;19(3):353–63.

[14] Patel L, McNally RJ, Harrison E, et al. Geographical distribution of optic nerve hypoplasia and septo-optic dysplasia in Northwest England. J Pediatr 2006;148(1):85–8.

[15] Mohney BG, Young RC, Diehl N. Incidence and associated endocrine and neurologic abnormalities of optic nerve hypoplasia. JAMA Ophthalmol 2013;131(7):898–902.

[16] Garcia-Filion P, Fink C, Geffner ME, et al. Optic nerve hypoplasia in North America: a reappraisal of perinatal risk factors. Acta Ophthalmol 2010;88(5):527–34.

[17] Garcia-Filion P, Borchert M. Prenatal determinants of optic nerve hypoplasia: review of suggested correlates and future focus. Surv Ophthalmol 2013;58(6):610–9.

[18] Atapattu N, Ainsworth J, Willshaw H, et al. Septo-optic dysplasia: antenatal risk factors and clinical features in a regional study. Horm Res Paediatr 2012;78(2):81–7.

[19] Margalith D, Jan JE, McCormick AQ, et al. Clinical spectrum of congenital optic nerve hypoplasia: review of 51 patients. Dev Med Child Neurol 1984;26(3):311–22.

[20] Murray PG, Paterson WF, Donaldson MD. Maternal age in patients with septo-optic dysplasia. J Pediatr Endocrinol Metab 2005;18(5):471–6.

[21] Tornqvist K, Ericsson A, Kallen B. Optic nerve hypoplasia: Risk factors and epidemiology. Acta Ophthalmol Scand 2002;80(3):300–4.

[22] Webb EA, Dattani MT. Septo-optic dysplasia. Eur J Hum Genet 2010;18(4):393–7.

[23] Lubinsky MS. Hypothesis: septo-optic dysplasia is a vascular disruption sequence. Am J Med Genet 1997;69(3):235–6.

[24] Dominguez R, Aguirre Vila-Coro A, Slopis JM, et al. Brain and ocular abnormalities in infants with in utero exposure to cocaine and other street drugs. Am J Dis Child 1991;145(6):688–95.

[25] Ribeiro IM, Vale PJ, Tenedorio PA, et al. Ocular manifestations in fetal alcohol syndrome. Eur J Ophthalmol 2007;17(1):104–9.

[26] Stromland K. Ocular involvement in the fetal alcohol syndrome. Surv Ophthalmol 1987;31(4):277–84.

[27] Mellado C, Poduri A, Gleason D, et al. Candidate gene sequencing of LHX2, HESX1, and SOX2 in a large schizencephaly cohort. Am J Med Genet A 2010;152A(11):2736–42.

[28] McNay DE, Turton JP, Kelberman D, et al. HESX1 mutations are an uncommon cause of septooptic dysplasia and hypopituitarism. J Clin Endocrinol Metab 2007;92(2):691–7.

[29] Larson A, Nokoff NJ, Meeks NJ. Genetic causes of pituitary hormone deficiencies. Discov Med 2015;19(104):175–83.

[30] Cidis MB, Warshowsky JH, Goldrich SG, et al. Mirror-image optic nerve dysplasia with associated anisometropia in identical twins. J Am Optom Assoc 1997;68(5): 325–9.

[31] Benner JD, Preslan MW, Gratz E, et al. Septo-optic dysplasia in two siblings. Am J Ophthalmol 1990;109(6):632–7.

[32] Hackenbruch Y, Meerhoff E, Besio R, et al. Familial bilateral optic nerve hypoplasia. Am J Ophthalmol 1975;79(2):314–20.

[33] Thomas PQ, Dattani MT, Brickman JM, et al. Heterozygous HESX1 mutations associated with isolated congenital pituitary hypoplasia and septo-optic dysplasia. Hum Mol Genet 2001;10(1):39–45.

[34] Dattani MT, Martinez-Barbera JP, Thomas PQ, et al. Mutations in the homeobox gene HESX1/Hesx1 associated with septo-optic dysplasia in human and mouse. Nat Genet 1998;19(2):125–33.

[35] Cohen RN, Cohen LE, Botero D, et al. Enhanced repression by HESX1 as a cause of hypopituitarism and septooptic dysplasia. J Clin Endocrinol Metab 2003;88(10):4832–9.

[36] Tajima T, Hattorri T, Nakajima T, et al. Sporadic heterozygous frameshift mutation of HESX1 causing pituitary and optic nerve hypoplasia and combined pituitary hormone deficiency in a Japanese patient. J Clin Endocrinol Metab 2003;88(1):45–50.

[37] Gorbenko Del Blanco D, Romero CJ, Diaczok D, et al. A novel OTX2 mutation in a patient with combined pituitary hormone deficiency, pituitary malformation, and an underdeveloped left optic nerve. Eur J Endocrinol 2012;167(3):441–52.

[38] Raivio T, Avbelj M, McCabe MJ, et al. Genetic overlap in Kallmann syndrome, combined pituitary hormone deficiency, and septo-optic dysplasia. J Clin Endocrinol Metab 2012;97(4):E694–9.

[39] Vedin AM, Garcia-Filion P, Fink C, et al. Serum prolactin concentrations in relation to hypopituitarism and obesity in children with optic nerve hypoplasia. Horm Res Paediatr 2012;77(5):277–80.

[40] Haddad NG, Eugster EA. Hypopituitarism and neurodevelopmental abnormalities in relation to central nervous system structural defects in children with optic nerve hypoplasia. J Pediatr Endocrinol Metab 2005;18(9):853–8.

[41] Riedl SW, Mullner-Eidenbock A, Prayer D, et al. Auxological, ophthalmological, neurological and MRI findings in 25 Austrian patients with septo-optic dysplasia (SOD). Preliminary data. Horm Res 2002;58(Suppl 3):16–9.

[42] Rivkees SA, Fink C, Nelson M, et al. Prevalence and risk factors for disrupted circadian rhythmicity in children with optic nerve hypoplasia. Br J Ophthalmol 2010;94(10): 1358–62.

[43] Morishima A, Aranoff GS. Syndrome of septo-optic-pituitary dysplasia: the clinical spectrum. Brain Dev 1986;8(3):233–9.

[44] Ramakrishnaiah RH, Shelton JB, Glasier CM, et al. Reliability of magnetic resonance imaging for the detection of hypopituitarism in children with optic nerve hypoplasia. Ophthalmology 2014;121(1):387–91.

[45] Birkebaek NH, Patel L, Wright NB, et al. Endocrine status in patients with optic nerve hypoplasia: relationship to midline central nervous system abnormalities and appearance of the hypothalamic-pituitary axis on magnetic resonance imaging. J Clin Endocrinol Metab 2003;88(11):5281–6.

[46] Garcia ML, Ty EB, Taban M, et al. Systemic and ocular findings in 100 patients with optic nerve hypoplasia. J Child Neurol 2006;21(11):949–56.

[47] Roberts-Harry J, Green SH, Willshaw HE. Optic nerve hypoplasia: associations and management. Arch Dis Child 1990;65(1):103–6.

[48] Costin G, Murphree AL. Hypothalamic-pituitary function in children with optic nerve hypoplasia. Am J Dis Child 1985;139(3):249–54.

[49] Siatkowski RM, Sanchez JC, Andrade R, et al. The clinical, neuroradiographic, and endocrinologic profile of patients with bilateral optic nerve hypoplasia. Ophthalmology 1997;104(3):493–6.

[50] Phillips PH, Spear C, Brodsky MC. Magnetic resonance diagnosis of congenital hypopituitarism in children with optic nerve hypoplasia. J AAPOS 2001;5(5):275–80.

[51] Signorini SG, Decio A, Fedeli C, et al. Septo-optic dysplasia in childhood: the neurological, cognitive and neuro-ophthalmological perspective. Dev Med Child Neurol 2012;54(11): 1018–24.

[52] Ahmad T, Borchert M, Geffner M. Optic nerve hypoplasia and hypopituitarism. Pediatr Endocrinol Rev 2008;5(3):772–7.

[53] Borchert M. Reappraisal of the optic nerve hypoplasia syndrome. J Neuroophthalmol 2012;32(1):58–67.

[54] Brown R, Hobson RP, Lee A, et al. Are there "autistic-like" features in congenitally blind children? J Child Psychol Psychiatry 1997;38(6):693–703.

[55] Brodsky MC, Conte FA, Taylor D, et al. Sudden death in septo-optic dysplasia. Report of 5 cases. Arch Ophthalmol 1997;115(1):66–70.

[56] Humphreys P. Septo-optic-pituitary dysplasia. Handb Clin Neurol 2008;87:39–52.

[57] Cemeroglu AP, Coulas T, Kleis L. Spectrum of clinical presentations and endocrinological findings of patients with septo-optic dysplasia: a retrospective study. J Pediatr Endocrinol Metab 2015;28(9–10):1057–63.

[58] Cavarzere P, Biban P, Gaudino R, et al. Diagnostic pitfalls in the assessment of congenital hypopituitarism. J Endocrinol Invest 2014;37(12):1201–9.

[59] Bell JJ, August GP, Blethen SL, et al. Neonatal hypoglycemia in a growth hormone registry: incidence and pathogenesis. J Pediatr Endocrinol Metab 2004;17(4):629–35.

[60] Choo-Kang LR, Sun CC, Counts DR. Cholestasis and hypoglycemia: manifestations of congenital anterior hypopituitarism. J Clin Endocrinol Metab 1996;81(8):2786–9.

[61] Xinias I, Papadopoulou M, Papastavrou T, et al. Optic nerve hypoplasia and growth hormone deficiency in a cholestatic infant. Pediatr Neurol 2006;34(4):319–22.

[62] Spray CH, McKiernan P, Waldron KE, et al. Investigation and outcome of neonatal hepatitis in infants with hypopituitarism. Acta Paediatr 2000;89(8):951–4.

[63] Binder G, Martin DD, Kanther I, et al. The course of neonatal cholestasis in congenital combined pituitary hormone deficiency. J Pediatr Endocrinol Metab 2007;20(6):695–702.

[64] Torbenson M, Hart J, Westerhoff M, et al. Neonatal giant cell hepatitis: histological and etiological findings. Am J Surg Pathol 2010;34(10):1498–503.

[65] Schoenmakers N, Alatzoglou KS, Chatterjee VK, et al. Recent advances in central congenital hypothyroidism. J Endocrinol 2015;227(3):R51–71.

[66] Fink C, Vedin AM, Garcia-Filion P, et al. Newborn thyroid-stimulating hormone in children with optic nerve hypoplasia: associations with hypothyroidism and vision. J AAPOS 2012;16(5):418–23.

[67] Djermane A, Elmaleh M, Simon D, et al. Central diabetes insipidus in infancy with or without hypothalamic adipsic hypernatremia syndrome: early identification and outcome. J Clin Endocrinol Metab 2016;101(2):635–43.

[68] Ma NS, Fink C, Geffner ME, et al. Evolving central hypothyroidism in children with optic nerve hypoplasia. J Pediatr Endocrinol Metab 2010;23(1–2):53–8.

[69] Stewart C, Garcia-Filion P, Fink C, et al. Efficacy of growth hormone replacement on anthropometric outcomes, obesity, and lipids in children with optic nerve hypoplasia and growth hormone deficiency. Int J Pediatr Endocrinol 2016;2016:5.

[70] Mehta A, Hindmarsh PC, Mehta H, et al. Congenital hypopituitarism: clinical, molecular and neuroradiological correlates. Clin Endocrinol (Oxf) 2009;71(3):376–82.

[71] Fard MA, Wu-Chen WY, Man BL, et al. Septo-optic dysplasia. Pediatr Endocrinol Rev 2010;8(1):18–24.

[72] Hanna CE, Mandel SH, LaFranchi SH. Puberty in the syndrome of septo-optic dysplasia. Am J Dis Child 1989;143(2):186–9.

[73] Willnow S, Kiess W, Butenandt O, et al. Endocrine disorders in septo-optic dysplasia (De Morsier syndrome)—evaluation and follow up of 18 patients. Eur J Pediatr 1996;155(3): 179–84.

[74] Oatman OJ, McClellan DR, Olson ML, et al. Endocrine and pubertal disturbances in optic nerve hypoplasia, from infancy to adolescence. Int J Pediatr Endocrinol 2015;2015(1):8.

[75] Huseman CA, Kelch RP, Hopwood NJ, et al. Sexual precocity in association with septo-optic dysplasia and hypothalamic hypopituitarism. J Pediatr 1978;92(5):748–53.

[76] Nanduri VR, Stanhope R. Why is the retention of gonadotrophin secretion common in children with panhypopituitarism due to septo-optic dysplasia? Eur J Endocrinol 1999;140(1):48–50.

[77] Fink C, Borchert M. Optic nerve hypoplasia and autism: common features of spectrum diseases. J Vis Impair Blind 2011;105(6):334–8.

[78] Ek U, Fernell E, Jacobson L. Cognitive and behavioural characteristics in blind children with bilateral optic nerve hypoplasia. Acta Paediatr 2005;94(10):1421–6.

[79] Parr JR, Dale NJ, Shaffer LM, et al. Social communication difficulties and autism spectrum disorder in young children with optic nerve hypoplasia and/or septo-optic dysplasia. Dev Med Child Neurol 2010;52(10):917–21.

[80] Jordan MA, Montezuma SR. Septo-optic dysplasia associated with congenital persistent fetal vasculature, retinal detachment, and gastroschisis. Retin Cases Brief Rep 2015;9(2):123–6.

[81] Kavarodi AM, Zharani K, Ali el S, et al. Septo-optic Dysplasia Complex with Omphalocele, Pre-maxillary Agenesis and Encephalocele. J Maxillofac Oral Surg 2015;14(Suppl 1): 457–61.

[82] Burnell L, Verchere C, Pugash D, et al. Additional post-natal diagnoses following antenatal diagnosis of isolated cleft lip +/- palate. Arch Dis Child Fetal Neonatal Ed 2014;99(4): F286–90.

[83] Chinta S, Gupta A, Sachdeva V, et al. Persistent pupillary membrane, strabismus, and optic nerve hypoplasia in Donnai-Barrow syndrome. J AAPOS 2011;15(6):604–5.

[84] McCulloch DL, Garcia-Filion P, Fink C, et al. Clinical electrophysiology and visual outcome in optic nerve hypoplasia. Br J Ophthalmol 2010;94(8):1017–23.

[85] Mosier MA, Lieberman MF, Green WR, et al. Hypoplasia of the optic nerve. Arch Ophthalmol 1978;96(8):1437–42.

[86] Lenhart PD, Desai NK, Bruce BB, et al. The role of magnetic resonance imaging in diagnosing optic nerve hypoplasia. Am J Ophthalmol 2014;158(6):1164–71.e2.

[87] Fink C, Garcia-Filion P, Borchert M. Failure of stem cell therapy to improve visual acuity in children with optic nerve hypoplasia. J AAPOS 2013;17(5):490–3.

[88] Saranac L, Gucev Z. New insights into septo-optic dysplasia. Prilozi 2014;35(1):123–8.

[89] Bereket A, Lang CH, Geffner ME, et al. Normal growth in a patient with septo-optic dysplasia despite both growth hormone and IGF-I deficiency. J Pediatr Endocrinol Metab 1998;11(1):69–75.

[90] De Buyst J, Massa G, Christophe C, et al. Clinical, hormonal and imaging findings in 27 children with central diabetes insipidus. Eur J Pediatr 2007;166(1):43–9.

[91] Rivkees SA. Arrhythmicity in a child with septo-optic dysplasia and establishment of sleep-wake cyclicity with melatonin. J Pediatr 2001;139(3):463–5.

Advances in Pediatrics 63 (2016) 147–171

ADVANCES IN PEDIATRICS

Update on Pediatric Human Immunodeficiency Virus Infection
Paradigms in Treatment and Prevention

Christiana Smith, MD, Elizabeth J. McFarland, MD*

Section of Infectious Diseases, Department of Pediatrics, Children's Hospital Colorado, University of Colorado School of Medicine, 13123 East 16th Avenue, Box 055, Aurora, CO 80045, USA

Keywords
• HIV • AIDS • Antiretroviral • Viral reservoir • PrEP • Pediatric • Perinatal

Key points
- Potent antiretroviral therapy allows the control of viremia and improved prognosis; however despite treatment, HIV infection is associated with global immune activation and associated metabolic complications, including cardiovascular disease.
- Research is ongoing to find a cure for HIV, and potential strategies will require eradication of the latent viral reservoir.
- Prevention strategies to decrease behavioral transmission of HIV include the use of preexposure prophylaxis and the concept of treatment as prevention.

INTRODUCTION
Since the first description of patients with an unusual acquired immunodeficiency in 1981, human immunodeficiency virus (HIV) has changed from a fatal diagnosis to a manageable chronic disease. Potent antiretroviral therapy (ART) has improved the life expectancy of those infected with HIV. Antiretroviral therapy also helps to prevent both perinatal and behavioral transmission of HIV. However, access to HIV testing and treatment is insufficient in many parts of the world. In addition, although ART can control HIV, it cannot eradicate the virus because of the development of latent reservoirs. Individuals infected with HIV also experience the consequences of chronic inflammation

---

Conflicts of Interest: Dr E.J. McFarland receives research funds from Gilead Sciences, Inc. Dr C. Smith has no conflicts of interest to disclose.

*Corresponding author. E-mail address: Betsy.McFarland@ucdenver.edu

0065-3101/16/$ – see front matter
http://dx.doi.org/10.1016/j.yapd.2016.04.007

and immune activation, which include an increased risk for cardiovascular disease. Current research into HIV prevention and cure offers hope for the future.

EPIDEMIOLOGY OF HUMAN IMMUNODEFICIENCY VIRUS IN THE UNITED STATES

At the end of 2013, an estimated 933,941 persons in the United States were living with diagnosed HIV infection, and approximately 50,000 new infections occur each year [1,2]. An estimated 2500 children less than 13 years of age are living with HIV in the United States; 174 children were newly diagnosed in 2014 [1,2]. Rates of perinatal transmission in the United States have declined more than 90% since the mid-1990s, because of the development of effective ART and other methods of preventing perinatal transmission. During 2008 to 2011, overall, only 3.1% of infants born to mothers infected with HIV acquired HIV. However, among mothers infected with HIV who did not receive ART, 13.3% of infants were infected with HIV [1]. These statistics show the importance of early testing and treatment of pregnant women.

Youth aged 13 to 24 years accounted for 21% of new HIV infections in the United States in 2013 [1]. Sexual contact is the most common route of transmission in youth. Male-to-male sexual contact and heterosexual contact accounted for 92% and 87% of new HIV infections among male and female youth, respectively, between 2010 and 2014 [1]. Intravenous drug use accounts for only 3% of new infections in youth. Men who have sex with men (MSM) are the population at highest risk of acquiring HIV, and rates of new HIV diagnoses among young MSM continue to increase. Between 2010 and 2014, new HIV infections increased 10% among MSM aged 13 to 24 years, and 27% among MSM aged 25 to 34 years, whereas numbers of new infections in older men (35–54 years) were stable or decreased (Fig. 1) [1]. The incidence of HIV infections in youth is highest in the southeastern United States, including District of Columbia, Louisiana, Maryland, Georgia, Mississippi, and Florida. Factors that contribute to increasing rates of new HIV infections in youth include inadequate education, low perception of risk, and behaviors such as substance use and low rates of condom use.

African Americans are disproportionately affected by HIV. African American infants consistently have the highest perinatal HIV acquisition rate in the United States, as high as 9.9 per 100,000 live births in 2009, compared with 1.7 and 0.1 per 100,000 live births in Hispanic/Latino and white infants, respectively [1]. Likewise, in youth, more than 55% of new HIV diagnoses have been in African Americans, compared with 20% in Hispanic/Latino youth, and 17% in white youth since 2009 [1]. Health and socioeconomic disparities in African American communities contribute to this increased risk of HIV [1].

Although the number of new HIV infections has remained stable since 1999, the annual number of people newly classified with AIDS in the United States has been steadily declining since 1993, reflecting the improved health of individuals infected with HIV following the introduction of combination ART in the mid-1990s [1,3]. Before effective ART was available, infants perinatally infected with HIV routinely developed AIDS in early childhood. New AIDS

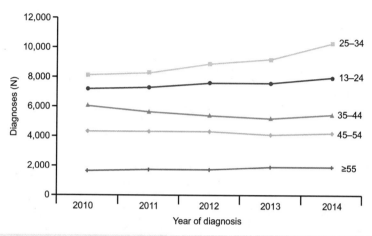

Fig. 1. Diagnoses of HIV infection among MSM. The number of HIV diagnoses reported in United States and 6 dependent areas during the years 2010 to 2014 are shown by age group. (*Adapted from* Centers for Disease Control and Prevention, HIV surveillance – men who have sex with men (MSM) (through 2014) slide set. Available at: http://www.cdc.gov/hiv/library/slidesets/index.html. Accessed December 13, 2015.)

classifications in perinatally infected children peaked in 1992 with more than 900 diagnoses per year, and have steadily declined since then, with fewer than 50 pediatric AIDS diagnoses per year since 2009 in the United States (Fig. 2) [1]. By contrast, youth are over-represented among those with new AIDS classifications because of diagnosis after disease progression. Youth represented 4.4% of people living with HIV but 10% of the 26,688 AIDS classifications in 2013 [1,4].

EPIDEMIOLOGY OF HUMAN IMMUNODEFICIENCY VIRUS WORLDWIDE

The HIV/AIDS epidemic tells a different story outside the United States, where access to testing and treatment is inadequate in many resource-limited settings (RLS), resulting in high rates of AIDS diagnoses and deaths, and ongoing transmission of HIV within communities. As of 2014, 36.9 million people were living with HIV worldwide, of whom 2.6 million were children less than 15 years of age [5]. Most of those infected with HIV (25.8 million, including 2.3 million children) reside in sub-Saharan Africa [5]. There were an estimated 220,000 new HIV infections and 150,000 AIDS-related deaths among children, representing more than 10% of total new infections and AIDS deaths in 2014 [5].

UPDATES ON HUMAN IMMUNODEFICIENCY VIRUS IMMUNOPATHOGENESIS

Immunopathogenesis of acute and chronic human immunodeficiency virus infection

The CD4 T-cell surface molecule is the main receptor for HIV; coreceptors include CC-chemokine receptor 5 (CCR5) and CXC-chemokine receptor 4

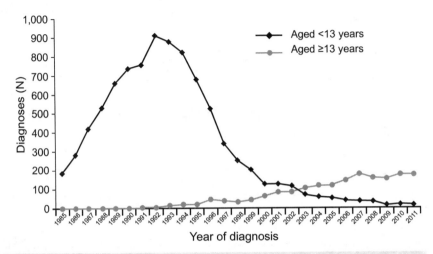

Fig. 2. AIDS classifications among perinatally infected people. The number of AIDS diagnoses reported in the United States and 6 dependent areas during the years 1985 to 2011 are shown. People aged less than 13 years at the time of AIDS classification are shown in black; people aged 13 years or more at the time of AIDS classification are shown in grey. (*Adapted from* Centers for Disease Control and Prevention, pediatric HIV surveillance (through 2011) slide set. Available at: http://www.cdc.gov/hiv/library/slideSets/index.html. Accessed December 13, 2015.)

(CXCR4). Binding of the virus to the CD4 molecule and one of these chemokine receptors results in conformational changes that allow HIV to enter the cell. HIV can be R5-tropic (requiring CCR5), X4-tropic (requiring CXCR4), or have dual/mixed tropism [6]. Of note, individuals with the homozygous CCR5Δ32 mutation are resistant to HIV infection because most transmitted virus is R5-tropic. Once inside the T cell, the retroviral genome undergoes reverse transcription and then integration into host DNA in a permissive cell. In addition, HIV takes advantage of host cell machinery to replicate and produce new virions capable of infecting other cells, thus establishing a productive infection.

During acute HIV infection, before the detection of HIV in circulating blood, there is an initial burst of replication in activated CD4 T cells in mucosal tissues. HIV disseminates rapidly throughout the gut-associated lymphoid tissue (GALT), resulting in depletion of up to 60% of the GALT's CD4 T cells within the first days to weeks of acute HIV infection [7]. Despite years of ART, CD4 T-cell populations within the GALT can only partially be restored [8]. In the GALT, Th17 CD4 T cells, which are critical for mucosal defense against bacteria and fungi, seem to be preferentially targeted. Loss of Th17 cells results in translocation of microbial pathogens and microbial products such as lipopolysaccharide across the gut mucosa; this contributes to chronic immune activation [9]. HIV infection also alters the gut microbiome, and these changes have been associated with increased mucosal and systemic immune activation [10,11]. Regulatory T cells (Tregs), which induce tolerance and limit the activation of other T cells, also play an important role in gut homeostasis. The expansion of Treg activity may dampen the immune response to HIV and other pathogens, thus allowing these infections to propagate [12].

HIV destroys CD4 T cells through both direct and indirect effects [13]. Indirect effects result in the apoptotic death of uninfected cells resulting from overexpression of death ligands, cytotoxicity of soluble HIV proteins, and activation-induced cell death [14]. The loss of infected, activated CD4 T cells also results from apoptosis triggered by HIV replication [13]. Recently, an additional mechanism of cell death has been identified for resting CD4 T cells in which HIV does not establish productive infection [15]. Viral DNA transcripts accumulate within the resting cells but do not integrate into the host genome. The viral DNA fragments elicit an intracellular innate immune response characterized by type I interferon production, which triggers pyroptosis, a highly inflammatory form of cell death in which cytoplasmic contents and inflammatory cytokines, such as interleukin (IL)-1β, are released into the environment [15]. These proinflammatory cytokines recruit activated T cells, which provide fuel for ongoing HIV infection and replication.

Immune abnormalities resulting from human immunodeficiency virus

The immune response to HIV infection affects nearly every cellular component of the host immune system (Table 1). Viral RNA directly stimulates toll-like receptors 7 and 9 on innate immune cells, resulting in a cascade of inflammation that includes the release of interferon-alfa from plasmacytoid dendritic cells [16]. This massive immune activation triggers cytotoxic responses from CD8 T lymphocytes and natural killer cells, which play an important role in the early control of viral replication [17,18]. Thereafter, the adaptive immune response results in proliferation of HIV-specific T cells. Ongoing immune activation leads to accumulation of these differentiated CD4 and CD8 T cells and, accordingly, shrinking of the naive T-cell repertoire. As T cells become further differentiated, they are subjected to senescence, losing their proliferative and functional cellular responses and eventually beginning a process of programmed cell death [19]. Senescent T cells produce large amounts of proinflammatory cytokines, thus contributing to ongoing immune activation [20]. B cells also show excessive activation, proliferation, differentiation, and senescence in the setting of HIV infection [21]. The downstream effects of this B-cell dysfunction include nonspecific hypergammaglobulinemia and impaired specific humoral immunity [22]. Natural killer cells, dendritic cells, and neutrophils also show increased markers of activation and apoptosis [23]. Unfortunately, many of these altered cellular immune functions are not fully restored even after years of virologic suppression in response to ART.

Elite controllers

A rare minority of adults and children infected with HIV (<1%), termed elite controllers, are able to maintain normal CD4 T-cell counts and an undetectable viral load for years in the absence of ART [24]. Several human leukocyte antigen (HLA) alleles, including HLA-B*57, HLA-B*27, and HLA-B*13, have been

Table 1
Effect of HIV infection on host immune cells

Cell type	Effect of HIV infection
T Cells	
CD4	↑ Differentiation and proliferation of HIV-specific cells
	↑ Markers of activation
	↑ Senescence and apoptosis
CD8	↑ Differentiation and proliferation of HIV-specific cells
	↑ Cytotoxicity
	↑ Senescence and apoptosis
B cells	↑ Proliferation
	↑ Markers of activation
	↑ Nonspecific immunoglobulin production
	↓ Specific humoral immunity
	↑ Apoptosis
	↑ Frequency of B-cell malignancies
Natural killer cells	↑ Proliferation
	↑ Markers of activation
	↓ Cytotoxicity
	↑ Senescence and apoptosis
Dendritic Cells	
Plasmacytoid	↑ Markers of activation
	↑ Production of type I interferons
Myeloid	↑ Markers of activation
	↑ Production of inflammatory cytokines
Neutrophils	↑ Markers of activation
	↑ Production of inflammatory cytokines
	↑ Apoptosis
Monocytes and macrophages	↑ Markers of activation
	↑ Production of inflammatory cytokines and chemokines
	↓ Chemotaxis and phagocytosis
	↑ Apoptosis
Endothelial cells	↑ Production of inflammatory cytokines and chemokines

associated with viral control [25,26]. These individuals have strong CD8 cellular immune responses, particularly cells with multiple antiviral functions, which likely help to control viremia [27]. However, elite controllers may still experience high levels of T-cell activation and increased cardiovascular morbidity, and some patients progress to AIDS despite maintaining an undetectable viral load [28].

PERSISTENCE, CONTROL, AND ERADICATION OF HUMAN IMMUNODEFICIENCY VIRUS: EFFORTS TOWARDS CURE

Human immunodeficiency virus persistence and the latent reservoir

The pursuit of a cure for HIV is hampered by the early formation of the latent viral reservoir. Within days of acute HIV infection, a pool of replication-competent but latent provirus is established within long-lived memory CD4 T cells. Other cells may contribute to this reservoir, including hematopoietic progenitor cells, macrophages, dendritic cells, and brain astrocytes or microglia [29]. Low-level viral replication and/or homeostatic proliferation of the resting cells might contribute to the maintenance of the latent reservoir (Fig. 3) [30]. On reactivation, the viral DNA integrated into the cellular genome can resume replication and, in the absence of ART, initiate new rounds of infection. The reservoir is not destroyed by ART or by host immune responses. The assays used for monitoring viral replication for clinical care (HIV RNA in plasma) do not detect the cellular proviral DNA of latent virus. Thus undetectable plasma HIV RNA does not indicate absence of a latent reservoir. Measures of latent virus used in research studies include sensitive techniques that quantify cell-associated DNA and the viral outgrowth assay that detects replication-competent virus in resting CD4 T cells [29].

The size of the latent viral reservoir, and therefore the time until viral rebound after ART is stopped [31], can be modified via early control of viral replication. The so-called Mississippi baby showed this concept: an infant infected with HIV received ART from 30 hours of life until 18 months of age, then had no detectable plasma HIV RNA for 27 months despite ART interruption, although the child eventually experienced viral rebound [32,33]. Additional studies of perinatally infected children showed that early initiation of ART correlated with smaller reservoir size [34]. In addition, the VISCONTI (viroimmunologic sustained control after treatment interruption) cohort showed that several adults infected with HIV could control viremia for years after interruption of ART [35]. Both posttreatment controllers and elite controllers share the finding of a small viral reservoir, suggesting that control of HIV (a functional cure) might be possible if reservoir formation is restricted [36].

Cure strategies

Any chance of achieving a sterilizing cure for HIV requires eradication of the latent viral reservoir. Thus far, a durable cure has only been shown in the so-called Berlin patient, an individual infected with HIV who required a bone marrow transplant for acute myeloid leukemia. His viral reservoir was significantly reduced by cytotoxic chemotherapy, before transplant with HIV-resistant stem cells from a donor homozygous for CCR5Δ32 [37]. The patient has had no signs of viral rebound for 8 years. In contrast, the Boston patients also required bone marrow transplants for lymphoma, and also received aggressive chemotherapy, but were transplanted with stem cells from donors with wild-type CCR5 [38]. Both of these patients experienced viral rebound within months of stopping ART, showing that their latent viral reservoirs were not eradicated with chemotherapy and that their wild-type donor cells were easily infected [38].

Recent cure efforts have focused on methods to identify and destroy latently infected cells, a so-called kick-and-kill approach. There are no known cellular biomarkers that distinguish latently infected resting T cells from uninfected cells. However, activating these cells results in cellular expression of viral proteins that can be targeted. Thus far, drugs that sufficiently activate all latently infected cells have not been identified. Importantly, the expression of provirus alone is not likely to be sufficient to result in cell death. To address this issue,

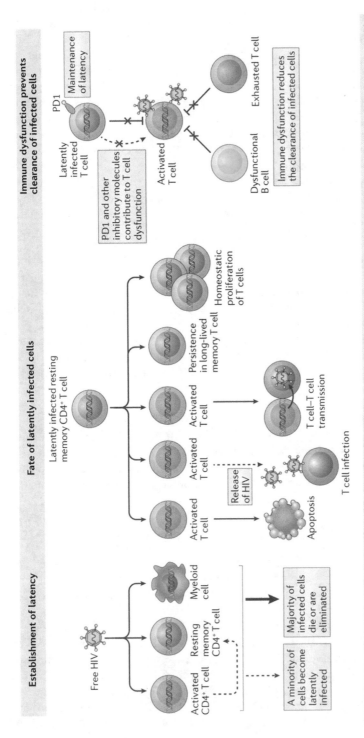

Fig. 3. Mechanisms of persistence of the latent viral reservoir. (*Left*) The establishment of latency within T cells and other immune cells. (*Center*) The possible outcomes of latently infected cells. (*Right*) How the latent reservoir escapes immune detection. (*Reprinted from International Aids Society Scientific Working Group on HIV Cure. Towards an HIV Cure: a global scientific strategy. Nat Rev Immunol 2012;12(8):610; with permission Macmillan Publishers Ltd.)

several strategies are being developed to enhance the CD8 T-cell and innate responses to activated cells expressing viral antigens; these include therapeutic vaccines, monoclonal antibodies, and genetic modification of the T-cell receptor [39–41]. In addition, other cure efforts have focused on using gene modification approaches to delete the HIV genome from latently infected cells, or introduce mutations within genes encoding cellular targets for HIV, such as CCR5 [42]. These novel gene modification strategies create many logistical and ethical dilemmas.

HUMAN IMMUNODEFICIENCY VIRUS DIAGNOSIS: FOCUS ON EARLY HUMAN IMMUNODEFICIENCY VIRUS INFECTION

Diagnosis of HIV infection in perinatally exposed infants aged less than 18 months relies on HIV nucleic acid tests (NATs) that detect RNA in plasma or DNA in cells, because transplacental maternal antibody, present throughout infancy, confounds serologic diagnosis. Testing as soon as possible after birth allows for the early initiation of ART for in utero infection. Infants who acquire HIV infection in the peripartum period typically have detectable HIV nucleic acid by 2 weeks of age. Therefore, in the absence of breast milk exposure, perinatal HIV infection can be presumptively excluded by 2 negative HIV NATs determined at ages 2 and 4 weeks, and definitively excluded with 2 negative HIV NATs determined at ages 1 and 4 months [43]. Many providers continue to obtain HIV antibody testing at ages greater than 18 months to confirm conversion to seronegativity, which is particularly important if there may have been undisclosed breastfeeding or feeding of premasticated food after the early testing dates, because these exposures may result in transmission [44].

The Centers for Disease Control and Prevention (CDC) revised the HIV diagnostic algorithm for behavioral infection in 2014 to take advantage of new testing methods that improve sensitivity for diagnosis in the early days after acute infection. Early treatment of HIV has important public health benefits, because 10% to 50% of all HIV transmissions are thought to originate from individuals with acute HIV infection [45]. Early treatment also has important implications for the individual, because it may lower the viral set point [46], reduce the size of the latent viral reservoir [47], decrease the viral mutation rate [48], and slow disease progression [49].

In recent years, new generations of HIV immunoassays have become available, with each generation showing improved sensitivity during early stages of infection. First-generation and second-generation immunoassays detect immunoglobulin (Ig) G antibodies only. Third-generation immunoassays also detect IgM antibodies, which allows diagnosis early during seroconversion. Fourth-generation immunoassays detect HIV p24 antigen in addition to IgM and IgG antibodies. During acute infection, the HIV p24 antigen can be detected in plasma 3 to 5 days before the detection of IgM antibodies (Fig. 4). The earliest marker of HIV infection is RNA, which can be detected in plasma as soon as 10 days after an acute infection, and 4 to 10 days before p24 antigen is detectable.

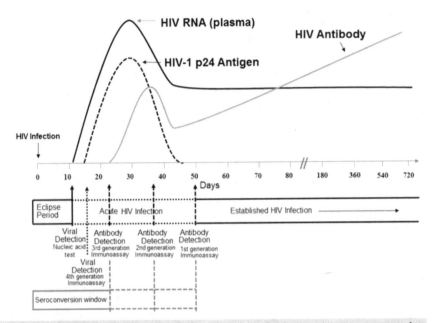

Fig. 4. Laboratory markers of HIV infection. Laboratory markers detected during acute HIV infection are shown by time of appearance. Units are not noted on the vertical axis because they differ for the various laboratory markers. (*Reprinted from* Centers for Disease Control and Prevention and Association of Public Health Laboratories. Laboratory testing for the diagnosis of HIV Infection: updated recommendations. Available at: http://dx.doi.org/10.15620/cdc.23447. Accessed December 17, 2015.)

The new algorithm begins with a fourth-generation immunoassay; if reactive, testing proceeds to a third-generation immunoassay that confirms the presence of antibodies and differentiates HIV-1 from HIV-2 infection (Fig. 5). Tests that are positive for the initial immunoassay, but negative or indeterminate by the HIV-1/HIV-2 antibody differentiation immunoassay, may be consistent with early HIV infection with the presence of p24 antigen preceding appearance of circulating antibody. These samples undergo nucleic acid testing for HIV-1 RNA. A reactive NAT result confirms an acute HIV-1 infection before development of an antibody response. A negative NAT result indicates a false-positive result on the initial antibody/antigen immunoassay. The new testing algorithm detects acute HIV infection days to weeks before seroconversion occurs.

Patients who present with suspected acute retroviral syndrome should be tested for HIV using RNA PCR, because the fourth-generation immunoassay may not detect the p24 antigen during very early infection. Symptoms of acute retroviral syndrome begin within days of HIV exposure and typically include fever (53%–90%), weight loss/anorexia (46%–76%), fatigue (26%–90%), gastrointestinal upset (31%–68%), rash (9%–80%), headache (32%–70%), and lymphadenopathy (7%–75%) [50]. Other findings can include pharyngitis, myalgia or arthralgia, aseptic meningitis, and oral ulcers.

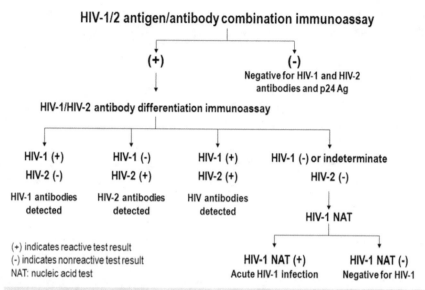

Fig. 5. HIV testing algorithm recommended in the United States. The recommended laboratory testing algorithm for HIV begins with a fourth-generation immunoassay, which detects HIV-1/HIV-2 antibodies and p24 antigen. If positive, the test proceeds to a confirmatory HIV-1/HIV-2 antibody differentiation immunoassay. If negative or indeterminate, the test proceeds to an HIV-1 nucleic acid test. Several potential combinations of test results are shown. (*Reprinted from* Centers for Disease Control and Prevention and Association of Public Health Laboratories. Laboratory testing for the diagnosis of HIV infection: updated recommendations. Available at: http://dx.doi.org/10.15620/cdc.23447. Accessed December 17, 2015.)

REVISED HUMAN IMMUNODEFICIENCY VIRUS DISEASE STAGING

HIV disease staging is based on clinical and CD4 T-cell parameters and is used for surveillance statistics and disease management. Individuals who are diagnosed with HIV should have additional screening laboratory tests, including a quantitative HIV plasma RNA (viral load), CD4 T-cell count, and antiretroviral resistance assay. These tests allow for staging of HIV disease and selection of an initial ART regimen. The revised staging system published by the CDC in 2014 uses a single case definition for the staging of infants, children, and adults infected with HIV (Table 2) [43]. Stage 0 indicates infection within the last 180 days. Stages 1 to 3 are classified by CD4 T-cell count. Individuals with an AIDS-defining illness are also classified as stage 3 [43].

PARADIGMS IN HUMAN IMMUNODEFICIENCY VIRUS TREATMENT

HIV is now a chronic condition that can be controlled with drug treatment for an indefinite number of years. The mortality among children with access to combination ART is reduced by 76% compared with children receiving older

Table 2
HIV infection stage, based on age-specific CD4 T-cell count

	Age on date of CD4 T-cell test					
	<1 y		1–5 y		6 y to adult	
Stage[a]	Cells/μL	%	Cells/μL	%	Cells/μL	%
1	≥1500	≥34	≥1000	≥30	≥500	≥26
2	750–1499	26–33	500–999	22–29	200–499	14–25
3	<750	<26	<500	<22	<200	<14

[a]The CD4+ T-cell count takes precedence over the CD4 T-lymphocyte percentage, and the percentage is considered only if the count is missing.

Adapted from Centers for Disease Control and Prevention. Revised surveillance case definition for HIV infection–United States, 2014. MMWR Recomm Rep 2014;63:11; with permission.

regimens [51]. Treatment of HIV was transformed in the second half of the 1990s as a result of the development of drugs that could potently suppress viral replication and the recognition that combination ART was necessary to prevent the outgrowth of resistant virus. Continued rapid drug development since then has arisen out of an increased understanding of virology and pharmacology [52]. There are now 25 US Food and Drug Administration (FDA)–approved anti-HIV agents that are active at 4 distinct steps of the virus life cycle (Table 3) [53]. The new drugs coming to market within each drug class have improved characteristics compared with the earlier generations with respect to longer half-lives, better tolerability, and fewer toxicities. Although evaluation of new ART in children lags behind the studies in adults, most of the first-line drugs have been studied in children more than 3 years of age. Choices for younger children are more limited, but are gradually expanding with the addition in the past year of raltegravir and atazanavir [54–56].

The question of when to start ART has challenged clinicians for many years. For infants, immediate initiation of ART has been standard of care, based first on observational data, and then supported with a randomized clinical trial that showed higher mortality for infants with deferred treatment [57,58]. Starting ART in early infancy has now been shown to result in a lower frequency of cells with latent virus, which may have benefits in the future related to potential cure strategies [34]. However, for older children, who have survived infancy before diagnosis, clinical manifestations may not appear for many years [59], and data for when to initiate treatment have been mixed [60–62]. The paradigm is shifting to early initiation of treatment based on several recent studies in adults [49,63,64]. The Strategic Timing of Antiretroviral Therapy (START) study randomized adults to immediate versus deferred treatment (ART start based on CD4 T- cell parameters) and showed more than a 50% reduction in serious events and death in the immediate treatment group [49]. Moreover, two-thirds of the events occurred when the participants had CD4 T-cell counts that were greater than the usual threshold for treatment. These data have led to current US guidelines that recommend starting treatment as soon as feasible

Table 3
FDA-approved antiretroviral drug class, mechanism of action, and specific drugs within each class

Drug class	Mechanism of action	Drugs within class
Nucleoside/nucleotide reverse transcriptase inhibitors	Chain termination of HIV DNA	Abacavir[a] Didanosine[a] Emtricitabine[a] Lamivudine[a] Stavudine[a] Tenofovir[a] Zidovudine[a]
Non-nucleoside reverse transcriptase inhibitors	Synthesis of HIV DNA inhibited	Efavirenz[a] Etravirine Nevirapine[a] Rilpivirine
Protease inhibitors	Production of noninfectious virions	Atazanavir[a] Darunavir[a] Fosamprenavir[a] Indinavir Lopinavir[a] Nelfinavir[a] Saquinavir Tipranavir[a]
Integrase inhibitor	Integration of viral nucleic acid in host genome prevented	Dolutegravir[a] Elvitegravir Raltegravir[a]
Entry inhibitors	Viral entry prevented by inhibition of virus–cell membrane fusion or blocking coreceptor	Enfuvirtide[a] Maraviroc
Pharmacokinetic enhancers	Interacts with P450 cytochrome enzymes to increase levels of selected antiretroviral drugs	Cobicistat Ritonavir[a]

[a]FDA-approved drug for use in some pediatric populations.

after diagnosis, even among those adults and adolescents with no evidence of disease progression [63]. The World Health Organization (WHO) updated guidelines also recommend universal treatment of adults and children [65]. However, similar high-quality data regarding when to start treatment of children more than 2 years of age are few. The US pediatric guidelines provide an option for deferring treatment of a particular child if there are psychosocial or clinical concerns, but only if the child has a low viral load, normal CD4 T-cell count, and no clinical progression [53]. However, many experts favor early initiation of treatment for all children.

COMPLICATIONS OF HUMAN IMMUNODEFICIENCY VIRUS AND TREATMENT

Although ART has radically changed the prognosis of HIV infection, there is ongoing concern that the complications of antiretroviral drugs and HIV, despite viral suppression, will shorten the life expectancy of children infected with HIV. Metabolic, cardiovascular, cerebrovascular, and bone toxicities are particularly concerning adverse outcomes associated with pediatric HIV (reviewed in Refs. [66,67]). In the current era, much of the morbidity experienced by children infected with HIV over their lifetime is likely to be a result of metabolic complications. Therefore, it is important to carefully monitor lipid profiles and fasting glucose levels, and to counsel patients to avoid smoking and make other healthy lifestyle choices.

Dyslipidemia and insulin resistance

Insulin resistance observed in children infected with HIV and overt type 2 diabetes mellitus observed in adults infected with HIV are associated with the use of protease inhibitors and thymidine analogue nucleoside reverse transcriptase inhibitors (NRTIs) [66]. Dyslipidemia is common in HIV infection, characterized by hypertriglyceridemia, low high-density lipoprotein (HDL) cholesterol, and a predominance of low-density lipoprotein (LDL) and very-low-density lipoprotein. Protease inhibitors, especially with ritonavir boosting, stavudine and efavirenz contribute to dyslipidemia [66], whereas tenofovir reduces levels of LDL and total cholesterol, and nevirapine increases levels of HDL [68,69].

Cardiovascular and cerebrovascular risk

Early onset of cardiovascular and cerebrovascular disease is well described among adults living with HIV [70]. A meta-analysis reported that the incidence of cardiovascular disease is 1.5-fold to 2-fold higher in adults infected with HIV compared with their age-matched peers [71]. This risk is attributed both to the ongoing inflammation resulting from HIV [72] and to the metabolic effects of ART [73]. Endothelial cells are affected by chronic immune activation, and can themselves produce inflammatory cytokines and chemokines [74]. Inflammation of vascular endothelium results in an adherent lumen, which may increase the risk of thromboses. Proinflammatory cytokines interact with the coagulation cascade to further increase the hypercoagulable state. Thus, the chronic inflammation characteristic of HIV infection contributes in multiple ways to an increased risk for cardiovascular events.

There is now mounting evidence of this disorder in children infected with HIV. A study applying the Pathobiological Determinants of Atherosclerosis in Youth score to adolescents infected with HIV described increased coronary disease risk in 48% of the youth [75]. Abnormal coronary arteries were found by cardiac magnetic resonance techniques in a cohort of mostly vertically infected young adults [76] as well as altered carotid intima-media thickness and arterial stiffness [77]. Biomarkers of endothelial dysfunction are associated with viral replication and metabolic abnormalities in children infected with HIV [78]. Although these abnormalities in children have been subclinical, there is mounting concern for early onset of symptomatic cardiovascular and cerebrovascular disease as these vertically infected children reach adult age.

Bone health

Low bone mineral density is commonly observed among children infected with HIV compared with their uninfected peers, with rates ranging from 7% to 32% [67]. Associated risk factors include time on ART, treatment with tenofovir and protease inhibitors, advanced HIV disease, and delayed puberty. Initial studies have not found a higher rate of fractures [79] but the long-term effects as these children age into adulthood are unknown and higher fracture risk has been observed in adults infected with HIV [80].

Lipodystrophy

Lipodystrophy is a term that describes body composition changes that may be seen in individuals infected with HIV, including both peripheral subcutaneous lipoatrophy and central lipohypertrophy. Lipoatrophy is often most apparent in the face, including the malar, buccal, and temporal regions. The peripheral extremities and buttocks can also be involved. This characteristic appearance is associated with increased stigma, reduced quality of life, and compromised adherence to ART [81]. Use of the thymidine analogue NRTIs, particularly stavudine, cause lipoatrophy via mitochondrial dysfunction that leads to apoptosis of adipocytes [82]. Switching to alternative NRTIs after the changes occur may not fully restore fat mass. Lipohypertrophy refers to the accumulation of excess adipose tissue in the visceral compartment of the abdomen. The pathogenesis of lipohypertrophy is unclear, but it seems to be linked to other metabolic disorders, including insulin resistance and dyslipidemia.

PREVENTION

Prevention of vertical human immunodeficiency virus transmission

The discovery that antiretroviral drugs (ARV) could reduce the risk of perinatal HIV transmission was a landmark event in HIV prevention. Not long after the original study of zidovudine monotherapy, combination ART regimens that also benefit the mother's health became available in well-resourced countries and are now recommended during pregnancy [83]. The risk of in utero and peripartum transmission is estimated at less than 1% with initiation of ART early in pregnancy, effective viral suppression, infant prophylaxis, and avoidance of breastfeeding [84].

Initially the recommended course of zidovudine monotherapy was considered infeasible in RLS, and studies identified several limited ART regimens that also reduced transmission in utero and peripartum [83]. Transmission via breastfeeding was another major challenge, with an added risk of transmission of 15% in the absence of intervention [85]. Women living with HIV in RLS faced a difficult dilemma because breastfeeding had the inherent risk of HIV transmission but replacement feeding placed the infant at significant risk of mortality caused by malnutrition, diarrhea, and other diseases [86]. This challenge was addressed with studies that showed reduced HIV transmission during breastfeeding with either extended infant ART prophylaxis or maternal ART to suppress maternal viral load in plasma and breast milk [85].

The 2010 WHO guidelines offered 2 options in RLS for women with HIV during pregnancy whose HIV disease stage did not qualify them for lifelong ART: option A, maternal zidovudine during pregnancy with extended infant nevirapine throughout breastfeeding; and option B, maternal ART during pregnancy and breastfeeding with 4 to 6 weeks of infant nevirapine. A head-to-head comparison of these approaches was recently completed in a large study, Promoting Maternal and Infant Survival Everywhere (PROMISE). PROMISE showed a lower rate of transmission for the combined outcome of in utero and peripartum transmission for the option B versus option A treatment (0.5% vs 1.8%) [87]. The study is continuing in order to compare postpartum transmission rates during breastfeeding.

Both options A and B stopped ART for the mother either after delivery or at cessation of breastfeeding unless her HIV disease stage qualified her for ongoing ART. This required assessment of CD4 T-cell count or other clinical evidence of HIV disease progression to determine whether the woman should remain on treatment. In an effort to simplify ART management, improve uptake, and reduce the risk of loss to follow-up (LTFU) and the potential for unmonitored disease progression, the WHO initiated recommendations for lifelong ART for pregnant women living with HIV [88]. This recommendation, known as option B+, has been widely implemented and is in line with new guidelines supporting universal HIV treatment.

Effects of antiretroviral and human immunodeficiency virus exposure during pregnancy and early infancy

Each year there are approximately 1 million infants exposed to ARV in utero and during infancy. These infants are also exposed to maternal HIV and associated abnormal maternal immune activation and inflammation. The clinical consequences of this exposure are an area of active investigation. In the short term, the main concerns have been effects on prematurity. Although there is ongoing controversy, combination ART, especially regimens containing protease inhibitors, may increase the risk of adverse birth outcomes such as prematurity, low birth weight, and small for gestational age [89–92]. Several studies have found small increased risks for congenital anomalies, mostly minor, associated with first-trimester exposure to particular ARV [93–95]. Concern has been raised for mitochondrial toxicity resulting from NRTI exposure [96]. Although the possibility of mitochondria-related adverse events continues to be investigated, the potential events seem to be at least very rare or subtle and do not outweigh the benefits of ART for prevention of vertical transmission and maternal health [83]. However, it will be important to continue to search for drug regimens that have the best possible safety profile.

Perinatal exposure to maternal HIV also seems to affect the immune system of uninfected infants [97]. Compared with their HIV-unexposed peers, these exposed infants have lower CD4 T-cell counts and CD4 and CD8 T cells with increased markers of activation, differentiation, memory, and senescence [98,99], and dendritic cells and natural killer cells show dysfunctional responses in vitro [100–102]. These cellular changes might be triggered by in utero exposure to HIV proteins or subviral particles that are not capable of establishing a productive infection but can stimulate an immune response nonetheless. Alternatively, exposure to the hyperinflammatory cytokine milieu of a mother infected with HIV may trigger immune responses in these infants. HIV-exposed, uninfected infants have higher rates of hospitalization, treatment failure, and death from respiratory infections and sepsis than unexposed infants, likely as a result of these immune dysfunctions [103,104].

Prevention of behavioral human immunodeficiency virus transmission

New HIV infections of adolescents and young adults continue to occur, particularly among young MSM, despite years of interventions aimed to reduce sexual risk behavior [1]. Preexposure prophylaxis (PrEP) with ARV offers a biomedical prevention intervention shown to reduce HIV transmission [105]. Landmark studies showing that PrEP using a daily fixed dose of tenofovir/emtricitabine, provided in combination with behavioral counseling and condoms, substantially reduced the risk of HIV acquisition among MSM, heterosexual discordant couples, young African heterosexuals, and injecting drug users [105]. These studies led to an FDA indication for the use of tenofovir/emtricitabine for PrEP, and to CDC PrEP guidelines [106]. Efficacy has been shown to correlate highly with adherence, which was suboptimal in some randomized trials. An analysis of blood intracellular tenofovir diphosphate levels (which are correlated with the number of doses taken per week) found a 76% versus 96% reduction in HIV acquisition with 2 versus 4 doses per week, respectively [107]. Recent demonstration projects using open-label PrEP among adult MSM found a 78% retention in the program and more than 80% protective blood levels, suggesting that PrEP in clinical practice may be associated with acceptable adherence, at least among adult MSM [108]. For young MSM, Project PrEPare showed acceptability and feasibility of prescribing PrEP, although there are concerns regarding adherence [109]. A larger open-label study of PrEP in this population investigating safety and adherence is approaching completion. Evidence on which to base PrEP recommendation for young MSM is urgently needed for this high-risk group.

The continuum of care: treatment as prevention

The continuum of care (CoC) has become the dominant paradigm for assessment of outcomes related to both treatment and prevention in the United States and worldwide with incorporation into the National AIDS Strategy (https://www.aids.gov/federal-resources/national-hiv-aids-strategy/overview), supported by a presidential executive order (https://federalregister.gov/a/2013-17478), and into WHO guidance [65]. The concept of the CoC, a set of steps leading to successful HIV care, also referred to as the HIV treatment cascade, reached prominence in 2011 when Gardner and colleagues [110] estimated that only 19% of people living with HIV in the United States had achieved viral suppression. The cascade describes the proportion of individuals living with HIV at each step of a continuum leading to full suppression of plasma viremia (Fig. 6). In the optimal scenario, 100% of people living with HIV would achieve each step. Analysis of the proportion of a specified population at each step allows programs to determine where efforts are needed to increase success rates. These steps are necessary to improve the health of individual patients, but success on the CoC is also a prevention strategy [111]. The power of treatment as prevention became fully evident based on a large study among discordant couples living in Africa in whom there was a 96% decrease in transmission when the partners infected with HIV were treated with effective ART [112]. The CDC estimates that 91% of new infections in the United States result from people living with HIV who are either not diagnosed or are diagnosed but not engaged in care [111]. Thus, success in helping patients move through the CoC is a strategy to reduce HIV infections and improve the health of communities.

The CoC concept may be applied to particular patient populations and care systems at any level ranging from individual clinics to cross-continent populations. With respect to pediatric HIV, the CoC can be evaluated for pregnant women, children, and youth. There has been considerable progress on the cascade for pregnant women, with greater than 70% of pregnant women living with HIV globally receiving HIV treatment to prevent infant transmission [5]. Implementation of option B+ as described earlier has streamlined steps along the CoC and has been associated with increased enrollment in ART and shorter times to ART initiation [113]. However, there remain challenges in long-term retention, with a study in Malawi finding 17% LFTU at 6 months and the rate of LTFU higher among women started on ART for pregnancy versus for their own health [114]. The cascade statistics among perinatally infected children

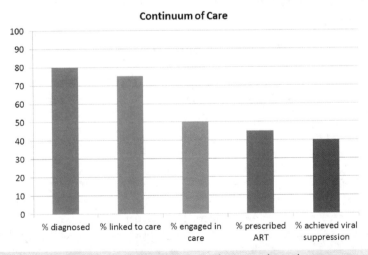

Fig. 6. The CoC, also known as the treatment cascade. Bars indicate the percentage of the total patients living with HIV who have achieved each step of the cascade; data are for illustrative purposes only.

have much room for improvement, with studies reporting only 33% to 63% of exposed infants receiving diagnostic testing in the early weeks of life [115]. After initiation of ART, retention in care among children in RLS was only 67% at 36 months in a large systematic review [116]. Leaders in the field recommend reconceptualizing the CoC for mothers and infants into 2 interlinked continua that include the step of maternal transfer from antenatal to adult care and use a stringent, combined outcome of both infant HIV-free survival and maternal sustained viral load suppression [117]. Adolescents with HIV are less likely to be engaged in care than either children or adults. A study of retention across 4 African countries found 48% LTFU among youth aged 15 to 24 years [118]. In the United States, the fraction of youth achieving the cascade milestones was low at every step [119]. Even among those in care, viral suppression was found in only 46% and 64% of perinatally and behaviorally infected youth [120]. It is clear that significant improvement and rigorous evaluation are needed to improve the CoC outcomes for mothers, children, and youth.

SUMMARY

HIV is now a chronic infection managed with ART, but ongoing inflammation despite viral suppression raises concerns for premature cardiovascular and other metabolic morbidities. Perinatal transmission has been significantly reduced, but gaps in the CoC result in ongoing transmission. Early diagnosis and recognition of acute infection is important for individual health and for prevention. Rare patients with sustained viral suppression without ART have spurred research into cure strategies informed by advances in understanding of virology and host immune responses. Much has been accomplished but much remains to be done.

References

[1] Centers for Disease Control and Prevention. HIV/AIDS. Available at: http://www.cdc.gov/hiv/statistics/index.html. Accessed December 13, 2015.

[2] Centers for Disease Control and Prevention. HIV surveillance report, 2015. vol. 26. 2015. Available at: http://www.cdc.gov/hiv/library/reports/surveillance/. Accessed December 29, 2015.

[3] Hall HI, Song R, Rhodes P, et al. Estimation of HIV incidence in the United States. JAMA 2008;300(5):520–9.

[4] Centers for Disease Control and Prevention. HIV surveillance report, 2013. vol. 25. 2015. Available at: http://www.cdc.gov/hiv/library/reports/surveillance/. Accessed December 19, 2015.

[5] World Health Organization. HIV/AIDS. Available at: www.who.int/hiv/. Accessed December 13, 2015.

[6] Weiss RA. Thirty years on: HIV receptor gymnastics and the prevention of infection. BMC Biol 2013;11:57.

[7] Brenchley JM, Schacker TW, Ruff LE, et al. CD4+ T cell depletion during all stages of HIV disease occurs predominantly in the gastrointestinal tract. J Exp Med 2004;200(6):749–59.

[8] Mehandru S, Poles MA, Tenner-Racz K, et al. Lack of mucosal immune reconstitution during prolonged treatment of acute and early HIV-1 infection. PLoS Med 2006;3(12):e484.

[9] Prendergast A, Prado JG, Kang YH, et al. HIV-1 infection is characterized by profound depletion of CD161+ Th17 cells and gradual decline in regulatory T cells. AIDS 2010;24(4):491–502.

[10] Dillon SM, Lee EJ, Kotter CV, et al. An altered intestinal mucosal microbiome in HIV-1 infection is associated with mucosal and systemic immune activation and endotoxemia. Mucosal Immunol 2014;7(4):983–94.

[11] Dinh DM, Volpe GE, Duffalo C, et al. Intestinal microbiota, microbial translocation, and systemic inflammation in chronic HIV infection. J Infect Dis 2015;211(1):19–27.

[12] Kanwar B, Favre D, McCune JM. Th17 and regulatory T cells: implications for AIDS pathogenesis. Curr Opin HIV AIDS 2010;5(2):151–7.

[13] Cummins NW, Badley AD. Making sense of how HIV kills infected CD4 T cells: implications for HIV cure. Mol Cell Ther 2014;2:20.

[14] Cummins NW, Badley AD. Mechanisms of HIV-associated lymphocyte apoptosis: 2010. Cell Death Dis 2010;1:e99.

[15] Doitsh G, Galloway NL, Geng X, et al. Cell death by pyroptosis drives CD4 T-cell depletion in HIV-1 infection. Nature 2014;505(7484):509–14.

[16] Beignon AS, McKenna K, Skoberne M, et al. Endocytosis of HIV-1 activates plasmacytoid dendritic cells via Toll-like receptor-viral RNA interactions. J Clin Invest 2005;115(11):3265–75.

[17] Alter G, Heckerman D, Schneidewind A, et al. HIV-1 adaptation to NK-cell-mediated immune pressure. Nature 2011;476(7358):96–100.

[18] Ndhlovu ZM, Kamya P, Mewalal N, et al. Magnitude and kinetics of CD8+ T cell activation during hyperacute HIV infection impact viral set point. Immunity 2015;43(3):591–604.

[19] Appay V, Rowland-Jones SL. Premature ageing of the immune system: the cause of AIDS? Trends Immunol 2002;23(12):580–5.

[20] Effros RB, Cai Z, Linton PJ. CD8 T cells and aging. Crit Rev Immunol 2003;23(1–2):45–64.

[21] Moir S, Fauci AS. B-cell exhaustion in HIV infection: the role of immune activation. Curr Opin HIV AIDS 2014;9(5):472–7.

[22] De Milito A, Nilsson A, Titanji K, et al. Mechanisms of hypergammaglobulinemia and impaired antigen-specific humoral immunity in HIV-1 infection. Blood 2004;103(6):2180–6.

[23] Younas M, Psomas C, Reynes J, et al. Immune activation in the course of HIV-1 infection: Causes, phenotypes and persistence under therapy. HIV Med 2015;17(2):89–105.

[24] Deeks SG, Walker BD. Human immunodeficiency virus controllers: mechanisms of durable virus control in the absence of antiretroviral therapy. Immunity 2007;27(3):406–16.

[25] Migueles SA, Sabbaghian MS, Shupert WL, et al. HLA B*5701 is highly associated with restriction of virus replication in a subgroup of HIV-infected long term nonprogressors. Proc Natl Acad Sci U S A 2000;97(6):2709–14.

[26] Martin MP, Gao X, Lee JH, et al. Epistatic interaction between KIR3DS1 and HLA-B delays the progression to AIDS. Nat Genet 2002;31(4):429–34.

[27] Migueles SA, Connors M. Success and failure of the cellular immune response against HIV-1. Nat Immunol 2015;16(6):563–70.

[28] Hunt PW, Brenchley J, Sinclair E, et al. Relationship between T cell activation and CD4+ T cell count in HIV-seropositive individuals with undetectable plasma HIV RNA levels in the absence of therapy. J Infect Dis 2008;197(1):126–33.

[29] Archin NM, Sung JM, Garrido C, et al. Eradicating HIV-1 infection: seeking to clear a persistent pathogen. Nat Rev Microbiol 2014;12(11):750–64.

[30] International Aids Society Scientific Working Group on HIV Cure. Towards an HIV cure: a global scientific strategy. Nat Rev Immunol 2012;12(8):607–14.

[31] Williams JP, Hurst J, Stohr W, et al. HIV-1 DNA predicts disease progression and post-treatment virological control. ELife 2014;3:e03821.

[32] Persaud D, Gay H, Ziemniak C, et al. Absence of detectable HIV-1 viremia after treatment cessation in an infant. N Engl J Med 2013;369(19):1828–35.

[33] Luzuriaga K, Gay H, Ziemniak C, et al. Viremic relapse after HIV-1 remission in a perinatally infected child. N Engl J Med 2015;372(8):786–8.

[34] Persaud D, Patel K, Karalius B, et al. Influence of age at virologic control on peripheral blood human immunodeficiency virus reservoir size and serostatus in perinatally infected adolescents. JAMA Pediatr 2014;168(12):1138–46.

[35] Saez-Cirion A, Bacchus C, Hocqueloux L, et al. Post-treatment HIV-1 controllers with a long-term virological remission after the interruption of early initiated antiretroviral therapy ANRS VISCONTI Study. PLoS Pathog 2013;9(3):e1003211.

[36] Rainwater-Lovett K, Uprety P, Persaud D. Advances and hope for perinatal HIV remission and cure in children and adolescents. Curr Opin Pediatr 2016;28(1):86–92.

[37] Hutter G, Nowak D, Mossner M, et al. Long-term control of HIV by CCR5 Delta32/Delta32 stem-cell transplantation. N Engl J Med 2009;360(7):692–8.

[38] Henrich TJ, Hanhauser E, Marty FM, et al. Antiretroviral-free HIV-1 remission and viral rebound after allogeneic stem cell transplantation: report of 2 cases. Ann Intern Med 2014;161(5):319–27.

[39] Garcia F, Leon A, Gatell JM, et al. Therapeutic vaccines against HIV infection. Hum Vaccin Immunother 2012;8(5):569–81.

[40] Stephenson KE, Barouch DH. Broadly neutralizing antibodies for HIV eradication. Curr HIV/AIDS Rep 2016;13(1):31–7.

[41] Varela-Rohena A, Molloy PE, Dunn SM, et al. Control of HIV-1 immune escape by CD8 T cells expressing enhanced T-cell receptor. Nat Med 2008;14(12):1390–5.

[42] Tebas P, Stein D, Tang WW, et al. Gene editing of CCR5 in autologous CD4 T cells of persons infected with HIV. N Engl J Med 2014;370(10):901–10.

[43] Centers for Disease Control and Prevention. Revised surveillance case definition for HIV infection—United States, 2014. MMWR Recomm Rep 2014;63(RR–03):1–10.

[44] Ivy W 3rd, Dominguez KL, Rakhmanina NY, et al. Premastication as a route of pediatric HIV transmission: case-control and cross-sectional investigations. J Acquir Immune Defic Syndr 2012;59(2):207–12.

[45] Centers for Disease Control and Prevention and Association of Public Health Laboratories. Laboratory testing for the diagnosis of HIV infection: updated recommendations. 2014. Available at: http://dx.doi.org/10.15620/cdc.23447. Accessed December 17, 2015.

[46] Steingrover R, Garcia EF, van Valkengoed IG, et al. Transient lowering of the viral set point after temporary antiretroviral therapy of primary HIV type 1 infection. AIDS Res Hum Retroviruses 2010;26(4):379–87.

[47] Buzon MJ, Martin-Gayo E, Pereyra F, et al. Long-term antiretroviral treatment initiated at primary HIV-1 infection affects the size, composition, and decay kinetics of the reservoir of HIV-1-infected CD4 T cells. J Virol 2014;88(17):10056–65.

[48] Kearney MF, Spindler J, Shao W, et al. Lack of detectable HIV-1 molecular evolution during suppressive antiretroviral therapy. PLoS Pathog 2014;10(3):e1004010.

[49] INSIGHT START Study Group, Lundgren JD, Babiker AG, Gordin F, et al. Initiation of antiretroviral therapy in early asymptomatic HIV Infection. N Engl J Med 2015;373(9):795–807.

[50] Richey LE, Halperin J. Acute human immunodeficiency virus infection. Am J Med Sci 2013;345(2):136–42.

[51] Patel K, Hernan MA, Williams PL, et al. Long-term effectiveness of highly active antiretroviral therapy on the survival of children and adolescents with HIV infection: a 10-year follow-up study. Clin Infect Dis 2008;46(4):507–15.

[52] Tseng A, Seet J, Phillips EJ. The evolution of three decades of antiretroviral therapy: challenges, triumphs and the promise of the future. Br J Clin Pharmacol 2015;79(2):182–94.

[53] Panel on Antiretroviral Therapy and Medical Management of HIV Infected Children. Guidelines for the use of antiretroviral agents in pediatric HIV infections. 2015. Available at: https://aidsinfo.nih.gov/guidelines/html/2/pediatric-treatment-guidelines/0#. Accessed February 16, 2016.

[54] Nachman S, Zheng N, Acosta EP, et al. Pharmacokinetics, safety, and 48-week efficacy of oral raltegravir in HIV-1-infected children aged 2 through 18 years. Clin Infect Dis 2014;58(3):413–22.

[55] Flynn P, Komar S, Blanche S, et al. Efficacy and safety of darunavir/ritonavir at 48 weeks in treatment-naive, HIV-1-infected adolescents: results from a phase 2 open-label trial (DI-ONE). Pediatr Infect Dis J 2014;33(9):940–5.

[56] Rutstein RM, Samson P, Fenton T, et al. Long-term safety and efficacy of atazanavir-based therapy in HIV-infected infants, children and adolescents: the Pediatric AIDS Clinical Trials Group Protocol 1020A. Pediatr Infect Dis J 2015;34(2):162–7.

[57] Violari A, Cotton MF, Gibb DM, et al. Early antiretroviral therapy and mortality among HIV-infected infants. N Engl J Med 2008;359(21):2233–44.

[58] Penazzato M, Prendergast A, Tierney J, et al. Effectiveness of antiretroviral therapy in HIV-infected children under 2 years of age. Cochrane Database Syst Rev 2012;(7):CD004772.

[59] Dunn D, Woodburn P, Duong T, et al. Current CD4 cell count and the short-term risk of AIDS and death before the availability of effective antiretroviral therapy in HIV-infected children and adults. J Infect Dis 2008;197(3):398–404.

[60] Puthanakit T, Saphonn V, Ananworanich J, et al. Early versus deferred antiretroviral therapy for children older than 1 year infected with HIV (PREDICT): a multicentre, randomised, open-label trial. Lancet Infect Dis 2012;12(12):933–41.

[61] Sturt AS, Halpern MS, Sullivan B, et al. Timing of antiretroviral therapy initiation and its impact on disease progression in perinatal human immunodeficiency virus-1 infection. Pediatr Infect Dis J 2012;31(1):53–60.

[62] Picat MQ, Lewis J, Musiime V, et al. Predicting patterns of long-term CD4 reconstitution in HIV-infected children starting antiretroviral therapy in sub-Saharan Africa: a cohort-based modelling study. PLoS Med 2013;10(10):e1001542.

[63] Panel on Antiretroviral Guidelines for Adults and Adolescents. Guidelines for the use of antiretroviral agents in HIV-1-infected adults and adolescents. 2016. Available at: https://aidsinfo.nih.gov/guidelines/html/1/adult-and-adolescent-treatment-guidelines/0. Accessed February 16, 2016.

[64] Danel C, Moh R, Gabillard D, et al. A trial of early antiretrovirals and isoniazid preventive therapy in Africa. N Engl J Med 2015;373(9):808–22.

[65] World Health Organization. Guideline on when to start antiretroviral therapy and on pre-exposure prophylaxis. 2015. Available at: http://apps.who.int/iris/bitstream/10665/186275/1/9789241509565_eng.pdf. Accessed February 13, 2016.

[66] Fortuny C, Deya-Martinez A, Chiappini E, et al. Metabolic and renal adverse effects of antiretroviral therapy in HIV-infected children and adolescents. Pediatr Infect Dis J 2015;34(5 Suppl 1):S36–43.

[67] Puthanakit T, Siberry GK. Bone health in children and adolescents with perinatal HIV infection. J Int AIDS Soc 2013;16:18575.

[68] van Leth F, Phanuphak P, Stroes E, et al. Nevirapine and efavirenz elicit different changes in lipid profiles in antiretroviral-therapy-naive patients infected with HIV-1. PLoS Med 2004;1(1):e19.

[69] Tungsiripat M, Kitch D, Glesby MJ, et al. A pilot study to determine the impact on dyslipidemia of adding tenofovir to stable background antiretroviral therapy: ACTG 5206. AIDS 2010;24(11):1781–4.

[70] Post WS, Budoff M, Kingsley L, et al. Associations between HIV infection and subclinical coronary atherosclerosis. Ann Intern Med 2014;160(7):458–67.

[71] Islam FM, Wu J, Jansson J, et al. Relative risk of cardiovascular disease among people living with HIV: a systematic review and meta-analysis. HIV Med 2012;13(8):453–68.

[72] Kuller LH, Tracy R, Belloso W, et al. Inflammatory and coagulation biomarkers and mortality in patients with HIV infection. PLoS Med 2008;5(10):e203.

[73] Bavinger C, Bendavid E, Niehaus K, et al. Risk of cardiovascular disease from antiretroviral therapy for HIV: a systematic review. PLoS One 2013;8(3):e59551.

[74] Arildsen H, Sorensen KE, Ingerslev JM, et al. Endothelial dysfunction, increased inflammation, and activated coagulation in HIV-infected patients improve after initiation of highly active antiretroviral therapy. HIV Med 2013;14(1):1–9.

[75] Patel K, Wang J, Jacobson DL, et al. Aggregate risk of cardiovascular disease among adolescents perinatally infected with the human immunodeficiency virus. Circulation 2014;129(11):1204–12.

[76] Mikhail IJ, Purdy JB, Dimock DS, et al. High rate of coronary artery abnormalities in adolescents and young adults infected with human immunodeficiency virus early in life. Pediatr Infect Dis J 2011;30(8):710–2.

[77] Sainz T, Alvarez-Fuente M, Navarro ML, et al. Subclinical atherosclerosis and markers of immune activation in HIV-infected children and adolescents: the CaroVIH Study. J Acquir Immune Defic Syndr 2014;65(1):42–9.

[78] Miller TL, Borkowsky W, DiMeglio LA, et al. Metabolic abnormalities and viral replication are associated with biomarkers of vascular dysfunction in HIV-infected children. HIV Med 2012;13(5):264–75.

[79] Siberry GK, Li H, Jacobson D. Fracture risk by HIV infection status in perinatally HIV-exposed children. AIDS Res Hum Retroviruses 2012;28(3):247–50.

[80] Guerri-Fernandez R, Vestergaard P, Carbonell C, et al. HIV infection is strongly associated with hip fracture risk, independently of age, gender, and comorbidities: a population-based cohort study. J Bone Miner Res 2013;28(6):1259–63.

[81] Santos CP, Felipe YX, Braga PE, et al. Self-perception of body changes in persons living with HIV/AIDS: prevalence and associated factors. AIDS 2005;19(Suppl 4):S14–21.

[82] Cherry CL, Nolan D, James IR, et al. Tissue-specific associations between mitochondrial DNA levels and current treatment status in HIV-infected individuals. J Acquir Immune Defic Syndr 2006;42(4):435–40.

[83] Panel on Treatment of HIV Infected Pregnant Women and Prevention of Perinatal Transmission. Recommendations for use of antiretroviral drugs in pregnant HIV-1-infected women for maternal health and interventions to reduce perinatal HIV transmission in the United States. Available at: http://aidsinfo.nih.gov/contentfiles/lvguidelines/PerinatalGL.pdf. Accessed February 13, 2016.

[84] Townsend CL, Byrne L, Cortina-Borja M, et al. Earlier initiation of ART and further decline in mother-to-child HIV transmission rates, 2000-2011. AIDS 2014;28(7):1049–57.

[85] Mofenson LM. Antiretroviral drugs to prevent breastfeeding HIV transmission. Antivir Ther 2010;15(4):537–53.

[86] Kuhn L, Aldrovandi GM, Sinkala M, et al. Effects of early, abrupt weaning on HIV-free survival of children in Zambia. N Engl J Med 2008;359(2):130–41.

[87] Fowler MG, Qin M, Fiscus SA, et al. Promise: efficacy and safety of 2 strategies to prevent perinatal HIV transmission. Seattle (WA): CROI; 2015 [Abstract 31LB].

[88] World Health Organization. Consolidated guidelines on the use of antiretroviral drugs for treating and preventing HIV infection: recommendations for a public health approach. 2013. Available at: http://apps.who.int/iris/bitstream/10665/85321/1/9789241505727_eng.pdf?ua=1. Accessed February 16, 2016.

[89] Ford N, Mofenson L, Shubber Z, et al. Safety of efavirenz in the first trimester of pregnancy: an updated systematic review and meta-analysis. AIDS 2014;28(Suppl 2):S123–31.

[90] Chen JY, Ribaudo HJ, Souda S, et al. Highly active antiretroviral therapy and adverse birth outcomes among HIV-infected women in Botswana. J Infect Dis 2012;206(11):1695–705.

[91] Jao J, Abrams EJ. Metabolic complications of in utero maternal HIV and antiretroviral exposure in HIV-exposed infants. Pediatr Infect Dis J 2014;33(7):734–40.

[92] Papp E, Mohammadi H, Loutfy MR, et al. HIV protease inhibitor use during pregnancy is associated with decreased progesterone levels, suggesting a potential mechanism contributing to fetal growth restriction. J Infect Dis 2015;211(1):10–8.

[93] Williams PL, Crain MJ, Yildirim C, et al. Congenital anomalies and in utero antiretroviral exposure in human immunodeficiency virus-exposed uninfected infants. JAMA Pediatr 2015;169(1):48–55.

[94] Knapp KM, Brogly SB, Muenz DG, et al. Prevalence of congenital anomalies in infants with in utero exposure to antiretrovirals. Pediatr Infect Dis J 2012;31(2):164–70.

[95] Brogly SB, Abzug MJ, Watts DH, et al. Birth defects among children born to human immunodeficiency virus-infected women: pediatric AIDS clinical trials protocols 219 and 219C. Pediatr Infect Dis J 2010;29(8):721–7.

[96] Williams PL, Hazra R, Van Dyke RB, et al. Antiretroviral exposure during pregnancy and adverse outcomes in HIV-exposed uninfected infants and children using a trigger-based design. AIDS 2016;30(1):133–44.

[97] Mofenson LM. Editorial commentary: New challenges in the elimination of pediatric HIV infection: the expanding population of HIV-exposed but uninfected children. Clin Infect Dis 2015;60(9):1357–60.

[98] Miles DJ, Gadama L, Gumbi A, et al. Human immunodeficiency virus (HIV) infection during pregnancy induces CD4 T-cell differentiation and modulates responses to Bacille Calmette-Guerin (BCG) vaccine in HIV-uninfected infants. Immunology 2010;129(3):446–54.

[99] Ono E, Nunes dos Santos AM, de Menezes Succi RC, et al. Imbalance of naive and memory T lymphocytes with sustained high cellular activation during the first year of life from uninfected children born to HIV-1-infected mothers on HAART. Braz J Med Biol Res 2008;41(8):700–8.

[100] Reikie BA, Adams RC, Leligdowicz A, et al. Altered innate immune development in HIV-exposed uninfected infants. J Acquir Immune Defic Syndr 2014;66(3):245–55.

[101] Velilla PA, Montoya CJ, Hoyos A, et al. Effect of intrauterine HIV-1 exposure on the frequency and function of uninfected newborns' dendritic cells. Clin Immunol 2008;126(3): 243–50.

[102] Smith C, Jalbert E, de Almeida V, et al, for the NISDI-LILAC Protocol. Natural killer cell dysfunction in HIV-exposed uninfected infants. IDWeek 2015 [abstract 51621].

[103] Slogrove A, Reikie B, Naidoo S, et al. HIV-exposed uninfected infants are at increased risk for severe infections in the first year of life. J Trop Pediatr 2012;58(6):505–8.

[104] Kelly MS, Wirth KE, Steenhoff AP, et al. Treatment failures and excess mortality among HIV-exposed, uninfected children with pneumonia. J Pediatr Infect Dis Soc 2015;4(4): e117–26.

[105] Krakower DS, Jain S, Mayer KH. Antiretrovirals for primary HIV prevention: the current status of pre- and post-exposure prophylaxis. Curr HIV/AIDS Rep 2015;12(1):127–38.

[106] Smith DK, Koenig LJ, Martin M, et al. Preexposure prophylaxis for the prevention of HIV infection in the United States –2014 clinical practice guideline. 2014. Available at: http://stacks.cdc.gov/view/cdc/23109#jump-here. Accessed April 30, 2016.

[107] Anderson PL, Glidden DV, Liu A, et al. Emtricitabine-tenofovir concentrations and pre-exposure prophylaxis efficacy in men who have sex with men. Sci Transl Med 2012;4(151):151ra125.

[108] Liu AY, Cohen SE, Vittinghoff E, et al. Preexposure prophylaxis for HIV infection integrated with municipal- and community-based sexual health services. JAMA Intern Med 2016;176(1):75–84.

[109] Hosek SG, Siberry G, Bell M, et al. The acceptability and feasibility of an HIV preexposure prophylaxis (PrEP) trial with young men who have sex with men. J Acquir Immune Defic Syndr 2013;62(4):447–56.

[110] Gardner EM, McLees MP, Steiner JF, et al. The spectrum of engagement in HIV care and its relevance to test-and-treat strategies for prevention of HIV infection. Clin Infect Dis 2011;52(6):793–800.

[111] Skarbinski J, Rosenberg E, Paz-Bailey G, et al. Human immunodeficiency virus transmission at each step of the care continuum in the United States. JAMA Intern Med 2015;175(4):588–96.

[112] Cohen MS, Chen YQ, McCauley M, et al. Prevention of HIV-1 infection with early antiretroviral therapy. N Engl J Med 2011;365(6):493–505.

[113] Kim MH, Ahmed S, Hosseinipour MC, et al. Implementation and operational research: the impact of option B+ on the antenatal PMTCT cascade in Lilongwe, Malawi. J Acquir Immune Defic Syndr 2015;68(5):e77–83.

[114] Tenthani L, Haas AD, Tweya H, et al. Retention in care under universal antiretroviral therapy for HIV-infected pregnant and breastfeeding women ('Option B+') in Malawi. AIDS 2014;28(4):589–98.

[115] Feinstein L, Edmonds A, Okitolonda V, et al. Implementation and operational research: maternal combination antiretroviral therapy is associated with improved retention of HIV-exposed infants in Kinshasa, Democratic Republic of Congo. J Acquir Immune Defic Syndr 2015;69(3):e93–9.

[116] Fox MP, Rosen S. Systematic review of retention of pediatric patients on HIV treatment in low and middle-income countries 2008-2013. AIDS 2015;29(4):493–502.

[117] McNairy ML, Teasdale CA, El-Sadr WM, et al. Mother and child both matter: reconceptualizing the prevention of mother-to-child transmission care continuum. Curr Opin HIV AIDS 2015;10(6):403–10.

[118] Lamb MR, Fayorsey R, Nuwagaba-Biribonwoha H, et al. High attrition before and after ART initiation among youth (15-24 years of age) enrolled in HIV care. AIDS 2014;28(4): 559–68.

[119] Zanoni BC, Mayer KH. The adolescent and young adult HIV cascade of care in the United States: exaggerated health disparities. AIDS Patient Care STDs 2014;28(3):128–35.

[120] Kahana SY, Fernandez MI, Wilson PA, et al. Rates and correlates of antiretroviral therapy use and virologic suppression among perinatally and behaviorally HIV-infected youth linked to care in the United States. J Acquir Immune Defic Syndr 2015;68(2):169–77.

Advances in Pediatrics 63 (2016) 173–194

ADVANCES IN PEDIATRICS

Chronic Hepatitis C Infection in Children

Yen H. Pham, MD[a],*, Philip Rosenthal, MD[b]

[a]Texas Children's Hospital, Baylor College of Medicine, 18200 Katy Freeway, Suite 250, Houston, TX 77094, USA; [b]UCSF Benioff Children's Hospital, University of California San Francisco, 550 16th Street, 5th Floor, San Francisco, CA 94143, USA

Keywords

- Hepatitis C virus • Chronic hepatitis C • Children • Treatment
- Pegylated interferon • Ribavirin • Direct-acting antivirals

Key points

- Perinatal transmission is now the most common mode of hepatitis C virus (HCV) infection in children in developed countries.
- Spontaneous resolution may occur, but most children progress to chronic hepatitis C infection.
- Severe liver disease and hepatocellular carcinoma are uncommon in children, but have been reported.
- In anticipation of new interferon-free regimen with direct acting antivirals, it is reasonable to defer treatment in children with clinically stable disease.

INTRODUCTION

Chronic infection with the hepatitis C virus (HCV) is a major health problem globally. It is estimated to affect more than 180 million individuals worldwide [1,2]. The majority of children infected with the virus will go on to develop chronic hepatitis C (CHC) and are at risk for developing HCV-related complications including cirrhosis, liver cancer, and death. HCV in the pediatric population differs from adults in its modes of transmission, rates of clearance, progression of fibrosis, and duration of potential chronic infection when acquired at birth. The presence of severe liver disease and hepatocellular

Disclosures: Y.H. Pham reports no relevant financial disclosures. P. Rosenthal reports associations with AbbVie, Bristol-Myers Squibb, Genentech/Roche, Gilead, Merck, and Vertex.

*Corresponding author. *E-mail address:* Yen.Pham@bcm.edu

0065-3101/16/$ – see front matter
http://dx.doi.org/10.1016/j.yapd.2016.04.019

carcinoma (HCC) in children is less common than in adults, but HCV infection in children is not entirely benign, with reports of decompensated cirrhosis in young children with CHC. Children with HCV infection also have impaired quality of life, developmental delay, learning disorders, and cognitive deficits [3–6]. Despite advances in the understanding of the virology and natural history of CHC in children, the current recommended treatment regimen for children has an undesirable side effect profile and less than ideal cure rate. New therapies with significantly better cure rates with safer side effect profiles have been developed and approved for adults with CHC, which will hopefully prove to be just as efficacious and safe in children in the near future.

EPIDEMIOLOGY
Reports from 87 countries estimate the total global anti-HCV prevalence to be 1.6% (range, 1.3%–2.1%) [1,2] with approximately 3 to 4 million new cases and 350,000 deaths every year owing to HCV-related disorders [1,2]. Hepatitis C affects more than 4 million people in the United States. An estimation of the prevalence of HCV infection in children varies from 0.05% to 0.36% in the United States and Europe, and up to 1.8% to 5.8% in some developing countries [7]. In the United States, approximately 0.1% to 2% children are affected by the virus [8]. CHC is estimated to affect 23,000 to 46,000 children in the United States, with approximately 7500 new cases every year from vertical transmission. There is a 26-fold increased risk of liver-related death associated with CHC acquired in childhood [9]. The 10-year costs associated with HCV in children is estimated to be $199 to $336 million [10], contributing to a significant economic and health burden in the United States and worldwide.

VIROLOGY AND PATHOGENESIS
HCV is a single-stranded, positive sense RNA virus of the *Flaviviridae* family, a hepacivirus genus that was discovered in 1989. There are 6 recognized genotypes identified by numbers 1 to 6 and as many as 100 subtypes identified by lower-case letters. Genotypes vary in geographic distribution, and confer varying metabolic effects and susceptibility to antiviral drugs [11]. The most common, genotype 1, has worldwide distribution but predominates in North America (HCV 1a) and Europe (HCV 1b). Genotypes 2 and 3 also have a worldwide distribution, whereas genotype 4 is predominantly in North Africa and the Middle East, 5 in South Africa, and 6 in Asia [7].

Approximately 10^{10} to 10^{12} viral genomes are produced each day in a chronically infected person. Viral genomes encode 9 proteins, including their own RNA polymerase. This process is greatly error prone, leading to many variant viruses known as "quasispecies," providing HCV with a survival advantage. Variation in the composition of an individual's quasispecies leads to variation in the natural history of an individual's liver disease [12].

Other factors have also been found to affect an individual's disease progression. The 2 genes DDX5 and CPT1A are associated with increased susceptibility to liver fibrosis in adults with CHC [13]. Various other genes related to

HCV clearance or persistence are being studied [14]. Infants with HLA DR13 are significantly less likely to develop CHC after mother-to-infant transmission [15], and additional HLA loci may influence disease transmission [16,17]. Infants with Rs12979860 CC genotype for the interleukin (IL) 28B polymorphism may also be more likely to have spontaneous resolution of their vertical HCV infection [18].

The pattern of clinical presentation associated with the virus varies, and differs between children and adults. Acute hepatitis C infection is frequently asymptomatic and usually not identified in children. Fulminant hepatitis C is uncommon in children. Patients acutely infected with HCV should be monitored for up to 2 months for spontaneous resolution before treatment is considered.

Neonates born to HCV-infected mothers can have transient perinatal viremia (HCV RNA detected in peripheral blood within 0–5 days of birth) [19,20]. Persistent neonatal HCV infection is defined as having a detectable serum HCV RNA in the first 1 to 6 months of life, usually in the setting of maternal-to-infant transmission of the virus. Spontaneous resolution of CHC (2 negative RNA tests $\geq$6 months apart) may occur spontaneously or with treatment [21]. The majority of children go on to develop CHC. The definition of CHC, having evidence of active viral infection with detectable RNA for at least 6 months is the same in children and adults. This designation implies ongoing liver injury.

TRANSMISSION

HCV is transmitted via contaminated blood or body fluids. HCV infection previously accounted for the majority of transfusion-associated hepatitis cases. The risk of acquiring HCV infection by transfusion of blood or blood products is now negligible owing to stringent screening protocols [22]. Vertical transmission has become the most common cause of HCV infection among children in developed countries.

The prevalence of CHC among pregnant women (both anti-HCV and HCV RNA positive during pregnancy) is approximately 0.75% (0.49%–1.7%) [23–29]. The risk of vertical transmission is estimated at approximately 5% (3%–10%), 1.7% per pregnancy if mother had detectable anti-HCV antibodies, 4.3% if detectable HCV RNA, and 7.1% if mother tested positive for HCV RNA at least twice during pregnancy or around time of delivery [30]. There is a small risk even if RNA levels are undetectable (presumably because viral load can vary during pregnancy) [31,32]. Concomitant human immunodeficiency virus (HIV) infection increases the risk of transmission by 2- to 3-fold [30]. We currently do not have methods to prevent vertical transmission of HCV infection other than early identification and effective treatment in young women before conception. Recent advances in newer direct-acting antivirals with safe side effect profiles may lead to development of a regimen to prevent the transmission of HCV infection from mother to child.

During pregnancy, various components of the innate immune system such as natural killer and T cells, operate within the placenta to eradicate HCV [33]. It is not known exactly when transmission of the virus takes place, but several factors have been shown to affect the risk of HCV transmission [34]. High viral load (>600,000 IU/mL) favors transmission [35–38], and internal monitoring of the fetus (fetal scalp vein monitoring), episiotomies, prolonged rupture, and fetal anoxia around time of delivery (indicated by decreased cord blood pH) may enhance transmission [19,32,37,39]. It is not certain whether amniocentesis is associated with an increased risk of transmission [40,41]. Interestingly, elective cesarean section has not been found to consistently reduce the rate of transmission, but attention to avoiding large tears with vaginal delivery is recommended. Similarly, breast feeding does not promote transmission, but mothers may want to avoid breastfeeding if there is bleeding at the nipples, mastitis, or flare of hepatitis with jaundice postpartum [30,32,37,42,43].

The second most common route of transmission in children, mainly in adolescents, is intravenous drug use with sharing of contaminated needles. Tattooing and body piercing are potential modes, although the risk is not increased if done at a reputable tattoo store. There is an extremely small risk with household contact (<2%), and the risk associated with sexual intercourse in a stable relationship is negligible [44–47]. Recommendations for HCV screening in children are summarized in (Box 1).

NATURAL HISTORY

Perinatally acquired HCV infections can have several patterns of outcomes. Spontaneous resolution of the infection can be seen in very early infancy,

---

Box 1: Children for whom screening is recommended

Children who are or were IV drug users (even if only once in past)

Children with HIV infection

Children who have ever been on dialysis

Children with unexplained or chronically elevated aminotransferase levels

Children born to HCV-infected mothers

Sexual partners of an HCV-infected person

Children from region with high prevalence of HCV infection

Abbreviations: HCV, hepatitis C virus; HIV, human immunodeficiency virus; IV, intravenous.

Adapted from Recommendations for prevention and control of hepatitis C virus (HCV) infection and HCV-related chronic disease. Centers for disease control and prevention. MMWR Recomm Rep 1998;47(RR-19):1–39; and Mack CL, Gonzalez-Peralta RP, Gupta N, et al. NASPGHAN practice guidelines: diagnosis and management of hepatitis C infection in infants, children, and adolescents J Pediatr Gastroenterol Nutr 2012;54(6):838–55.

which some authors may refer to as resolution of neonatal acute hepatitis C infection or transient perinatal viremia [19,20,32,48,49]. The rate of spontaneous resolution in infants is 25% to 40%, and is lower in older children, at 6% to 12% [21,44,50,51]. Spontaneous resolution can occur up to 7 to 8 years, but is rare after 3 years of age [21,44,52,53].

The majority of children go on to develop CHC (54%–86%) [7]. Children with CHC generally seem to be well clinically, with normal or near normal serum aminotransferases and little inflammation on biopsy [54]. Only 14% are mildly symptomatic [44]. CHC in children is usually a slowly progressing disease with accumulating liver damage. The degree of liver injury generally correlates with age and duration of infection [55–57]. Cirrhosis occurs in children rarely, and is found in only 1% to 2% of liver biopsies from children with CHC. Liver transplantation is rarely needed for CHC in children. From 1988 to 2009, 133 children were transplanted for chronic liver failure owing to CHC in the United States. There have only been a handful of cases of HCC in children with CHC [58,59]. However, CHC in children is not entirely benign. Bridging fibrosis can be found in 12% of biopsies [60,61], and there have been reports of decompensated cirrhosis in children as young as 4 to 11 years old [53,62]. Furthermore, HCC has been reported in adults with HCV in the absence of cirrhosis [63,64].

Various biological factors have been found to affect the natural history of CHC in children and adolescents. Patients with HCV genotype 3 and infants with higher alanine aminotransferase levels in the first 2 years of life may be more likely to clear spontaneously [53,65]. Individuals with the favorable IL-28B single nucleotide polymorphism CC rs12979860 have been shown in several studies to have an increased chance of spontaneous clearance or sustained virologic response (SVR) achievement. This association is better appreciated for genotypes 1 and 4 than for genotypes 2 and 3, and does not seem relevant when considering treatment with new direct-acting antiviral regimens [18]. Certain medical conditions are associated with increased risk of more severe disease, including obesity, survivors of childhood cancer, congenital anemias requiring chronic transfusions, and coinfection with HIV or hepatitis B virus (HBV) infection [56,66,67].

Social factors may also affect the disease progression. Risky behaviors such as intravenous drug use and alcohol use are associated with more severe disease. Homeless and incarcerated teens are at increased risk for poor outcomes [68–72].

Regression of cirrhosis after treatment has been reported in adults with CHC. Adult studies also report extrahepatic disorders such as glomerulonephritis (typically membranoproliferative), which may occur in children with CHC. Lymphoma has not been reported in children. HCV infection in the central nervous system has been shown to cause cognitive impairment in some adults [73]. Children with HCV infection have impaired quality of life, developmental delay, learning disorders, and cognitive deficits [3–6].

DIAGNOSIS AND TESTING

Diagnosis of HCV infection is determined by immunoassays and RNA polymerase chain reaction assays. Antibody-based (immunoglobulin [Ig]G) assays have the benefit of being inexpensive, automated, and easy to perform with low variability. Later generations of enzyme immunoassays can be performed on plasma or serum, and uses recombinant antigens from core (c22) and nonstructural proteins 3 (c33), 4 (c100), and 5 with specificity and sensitivity in patients with chronic liver disease owing to HCV infection greater than 98% and 97%, respectively [74]. Unfortunately, antibody-based tests cannot distinguish acute from chronic infection. These enzyme immunoassays generally become positive about 6 to 8 weeks after acquisition of infection. Anti-HCV IgG antibodies are usually negative during the acute phase, when only HCV RNA can be used to detect infection [75]. Anti-HCV IgM is not useful for distinguishing between acute and chronic HCV infection, and measuring HCV IgM is not recommended. Quantitative HCV RNA by reverse transcription-polymerase chain reaction tests are now recommended for diagnosis in patients with positive anti-HCV antibody tests [76]. HCV RNA can be detected in serum or plasma as early as 1 to 2 weeks after exposure to the virus and weeks before antibody tests become positive or serum transaminases become elevated [75]. Determination of the HCV genotype is useful for prediction of likelihood of response to antiviral agents and determination of optimal duration of therapy.

In cases of vertical transmission, anti-HCV IgG crosses the placenta, making antibody testing not informative until 18 months of age. Infants at risk for vertical transmission of HCV infection should be tested for anti-HCV IgG at 18 months, followed by HCV RNA to determine active infection if the anti-HCV is positive. Before 18 months of age, RNA testing can be obtained at the request of families, but the patient should be at least 2 months of age. If RNA test is positive, it needs to be rechecked after 12 months of age to determine CHC [77,78]. Infants with detectable RNA should be monitored periodically for spontaneous viral clearance, which may occur in early childhood, particularly with genotype 3 [55].

Histologic findings in children are generally not as severe as in adults. In many children, liver biopsy shows no obvious histologic changes or only mild inflammation and fibrosis, although significant fibrosis or cirrhosis may occur [60]. Liver biopsy remains the gold standard for determining the degree of liver injury in CHC. However, it is generally not recommended for the diagnosis of HCV infection in children owing to the risk of complications. Liver biopsy may be considered if it may influence medical decision making (such as starting antiviral therapy), or to aid in the investigation of unexplained clinical hepatic decompensation in a previously stable patient with CHC. Some may elect to forgo the liver biopsy in genotypes 2 and 3 who have a high (>80%) probability of achieving virologic cure with current treatment [75,79].

Studies are underway to explore potential noninvasive tests for the assessment of hepatic fibrosis and inflammatory activity in CHC pediatric patients.

Preliminary data for FibroTest and ActiTest show limited prognostic potential [80–82]. Recent pediatric and adult studies looking at complement C4a and inter–alpha-trypsin inhibitor heavy chain 4 may be useful for the detection of significant fibrosis, but still have too many limitations to replace liver biopsies in practice [79,83–86].

In pediatric patients with CHC who are being followed without treatment, periodic evaluation and education are recommended. Serum RNA level, complete blood count with platelets, serum aminotransferases, bilirubin, albumin, and International Normalized Ratio (if cirrhosis is present) should be monitored. Although HCC is rare in children, it is generally recommended that abdominal ultrasound and serum alpha fetoprotein be considered yearly, especially if cirrhosis is present.

TREATMENT

The goal for treatment is to eradicate the virus, prevent disease progression and future complications, remove the stigma associated with HCV infection, and decrease the global burden of disease. An ideal treatment regimen would be one that would treat all genotypes, have as few side effects as possible, and be universally affordable.

Who needs treatment?

Liver disease in children with CHC has a slow progression with severe disease rarely seen. Treatment during childhood does not achieve a better response rate than in adults. Adverse events are frequent and can be severe in some cases. With the development of multiple treatment regimens with safe side effect profiles, shorter courses and higher cure rates in adults with CHC, it is reasonable to wait until adulthood or until these drugs are available to use in children. Children with persistently elevated enzymes and those with progressive diagnosis (fibrosis on history) may be considered for treatment. In adults, evidence of bridging fibrosis on biopsy is an important predictor of progression to cirrhosis, but this finding has not been confirmed in children [87–89]. Adolescents and young adults may be less compliant with medications, so treating at a younger age may achieve better compliance owing to caregiver's motivation.

Currently approved treatment in children

The current US Food and Drug Administration–approved treatment for HCV in children over the age of 3 years is the combination of weekly injections of pegylated interferon (IFN) and twice-daily oral ribavirin, with response to treatment similar to that seen in adults (Tables 1–2). Side effects of treatment are slightly better tolerated than in adults, but symptoms including fatigue, depression, irritability, or nausea almost invariably occur. IFN can also have effects on growth, weight loss, and neutropenia.

Systematic review with metaanalysis by El Sherbini and colleagues [90] of 23 peer-reviewed articles of single-center and large blinded multicenter studies show that combination treatment with pegylated INF-α in pediatric patients

Table 1
Definitions of virologic response

Rapid virologic response (RVR)	Undetectable HCV RNA (<50 IU/mL) after 4 wk of treatment
Early virologic response (EVR)	Undetectable or ≥ 2 $\log_{10}$ reduction in HCV after 12 wk of treatment
End-of-treatment response (ETR)	Undetectable HCV RNA (<50 IU/mL) at conclusion of treatment
Sustained virologic response (SVR)	Undetectable HCV RNA (<50 IU/mL) at 24 wk after end of treatment

with compensated CHC was superior in achieving SVR over INF-α alone [91–99]. SVR is seen in up to 30% to 50% of children with genotype 1 HCV after 48 weeks of treatment, and 80% in genotypes 2 and 3 with 24 weeks of treatment [90]. Higher response with genotype 2 and 3 and with lower viral load in genotype 1 (<600,000 IU/mL or $<2 \times 10^6$ copies/mL) have been observed [91,92,94].

The goal of treatment is to achieve SVR once treatment is discontinued. SVR is affected by genotype, age, viral load, fibrosis score, and compliance. Rapid virologic response is considered the strongest predictor of SVR. In pediatric CHC patients being treated with combination pegylated INF-α and ribavirin therapy, discontinuation of treatment is recommended if RNA does not become undetectable at 24 weeks. Continued treatment has not been shown to improve clinical outcome (cirrhosis, HCC, SVR) [100].

Interferon
INF-α is a cytokine with broad mechanism of action including increasing antigen presentation of viral peptides, stimulating action of CD8$^+$ T cells and natural killer cells, and inducing the synthesis of several key antiviral protein mediators. IFN can be pegylated by covalent attachment of a large molecule of polyethylene glycol to the recombinant INF-α. Pegylated INF-α carries a longer half-life with a better pharmacokinetic profile and better rate of virologic response [101–104]. Two pegylated INF-α have been approved by the US Food and Drug Administration for the treatment of CHC. Pegylated IFN-a-2b (PegIntron; Merck & Co, Inc, Whitehouse Station, NJ) contains a 12-kDa pegylated moiety with recommended dose 60 µg/m [2] weekly subcutaneous

Table 2
Recommended treatment regimen for CHC in children

Genotype	Duration	Regimen[a]	
1 and 4	48 wk	Ribavirin 15 mg/kg/d divided BID	AND Pegylated IFN-α-2a 180 µg/1.73 m^2 weekly OR Pegylated IFN-α-2b 60 µg/m^2 weekly
2 and 3	24 wk		

[a]Discontinue if RNA does not become undetectable at 24 wks.

injection. Pegylated IFN-α-2a (Pegasys; Genentech/Roche, San Francisco, CA) contains a larger, 40-kDa pegylated moiety, and recommended dose is 180 μg/ 1.73 m^2 to be given subcutaneously once a week. Multiple studies have not been able to demonstrate a significant difference in efficacy between the 2 formulations [105–108].

Ribavirin

Ribavirin is a guanosine analog that interferes with HCV RNA polymerase, leading to rapid and lethal mutations of virions and depletion of intracellular GTP, which is necessary for viral RNA synthesis [109–111]. The addition of ribavirin to INF-α dramatically improves the SVR and end-of-treatment response and decreases the relapse rate and development of viral resistance in adults and children with CHC [92,96,112,113].

Side effects

Several large multicenter trials have evaluated the safety and efficacy of combination pegylated INF-α and ribavirin for the treatment of CHC in children [90,92,94]. Constitutional symptoms are almost universal in children undergoing therapy and are described as "flulike." Symptoms including fever, fatigue, myalgia, arthralgia, headaches, and nausea are predominantly side effects of IFN-α. They are most severe within 24 hours of the IFN injection, and many will wane or resolve after the first few months of therapy [93,114] Children are susceptible to deficits in growth while on treatment. Both pegylated IFN-α and ribavirin can be associated with anorexia, nausea, weight loss, and reduction in height velocity, with most patients experiencing compensatory weight gain after completion of treatment. Dose adjustments may be needed for weight or a reduction in body mass index of 10% or more [94,115].

INF-α induces bone marrow suppression in approximately one-third of patients, as evidenced by a decrease in the total white blood cells and absolute neutrophil count, and to a lesser extent platelets and red cells. Neutropenia usually reaches its nadir by 8 weeks, and returns to baseline within weeks after cessation of treatment. The neutropenia has not been found to be associated with increased bacterial infections. Dose reduction in 12% to 38% of patients owing to neutropenia was needed in the 2 large multicenter studies in North America and Europe [92,94,115]. Neutropenia is the most common cause of dose reduction (up to 25%) in adult CHC treatment, and granulocyte colony stimulating factor has been shown to be effective in normalizing absolute neutrophil count, well-tolerated, and improves SVR [116,117]. However, there are currently no dosing recommendations or data for the use of granulocyte colony stimulating factor for children in the context HCV therapy. Furthermore, the neutropenia was managed easily with dose reduction in the North American trial making treatment with granulocyte colony stimulating factor unnecessary. The decrease in platelets is usually asymptomatic, occurring within the first 8 weeks of treatment, and stabilizing for the duration of therapy. Only 1 patient in the European study required discontinuation of therapy at week 42 owing to thrombocytopenia (platelet count of 45,000 cells/mm^3)

[118–120]. Ribavirin contributes to the hematologic complications of the combined pegylated INF-α and ribavirin by causing hemolytic anemia in some patients, which usually occurs in the first month of treatment, reaching nadir by week 4 [114,115]. The mechanism by which ribavirin causes hemolytic anemia is thought to involve ribavirin metabolites that impair antioxidant defenses and promote red cell oxidative damage [121]. Frequent complete blood count assessment is recommended for the monitoring of hematologic complications during treatment for CHC in children.

INF-α is also associated with neuropsychiatric side effects, including depression, anxiety, and suicidal ideation. Baseline neuropsychiatric evaluation and screening for depression before starting treatment is recommended. Onset of neuropsychiatric symptoms may not occur until 3 to 6 months into treatment, and suicidal ideation would be an indication to discontinue treatment prematurely [122].

The recommended treatment regimen of pegylated INF-α and ribavirin may also cause side effects in other organ systems. Thyroid disorders can occur at any time during treatment owing to direct inhibition of thyroid synthetic functions and secretion or development of antithyroid peroxidase or antithyroglobulin autoantibodies. Hypothyroidism has been found in 2% to 3% of children undergoing treatment for CHC, and the majority of those patients required thyroxine supplementation. New onset of type 1 diabetes was observed in 1 patient on pegylated IFN-α and ribavirin [92,94]. Visual disturbance or complaints should prompt immediate ophthalmologic examination for retinopathy or optic neuritis. Cutaneous reactions are seen in 20% of patients, ranging from local injection site reactions to alopecia. Ribavirin is teratogenic, and a urine pregnancy test should be obtained before initiating treatment and while on treatment. Side effects of interferon and ribavirin therapy are summarized in (Table 3).

Special populations
Significant side effect profiles of current recommended treatment with combined with pegylated INF-α and ribavirin requires especially careful consideration and monitoring in certain children with other comorbidities. Treatment is generally not recommended for children under 3 years of age, because spontaneous resolution may occur and there is currently no approved treatment

Table 3
Side effects associated with interferon + ribavirin treatment regimen

Constitutional	"Flulike" symptoms, arthralgia, myalgia, fever, fatigue, headache
Hematologic	Anemia (marrow suppression and hemolytic), thrombocytopenia, neutropenia
Gastrointestinal	Anorexia, weight loss, reduced growth velocity, nausea/vomiting, abdominal pain, diarrhea
Endocrine	Hypothyroidism
Ophthalmologic	Retinopathy, optic neuropathy/neuritis
Neuropsychiatric	Mood change, irritability, insomnia, depression, suicidal ideation
Dermatologic	Dermatitis, pruritus, alopecia, injection site reaction

regimen to date in this age group. Patients with psychiatric illness will require close monitoring and evaluation by a trained psychiatrist owing to the neuropsychiatric side effects that may occur with treatment. Suicidal ideation or gesture would be an indication to discontinue treatment prematurely. Adolescents who are incarcerated are good candidates for treatment to prevent spread of HCV and for close monitoring while incarcerated, but compliance may be poor if released before completion of the treatment course.

Children with HIV co-infection have higher rates of viral persistence, lower rates of spontaneous resolution, increased viral load, more rapid progression to end-stage liver disease, and may warrant earlier and more aggressive treatment [123]. SVR to treatment with pegylated INF-α and ribavirin is 15% to 50% lower in patients with CHC and HIV co-infection, and should they receive 48 weeks of treatment regardless of genotype [124–126]. HBV was previously thought to have a negative effect on the natural history of HCV [127], but a recent study in Polish children suggests that HBV/HCV co-infection did not enhance fibrosis compared with patients who have HCV or HBV monoinfections. Liver biopsies did show moderate to severe necroinflammation irrespective of age at biopsy or duration of infection, significantly more than in patients with HCV monoinfection [128]. A full treatment course of pegylated INF-α and ribavirin is also recommended regardless of genotype [75].

Patients with hematologic disorders such as sickle cell anemia and thalassemia usually have a history of multiple blood transfusions. The associated hepatic iron overload may accelerate progression of cirrhosis and risk for HCC. Treatment may be effective, but concern for hemolysis with ribavirin, use of injections, and iron overload need to be considered in the decision to treat [129].

In patients with decompensated cirrhosis, the risk and benefit of treatment must be weighed. A low accelerating dose protocol may be helpful. It has been shown to achieve end-of-treatment response in 46% and SVR in 24% of adult patients with advanced disease (30% and 13% in genotype 1, 82% and 50% in nongenotype 1, respectively) [130,131]. CHC is the leading indication for liver transplantation in adults in the United States. Graft reinfection is almost universal and development of chronic HCV, cirrhosis, and death occur in one-third of adult liver transplant recipients [132]. Liver transplantation for CHC in children is rare. Risk for recurrence of HCV in pediatric orthotopic liver transplantation is high and associated with a high rate of retransplantation. Up to 31% of children transplanted for CHC required relisting, and 19% were retransplanted for HCV recurrence [133]. Pediatric patient and graft survival rates are 72% and 55% at 5 years, respectively, but decrease to 55% and 34% on retransplantation for end-stage liver disease owing to CHC. A large review of the United Network for Organ Sharing database looking at 506 children and young adults age 8 to 35 years who underwent liver transplantation for HCV from 1989 to 2012 showed a 42.8% mortality and a 65.7% rate of retransplantation owing to HCV. These poor outcomes suggest that better treatment regimens and more aggressive evaluation and treatment for HCV in children are needed [134].

Renal transplant recipients with CHC have similar patient and graft survival as those without CHC. Antiviral treatment after renal transplant is generally not considered to be safe, and treatment is recommended before transplantation. Treatment of HCV with INF-α after renal transplant is associated with increased risk of irreversible renal graft rejection in 15% to 64% by promoting cytotoxic action of T lymphocytes and monocytes, cytokines, and HLA antigen production. Extremely close monitoring is required if treatment is initiated [135–139].

Future therapies

An ideal treatment regimen will be one that will treat all genotypes, have as few side effects as possible, and is universally affordable, and recent advances in adult clinical trials may soon realize this goal.

The recently introduced direct-acting antivirals target the nonstructural proteins of HCV. HCV RNA is translated into a single polyprotein that is cleaved by viral and cellular proteases into structural and nonstructural individual proteins. The nonstructural proteins are designated NS2, NS3, NS4A, NS4B, NS5A, and NS5B. NS2 and NS3 are proteases. NS4A is a cofactor for NS3. NS4B creates changes in the cellular membrane that allows viral replication. NS5A is essential for regulation of viral replication. NS5B is an RNA polymerase [140].

Telaprevir and boceprevir were the first 2 direct-acting antivirals to receive approval from the US Food and Drug Administration in 2011. The successes of telaprevir and boceprevir, which offered improved SVR rates for genotype 1 HCV infections when used in triple therapy with pegylated IFN-α and RBV, were tempered by additional adverse effects, multiple drug interactions, and increased susceptibility to early viral resistance. Both protease inhibitors are inhibitors of the cytochrome (Cyp) 3A4/5 enzyme and P-glycoprotein transporter, resulting in a large number of interactions with medications. Boceprevir and telaprevir are associated with anemia, neutropenia, and dysguesia. Telaprevir is also associated with anorectal discomfort and skin rashes [141–144]. Newer protease inhibitors including simeprevir, asunaprevir, and ABT-450 + ritonavir, offer the potential advantages of broader genotype activity, and improved tolerability and resistance profiles.

The recent successes with direct-acting antivirals have led to the development of multiple IFN-free treatment regimens with SVR of 95% to 99% for genotype 1, 94% for genotype 2, and 84% for genotype 3 in adults with CHC (Table 4). Sofosbuvir was the first available nucleoside inhibitor and is well-tolerated, associated with a low probability of drug resistance, and has fewer drug interactions than protease inhibitors. Sofosbuvir plus ledipasvir (Gilead) has been shown to provide 95% or more SVR in HCV genotype 1 patients irrespective of the treatment history or presence of compensated cirrhosis [145,146]. Sofosbuvir in combination with RBV has demonstrated approximately 90% SVR with 12 weeks of treatment in genotype 2, but only 85% at 24 weeks for genotype 3 [147–149]. The NS5A inhibitor daclatasvir

Table 4
Recommended regimens for adults with chronic hepatitis C virus infection

Genotype	Regimen
1	Ledipasvir/sofosbuvir for 12 wk OR
	Paritaprevir/ritonavir/ombitasvir plus dasabuvir and ribavirin for 12 wk (24 wk in cirrhosis) OR
	Sofosbuvir plus simeprevir ± ribavirin for 12 wk (24 wk in cirrhosis)
2	Sofosbuvir and ribavirin for 12 wk (16 wk with cirrhosis)
3	Sofosbuvir and ribavirin for 24 wk

Data from AASLD/IDSA HCV Guidance Panel. Hepatitis C guidance: AASLD-IDSA recommendations for testing, managing, and treating adults infected with hepatitis C virus. Hepatology 2015;62(3):932–54.

(Bristol-Myers Squibb) produced best results in combination with sofosbuvir, with 98% SVR rate in treatment-naïve genotype 1 patients after 12 weeks of treatment [150]. Additional study looking at an all-BMS combination of daclatasvir with asunaprevir (NS3 protease inhibitor) and BMS-791325 (nonnucleoside NS5B inhibitor) yielded a cure rate of more than 90% in the same patient category [151]. AbbVie's "3D" combination, which includes ABT-333 (dasabuvir), ABT-450/ritonavir and ABT-267 (ombitasvir), yielded an impressively high SVR rate (>95%) in genotype 1a and 1b, including patients previously treated with pegylated IFN and ribavirin [152]. For genotype 4, ribavirin is used instead of ABT-333 (because it is only effective against genotype 1), with 100% SVR with ribavirin and 91% without, after 12 weeks treatment. Recently, AbbVie's regimen has been contraindicated in patients with moderate to severe hepatic impairment (Child-Pugh classes B and C) owing to risk of potential toxicity [153].

The combination of Merck's MK-5172 (NS3/4A protease inhibitor) and MK-8742 (NS5A inhibitor) with broader genotype coverage achieved 94% to 100% SVR rate with or without ribavirin in patients with genotype 1 after 12 weeks of treatment. Newer drugs in various phases of investigation including the NS3/4A protease inhibitor sovaprevir (ACH-1625), uridine-based nucleotide prodrugs IDX 21459 and IDX 21437 (Idenix), nucleotide NS5B polymerase inhibitor ACH-3422 (Achillion), and NS5A inhibitor samatasvir (Idenix) promise hope of a pangenotypic cure. Interestingly, HCV genotypes 2 and 3, which achieved higher SVR rates than genotype 1 with previous INF treatment regimens, are now lagging behind genotype 1 in SVR to newer all-oral IFN-free regimens.

The advent of direct-acting antivirals and newer agents in the treatment of CHC in adults gives hope that pediatric CHC may also achieve higher virologic cure rates with safer treatment side effect profiles and shorter treatment duration in the near future. Recently. a phase II open-label study of the effect of telaprevir in combination with pegylated INF-α and ribavirin for children with CHC genotype 1 (Vertex Pharmaceuticals, clinicaltrials.gov, NCT01701063) was completed with results pending. Of note, telaprevir was withdrawn from the US market in October 2015. A second clinical trial of triple therapy, with boceprevir, for the treatment of children ages 3 to 17 with genotype 1 (Merck Sharp & Dohme, clinicaltrials.gov, NCT01590225) was withdrawn in anticipation that newer all-oral therapies would supplant use of this drug by the time the trial was concluded. As of December 2015, 3 multicenter clinical trials looking at the safety and efficacy of all oral, IFN-free regimen in children with CHC are currently recruiting (Tables 5 and 6). It

Table 5
Active clinical trials for interferon-free treatment in children with CHC[a]

Clinical trial	Regimen	Duration
Gilead NCT02175758 Phase 2 SOF + RBV Age 3–17 y	Genotype 2 3–11 y - SOF + RBV dose based on lead-in results 12–17 y - SOF (400 mg: 1 × 400 mg, or 4 × 100 mg) + RBV	Genotype 2 12 wk
	Genotype 3 3–11 y - SOF + RBV dose based on lead-in results 12–17 y - SOF (200 mg: 2 × 100 mg) + RBV	Genotype 3 24 wk
Gilead NCT02249182 Phase 2 LDV/SOF fixed dose ± RBV Age 3–17 y	Genotype 1 or 4 3 to <12 y (wt 17–45 kg) LDV/SOF FDC 2 × 22.5 mg/100 mg (adjustments depending on lead-in phase results) 12 to <18 y (≥45 kg) LDV/SOF FDC 90 mg/400 mg	Genotype 1 or 4 12 wk (treatment naïve with or without cirrhosis; treatment-experienced without cirrhosis) OR 24 wk (treatment-experienced with cirrhosis)
	Genotype 3 LDV/SOF FDC + RBV	Genotype 3 24 wk (treatment-experienced with or without cirrhosis)
AbbVie NCT02486406 Phase 3 OBV/PTV/RTV ± DSV ± RBV Age 3–17 y	Genotype 1b without cirrhosis OBV + PTV + RTV + DSV	Genotype 1b without cirrhosis 12 wk
	Genotype 1a without cirrhosis OBV + PTV + RTV + DSV + RBV	Genotype 1a without cirrhosis 12 wk
	Genotype 1b with compensated cirrhosis OBV + PTV + RTV + DSV + RBV	Genotype 1b with compensated cirrhosis 12 wk
	Genotype 1a with compensated cirrhosis OBV + PTV + RTV + DSV + RBV	Genotype 1a with compensated cirrhosis 24 wk
	Genotype 4 without cirrhosis OBV + PTV + RTV + RBV	Genotype 4 without cirrhosis 12 wk
	Genotype 4, with compensated cirrhosis OBV + PTV + RTV + RBV	Genotype 4, with compensated cirrhosis 24 wk

Abbreviations: DSV, dasabuvir; LDV, ledipasvir; OBV, ombitasvir; PTV, paritaprevir; RBV, ribavirin; RTV, ritonavir; SOF, sofosbuvir.
[a]As of December 2015.

Table 6
Direct acting antivirals

Drug	Manufacturer	Action	Target
Boceprevir	Merck	Inhibitor of serine protease	NS3
Telaprevir	Vertex, Janssen	Inhibitor of serine protease	NS3/NS4A
Simeprevir	Janssen	Inhibitor of serine protease	NS3/NS4A
Asunaprevir	Bristol-Myers Squibb (BMS)	Inhibitor of serine protease	NS3/NS4A
Paritaprevir (ABT-450)	AbbVie	Inhibitor of serine protease	NS3/NS4A
Sofosbuvir	Gilead	RNA polymerase inhibitor	NS5B
Dasabuvir	AbbVie	RNA polymerase inhibitor	NS5B
Ledipasvir	Gilead	Inhibitor of replication, assembly, and secretion	NS5A
Daclatasvir	Bristol-Myers Squibb (BMS)	Blocks RNA synthesis, viral assembly, and secretion	NS5A
Ombitasvir	AbbVie	Inhibitor of replication, assembly, and secretion	NS5A

is expected that the same excellent efficacy and safety profiles for these all-oral regimens in adults will occur in children.

References

[1] Webster DP, Klenerman P, Dusheiko GM. Hepatitis C. Lancet 2015;385(9973):1124–35.
[2] Gower E, Estes C, Blach S, et al. Global epidemiology and genotype distribution of the hepatitis C virus infection. J Hepatol 2014;61(1 Suppl):S45–57.
[3] Abu Faddan NH, Shehata GA, Abd Elhafeez HA, et al. Cognitive function and endogenous cytokine levels in children with chronic hepatitis C. J Viral Hepat 2015;22(8):665–70.
[4] Rodrigue JR, Balistreri W, Haber B, et al. Impact of hepatitis C virus infection on children and their caregivers: quality of life, cognitive, and emotional outcomes. J Pediatr Gastroenterol Nutr 2009;48(3):341–7.
[5] Nydegger A, Srivastava A, Wake M, et al. Health-related quality of life in children with hepatitis C acquired in the first year of life. J Gastroenterol Hepatol 2008;23(2):226–30.
[6] Foster GR. Quality of life considerations for patients with chronic hepatitis C. J Viral Hepat 2009;16(9):605–11.
[7] El-Shabrawi MH, Kamal NM. Burden of pediatric hepatitis C. World J Gastroenterol 2013;19(44):7880–8.
[8] Hepatitis C virus infection. American academy of pediatrics. Committee on infectious diseases. Pediatrics 1998;101(3 Pt 1):481–5.
[9] Omland LH, Krarup H, Jepsen P, et al. Mortality in patients with chronic and cleared hepatitis C viral infection: a nationwide cohort study. J Hepatol 2010;53(1):36–42.
[10] Jhaveri R, Grant W, Kauf TL, et al. The burden of hepatitis C virus infection in children: estimated direct medical costs over a 10-year period. J Pediatr 2006;148(3):353–8.
[11] Nainan OV, Alter MJ, Kruszon-Moran D, et al. Hepatitis C virus genotypes and viral concentrations in participants of a general population survey in the united states. Gastroenterology 2006;131(2):478–84.
[12] Sullivan DG, Bruden D, Deubner H, et al. Hepatitis C virus dynamics during natural infection are associated with long-term histological outcome of chronic hepatitis C disease. J Infect Dis 2007;196(2):239–48.

[13] Huang H, Shiffman ML, Cheung RC, et al. Identification of two gene variants associated with risk of advanced fibrosis in patients with chronic hepatitis C. Gastroenterology 2006;130(6):1679–87.

[14] Mosbruger TL, Duggal P, Goedert JJ, et al. Large-scale candidate gene analysis of spontaneous clearance of hepatitis C virus. J Infect Dis 2010;201(9):1371–80.

[15] Bosi I, Ancora G, Mantovani W, et al. HLA DR13 and HCV vertical infection. Pediatr Res 2002;51(6):746–9.

[16] Martinetti M, Pacati I, Cuccia M, et al. Hierarchy of baby-linked immunogenetic risk factors in the vertical transmission of hepatitis C virus. Int J Immunopathol Pharmacol 2006;19(2): 369–78.

[17] Bevilacqua E, Fabris A, Floreano P, et al. Genetic factors in mother-to-child transmission of HCV infection. Virology 2009;390(1):64–70.

[18] Ruiz-Extremera A, Munoz-Gamez JA, Salmeron-Ruiz MA, et al. Genetic variation in interleukin 28B with respect to vertical transmission of hepatitis C virus and spontaneous clearance in HCV-infected children. Hepatology 2011;53(6):1830–8.

[19] Mast EE, Hwang LY, Seto DS, et al. Risk factors for perinatal transmission of hepatitis C virus (HCV) and the natural history of HCV infection acquired in infancy. J Infect Dis 2005;192(11):1880–9.

[20] Shebl FM, El-Kamary SS, Saleh DA, et al. Prospective cohort study of mother-to-infant infection and clearance of hepatitis C in rural Egyptian villages. J Med Virol 2009;81(6): 1024–31.

[21] Yeung LT, To T, King SM, et al. Spontaneous clearance of childhood hepatitis C virus infection. J Viral Hepat 2007;14(11):797–805.

[22] Luban NL, Colvin CA, Mohan P, et al. The epidemiology of transfusion-associated hepatitis C in a children's hospital. Transfusion 2007;47(4):615–20.

[23] Zanetti AR, Tanzi E, Paccagnini S, et al. Mother-to-infant transmission of hepatitis C virus. Lombardy Study Group on Vertical HCV Transmission. Lancet 1995;345(8945): 289–91.

[24] Okamoto M, Nagata I, Murakami J, et al. Prospective reevaluation of risk factors in mother-to-child transmission of hepatitis C virus: high virus load, vaginal delivery, and negative anti-NS4 antibody. J Infect Dis 2000;182(5):1511–4.

[25] Resti M, Azzari C, Mannelli F, et al. Mother to child transmission of hepatitis C virus: prospective study of risk factors and timing of infection in children born to women seronegative for HIV-1. Tuscany study group on hepatitis C virus infection. BMJ 1998;317(7156): 437–41.

[26] Moriya T, Sasaki F, Mizui M, et al. Transmission of hepatitis C virus from mothers to infants: its frequency and risk factors revisited. Biomed Pharmacother 1995;49(2): 59–64.

[27] Conte D, Fraquelli M, Prati D, et al. Prevalence and clinical course of chronic hepatitis C virus (HCV) infection and rate of HCV vertical transmission in a cohort of 15,250 pregnant women. Hepatology 2000;31(3):751–5.

[28] Claret G, Noguera A, Esteva C, et al. Mother-to-child transmission of hepatitis C virus infection in Barcelona, Spain: a prospective study. Eur J Pediatr 2007;166(12):1297–9.

[29] Mast EE. Mother-to-infant hepatitis C virus transmission and breastfeeding. Adv Exp Med Biol 2004;554:211–6.

[30] Yeung LT, King SM, Roberts EA. Mother-to-infant transmission of hepatitis C virus. Hepatology 2001;34(2):223–9.

[31] Granovsky MO, Minkoff HL, Tess BH, et al. Hepatitis C virus infection in the mothers and infants cohort study. Pediatrics 1998;102(2 Pt 1):355–9.

[32] European Paediatric Hepatitis C Virus Network. A significant sex–but not elective cesarean section–effect on mother-to-child transmission of hepatitis C virus infection. J Infect Dis 2005;192(11):1872–9.

[33] Hurtado CW, Golden-Mason L, Brocato M, et al. Innate immune function in placenta and cord blood of hepatitis C–seropositive mother-infant dyads. PLoS One 2010;5(8):e12232.
[34] Yeung CY, Lee HC, Chan WT, et al. Vertical transmission of hepatitis C virus: current knowledge and perspectives. World J Hepatol 2014;6(9):643–51.
[35] Ohto H, Terazawa S, Sasaki N, et al. Transmission of hepatitis C virus from mothers to infants. the vertical transmission of hepatitis C virus collaborative study group. N Engl J Med 1994;330(11):744–50.
[36] Tajiri H, Miyoshi Y, Funada S, et al. Prospective study of mother-to-infant transmission of hepatitis C virus. Pediatr Infect Dis J 2001;20(1):10–4.
[37] Steininger C, Kundi M, Jatzko G, et al. Increased risk of mother-to-infant transmission of hepatitis C virus by intrapartum infantile exposure to maternal blood. J Infect Dis 2003;187(3):345–51.
[38] Indolfi G, Azzari C, Resti M. Perinatal transmission of hepatitis C virus. J Pediatr 2013;163(6):1549–52.e1.
[39] Garcia-Tejedor A, Maiques-Montesinos V, Diago-Almela VJ, et al. Risk factors for vertical transmission of hepatitis C virus: a single center experience with 710 HCV-infected mothers. Eur J Obstet Gynecol Reprod Biol 2015;194:173–7.
[40] Minola E, Maccabruni A, Pacati I, et al. Amniocentesis as a possible risk factor for mother-to-infant transmission of hepatitis C virus. Hepatology 2001;33(5):1341–2.
[41] Ducarme G, Ceccaldi PF, Bernuau J, et al. Amniocentesis and viral risk (hepatitis B, C virus and HIV). J Gynecol Obstet Biol Reprod (Paris) 2009;38(6):469–73.
[42] Shiraki K, Ohto H, Inaba N, et al. Guidelines for care of pregnant women carrying hepatitis C virus and their infants. Pediatr Int 2008;50(1):138–40.
[43] Ferrero S, Lungaro P, Bruzzone BM, et al. Prospective study of mother-to-infant transmission of hepatitis C virus: a 10-year survey (1990-2000). Acta Obstet Gynecol Scand 2003;82(3):229–34.
[44] Jara P, Resti M, Hierro L, et al. Chronic hepatitis C virus infection in childhood: clinical patterns and evolution in 224 white children. Clin Infect Dis 2003;36(3):275–80.
[45] Ackerman Z, Ackerman E, Paltiel O. Intrafamilial transmission of hepatitis C virus: a systematic review. J Viral Hepat 2000;7(2):93–103.
[46] Tohme RA, Holmberg SD. Is sexual contact a major mode of hepatitis C virus transmission? Hepatology 2010;52(4):1497–505.
[47] Mohamed MK, Magder LS, Abdel-Hamid M, et al. Transmission of hepatitis C virus between parents and children. Am J Trop Med Hyg 2006;75(1):16–20.
[48] Ketzinel-Gilad M, Colodner SL, Hadary R, et al. Transient transmission of hepatitis C virus from mothers to newborns. Eur J Clin Microbiol Infect Dis 2000;19(4):267–74.
[49] Ceci O, Margiotta M, Marello F, et al. Vertical transmission of hepatitis C virus in a cohort of 2,447 HIV-seronegative pregnant women: a 24-month prospective study. J Pediatr Gastroenterol Nutr 2001;33(5):570–5.
[50] Iorio R, Giannattasio A, Sepe A, et al. Chronic hepatitis C in childhood: an 18-year experience. Clin Infect Dis 2005;41(10):1431–7.
[51] Vogt M, Lang T, Frosner G, et al. Prevalence and clinical outcome of hepatitis C infection in children who underwent cardiac surgery before the implementation of blood-donor screening. N Engl J Med 1999;341(12):866–70.
[52] Rerksuppaphol S, Hardikar W, Dore GJ. Long-term outcome of vertically acquired and post-transfusion hepatitis C infection in children. J Gastroenterol Hepatol 2004;19(12):1357–62.
[53] Bortolotti F, Verucchi G, Camma C, et al. Long-term course of chronic hepatitis C in children: from viral clearance to end-stage liver disease. Gastroenterology 2008;134(7):1900–7.

[54] Casiraghi MA, De Paschale M, Romano L, et al. Long-term outcome (35 years) of hepatitis C after acquisition of infection through mini transfusions of blood given at birth. Hepatology 2004;39(1):90–6.

[55] Guido M, Rugge M, Jara P, et al. Chronic hepatitis C in children: the pathological and clinical spectrum. Gastroenterology 1998;115(6):1525–9.

[56] Cesaro S, Bortolotti F, Petris MG, et al. An updated follow-up of chronic hepatitis C after three decades of observation in pediatric patients cured of malignancy. Pediatr Blood Cancer 2010;55(1):108–12.

[57] Indolfi G, Guido M, Azzari C, et al. Histopathology of hepatitis C in children, a systematic review: implications for treatment. Expert Rev Anti Infect Ther 2015;13(10):1225–35.

[58] Gonzalez-Peralta RP, Langham MR Jr, Andres JM, et al. Hepatocellular carcinoma in 2 young adolescents with chronic hepatitis C. J Pediatr Gastroenterol Nutr 2009;48(5): 630–5.

[59] Strickland DK, Jenkins JJ, Hudson MM. Hepatitis C infection and hepatocellular carcinoma after treatment of childhood cancer. J Pediatr Hematol Oncol 2001;23(8):527–9.

[60] Rumbo C, Fawaz RL, Emre SH, et al. Hepatitis C in children: a quaternary referral center perspective. J Pediatr Gastroenterol Nutr 2006;43(2):209–16.

[61] Mohan P, Colvin C, Glymph C, et al. Clinical spectrum and histopathologic features of chronic hepatitis C infection in children. J Pediatr 2007;150(2):168–74, 174.e1.

[62] Birnbaum AH, Shneider BL, Moy L. Hepatitis C in children. N Engl J Med 2000;342(4): 290–1.

[63] Madhoun MF, Fazili J, Bright BC, et al. Hepatitis C prevalence in patients with hepatocellular carcinoma without cirrhosis. Am J Med Sci 2010;339(2):169–73.

[64] Lok AS, Seeff LB, Morgan TR, et al. Incidence of hepatocellular carcinoma and associated risk factors in hepatitis C-related advanced liver disease. Gastroenterology 2009;136(1): 138–48.

[65] Garazzino S, Calitri C, Versace A, et al. Natural history of vertically acquired HCV infection and associated autoimmune phenomena. Eur J Pediatr 2014;173(8):1025–31.

[66] Delgado-Borrego A, Healey D, Negre B, et al. Influence of body mass index on outcome of pediatric chronic hepatitis C virus infection. J Pediatr Gastroenterol Nutr 2010;51(2): 191–7.

[67] Delgado-Borrego A, Jordan SH, Negre B, et al. Reduction of insulin resistance with effective clearance of hepatitis C infection: results from the HALT-C trial. Clin Gastroenterol Hepatol 2010;8(5):458–62.

[68] Page K, Hahn JA, Evans J, et al. Acute hepatitis C virus infection in young adult injection drug users: a prospective study of incident infection, resolution, and reinfection. J Infect Dis 2009;200(8):1216–26.

[69] Serra MA, Escudero A, Rodriguez F, et al. Effect of hepatitis C virus infection and abstinence from alcohol on survival in patients with alcoholic cirrhosis. J Clin Gastroenterol 2003;36(2):170–4.

[70] Wise M, Finelli L, Sorvillo F. Prognostic factors associated with hepatitis C disease: a case-control study utilizing U.S. multiple-cause-of-death data. Public Health Rep 2010;125(3): 414–22.

[71] Beech BM, Myers L, Beech DJ. Hepatitis B and C infections among homeless adolescents. Fam Community Health 2002;25(2):28–36.

[72] Murray KF, Richardson LP, Morishima C, et al. Prevalence of hepatitis C virus infection and risk factors in an incarcerated juvenile population: a pilot study. Pediatrics 2003;111(1): 153–7.

[73] Forton DM, Thomas HC, Murphy CA, et al. Hepatitis C and cognitive impairment in a cohort of patients with mild liver disease. Hepatology 2002;35(2):433–9.

[74] de Leuw P, Sarrazin C, Zeuzem S. How to use virological tools for the optimal management of chronic hepatitis C. Liver Int 2011;31(Suppl 1):3–12.

[75] Mack CL, Gonzalez-Peralta RP, Gupta N, et al. NASPGHAN practice guidelines: diagnosis and management of hepatitis C infection in infants, children, and adolescents. J Pediatr Gastroenterol Nutr 2012;54(6):838–55.
[76] Ghany MG, Strader DB, Thomas DL, et al. American Association for the Study of Liver Diseases. Diagnosis, management, and treatment of hepatitis C: an update. Hepatology 2009;49(4):1335–74.
[77] England K, Pembrey L, Tovo PA, et al, European Paediatric HCV Network. Excluding hepatitis C virus (HCV) infection by serology in young infants of HCV-infected mothers. Acta Paediatr 2005;94(4):444–50.
[78] Polywka S, Pembrey L, Tovo PA, et al. Accuracy of HCV-RNA PCR tests for diagnosis or exclusion of vertically acquired HCV infection. J Med Virol 2006;78(2):305–10.
[79] Pokorska-Spiewak M, Kowalik-Mikolajewska B, Aniszewska M, et al. Is liver biopsy still needed in children with chronic viral hepatitis? World J Gastroenterol 2015;21(42): 12141–9.
[80] de Ledinghen V, Wong VW, Vergniol J, et al. Diagnosis of liver fibrosis and cirrhosis using liver stiffness measurement: comparison between M and XL probe of FibroScan(R). J Hepatol 2012;56(4):833–9.
[81] Poynard T, de Ledinghen V, Zarski JP, et al. Performances of elasto-FibroTest((R)), a combination between FibroTest((R)) and liver stiffness measurements for assessing the stage of liver fibrosis in patients with chronic hepatitis C. Clin Res Hepatol Gastroenterol 2012;36(5):455–63.
[82] El-Shabrawi MH, Mohsen NA, Sherif MM, et al. Noninvasive assessment of hepatic fibrosis and necroinflammatory activity in Egyptian children with chronic hepatitis C virus infection using FibroTest and ActiTest. Eur J Gastroenterol Hepatol 2010;22(8):946–51.
[83] Pawlowska M, Domagalski K, Pniewska A, et al. What's new in hepatitis C virus infections in children? World J Gastroenterol 2015;21(38):10783–9.
[84] Sira MM, Behairy BE, Abd-Elaziz AM, et al. Serum inter-alpha-trypsin inhibitor heavy chain 4 (ITIH4) in children with chronic hepatitis C: relation to liver fibrosis and viremia. Hepat Res Treat 2014;2014:307942.
[85] Yang L, Rudser KD, Higgins L, et al. Novel biomarker candidates to predict hepatic fibrosis in hepatitis C identified by serum proteomics. Dig Dis Sci 2011;56(11):3305–15.
[86] Behairy BE, El-Mashad GM, Abd-Elghany RS, et al. Serum complement C4a and its relation to liver fibrosis in children with chronic hepatitis C. World J Hepatol 2013;5(8): 445–51.
[87] NIH consensus statement on management of hepatitis C: 2002. NIH Consens State Sci Statements 2002;19(3):1–46.
[88] Camarero C, Ramos N, Moreno A, et al. Hepatitis C virus infection acquired in childhood. Eur J Pediatr 2008;167(2):219–24.
[89] Goodman ZD, Makhlouf HR, Liu L, et al. Pathology of chronic hepatitis C in children: liver biopsy findings in the PEDS-C trial. Hepatology 2008;47(3):836–43.
[90] El Sherbini A, Mostafa S, Ali E. Systematic review with meta-analysis: comparison between therapeutic regimens for paediatric chronic hepatitis C. Aliment Pharmacol Ther 2015;42(1):12–9.
[91] Gonzalez-Peralta RP, Kelly DA, Haber B, et al. Interferon alfa-2b in combination with ribavirin for the treatment of chronic hepatitis C in children: efficacy, safety, and pharmacokinetics. Hepatology 2005;42(5):1010–8.
[92] Schwarz KB, Gonzalez-Peralta RP, Murray KF, et al. The combination of ribavirin and peginterferon is superior to peginterferon and placebo for children and adolescents with chronic hepatitis C. Gastroenterology 2011;140(2):450–8.e1.
[93] Wirth S, Pieper-Boustani H, Lang T, et al. Peginterferon alfa-2b plus ribavirin treatment in children and adolescents with chronic hepatitis C. Hepatology 2005;41(5):1013–8.

[94] Wirth S, Ribes-Koninckx C, Calzado MA, et al. High sustained virologic response rates in children with chronic hepatitis C receiving peginterferon alfa-2b plus ribavirin. J Hepatol 2010;52(4):501–7.

[95] Wirth S, Lang T, Gehring S, et al. Recombinant alfa-interferon plus ribavirin therapy in children and adolescents with chronic hepatitis C. Hepatology 2002;36(5):1280–4.

[96] Christensson B, Wiebe T, Akesson A, et al. Interferon-alpha and ribavirin treatment of hepatitis C in children with malignancy in remission. Clin Infect Dis 2000;30(3):585–6.

[97] Schwarz KB, Mohan P, Narkewicz MR, et al. Safety, efficacy and pharmacokinetics of peginterferon alpha2a (40 kd) in children with chronic hepatitis C. J Pediatr Gastroenterol Nutr 2006;43(4):499–505.

[98] Tsunoda T, Inui A, Etani Y, et al. Efficacy of pegylated interferon-alpha2a monotherapy in Japanese children with chronic hepatitis C. Hepatol Res 2011;41(5):399–404.

[99] Lackner H, Moser A, Deutsch J, et al. Interferon-alpha and ribavirin in treating children and young adults with chronic hepatitis C after malignancy. Pediatrics 2000;106(4):E53.

[100] Di Bisceglie AM, Shiffman ML, Everson GT, et al. Prolonged therapy of advanced chronic hepatitis C with low-dose peginterferon. N Engl J Med 2008;359(23):2429–41.

[101] Feld JJ, Hoofnagle JH. Mechanism of action of interferon and ribavirin in treatment of hepatitis C. Nature 2005;436(7053):967–72.

[102] Bekisz J, Schmeisser H, Hernandez J, et al. Human interferons alpha, beta and omega. Growth Factors 2004;22(4):243–51.

[103] Zeuzem S, Feinman SV, Rasenack J, et al. Peginterferon alfa-2a in patients with chronic hepatitis C. N Engl J Med 2000;343(23):1666–72.

[104] Lindsay KL, Trepo C, Heintges T, et al. A randomized, double-blind trial comparing pegylated interferon alfa-2b to interferon alfa-2b as initial treatment for chronic hepatitis C. Hepatology 2001;34(2):395–403.

[105] Ascione A, De Luca M, Tartaglione MT, et al. Peginterferon alfa-2a plus ribavirin is more effective than peginterferon alfa-2b plus ribavirin for treating chronic hepatitis C virus infection. Gastroenterology 2010;138(1):116–22.

[106] McHutchison JG, Lawitz EJ, Shiffman ML, et al. Peginterferon alfa-2b or alfa-2a with ribavirin for treatment of hepatitis C infection. N Engl J Med 2009;361(6):580–93.

[107] Rumi MG, Aghemo A, Prati GM, et al. Randomized study of peginterferon-alpha2a plus ribavirin vs peginterferon-alpha2b plus ribavirin in chronic hepatitis C. Gastroenterology 2010;138(1):108–15.

[108] Sporea I, Danila M, Sirli R, et al. Comparative study concerning the efficacy of peg-IFN alpha-2a versus peg-IFN alpha-2b on the early virological response (EVR) in patients with chronic viral C hepatitis. J Gastrointest Liver Dis 2006;15(2):125–30.

[109] Lau JY, Tam RC, Liang TJ, et al. Mechanism of action of ribavirin in the combination treatment of chronic HCV infection. Hepatology 2002;35(5):1002–9.

[110] Maag D, Castro C, Hong Z, et al. Hepatitis C virus RNA-dependent RNA polymerase (NS5B) as a mediator of the antiviral activity of ribavirin. J Biol Chem 2001;276(49):46094–8.

[111] Crotty S, Maag D, Arnold JJ, et al. The broad-spectrum antiviral ribonucleoside ribavirin is an RNA virus mutagen. Nat Med 2000;6(12):1375–9.

[112] McHutchison JG, Gordon SC, Schiff ER, et al. Interferon alfa-2b alone or in combination with ribavirin as initial treatment for chronic hepatitis C. hepatitis interventional therapy group. N Engl J Med 1998;339(21):1485–92.

[113] Poynard T, Marcellin P, Lee SS, et al. Randomised trial of interferon alpha2b plus ribavirin for 48 weeks or for 24 weeks versus interferon alpha2b plus placebo for 48 weeks for treatment of chronic infection with hepatitis C virus. International hepatitis interventional therapy group (IHIT). Lancet 1998;352(9138):1426–32.

[114] Sung H, Chang M, Saab S. Management of hepatitis C antiviral therapy adverse effects. Curr Hepat Rep 2011;10(1):33–40.

[115] Abdel-Aziz DH, Sabry NA, El-Sayed MH, et al. Efficacy and safety of pegylated interferon in children and adolescents infected with chronic hepatitis C: a preliminary study. J Pharm Pract 2011;24(2):203–10.

[116] Ong JP, Younossi ZM. Managing the hematologic side effects of antiviral therapy for chronic hepatitis C: anemia, neutropenia, and thrombocytopenia. Cleve Clin J Med 2004;71(Suppl 3):S17–21.

[117] Sulkowski MS. Management of the hematologic complications of hepatitis C therapy. Clin Liver Dis 2005;9(4):601–16, vi.

[118] Yamane A, Nakamura T, Suzuki H, et al. Interferon-alpha 2b-induced thrombocytopenia is caused by inhibition of platelet production but not proliferation and endomitosis in human megakaryocytes. Blood 2008;112(3):542–50.

[119] Pockros PJ, Duchini A, McMillan R, et al. Immune thrombocytopenic purpura in patients with chronic hepatitis C virus infection. Am J Gastroenterol 2002;97(8):2040–5.

[120] Dourakis SP, Deutsch M, Hadziyannis SJ. Immune thrombocytopenia and alpha-interferon therapy. J Hepatol 1996;25(6):972–5.

[121] De Franceschi L, Fattovich G, Turrini F, et al. Hemolytic anemia induced by ribavirin therapy in patients with chronic hepatitis C virus infection: role of membrane oxidative damage. Hepatology 2000;31(4):997–1004.

[122] Al-Huthail YR. Neuropsychiatric side-effects of interferon alfa therapy for hepatitis C and their management: a review. Saudi J Gastroenterol 2006;12(2):59–67.

[123] Indolfi G, Bartolini E, Serranti D, et al. Hepatitis C in children co-infected with human immunodeficiency virus. J Pediatr Gastroenterol Nutr 2015;61(4):393–9.

[124] Mofenson LM, Brady MT, Danner SP, et al. Guidelines for the prevention and treatment of opportunistic infections among HIV-exposed and HIV-infected children: recommendations from CDC, the National Institutes of Health, the HIV Medicine Association of the Infectious Diseases Society of America, the Pediatric Infectious Diseases Society, and the American Academy of Pediatrics. MMWR Recomm Rep 2009;58(RR-11):1–166.

[125] Soriano V, Puoti M, Sulkowski M, et al. Care of patients coinfected with HIV and hepatitis C virus: 2007 updated recommendations from the HCV-HIV international panel. AIDS 2007;21(9):1073–89.

[126] Tural C, Galeras JA, Planas R, et al. Differences in virological response to pegylated interferon and ribavirin between hepatitis C virus (HCV)-monoinfected and HCV-HIV-coinfected patients. Antivir Ther 2008;13(8):1047–55.

[127] Zampino R, Marrone A, Merola A, et al. Long-term outcome of hepatitis B and hepatitis C virus co-infection and single HBV infection acquired in youth. J Med Virol 2009;81(12):2012–20.

[128] Pokorska-Spiewak M, Kowalik-Mikolajewska B, Aniszewska M, et al. The influence of hepatitis B and C virus coinfection on liver histopathology in children. Eur J Pediatr 2015;174(3):345–53.

[129] Harmatz P, Jonas MM, Kwiatkowski JL, et al. Safety and efficacy of pegylated interferon alpha-2a and ribavirin for the treatment of hepatitis C in patients with thalassemia. Haematologica 2008;93(8):1247–51.

[130] Vezali E, Aghemo A, Colombo M. A review of the treatment of chronic hepatitis C virus infection in cirrhosis. Clin Ther 2010;32(13):2117–38.

[131] Everson GT, Trotter J, Forman L, et al. Treatment of advanced hepatitis C with a low accelerating dosage regimen of antiviral therapy. Hepatology 2005;42(2):255–62.

[132] Ferrell LD, Wright TL, Roberts J, et al. Hepatitis C viral infection in liver transplant recipients. Hepatology 1992;16(4):865–76.

[133] Barshes NR, Udell IW, Lee TC, et al. The natural history of hepatitis C virus in pediatric liver transplant recipients. Liver Transpl 2006;12(7):1119–23.

[134] Mohamad B, Hanouneh IA, Zein NN, et al. Liver transplant in young adults with chronic hepatitis C virus: an argument for hepatitis C treatment in childhood. Exp Clin Transplant 2016;14(2):201–6.

[135] Arango J, Arbelaez M, Henao J, et al. Kidney graft survival in patients with hepatitis C: a single center experience. Clin Transplant 2008;22(1):16–9.

[136] Pereira BJ, Natov SN, Bouthot BA, et al. Effects of hepatitis C infection and renal transplantation on survival in end-stage renal disease. The new England organ bank hepatitis C study group. Kidney Int 1998;53(5):1374–81.

[137] Schmitz V, Kiessling A, Bahra M, et al. Peginterferon alfa-2b plus ribavirin for the treatment of hepatitis C recurrence following combined liver and kidney transplantation. Ann Transplant 2007;12(3):22–7.

[138] Baid S, Cosimi AB, Tolkoff-Rubin N, et al. Renal disease associated with hepatitis C infection after kidney and liver transplantation. Transplantation 2000;70(2):255–61.

[139] Baid S, Tolkoff-Rubin N, Saidman S, et al. Acute humoral rejection in hepatitis C-infected renal transplant recipients receiving antiviral therapy. Am J Transplant 2003;3(1):74–8.

[140] Bell TW. Drugs for hepatitis C: unlocking a new mechanism of action. ChemMedChem 2010;5(10):1663–5.

[141] Bacon BR, Gordon SC, Lawitz E, et al. Boceprevir for previously treated chronic HCV genotype 1 infection. N Engl J Med 2011;364(13):1207–17.

[142] Jacobson IM, Pawlotsky JM, Afdhal NH, et al. A practical guide for the use of boceprevir and telaprevir for the treatment of hepatitis C. J Viral Hepat 2012;19(Suppl 2):1–26.

[143] Susser S, Welsch C, Wang Y, et al. Characterization of resistance to the protease inhibitor boceprevir in hepatitis C virus-infected patients. Hepatology 2009;50(6):1709–18.

[144] Chou R, Hartung D, Rahman B, et al. Comparative effectiveness of antiviral treatment for hepatitis C virus infection in adults: a systematic review. Ann Intern Med 2013;158(2):114–23.

[145] Reddy KR, Bourliere M, Sulkowski M, et al. Ledipasvir and sofosbuvir in patients with genotype 1 hepatitis C virus infection and compensated cirrhosis: an integrated safety and efficacy analysis. Hepatology 2015;62(1):79–86.

[146] Afdhal N, Reddy KR, Nelson DR, et al. Ledipasvir and sofosbuvir for previously treated HCV genotype 1 infection. N Engl J Med 2014;370(16):1483–93.

[147] Jacobson IM, Gordon SC, Kowdley KV, et al. Sofosbuvir for hepatitis C genotype 2 or 3 in patients without treatment options. N Engl J Med 2013;368(20):1867–77.

[148] Lawitz E, Jacobson IM, Nelson DR, et al. Development of sofosbuvir for the treatment of hepatitis C virus infection. Ann N Y Acad Sci 2015;1358(1):56–67.

[149] Zeuzem S, Dusheiko GM, Salupere R, et al. Sofosbuvir and ribavirin in HCV genotypes 2 and 3. N Engl J Med 2014;370(21):1993–2001.

[150] Sulkowski MS, Gardiner DF, Rodriguez-Torres M, et al. Daclatasvir plus sofosbuvir for previously treated or untreated chronic HCV infection. N Engl J Med 2014;370(3):211–21.

[151] Everson GT, Sims KD, Rodriguez-Torres M, et al. Efficacy of an interferon- and ribavirin-free regimen of daclatasvir, asunaprevir, and BMS-791325 in treatment-naive patients with HCV genotype 1 infection. Gastroenterology 2014;146(2):420–9.

[152] Zeuzem S, Jacobson IM, Baykal T, et al. Retreatment of HCV with ABT-450/r-ombitasvir and dasabuvir with ribavirin. N Engl J Med 2014;370(17):1604–14.

[153] Khatri A, Menon RM, Marbury TC, et al. Pharmacokinetics and safety of co-administered paritaprevir plus ritonavir, ombitasvir, and dasabuvir in hepatic impairment. J Hepatol 2015;63(4):805–12.

Advances in Pediatrics 63 (2016) 195–209

ADVANCES IN PEDIATRICS

ELSEVIER
MOSBY

Update on Youth-Onset Type 2 Diabetes

Lessons Learned from the Treatment Options for Type 2 Diabetes in Adolescents and Youth Clinical Trial

Rachelle Gandica, MD[a], Phil Zeitler, MD, PhD[b],*

[a]Naomi Berrie Diabetes Center, Columbia University Medical Center, 1150 Street Nicholas Avenue, 2nd Floor, New York, NY, USA; [b]Section of Endocrinology, Department of Pediatrics, University of Colorado School of Medicine, 13123 East 16th Avenue, Box 265, Aurora, CO, USA

Keywords
- Type 2 diabetes • Youth • Update • TODAY clinical trial

Key points
- Youth-onset type 2 diabetes is increasingly more prevalent and carries a high disease burden.
- Youth with type 2 diabetes who cannot lower their blood sugars to a non-diabetes range on metformin monotherapy should be followed closely for a rapid decline in glucose control.
- There is a high risk of vascular and pregnancy complications in teens with type 2 diabetes.

INTRODUCTION

Type 2 diabetes mellitus (T2D) in children and adolescents has become increasingly prevalent in parallel with increasing rates of childhood obesity. Before the late 1990s, T2D was a rare entity in children; an increase in

Disclosures: nothing to disclose (R. Gandica); consultant: Daiichi-Sankyo, Takeda Pharmaceuticals, Merck, Boehringer Ingelheim, and Bristol-Myers Squibb (P. Zeitler).

This work was completed with funding from NIDDK and the NIH Office of the Director through grants U01-DK61212, U01-DK61230, U01-DK61239, U01-DK61242, and U01-DK61254. The content is solely the responsibility of the authors and does not necessarily represent the official views of the National Institutes of Health.

*Corresponding author. *E-mail address*: Philip.Zeitler@childrenscolorado.org

0065-3101/16/$ – see front matter
http://dx.doi.org/10.1016/j.yapd.2016.04.013

prevalence was first described in urban minority youth in 1996 [1,2]. Now youth-onset T2D spans across continents and affects children of all ethnicities and socioeconomic backgrounds. However, youth-onset T2D disproportionately affects disadvantaged families of minority, indigenous, or migrant communities. The SEARCH for Diabetes in Youth, a registry-based study in the United States, has shown that the overall prevalence of T2D in 2009, the latest year for which data are available, was 0.46 per 1000 youths younger than 18 years, a 30.5% increase in comparison with 2001 [3,4]. Yet, despite the increase over time, T2D remains much less prevalent in adolescents than in adults; T2D is present in 120 to 140 per 1000 adults in the United States, based on National Health and Nutrition Examination Survey data [5]. Between 2001 and 2009, a significant increase in childhood T2D was seen in non-Hispanic whites, African Americans, and Hispanics but not among Asian Pacific Islanders and American Indians [3,4], who already had high rates of T2D. In children 10 years of age or older, T2D is now responsible for 3% of all cases of diabetes among Caucasians, 23% in Hispanics, 25% in African Americans, and 64% in American Indians [4].

The Treatment Options for Type 2 Diabetes in Adolescents and Youth (TODAY) study cohort consists of racially/ethnically diverse participants with youth-onset T2D who have been rigorously characterized and followed longitudinally to better understand the clinical course of complications and comorbidities of diabetes [6]. The initial results of the TODAY intervention trial have been published and reviewed in many publications and are summarized in the next few paragraphs. The remainder of this article focuses on the more recent findings from the TODAY study.

TREATMENT OPTIONS FOR TYPE 2 DIABETES IN ADOLESCENTS AND YOUTH TRIAL RESULTS

The TODAY trial began recruiting subjects in 2004 [6]. Subjects eligible for participation were 10 to 17 years old with T2D (based on established criteria from the American Diabetes Association) for less than 2 years. They also had a body mass index (BMI) of 85% or greater and a fasting C peptide greater than 0.6 ng/mL without demonstrable pancreatic islet autoantibodies [6]. Exclusion criteria included renal insufficiency, uncontrolled hypertension, liver disease, and uncontrolled hyperlipidemia [6]. A total of 699 subjects were randomized to receive one of 3 treatments: metformin monotherapy, metformin plus rosiglitazone, and metformin plus an intensive lifestyle intervention [6]. The primary outcome was the length of time to glycemic failure, defined as a hemoglobin A1c (HbA1c) 8% or greater for at least 6 months or the inability to wean from insulin injections for at least 3 months after acute metabolic decompensation [6].

Nearly half (45.6%) of all TODAY participants reached glycemic failure over an average time of 3.86 years [7]. Failure rates for each of the 3 treatment arms were 51.7% in the metformin monotherapy group, 46.6% for the metformin plus lifestyle group, and 38.6% for the metformin plus rosiglitazone group (Fig. 1). The difference between the metformin monotherapy and metformin

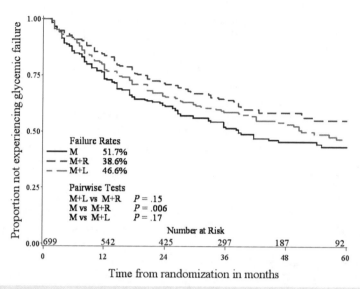

Fig. 1. TODAY primary outcome results. M, metformin alone treatment arm; M + L, metformin plus intensive lifestyle changes treatment arm; M + R, metformin plus rosiglitazone treatment arm.

plus rosiglitazone arms was statistically significant, suggesting that adding a second oral medication early in the disease process of youth-onset T2D may help to promote durable glycemic control [7]. These differences were not the result of differences in medication adherence. The metformin plus lifestyle arm did not differ significantly from the other two treatment arms, illustrating the challenges in delivering an intensive lifestyle intervention as a supplement to metformin monotherapy in this patient population [7].

Sex and racial differences were also noted in the subgroup analyses of the TODAY study. The combination of metformin plus rosiglitazone proved to be more effective at preventing glycemic failure in girls (65% of the cohort) than in boys [7]; among girls, those in the metformin plus rosiglitazone group did better than girls in the other two treatment arms, whereas there were no treatment group differences in the boys [7]. Race/ethnicity had an impact on glycemic failure rates as well. Non-Hispanic blacks had the highest rates of glycemic failure (52.8%), followed by Hispanics (45%) and non-Hispanic whites (36.6%) [7]. Metformin monotherapy was least effective in non-Hispanic blacks compared with other racial/ethnic groups, whereas no significant differences were found in other treatment arms [7].

LESSONS FROM THE TREATMENT OPTIONS FOR TYPE 2 DIABETES IN ADOLESCENTS AND YOUTH RUN-IN

After subjects were screened for participation in the TODAY trial, they entered a run-in phase. The objectives of the run-in phase were to provide standard diabetes education, assess subjects' tolerance to metformin and adherence to study protocol, wean off other diabetes mediations while achieving an HbA1c less than 8% for at least 2 months, and establish a uniform study cohort before randomization.

Of the 927 participants who entered the run-in phase, 35.6% had an HbA1c of 8% or greater and 38% were on insulin; the mean HbA1c was 7.7% [8,9]. Of note, 90.9% of these subjects achieved an HbA1c less than 8% and nearly all subjects who had been on insulin at screening were able to lower their HbA1c on metformin to less than 8% after insulin discontinuation [8,9]. After the completion of the run-in phase, 223 were not eligible for randomization. The most common reasons for ineligibility were inability to lower HbA1c to less than 8%, failure to wean off insulin, and metformin intolerance [9]. The group of participants who were unable to be randomized had a mean HbA1c of 8.5% at screening, were more likely to be non-Hispanic black, and gain weight during the run-in phase. C peptide levels were not significantly different in the nonrandomized group [9].

DURABLE CONTROL

Given the high rate of loss of glycemic control on oral therapy in youth-onset T2D, the TODAY study examined whether specific clinical markers identified early in a patient's disease may be useful in predicting which subjects were more likely to develop glycemic failure on oral agents [10]. Participants were divided into 2 categories: those who met the primary outcome of glycemic failure in less than 48 months and those who achieved durable control and did not exhibit glycemic failure over this period of time. Table 1 highlights the differences between these two groups [10].

In multivariate analysis, HbA1c at screening and at randomization (after treatment with metformin for 2 to 6 months during run-in) and baseline insulinogenic index (the change in insulin in response to change in glucose during the oral glucose tolerance test) were the two metabolic factors that were significantly different between the group that had glycemic failure and the group that achieved metabolic goals over 48 months [10]; baseline HbA1c was lower (Fig. 2) and insulinogenic index higher in the group with durable control. Because HbA1c is more clinically accessible, HbA1c as a potential marker for risk was examined more closely. In receiver-operator curve analysis, an HbA1c of 6.3% or more after initiation of metformin was shown to be a predictor of eventual loss of glycemic control; for every 0.1% increase in HbA1c there was a 16% increase in risk of loss of glycemic control, with a median time to loss of control of approximately 11 months, irrespective of treatment arm [10]. Therefore, patients who do not lower their HbA1c to a nondiabetes range on metformin monotherapy are at increased risk for loss of glycemic control and should be followed closely for a more rapid decline in glucose control.

METABOLIC SYNDROME

Metabolic syndrome in patients with T2D heightens cardiovascular disease risk. In the LOOK AHEAD (Action for the Health in Diabetes) trial, 94% of adults with T2D had metabolic syndrome; lifestyle interventions in these adults did not

Table 1
Demographics and baseline characteristics affecting durability of glycemic control

Demographic and baseline characteristics by analysis group: mean (SD) or n (%)				
Characteristic		Group 1 no PO <48 mo (n = 172)	Group 2 PO <48 mo (n = 305)	P value
Treatment	Metformin	53 (30.8%)	116 (38.0%)	.2453
	Metformin + Rosiglitazone	58 (33.7%)	86 (28.2%)	—
	Metformin + Lifestyle	61 (35.5%)	103 (33.8%)	—
Sex	Female	111 (64.5%)	193 (63.3%)	.7845
	Male	61 (35.5%)	112 (36.7%)	—
Age (y)	—	13.8 (1.9)	14.1 (2.1)	.1825
Race-ethnicity	NHB	47 (27.3%)	117 (38.3%)	.0323
	H	70 (40.7%)	119 (39.0%)	—
	NHW	43 (25.0%)	48 (15.7%)	—
	Other	12 (7.0%)	21 (6.9%)	—
Months since diagnosis	—	8.1 (6.2)	8.7 (6.2)	.3752
Depressive symptoms	No	154 (91.1%)	251 (83.4%)	.0217
	Yes	15 (8.9%)	50 (16.6%)	—
Tanner stage	≥4	155 (90.1%)	271 (88.9%)	.6682
	≤3	17 (9.9%)	34 (11.1%)	—
Household income	Low (<$25,000)	62 (39.7%)	120 (45.0%)	.0512
	Mid ($25,000–$49,999)	46 (29.5%)	93 (34.8%)	—
	High (≥$50,000)	48 (30.8%)	54 (20.2%)	—
Household education	Less than HS	46 (27.1%)	80 (26.5%)	.4529
	HS, GED, or tech	37 (21.8%)	85 (28.1%)	—
	College no degree	57 (33.5%)	93 (30.8%)	—
	College degree	30 (17.6%)	44 (14.6%)	—
First-degree family history of diabetes	No	86 (50.6%)	100 (33.3%)	.0003
	Yes	84 (49.4%)	200 (66.7%)	—
BMI (kg/m^2)	—	34.0 (7.6)	35.1 (7.5)	.1189
Waist circumference (cm)	—	107.1 (16.2)	109.2 (17.0)	.1940
HbA1c at screening (%)	—	6.79 (1.64)	8.05 (2.07)	<.0001
(mmol/mol)	—	51 (17.9)	64 (22.6)	<.0001
HbA1c at randomization (%) (mmol/mol)	—	5.68 (0.55)	6.39 (0.80)	<.0001
	—	39 (6.0)	46 (8.7)	<.0001
C-peptide (ng/mL)	—	3.71 (1.55)	3.91 (1.64)	.1921
DXA fat mass (kg)	—	32.9 (10.0)	33.0 (9.8)	.9453
DXA lean mass (kg)	—	55.6 (12.4)	54.0 (11.0)	.2299
Insulin inverse (mL/μU)	—	0.045 (0.027)	0.047 (0.037)	.7956
Insulinogenic index (μU/mL per mg/dL)	—	2.04 (2.18)	1.12 (2.08)	<.0001

Abbreviations: DXA, dual-energy X-ray absorptiometry; GED, general equivalency diploma; H, Hispanic; HS, high school; NHB, non-Hispanic black; NHW, non-Hispanic white; PO, primary outcome.

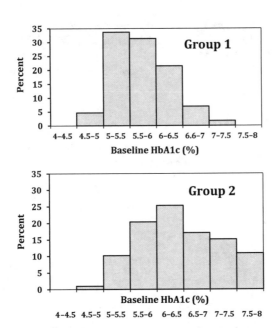

Fig. 2. Distribution of baseline HbA1c in Group 1 (no glycemic failure within 48 months) and Group 2 (glycemic failure within 48 months).

reduce cardiovascular events [11,12]. Metabolic syndrome in the TODAY study was defined using the Adult Treatment Panel III (ATP III) definition [13] and, because all subjects had diabetes, required at least 2 of the following 4 criteria: abdominal obesity (>102 cm in males and >88 cm in females), triglycerides greater than 150 mg/dL or on lipid-lowering treatment, low high-density lipoprotein (HDL) cholesterol (<40 in males and <50 in females), and high blood pressure (≥130/85 or on antihypertensive treatment).

The TODAY study found the prevalence of metabolic syndrome to be 75.8% at randomization [14]. Neither the overall prevalence nor incidence of metabolic syndrome significantly changed in first 2 years of the trial. Further there were no differences in the prevalence of metabolic syndrome among the 3 treatment arms [14]. Table 2 displays the prevalence of metabolic syndrome in TODAY subjects by sex, race/ethnicity, and glycemic status. Metabolic syndrome was more common in female subjects (83.1%) compared with their male counterparts (62.3%), and this difference persisted over time. The factors contributing to the difference between sexes were a higher likelihood of abdominal obesity and low HDL cholesterol in female subjects [14]. The prevalence of metabolic syndrome among subjects with different racial/ethnic backgrounds was similar at baseline and 6 months after the study began. However, after 2 years, 82.7% of Hispanics had metabolic syndrome, which was significantly higher than the rate observed in non-Hispanic blacks (72.7%) and non-Hispanic whites (67.5%). Low levels of

Table 2
Prevalence of metabolic syndrome by sex, race/ethnicity, and glycemic status

	Baseline (N = 679)			6 mo (N = 625)			24 mo (N = 545)		
	N and (%)		P value	N and (%)		P value	N and (%)		P value
Overall	515	(75.8)	—	472	(75.5)	—	418	(76.7)	—
Sex									
Female	368	(83.1)	<.0001	331	(81.5)	<.0001	293	(81.8)	<.0001
Male	147	(62.3)		141	(64.4)		125	(66.8)	
Race/ethnicity									
Non-Hispanic black	172	(76.4)	.7036	153	(75.7)	.4198	125	(72.7)	.0038[c]
Hispanic	205	(76.8)		190	(77.2)		187	(82.7)	
Non-Hispanic white	101	(73.2)		91	(71.1)		77	(67.5)	
Glycemic status[d]									
For those not reaching primary outcome by end of trial[a]									
HbA1c <6.0%	188	(74.6)	—	173	(72.1)	—	130	(70.7)	—
HbA1c <7%	264	(74.4)		228	(70.8)		204	(74.2)	
HbA1c 6.0%–7.9%	89	(75.4)		59	(68.6)		86	(83.5)	
Reached primary outcome at visit[a]	N/A[b]	N/A[b]		56	(83.6)		136	(79.5)	
Reached primary outcome by end of trial[a]	238	(77.0)		237	(80.3)		195	(78.3)	

Abbreviation: N/A, not applicable.

[a]Primary outcome: HbA1c greater than 8.0% over 6 months or inability to wean from temporary insulin therapy following acute metabolic decomposition.

[b]HbA1c less than 8.0% during prerandomization run-in period was an eligibility criteria so no possibility for having primary outcome at baseline.

[c]Non-Hispanic black versus Hispanic P value = .0164, Hispanic versus non-Hispanic white P value = .0017, non-Hispanic black versus non-Hispanic white P value = .3514.

[d]Only statistically significant difference is for the prevalence of metabolic syndrome in those who did not reach the primary outcome with HbA1c values of 6.0% to 7.9% versus other HbA1c values at 24 months (P = .0174).

triglycerides in non-Hispanic blacks and low HDL cholesterol levels in Hispanics contributed to these differences [14]. Subjects who reached glycemic failure in the study were more likely to have metabolic syndrome at 6 months and had higher rates of hypertriglyceridemia and hypertension [14].

PARENTAL DIABETES

Other studies have shown that having a parent with self-reported T2D greatly increases a child's risk for development of the disorder; exposure to T2D during pregnancy results in a 3-fold increased risk of diabetes in offspring compared with a sibling who was not exposed to high blood sugars in utero [15]. The maternal influence is known to be stronger than the paternal effect [16–20]. In addition to genetic factors, in utero exposure to diabetes may also affect offspring through an epigenetic process [21].

In the TODAY study, 50% of participants had a mother with diabetes, whereas 32% of the subjects' fathers were reported to have diabetes at the randomization visit [22]. Table 3 contrasts the effect of maternal versus paternal diabetes on demographic, anthropometric, parental, and metabolic measures. Participants with a maternal history of T2D and who were exposed to diabetes in utero were younger by 0.6 years at the time of diagnosis, more likely to be male, and were heavier at birth by approximately 400 g. BMI z score, percent body fat, and waist circumference were not associated with parental diabetes history [22]. Subjects whose mothers had diabetes during their pregnancy had a significantly higher (by 0.3%) HbA1c at baseline, and a maternal history of diabetes (either diagnosed during or after pregnancy) was also associated with a higher fasting and 2-hour glucose at the time of randomization. Insulin secretion (as measured by the C-peptide oral disposition index) was lower in subjects with a maternal history of diabetes; the lower oral disposition index was significant regardless of whether the mother's diabetes was diagnosed before, during, or after the pregnancy. Conversely, markers of insulin sensitivity were not associated with parental diabetes status [22].

PREGNANCY

Teen pregnancy carries a heightened risk to the mother and neonate. Pregnancy in individuals with diabetes poses additional risks to mother and baby, particularly when the mother's glycemic control is not optimal. The TODAY study provided an opportunity to assess the additional risks that face teens with T2D who become pregnant. Forty-six (10.8%) of the 452 female TODAY participants became pregnant during the study, a proportion in line with rates of pregnancy in the general teen population [23]. All female TODAY participants were counseled to use birth control at each visit; were advised against pregnancy because of the possible exposure to rosiglitazone, a pregnancy class C medication; and received a video-based program regarding pregnancy planning developed for girls with diabetes. However, only 13% of the participants who became pregnant recalled the recommendation to avoid pregnancy during the study [23].

Compared with the girls without pregnancy, subjects who became pregnant were more likely to be older, live outside of the parental home, and have a lower annual household income [23]. There was no difference in parental education, diabetes duration, BMI, smoking history, TODAY treatment group, HbA1c at baseline, or the percent losing glycemic control. Of all pregnancies in TODAY, 26.4% ended in a miscarriage, stillbirth, or intrauterine fetal demise. Of the live-born offspring, 20.5% had a major congenital anomaly: 50% with cardiac defects and the remaining with congenital kidney, intestinal, brain, or palate malformations. Maternal prenatal complications included 8.7%

Table 3
Parental diabetes

	Maternal diabetes status (n = 632)				Paternal diabetes status (n = 494)		
	During pregnancy (n = 215, 34%)	After pregnancy (n = 103, 16%)	Never (n = 314, 50%)	P value	Ever (n = 157, 32%)	Never (n = 337, 68%)	P value
Demographic							
Age at diagnosis (y)	13.3 ± 2.2	14.0 ± 2.1	13.9 ± 2.1	**.0021** D vs A, D vs N	13.6 ± 2.1	13.7 ± 2.2	.5978
Duration of diabetes (mo)	7.6 ± 5.7	8.4 ± 6.3	7.7 ± 5.8	.5603	8.4 ± 6.3	7.6 ± 5.8	.1638
% Male	42.3%	29.1%	31.8%	**.0189** D vs A, D vs N	28.0%	40.4%	**.0073**
Race/ethnicity (%)							
Non-Hispanic black	31.6%	30.1%	33.8%	.6333	30.6%	31.2%	.8833
Hispanic	40.5%	43.7%	37.3%	—	40.1%	38.9%	—
Non-Hispanic white	20.5%	17.5%	23.2%	—	21.0%	23.1%	—
Other	7.4%	8.7%	5.7%	—	8.3%	6.8%	—
Parental (self-report)							
Maternal BMI (kg/m^2)	34.5 ± 9.6	36.0 ± 9.6	33.6 ± 8.7	.0857	35.2 ± 9.7	33.6 ± 8.8	.0777
Maternal age at birth (y)	28.7 ± 6.0	26.3 ± 5.8	25.8 ± 5.7	**<.0001** D vs A, D vs N	27.9 ± 6.1	26.7 ± 5.7	**.0302**
Paternal age at birth (y)	31.7 ± 7.4	29.5 ± 6.8	28.6 ± 6.5	**<.0001** D vs A, D vs N	31.7 ± 8.0	29.1 ± 6.3	**.0001**
Anthropometric							
Birth weight at term (g)	3678 ± 788	3386 ± 660	3269 ± 629	**.0003** D vs N	3247 ± 765	3351 ± 820	.3190
BMI z-score	2.3 ± 0.5	2.2 ± 0.5	2.2 ± 0.5	.4571	2.2 ± 0.5	2.2 ± 0.5	.2543
% Body fat from DXA	37.5 ± 6.6	38.2 ± 6.2	37.6 ± 5.9	.7955	37.9 ± 6.3	37.4 ± 6.3	.6285
Waist circumference (cm)	107.5 ± 16.4	109.1 ± 15.3	109.5 ± 17.4	.8865	109.8 ± 18.2	107.9 ± 15.4	.0892
Metabolic							
HbA1c (%) [mmol/mol]	6.2 ± 0.8	6.1 ± 0.7	5.9 ± 0.7	**<.0001** D vs A, D vs N, A vs N	6.1 ± 0.8	6.0 ± 0.7	**.0241**
Fasting blood glucose (mg/dl)	116.1 ± 26.8	114.6 ± 25.9	105.4 ± 21.7	**<.0001** D vs N, A vs N	111.4 ± 25.4	110.1 ± 24.9	.5071
2-h Blood glucose (mg/dl)	217.3 ± 66.8	213.4 ± 60.5	190.4 ± 60.6	**<.0001** D vs N, A vs N	209.7 ± 61.7	199.2 ± 64.2	.1076

Abbreviations: A, after pregnancy; D, during pregnancy; N, never.

with preeclampsia, 10.9% with nephrotic-range proteinuria, and 21.7% with hypertension. In the women who had been pregnant and who had retinal photography after delivery (63% of total), 27.6% had mild nonproliferative diabetic retinopathy, compared with an overall rate of nonproliferative retinopathy of 13.7% in the cohort [23].

COMPLICATIONS

Microvascular and macrovascular complications of T2D are a main source of morbidity and mortality in adults, but less is known about youth-onset disease. Previous case series in children with T2D show higher rates of hypertension and microalbuminuria compared with youths with type 1 diabetes mellitus of similar age and duration of disease [24–26]. The TODAY trial provided an opportunity to examine the longitudinal prevalence of hypertension, microalbuminuria, retinopathy, and cardiovascular disease risk in children and adolescents with T2D.

Hypertension in the TODAY study was defined as either a blood pressure of 130/80 mm Hg or greater or 95th percentile or greater for age, sex, and height on 3 separate visits [27]. Dietary counseling restricting sodium consumption was initiated when high blood pressures first became apparent. Microalbuminuria was identified as an albumin-to-creatinine ratio of 30 µg/mg or greater in at least 2 urine samples collected over a 3-month time period [27]. Treatment of both hypertension and microalbuminuria began with an angiotensin-converting enzyme inhibitor followed by the sequential addition of antihypertensive agents (using a predefined algorithm) in order to reach goal blood pressure and urinary albumin excretion parameters [27].

The overall prevalence of hypertension increased from 11.6% at baseline to 33.8% by the end of the study [27]. These prevalences compare with less than 5% in the similarly aged nondiabetic, general population [28]. The factors associated with risk of hypertension were male sex, older age at baseline, and higher BMI. Boys were 81% more likely to be hypertensive compared with girls. Each year older at baseline conferred an additional 14% risk of hypertension. Each additional kilogram per square meter in BMI added an additional 6% risk of hypertension [27]. Treatment arm, race/ethnic background, HbA1c, and incidence of glycemic failure did not affected hypertension risk in the TODAY study.

Microalbuminuria among all participants increased from an overall prevalence of 6.3% at the start of the study to 16.6% by the end of the study [27]. Baseline and subsequent annual incidence rates of microalbuminuria were similar to those found in the adult UK Prospective Diabetes Study [29]. TODAY study participants who met the criteria for glycemic failure were more likely to develop microalbuminuria compared with those who did not (16.0% and 5.5%, respectively). HbA1c over time was significantly related to the risk of developing microalbuminuria; for every 1% increase in A1c, the risk increased by 17% [27]. However, rates of microalbuminuria did not differ among the TODAY study treatment arms, sex, or race/ethnic backgrounds.

In the final year of the TODAY trial, retinal examinations, including digital fundus photography, were obtained and read at a dedicated reading center at the University of Wisconsin. Retinopathy was defined as the minimum amount of retinal disease, including a microaneurysm, retinal hemorrhage, or cotton wool spot in at least one eye. The overall prevalence of retinopathy in TODAY participants with a mean diabetes duration of 4.5 ± 1.5 years was 13.7% [30]. All subjects with retinopathy were classified as mild nonproliferative diabetic retinopathy (NPDR); there were no participants with more advanced disease (ie, macular edema, advanced NPDR, proliferative retinopathy). Subjects who developed NPDR were older (19.1 vs 17.9 years), had higher A1c (8.3% vs 6.9%), and had diabetes for a longer duration (5.6 vs 4.7 years) [30]. The onset of retinopathy did not correlate with sex, ethnicity, TODAY treatment arm, blood pressure, smoking, pregnancy, microalbuminuria, or hyperlipidemia. Participants with the highest BMIs were least likely to develop retinopathy, suggesting that obesity and perhaps insulin resistance may play a protective role in the evolution of retinopathy in these patients [30]. Similar associations between obesity and lower risk for retinopathy have been reported in adults [31–34].

Cardiovascular disease is the leading cause of death in adults with T2D [2]. In the TODAY study there were no cardiovascular events. Lipid parameters (low-density lipoprotein [LDL], non-HDL, apolipoprotein B, LDL particle density, triglycerides, and HDL) and inflammatory markers (high-sensitivity C-reactive protein [CRP], homocysteine, plasminogen activator inhibitor-1, and nonesterified fatty acids) were assessed at baseline and then annually. Lipid goals were defined as LDL less than 100 mg/dL and triglycerides less than 150 mg/dL; if LDL was greater than 130 mg/dL and triglycerides greater than 300 mg/dL, nutrition counseling and dietary changes were attempted for 6 months before starting statin therapy [6]. The percentage of total subjects with an LDL greater than 130 mg/dL or who were taking a prescribed statin increased from 4.5% at baseline to 10.7% 3 years later [35]. Around half (55.9%) of the TODAY subjects remained at target LDL levels for the first 3 years of the study. Among the 3 TODAY treatment arms, LDL, triglycerides, apolipoprotein B, and non-HDL increased significantly in the first year after diagnosis and then stabilized for the next 2 years of observation. One notable exception was that triglycerides were considerably lower in the group receiving metformin plus an intensive lifestyle intervention [35]. Triglycerides levels were also significantly lower in the non-Hispanic blacks compared with the Hispanic and non-Hispanic white cohorts. Inflammatory markers high-sensitivity-CRP, homocysteine, and plasminogen activator inhibitor 1 all steadily increased throughout the first 3 years of the TODAY study [35].

Echocardiography was also performed on TODAY subjects during the last year of the trial. Mean left ventricular (LV) mass was high/normal in these subjects, and 16.2% of them had adverse LV geometry (8.1% concentric geometry, 4.5% LV hypertrophy, and 3.6% both) [36]. Factors that were positively associated with higher LV mass were male sex, non-Hispanic black race, BMI, systolic blood pressure, use of blood pressure medication, absence of glycemic failure, and smoking [36]. Longitudinal changes in BMI and blood pressure adversely affected LV mass, suggesting that control of these risk factors plays an important role in cardiovascular disease risk reduction in youth-onset T2D.

FUTURE RESEARCH

Youth-onset T2D has become more common, carries a high disease burden, and is associated with increased short-term and long-term morbidity and risk for earlier mortality. In 2013, Constantino and colleagues [37] compared rates of diabetes-related morbidity and mortality between 354 young adult subjects with T2D (average age of onset 25.6 years and average duration 11.6 years) and 470 subjects with type 1 diabetes (T1D) of similar diabetes duration. Subjects with T2D had 3 times the rate of albuminuria, 4 times the rate of stroke (4.3% vs 0.7%), nearly 6 times the rate of ischemic heart disease (12.6% vs 2.5%), and nearly 3 times the rate of any macrovascular disease [37]. Subjects with T2D had a mortality excess of 11% (vs 6.8% in patients with T1D) and a hazard ratio for death of 2.0 (95% confidence interval 1.2–3.2). Death occurred at a shorter disease duration of 27 years in subjects with T2D compared with 36.5 years in subjects with T1D [37]. However, although documenting the significant morbidity and mortality associated with youth-onset T2D, the study's cross-sectional and retrospective design limits our understanding of the causal relationships among treatment, metabolic control, β-cell function, and diabetes complications and comorbidities. The longitudinal follow-up of the well-characterized TODAY cohort in TODAY2, a long-term observational study of outcomes in the TODAY cohort, is well suited to help answer these questions.

The TODAY2 postintervention follow-up study will continue collecting data on diabetes outcomes on these subjects through the year 2021. To date, the retention rate in TODAY2 is high, as 72.1% of the original TODAY participants have consented to continue in TODAY2 and adherence to annual visits has been greater than 90%. Individuals in the cohort have been comprehensively characterized, including measures of glycemic control, insulin sensitivity, β-cell secretory capacity, body composition, fitness, physical activity, dietary intake, quality of life, hypertension, dyslipidemia, urinary albumin excretion, peripheral neuropathy, arterial stiffness (pulse wave velocity), cardiac function (echocardiography), retinal status, depression indicators, and eating disorders since soon after diagnosis. DNA has also been collected on these subjects to help determine what other genetic factors may contribute to the pathogenesis of youth-onset T2D. By following these well-characterized individuals as they transition to emerging adults, TODAY2 will expand our understanding of the nature and determinants of long-term outcomes in youth-onset T2D.

Acknowledgments

The TODAY Study Group thanks the following companies for donations in support of the study's efforts: Becton, Dickinson and Company; Bristol-Myers

Squibb; Eli Lilly and Company; GlaxoSmithKline; LifeScan; Pfizer; Sanofi Aventis. The authors also gratefully acknowledge the participation and guidance of the American Indian partners associated with the clinical center located at the University of Oklahoma Health Sciences Center, including members of the Absentee Shawnee Tribe, Cherokee Nation, Chickasaw Nation, Choctaw Nation of Oklahoma, and Oklahoma City Area Indian Health Service; the opinions expressed in this article are those of the authors and do not necessarily reflect the views of the respective Tribal and Indian Health Service Institution Review Boards or their members.

Materials developed and used for the TODAY standard diabetes education program and the intensive lifestyle intervention program are available to the public at https://today.bsc.gwu.edu/.

The authors thank the TODAY participants and members of the TODAY Study Group for their invaluable contributions and dedication.

References

[1] Pinhas-Hamiel O, Dolan LM, Daniels SR, et al. Increased incidence of non-insulin-dependent diabetes mellitus among adolescents. J Pediatr 1996;128(5 Pt 1):608–15.

[2] Tryggestad JB, Willi SM. Complications and comorbidities of T2DM in adolescents: findings from the TODAY clinical trial. J Diabet Complications 2015;29(2):307–12.

[3] Dabelea D. The accelerating epidemic of childhood diabetes. Lancet 2009;373(9680): 1999–2000.

[4] Dabelea D, Mayer-Davis EJ, Saydah S, et al. Prevalence of type 1 and type 2 diabetes among children and adolescents from 2001 to 2009. JAMA 2014;311(17):1778–86.

[5] Menke A, Casagrande S, Geiss L, et al. Prevalence of and trends in diabetes among adults in the United States, 1988-2012. JAMA 2015;314(10):1021–9.

[6] TODAY Study Group, Zeitler P, Epstein L, et al. Treatment options for type 2 diabetes in adolescents and youth: a study of the comparative efficacy of metformin alone or in combination with rosiglitazone or lifestyle intervention in adolescents with type 2 diabetes. Pediatr Diabetes 2007;8(2):74–87.

[7] TODAY Study Group, Zeitler P, Hirst K, et al. A clinical trial to maintain glycemic control in youth with type 2 diabetes. N Engl J Med 2012;366(24):2247–56.

[8] Kelsey MM, Geffner ME, Guandalini C, et al. Presentation and effectiveness of early treatment of type 2 diabetes in youth: lessons from the TODAY study. Pediatr Diabetes 2016;17(3):212–21.

[9] Laffel L, Chang N, Grey M, et al. Metformin monotherapy in youth with recent onset type 2 diabetes: experience from the prerandomization run-in phase of the TODAY study. Pediatr Diabetes 2012;13(5):369–75.

[10] Zeitler P, Hirst K, Copeland KC, et al. HbA1c after a short period of monotherapy with metformin identifies durable glycemic control among adolescents with type 2 diabetes. Diabetes Care 2015;38(12):2285–92.

[11] Ribisl PM, Lang W, Jaramillo SA, et al. Exercise capacity and cardiovascular/metabolic characteristics of overweight and obese individuals with type 2 diabetes: the Look AHEAD clinical trial. Diabetes Care 2007;30(10):2679–84.

[12] Look AHEAD Research Group, Wing RR, Bolin P, et al. Cardiovascular effects of intensive lifestyle intervention in type 2 diabetes. N Engl J Med 2013;369(2):145–54.

[13] National Cholesterol Education Program (NCEP) Expert Panel on Detection, Evaluation, and Treatment of High Blood Cholesterol in Adults (Adult Treatment Panel III). Treatment of High Blood Cholesterol in, Third Report of the National Cholesterol Education Program (NCEP) Expert Panel on Detection, Evaluation, and Treatment of High Blood Cholesterol in Adults (Adult Treatment Panel III) final report. Circulation 2002;106(25):3143–421.

[14] Weinstock RS, Drews KL, Caprio S, et al. Metabolic syndrome is common and persistent in youth-onset type 2 diabetes: results from the TODAY clinical trial. Obesity (Silver Spring) 2015;23(7):1357–61.

[15] Dabelea D, Hanson RL, Lindsay RS, et al. Intrauterine exposure to diabetes conveys risks for type 2 diabetes and obesity: a study of discordant sibships. Diabetes 2000;49(12): 2208–11.

[16] Franks PW, Looker HC, Kobes S, et al. Gestational glucose tolerance and risk of type 2 diabetes in young Pima Indian offspring. Diabetes 2006;55(2):460–5.

[17] McLean M, Chipps D, Cheung NW. Mother to child transmission of diabetes mellitus: does gestational diabetes program type 2 diabetes in the next generation? Diabet Med 2006;23(11):1213–5.

[18] Pettitt DJ, Lawrence JM, Beyer J, et al. Association between maternal diabetes in utero and age at offspring's diagnosis of type 2 diabetes. Diabetes Care 2008;31(11):2126–30.

[19] Singh R, Pearson E, Avery PJ, et al. Reduced beta cell function in offspring of mothers with young-onset type 2 diabetes. Diabetologia 2006;49(8):1876–80.

[20] Clausen TD, Mathiesen ER, Hansen T, et al. High prevalence of type 2 diabetes and prediabetes in adult offspring of women with gestational diabetes mellitus or type 1 diabetes: the role of intrauterine hyperglycemia. Diabetes Care 2008;31(2):340–6.

[21] Dabelea D, Mayer-Davis EJ, Lamichhane AP, et al. Association of intrauterine exposure to maternal diabetes and obesity with type 2 diabetes in youth: the SEARCH Case-Control Study. Diabetes Care 2008;31(7):1422–6.

[22] Chernausek SD, Arslanian S, Caprio S, et al. Relationship between parental diabetes and presentation of metabolic and glycemic function in youth with type 2 diabetes: baseline findings from the TODAY trial. Diabetes Care 2016;39(1):110–7.

[23] Klingensmith GJ, Pyle L, Nadeau KJ, et al. Pregnancy outcomes in youth with type 2 diabetes: the TODAY study experience. Diabetes Care 2016;39(1):122–9.

[24] Eppens MC, Craig ME, Cusumano J, et al. Prevalence of diabetes complications in adolescents with type 2 compared with type 1 diabetes. Diabetes Care 2006;29(6):1300–6.

[25] Maahs DM, Snively BM, Bell RA, et al. Higher prevalence of elevated albumin excretion in youth with type 2 than type 1 diabetes: the SEARCH for Diabetes in Youth study. Diabetes Care 2007;30(10):2593–8.

[26] Ettinger LM, Freeman K, DiMartino-Nardi JR, et al. Microalbuminuria and abnormal ambulatory blood pressure in adolescents with type 2 diabetes mellitus. J Pediatr 2005;147(1): 67–73.

[27] TODAY Study Group. Rapid rise in hypertension and nephropathy in youth with type 2 diabetes: the TODAY clinical trial. Diabetes Care 2013;36(6):1735–41.

[28] Falkner B. Hypertension in children and adolescents: epidemiology and natural history. Pediatr Nephrol 2010;25(7):1219–24.

[29] Retnakaran R, Cull CA, Thorne KI, et al. Risk factors for renal dysfunction in type 2 diabetes: U.K. Prospective Diabetes Study 74. Diabetes 2006;55(6):1832–9.

[30] TODAY Study Group. Retinopathy in youth with type 2 diabetes participating in the TODAY clinical trial. Diabetes Care 2013;36(6):1772–4.

[31] Klein R, Klein BE, Moss SE, et al. The Wisconsin epidemiologic study of diabetic retinopathy. III. Prevalence and risk of diabetic retinopathy when age at diagnosis is 30 or more years. Arch Ophthalmol 1984;102(4):527–32.

[32] Kohner EM, Aldington SJ, Stratton IM, et al. United Kingdom Prospective Diabetes Study, 30: diabetic retinopathy at diagnosis of non-insulin-dependent diabetes mellitus and associated risk factors. Arch Ophthalmol 1998;116(3):297–303.

[33] Nelson RG, Wolfe JA, Horton MB, et al. Proliferative retinopathy in NIDDM. Incidence and risk factors in Pima Indians. Diabetes 1989;38(4):435–40.

[34] Rajala U, Laakso M, Qiao Q, et al. Prevalence of retinopathy in people with diabetes, impaired glucose tolerance, and normal glucose tolerance. Diabetes Care 1998;21(10): 1664–9.

[35] TODAY Study Group. Lipid and inflammatory cardiovascular risk worsens over 3 years in youth with type 2 diabetes: the TODAY clinical trial. Diabetes Care 2013;36(6):1758–64.

[36] Levitt Katz L, Gidding SS, Bacha F, et al. Alterations in left ventricular, left atrial, and right ventricular structure and function to cardiovascular risk factors in adolescents with type 2 diabetes participating in the TODAY clinical trial. Pediatr Diabetes 2015;16(1):39–47.

[37] Constantino MI, Molyneaux L, Limacher-Gisler F, et al. Long-term complications and mortality in young-onset diabetes: type 2 diabetes is more hazardous and lethal than type 1 diabetes. Diabetes Care 2013;36(12):3863–9.

Advances in Pediatrics 63 (2016) 211–226

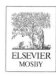

ADVANCES IN PEDIATRICS

Comorbidities of Thyroid Disease in Children

Janiel Pimentel, MD, Melissa Chambers, MD,
Madhia Shahid, MD, Reeti Chawla, MD,
Chirag Kapadia, MD*

Phoenix Children's Hospital, 1919 E Thomas Road, Phoenix, AZ 85016, USA

Keywords
• Thyroid comorbidities • Pediatric thyroid disease • Hypothyroidism

Key points

- Thyroid disease even when treated results in mild persistent issues in cognition, weight, and mood in a subset of the population.
- Outcomes in congenital hypothyroidism are good but mild brain development issues are present in a subset of patients; growth is fine in nearly all treated patients.
- Prolonged hypothyroidism or hyperthyroidism impairs and alters growth outcomes even after the disease is identified and treated.

INTRODUCTION: COMORBIDITIES OF THYROID DISEASE IN CHILDREN

Thyroid disease in the pediatric population is routinely managed by pediatric endocrinologists. The management of thyroid disease is well established. However, as with diabetes in the pediatric population, because comorbidities have been assumed to not be of concern until adulthood, there is insufficient clinical and research attention devoted to examination of thyroid comorbidities in children.

This review article first covers hypothyroidism, with focus on congenital hypothyroidism (CH), acquired hypothyroidism, and subclinical hypothyroidism (SH). We conclude with a review of comorbidities of treated Graves' disease.

The focus of the article is largely on comorbidities that occur in patients even when they are identified and under medical care. We identify

*Corresponding author. E-mail address: ckapadia@phoenixchildrens.com

0065-3101/16/$ – see front matter
http://dx.doi.org/10.1016/j.yapd.2016.04.016

neurologic/psychiatric impact, growth effects, weight effects and related complications, and cardiovascular risk for each disease.

CONGENITAL HYPOTHYROIDISM

CH is most commonly caused by abnormal thyroid glandular development and includes agenesis, dysgenesis, and ectopic gland formation. Less common etiologies include dyshormonogenesis and transient CH secondary to transplacental passage of maternal medication, maternal blocking antibodies, or iodine deficiency or excess. Rarely, central hypothyroidism from pituitary or hypothalamic dysfunction is seen [1]. In the developed world, permanent primary CH affects approximately 1 in every 3500 live births [2]. Lower cutoff points for thyrotropin (TSH) levels have been incorporated in screening programs allowing for detection of mild forms of the disease, which has led to an increase in the reported incidence of CH [2].

Neurologic/psychiatric impact

Before the implementation of newborn screen programs, significant morbidity existed secondary to delayed or untreated CH. However, with implementation of newborn screen programs, nearly all children in the United States and the developing world are screened for CH and therapy with thyroxine is implemented within the first 3 weeks of life. For this reason, we do not focus on comorbidities seen as a consequence of lack of or significantly delayed initiation of treatment, primarily impaired neurocognitive development and overt cretinism, as such clinical scenarios are rarely encountered in today's practice, and are already well described [2–4].

Despite early initiation of treatment within the first 3 weeks of life, multiple studies have reported subtle deficits in cognitive and motor development in young children treated for CH after that time [1,2]. In a meta-analysis of studies comparing patients with CH with controls, a statistically significant impairment in motor development (primarily balance and fine motor skills) along with IQ deficit was seen among patients with CH. The most important risk factor was the severity of CH at diagnosis. The investigators concluded that some degree of impaired brain development in patients with CH may occur in utero and may not be prevented by early postnatal initiation of thyroxine treatment [5].

Impairment of verbal and memory functioning has also been noted among patients with CH despite early initiation of treatment [2,6]. Furthermore, based on MRI assessment, Wheeler and colleagues [6] noted that patients with CH showed compromised hippocampal development, an area of the brain essential for learning and memory.

The effect of different thyroxine replacement doses on intellectual development among patients with CH has also been evaluated with results suggesting that higher treatment doses of thyroxine result in improvement in IQ scores [7]. In one study, 83 patients with CH started on treatment between 21 to 25 days of life were divided into 3 groups based on starting treatment doses (6–8 µg/kg per day, 8.1–10 µg/kg per day, and 10.1–15 µg/kg per day). IQ was assessed at 4 years of age and was significantly higher in the high-dose and middle-dose groups in comparison with the low-dose group. Additionally, even between mid-dose and high-dose groups, there was disparity, as the investigators found that the IQs were below normal range in 6 patients from the 8.1 to 10.0 µg/kg per day group but not in any patients in the 10.1 to 15.0 µg/kg per day group [7].

Conversely, as children get older, higher thyroxine levels may adversely impact attention. Rovet and Alvarez [8] measured distractibility and attention in 7-year-old children with CH on treatment and found that T4 levels accounted for more than 10% of the variance in attention.

These subtle cognitive and motor deficits may persist into adulthood. Kempers and colleagues [9] followed a cohort of 70 young adults with CH born in the first 2 years after the institution of newborn screening. The investigators observed greater cognitive deficits in verbal and performance domains in comparison with control subjects. Furthermore, deficits were also found in balance and fine motor skills. Similar to previous studies, they found that severity of CH influenced the degree of the deficits.

Thus, although it is common practice for parents of children with CH to be told that with treatment, the children will be cognitively normal, a more accurate statement would be to state that with actively and frequently monitored treatment, the risk of cognitive defects will be low, and that if they do occur, they are likely to be mild.

Growth effects

Early data suggested that patients with CH may have slightly impaired linear growth; however, more recent data suggest that height outcome is similar regardless of treatment dose, with genetics playing a larger role [2,7,10–12].

Among a cohort of approximately 100 Swedish and Norwegian infants with CH started on treatment between 15 to 20 days of life, Heyerdahl and colleagues [10] found that children with CH had reduced growth from 6 to 12 months, and increased growth after 12 months of age. Another early study suggested that the dose of thyroxine received during the first 6 months of treatment plays a role in influencing normal adult height [12].

However, subsequent studies did not support these early findings. In a retrospective analysis, Ng and colleagues [11] examined 125 patients with CH from birth to 3 years of age with treatment initiated at a mean age of 15 days. The investigators found no differences in linear growth at diagnosis among patients with CH and the general population independent of the etiology of CH. In another longitudinal study of patients with CH begun on thyroxine treatment at 25 ± 5 days of life followed from diagnosis until early adulthood, pubertal development and growth progressed normally in both boys and girls. Both sexes achieved final heights above the target height, with no relation to severity of CH or dose of thyroxine [13]. The same group later reported no differences in growth and bone age maturation at age 4 regardless of dose [7].

Thus clinicians can fairly state that CH, when treated, does not affect growth.

Weight effects and related complications

Patients with CH are at higher risk for being overweight and obese during childhood, predisposing to an increased risk of metabolic syndrome during adulthood [2]. An early study by Grant [14] examined growth parameters in a cohort of British children with CH identified on newborn screen and found that mean body mass index (BMI) values for children with CH were significantly greater than in controls yearly up to age 4 regardless of the severity of the CH at diagnosis. Salerno and colleagues [13] later reported that many patients with CH had BMI levels greater than the 95th percentile until 6 years of age. A possible mechanism for the observed increase in BMI among children with CH was proposed by Wong and colleagues. The investigators reported earlier adiposity rebound, with a higher nadir of BMI during childhood, among patients with CH. The subjects also showed a significantly higher risk of being overweight at 10 years of age [11].

Hence, even with treatment, there appears to be a higher obesity risk in CH, and patients and their families should be counseled accordingly.

Cardiovascular risk

An association between early cardiovascular disease and treatment of CH has been reported [15]. Long-term thyroxine treatment in young adults with CH is associated with impaired diastolic function, reduced exercise capacity, and reduced cardiopulmonary performance [16]. Oliviero and colleagues [15] noted impaired endothelial function in a cohort of 32 young adults with CH. The investigators suggested that high TSH levels inadequately corrected by thyroxine replacement therapy, particularly during puberty, is a risk factor for later endothelial dysfunction. However, although there is evidence of early indicators of increased cardiovascular risk, longer-term data are not clear.

Thus, at this time, routine screening for cardiac dysfunction in patients with CH is not indicated.

ACQUIRED AUTOIMMUNE HYPOTHYROIDISM (HASHIMOTO THYROIDITIS)

Neurologic/psychiatric impact

Deficits in memory, psychomotor slowing, visual perception, and construction skills can all be affected in hypothyroidism [17]. Hypothyroidism has been implicated in behavioral issues and emotional well-being [18]. Adolescent thyroid dysfunction is associated with difficulties in school performance when assessed by self-evaluation [18]. Deficits in executive function and memory are well established in hypothyroidism [19,20]. Generally, there is reversal of these deficits with levothyroxine therapy [19,20]. Thus, screening for thyroid disease in patients with psychiatric or cognitive disorders is warranted, as is treatment of overtly hypothyroid patients [20].

Hashimoto encephalopathy is a well-accepted but poorly understood condition in which acute or subacute encephalopathy is present in combination with positive thyroid autoantibodies without any other identifiable cause. It is thought to affect approximately 2.1 per 100,000 people [21], with peak incidence in people in their 40s, but occurrence in childhood and adolescence is reported as well [22]. The most common presenting symptoms include encephalopathy, seizures, cognitive decline with confusion, and behavioral changes including agitation, apathy, or restlessness, with psychosis, myoclonus, and tremors being described less commonly [23]. Thyroid function tests may be normal or abnormal at the time of the psychological or neurologic alterations. Electrocardiogram shows slow-wave abnormalities in more than 90% of cases [24]. Cerebrospinal fluid studies are abnormal in approximately 75% of cases, often with elevated protein level and mononuclear pleocytosis, with presence of antithyroid antibodies and normal glucose [25]. Steroids are effective treatment, although children and adolescents are more likely to have relapses or residual neurocognitive deficits than adults [23].

Growth effects

Poor linear growth velocity is the most common clinical manifestation of hypothyroidism, and is often the only symptom at diagnosis. This slowed growth velocity occurs gradually and often takes years to be identified. Thyroid hormone is a critical regulator of skeletal maturation; specifically longitudinal bone growth at the growth plate [26].

Hypothyroidism results in delayed bone age and reduces the thickness of the growth plate and long bone differentiation. This can be manifested as severe growth retardation and mechanical failure of the hip growth plate as seen with slipped capital femoral epiphysis [27]. Thyroid hormone also acts in a permissive way on growth hormone, and decreased production of thyroid hormone results in decreased growth hormone release from the pituitary [27,28].

Some studies have suggested that the duration of untreated hypothyroidism may be directly related to the amount of catch-up growth potential on restoration of thyroxine, with longer time period of untreated disease yielding permanent height deficit relative to expected height [26]. Many pediatric endocrinologists start slowly with thyroid replacement in profound, long-standing hypothyroidism, to avoid tachycardia and anxiety associated with rapid correction, and also to avoid a rapid bone age advance and hence compromise of height; however, data on this approach are lacking.

We and others have observed rapid pubertal tempo and skeletal maturation in children with long-standing hypothyroidism once treatment is begun, further compromising their final height. For those reasons, careful monitoring of pubertal progress and skeletal maturation should be part of the posttreatment regimen in these children, and appropriate use of gonadotropin agonists, such as depot leuprolide or implantable histrelin, should be considered.

Thus, in growth failure from compromised thyroid function, patients and their families should be counseled that thyroid therapy alone may not correct the height deficit in all cases.

Weight effects and related complications

Thyroid hormone modulates the metabolic rate. In the absence of thyroid hormone, basal thermogenesis and resting energy are reduced by 30% to 50% [29]. Hypothyroidism can alter the composition of the body and directly impact weight. Patients with overt hypothyroidism have higher body weight and lean body mass compared with euthyroid patients after thyroid replacement therapy, but it is due mostly to fluid excess [30].

When hypothyroidism is discovered in an obese child, there is often expectation that treatment will lead to weight loss, but this is not borne out in studies [29]. Consequently, practitioners should counsel families that they should not expect significant decreases in weight after treatment in most children with hypothyroidism. Lifestyle modifications are necessary to achieve improvement in weight and BMI.

Obstructive sleep apnea, on the other hand, can occur in hypothyroid patients and may be responsive to treatment. Potential mechanisms for this may be myopathy or decreased central ventilatory control [31,32]. Adult studies have shown incidence up to 25% and reversal of some symptoms with therapy [33]. A pediatric study found that routine thyroid screening in those with obstructive sleep apnea revealed a 6% to 11% incidence of thyroid disease, and recommended thyroid screening in those diagnosed with OSA [34].

Cardiovascular risk

The Framingham Heart study showed that left ventricular contractility is inversely related to TSH, thus hypothyroidism (elevated TSH) results in decreased contractility [35]. Cardiac myocytes rely on active T3 for proper calcium and ion fluxes [36,37]. Hypothyroidism, specifically low serum T3 levels, causes impaired diastolic function by suppressing the transcription of calcium cycling proteins, thus causing a decrease in cardiac output and heart rate, and this is seen in both adult and pediatric populations [37–39]. Patients with hypothyroidism also experience high systemic vascular resistance secondary to decreased release of endothelial-derived relaxation factor, which can cause varying degrees of diastolic hypertension [37,40].

Hypothyroidism also increases the risk of coronary artery disease, thought to be secondary to a combination of diastolic dysfunction, dyslipidemia, general inflammation, and endothelial dysfunction [41].

Fortunately, significant cardiac dysfunction is not common in children with hypothyroidism without underlying heart disease, as the peripheral oxygen demand is lower in children [42]. However, it should be considered as a potential etiology in those with unexplained pericardial effusion, pleural effusion, or edema. It should be noted that too-rapid correction of severe hypothyroidism in pediatric patients with heart disease poses risks, and hence, in this group, dosing should be started at 25% the expected dose and increased slowly every 6 to 8 weeks to goal [42].

It is well accepted that hypothyroidism can lead to secondary dyslipidemia in adults. Typical findings include a 30% elevation of total cholesterol and low-density lipoprotein, and marked increase in detrimental apolipoproteins and triglycerides [41,43–45]. Treatment with thyroid replacement often improves the lipid profile, but often patients still require lifestyle modifications and occasionally require the addition of lipid-lowering pharmacotherapy [41,43,46]. There is some evidence of a similar effect in children. The German Health Interview and Examination Survey for Children and Adolescents did find an association between higher TSH levels and less favorable lipid profiles in 6622 healthy children [47].

Subclinical hypothyroidism

Significance of, and need for treatment in, subclinical thyroid disease, in children, as in adults, remains a controversial area. For our purposes, SH refers to a normal Free T4 or T4 with TSH value above normal, but below 10 mIU/L [48,49].

The prevalence of SH in NHANES III was 4.3% in the adult population [50]. Incidence in pediatrics is thought to be somewhat lower (perhaps 2%) but data are more sparse [48]. In adults, the majority is associated with thyroid autoantibodies [51]. However, in children, the etiology is generally idiopathic in clinical settings. In research settings, thyroid morphologic abnormalities, autoimmunity, thyroid hormone synthesis defects, and TSHR gene mutations have been found to play a role [49,52,53].

Neurologic/psychiatric impact

In terms of mental health, in both children and adults, data on emotional well-being and correlation with SH are conflicting [54–62]. Generally, our recommendation is to avoid attributing severe psychiatric or cognitive dysfunction to SH [20,63,64].

Growth effects

SH does not cause impaired growth in most children. However, treatment can be considered in those with persistent SH and substantially compromised growth in whom other explanations for the poor growth have been ruled out [65,66].

Weight effects and related complications

In the pediatric population, defining SH is particularly problematic, as many children will have a mildly elevated TSH that resolves on repeat check or on weight loss, particularly in obesity [53,67–72]. Much of SH in children is seen as a referral when a TSH has been checked and found to be slightly abnormal in an obese child or adolescent.

Recent studies have reported that obesity is linked to mild elevations of TSH. The hypothesis is that elevated leptin levels may result in increased TSH levels, suggesting obesity as a possible cause of SH in some patients. Although the exact underlying mechanism is not understood, the observation that weight loss leads to decreased TSH levels implies that an increase in TSH in subjects with obesity is reversible and seems to be a consequence rather than a cause of obesity [73,74].

Cardiovascular risk

There has been speculation for years that SH would place obese individuals at further risk for cardiovascular disease, lipid abnormalities, or further weight gain. In fact, younger and middle-aged adults with subclinical thyroid dysfunction marked by TSH between 5 and 9 have a slight increase in cardiovascular risk overall, and adult literature is trending toward treatment if additional risk factors, such as hypertension, hyperlipidemia, obesity, or underlying heart dysfunction, are present [23,24].

In children and adolescents, there are no strong data indicating increased cardiovascular risk, or significant lipid abnormalities, in those with SH. A 2014 study evaluating CV risk factors in 49 children with SH showed higher waist-to-height ratio, atherogenic index, triglycerides-to–high-density lipoprotein–cholesterol (HDL-C) ratio, homocysteine levels, and lower HDL-C levels compared with controls. However, the abnormalities, although statistically significant, were not clearly of clinical significance, and other studies have had similar findings [71,75,76]. Just because treatment in middle age may improve cardiovascular outcome does not mean that treatment would improve the cardiac risk profile of adolescents; in fact, in some groups, such as the elderly, mild TSH elevation appears to be well tolerated [77–80].

Who to treat with subclinical hypothyroidism

We generally recommend against treating most pediatric patients with SH. Progression rates to overt hypothyroidism are generally 12.5% or less in most studies [81–86]. We do recommend to treat patients with repeated TSH greater than 10 mIU/L even if free T4 is normal [48,49,87], as these patients have a low rate of normalization of function [51,88]. Those with antibodies, or TSH greater than 7.5 at presentation, were the most likely to progress in various studies [48,81–86,89]. Thus, trials of treatment can be considered as well in those with apparent symptoms of thyroid disease and persistent TSH greater than 7.5 mIU/L, or those with persistent TSH elevation plus positive antibodies.

Treatment also can be considered in those with persistent SH and substantially compromised growth as noted previously, and in infants and toddlers younger than 3, when even SH may have impacts on cognitive function. It is also recommended to treat maternal SH [90,91] to ensure adequate transfer of thyroid hormone to the fetus throughout the pregnancy.

COMORBIDITIES ASSOCIATED WITH AUTOIMMUNE HYPERTHYROIDISM/GRAVES' DISEASE

Graves' disease is the most common cause of acquired hyperthyroidism in children and adolescents. It is caused by thyrotropin receptor-stimulating antibodies (TSHR-Ab), which activate the TSH receptor.

Neurologic/psychiatric impact

The presence of high levels of thyroid hormone in the central nervous system has been related to stimulation of α and β adrenergic receptors or changes in serotonin concentrations [92]. Children with hyperthyroidism tend to have greater mood swings and disturbances of behavior, as compared with adults. In a study involving children with Graves' disease, mood and behavior symptoms were present in 21% of subjects (and were the initial symptom in 6%) and included depression, anxiety, antisocial behavior, risk-taking behavior, hyperactivity, and declining performance in school [93]. Occasionally, children with hyperthyroidism may experience marked personality changes, agitation, depression, mania, or psychosis, which resolves with treatment of hyperthyroidism [94].

In younger preschool-aged children, cases of motor developmental delay and delayed speech and language skills in undiagnosed hyperthyroid children have been described in the literature. All cases showed significant improvement in development and speech skills after maintenance of euthyroid state [95].

Encephalopathy associated with autoimmune thyroid disease is similar in both Graves' and Hashimoto disease and manifests as described earlier [92,96].

Tremor and muscle weakness are common features of hyperthyroidism, but other involuntary movement disorders, such as chorea [97–101], choreoathetosis [102,103], ballism, and truncal flexion [101,104] have also been reported. Ataxia is rare in association with hyperthyroidism, but has also been reported [105,106]. Generally, the movement disorders resolved once euthyroid state was achieved.

Graves' disease in association with demyelinating disease has also been reported in the pediatric population [107]. Additionally, there has been a rare association of occurrence of generalized seizures in patients with Graves' disease described in literature. The underlying pathophysiology is not very well understood. Interestingly, the seizures occur not only in the thyrotoxic state, but also in euthyroid patients. Whether it is the direct effect of autoimmunity on neurons in such cases is unknown [108,109].

Thyrotoxic periodic paralysis (TPP) is a potentially lethal complication of hyperthyroidism characterized by varying degrees of muscle paralysis and hypokalemia. In North America, the incidence rate of TPP is reported to be 0.1% to 0.2% [110,111]. Many affected patients do not have obvious symptoms of thyrotoxicosis. Attacks usually first involve the lower limbs and progress to girdle muscles and subsequently the upper limbs. Sensation is intact and there is complete recovery between attacks. Attacks also can be precipitated by carbohydrate-rich meals, alcohol, and strenuous exercise [110,111]. Adequate control of underlying hyperthyroidism is the mainstay of therapy for TPP and prevents recurrence of paralysis. Immediate therapy with potassium supplementation and beta-adrenergic blockers can prevent serious cardiopulmonary complications [112].

Growth effects

In hyperthyroid children, acceleration of growth is accompanied by advancement of epiphyseal maturation. This acceleration depends on the duration of hyperthyroidism before diagnosis and may be more pronounced if hyperthyroidism presents in early childhood. Despite the advancement of bone age at presentation, there are no adverse effects on subsequent growth and final height in treated patients. With adequate treatment, growth velocity and bone age approach a more normal pattern and the final adult height is mostly normal, in fact, final adult height has been reported in some studies to be even slightly increased in the boys who were diagnosed during puberty [113]. In a report of children aged 3.4 to 7.5 years with Graves' disease, median final height was +1.25 SD, whereas BMI was −0.48 SDs [114].

The age of onset of puberty and attainment of pubertal stages does not appear to be altered by hyperthyroidism, but menstrual cycle disturbances may occur [113,115].

Studies in both adults and children with untreated hyperthyroidism demonstrated significantly decreased spinal (cancellous) and femoral neck (cortical) bone mineral density in untreated hyperthyroidism [116]. With adequate treatment of hyperthyroidism, cortical bone density normalizes in children and adolescents with hyperthyroidism approximately 1 to 2 years after a euthyroid state is achieved [117].

Weight effects and related complications
With treatment, lost weight is regained. However, studies in adults as well as children have reported weight gain in excess of the prediagnosis weight to occur once treatment is started, especially in the first 3 to 6 months [118,119]. Persistent increased appetite may play a role in this as well. Therefore, dietary counseling beginning at the initiation of treatment and careful monitoring of weight is necessary in this population [120].

Cardiovascular risk
Untreated hyperthyroidism can lead to cardiac hypertrophy through direct (eg, regulation of myocyte-specific gene and enhanced thyroid hormone receptor expression, increased cardiac contractility and lower systemic vascular resistance) and indirect effects (eg, enhanced adrenergic activity) of thyroid hormone [121].

Atrial fibrillation, which occurs in 10% to 15% of adults with hyperthyroidism, is rare in children [122]. Mitral valve prolapse is 2 to 3 times more prevalent in adult hyperthyroid patients than in healthy subjects, but not reported often in children [123].

References
[1] American Academy of Pediatrics, Rose SR, Section on Endocrinology and Committee on Genetics, et al. Update of newborn screening and therapy for congenital hypothyroidism. Pediatrics 2006;117(6):2290–303.
[2] Leger J. Congenital hypothyroidism: a clinical update of long-term outcome in young adults. Eur J Endocrinol 2015;172(2):R67–77.
[3] Delange F. Neonatal screening for congenital hypothyroidism: results and perspectives. Horm Res 1997;48(2):51–61.
[4] Grosse SD, Van Vliet G. Prevention of intellectual disability through screening for congenital hypothyroidism: how much and at what level? Arch Dis Child 2011;96(4):374–9.

[5] Derksen-Lubsen G, Verkerk PH. Neuropsychologic development in early treated congenital hypothyroidism: analysis of literature data. Pediatr Res 1996;39(3):561–6.

[6] Wheeler SM, Willoughby KA, McAndrews MP, et al. Hippocampal size and memory functioning in children and adolescents with congenital hypothyroidism. J Clin Endocrinol Metab 2011;96(9):E1427–34.

[7] Salerno M, Militerni R, Bravaccio C, et al. Effect of different starting doses of levothyroxine on growth and intellectual outcome at four years of age in congenital hypothyroidism. Thyroid 2002;12(1):45–52.

[8] Rovet J, Alvarez M. Thyroid hormone and attention in school-age children with congenital hypothyroidism. J Child Psychol Psychiatry 1996;37(5):579–85.

[9] Kempers MJ, van der Sluijs Veer L, Nijhuis-van der Sanden MW, et al. Intellectual and motor development of young adults with congenital hypothyroidism diagnosed by neonatal screening. J Clin Endocrinol Metab 2006;91(2):418–24.

[10] Heyerdahl S, Ilicki A, Karlberg J, et al. Linear growth in early treated children with congenital hypothyroidism. Acta Paediatr 1997;86(5):479–83.

[11] Ng SM, Wong SC, Didi M. Head circumference and linear growth during the first 3 years in treated congenital hypothyroidism in relation to aetiology and initial biochemical severity. Clin Endocrinol (Oxf) 2004;61(1):155–9.

[12] Dickerman Z, De Vries L. Prepubertal and pubertal growth, timing and duration of puberty and attained adult height in patients with congenital hypothyroidism (CH) detected by the neonatal screening programme for CH–a longitudinal study. Clin Endocrinol (Oxf) 1997;47(6):649–54.

[13] Salerno M, Micillo M, Di Maio S, et al. Longitudinal growth, sexual maturation and final height in patients with congenital hypothyroidism detected by neonatal screening. Eur J Endocrinol 2001;145(4):377–83.

[14] Grant DB. Growth in early treated congenital hypothyroidism. Arch Dis Child 1994;70(6):464–8.

[15] Oliviero U, Cittadini A, Bosso G, et al. Effects of long-term L-thyroxine treatment on endothelial function and arterial distensibility in young adults with congenital hypothyroidism. Eur J Endocrinol 2010;162(2):289–94.

[16] Salerno M, Oliviero U, Lettiero T, et al. Long-term cardiovascular effects of levothyroxine therapy in young adults with congenital hypothyroidism. J Clin Endocrinol Metab 2008;93(7):2486–91.

[17] Vasconcellos E, Piña-Garza JE, Fakhoury T, et al. Pediatric manifestations of Hashimoto's encephalopathy. Pediatr Neurol 1999;20(5):394–8.

[18] Gayatri NA, Whitehouse WP. Pilot survey of Hashimoto's encephalopathy in children. Dev Med Child Neurol 2005;47(8):556–8.

[19] Samuels MH. Cognitive function in untreated hypothyroidism and hyperthyroidism. Curr Opin Endocrinol Diabetes Obes 2008;15(5):429–33.

[20] Samuels MH. Thyroid disease and cognition. Endocrinol Metab Clin North Am 2014;43(2):529–43.

[21] Ferracci F, Bertiato G, Moretto G. Hashimoto's encephalopathy: epidemiologic data and pathogenetic considerations. J Neurol Sci 2004;217(2):165–8.

[22] Chong JY, Rowland LP, Utiger RD. Hashimoto encephalopathy: syndrome or myth? Arch Neurol 2003;60(2):164–71.

[23] Erol I, Saygi S, Alehan F. Hashimoto's encephalopathy in children and adolescents. Pediatr Neurol 2011;45(6):420–2.

[24] Mocellin R, Walterfang M, Velakoulis D. Hashimoto's encephalopathy: epidemiology, pathogenesis and management. CNS Drugs 2007;21(10):799–811.

[25] Chen HC, Marsharani U. Hashimoto's encephalopathy. South Med J 2000;93(5):504–6.

[26] Tarım Ö. Thyroid hormones and growth in health and disease. J Clin Res Pediatr Endocrinol 2011;3(2):51–5.

[27] Root AW, Shulman D, Root J, et al. The interrelationships of thyroid and growth hormones: effect of growth hormone releasing hormone in hypo- and hyperthyroid male rats. Eur J Endocrinol 1986;113(Suppl 4):S367–75.

[28] Gutch M, Philip R, Philip R, et al. Skeletal manifestations of juvenile hypothyroidism and the impact of treatment on skeletal system. Indian J Endocrinol Metab 2013;17(7):181.

[29] Lomenick JP, El-Sayyid M, Smith WJ. Effect of levo-thyroxine treatment on weight and body mass index in children with acquired hypothyroidism. J Pediatr 2008;152(1):96–100.

[30] Cerit ET, Akturk M, Altinova AE, et al. Evaluation of body composition changes, epicardial adipose tissue, and serum omentin-1 levels in overt hypothyroidism. Endocrine 2014;49(1):196–203.

[31] Grunstein RR, Sullivan CE. Sleep apnea and hypothyroidism: mechanisms and management. Am J Med 1988;85(6):775–9.

[32] Kapur VK, Koepsell TD, deMaine J, et al. Association of hypothyroidism and obstructive sleep apnea. Am J Respir Crit Care Med 1998;158(5):1379–83.

[33] Misiolek M, Marek B, Namyslowski G, et al. Sleep apnea syndrome and snoring in patients with hypothyroidism with relation to overweight. J Physiol Pharmacol 2007;58(Suppl 1):77–85.

[34] Sakellaropoulou AV, Hatzistilianou MN, Emporiadou MN, et al. Evaluation of thyroid gland function in children with obstructive apnea hypopnea syndrome. Int J Immunopathol Pharmacol 2011;24(2):377–86.

[35] Pearce EN, Yang Q, Benjamin EJ, et al. Thyroid function and left ventricular structure and function in the Framingham heart study. Thyroid 2010;20(4):369–73.

[36] Galli E, Pingitore A, Iervasi G. The role of thyroid hormone in the pathophysiology of heart failure: clinical evidence. Heart Fail Rev 2008;15(2):155–69.

[37] Iervasi G, Nicolini G. Thyroid hormone and cardiovascular system: from basic concepts to clinical application. Intern Emerg Med 2013;8(S1):71–4.

[38] Chowdhury D, Parnell VA, Ojamaa K, et al. Usefulness of triiodothyronine (T3) treatment after surgery for complex congenital heart disease in infants and children. Am J Cardiol 1999;84(9):1107–9.

[39] Mackie AS, Booth KL, Newburger JW, et al. A randomized, double-blind, placebo-controlled pilot trial of triiodothyronine in neonatal heart surgery. J Thorac Cardiovasc Surg 2005;130(3):810–6.

[40] Danzi S, Klein I. Thyroid disease and the cardiovascular system. Endocrinol Metab Clin North Am 2014;43(2):517–28.

[41] Duntas LH. Thyroid disease and lipids. Thyroid 2002;12(4):287–93.

[42] Klein I, Ojamaa K. Thyroid hormone and the cardiovascular system. N Engl J Med 2001;344:501–9.

[43] O'Brien T, Dinneen SF, O'Brien PC, et al. Hyperlipidemia in patients with primary and secondary hypothyroidism. Mayo Clin Proc 1993;68(9):860–6.

[44] Rizos CV. Effects of thyroid dysfunction on lipid profile. Open Cardiovasc Med J 2011;5(1):76–84.

[45] Thompson GR, Soutar AK, Spengel FA, et al. Defects of receptor-mediated low density lipoprotein catabolism in homozygous familial hypercholesterolemia and hypothyroidism in vivo. Proc Natl Acad Sci U S A 1981;78(4):2591–5.

[46] Nikkilä EA, Kekki M. Plasma triglyceride metabolism in thyroid disease. J Clin Invest 1972;51(8):2103–14.

[47] Witte T, Ittermann T, Thamm M, et al. Association between serum thyroid-stimulating hormone levels and serum lipids in children and adolescents: a population-based study of German youth. J Clin Endocrinol Metab 2015;100(5):2090–7.

[48] Bona G, Prodam F, Monzani A. Subclinical hypothyroidism in children: natural history and when to treat. J Clin Res Pediatr Endocrinol 2013;5(Suppl 1):23–8.

[49] O'Grady MJ, Cody D. Subclinical hypothyroidism in childhood. Arch Dis Child 2011;96(3):280–4.

[50] Hollowell JG, Staehling NW, Flanders WD, et al. Serum TSH, T(4), and thyroid antibodies in the United States population (1988 to 1994): National Health and Nutrition Examination Survey (NHANES III). J Clin Endocrinol Metab 2002;87(2):489–99.

[51] Cooper DS, Biondi B. Subclinical thyroid disease. Lancet 2012;379(9821):1142–54.

[52] Rapa A, Monzani A, Moia S, et al. Subclinical hypothyroidism in children and adolescents: a wide range of clinical, biochemical, and genetic factors involved. J Clin Endocrinol Metab 2009;94(7):2414–20.

[53] Aypak C, Türedi O, Yüce A, et al. Thyroid-stimulating hormone (TSH) level in nutritionally obese children and metabolic co-morbidity. J Pediatr Endocrinol Metab 2013;26(7–8):703–8.

[54] Holtmann M, Duketis E, Goth K, et al. Severe affective and behavioral dysregulation in youth is associated with increased serum TSH. J Affect Disord 2010;121(1–2):184–8.

[55] Almeida C, Brasil MA, Costa AJ, et al. Subclinical hypothyroidism: psychiatric disorders and symptoms. Rev Bras Psiquiatr 2007;29(2):157–9.

[56] Chueire VB, Romaldini JH, Ward LS. Subclinical hypothyroidism increases the risk for depression in the elderly. Arch Gerontol Geriatr 2007;44(1):21–8.

[57] Davis JD, Stern RA, Flashman LA. Cognitive and neuropsychiatric aspects of subclinical hypothyroidism: significance in the elderly. Curr Psychiatry Rep 2003;5(5):384–90.

[58] Demartini B, Ranieri R, Masu A, et al. Depressive symptoms and major depressive disorder in patients affected by subclinical hypothyroidism: a cross-sectional study. J Nerv Ment Dis 2014;202(8):603–7.

[59] Fjaellegaard K, Kvetny J, Allerup PN, et al. Well-being and depression in individuals with subclinical hypothyroidism and thyroid autoimmunity—a general population study. Nord J Psychiatry 2015;69(1):73–8.

[60] Joffe RT, Sullivan TB. The significance of an isolated elevated TSH level in a depressed patient: a clinical commentary. Int J Psychiatry Med 2014;48(3):167–73.

[61] Park YJ, Lee EJ, Lee YJ, et al. Subclinical hypothyroidism (SCH) is not associated with metabolic derangement, cognitive impairment, depression or poor quality of life (QoL) in elderly subjects. Arch Gerontol Geriatr 2010;50(3):e68–73.

[62] Zepf FD, Vloet TD, Polier GG, et al. No association between affective and behavioral dysregulation and parameters of thyroid function in youths. J Affect Disord 2011;134(1–3):478–82.

[63] Samuels MH. Cognitive function in subclinical hypothyroidism. J Clin Endocrinol Metab 2010;95(8):3611–3.

[64] Samuels MH, Schuff KG, Carlson NE, et al. Health status, mood, and cognition in experimentally induced subclinical hypothyroidism. J Clin Endocrinol Metab 2007;92(7):2545–51.

[65] Cetinkaya E, Aslan A, Vidinlisan S, et al. Height improvement by L-thyroxine treatment in subclinical hypothyroidism. Pediatr Int 2003;45(5):534–7.

[66] Eyal O, Blum S, Mueller R, et al. Improved growth velocity during thyroid hormone therapy in children with Fanconi anemia and borderline thyroid function. Pediatr Blood Cancer 2008;51(5):652–6.

[67] Bas VN, Aycan Z, Ağladıoğlu SY, et al. Prevalence of hyperthyrotropinemia in obese children before and after weight loss. Eat Weight Disord 2013;18(1):87–90.

[68] Gertig AM, Niechcial E, Skowronska B. Thyroid axis alterations in childhood obesity. Pediatr Endocrinol Diabetes Metab 2012;18(3):116–9.

[69] Ghergherehchi R, Hazhir N. Thyroid hormonal status among children with obesity. Ther Adv Endocrinol Metab 2015;6(2):51–5.

[70] Lobotkova D, Staníková D, Staník J, et al. Lack of association between peripheral activity of thyroid hormones and elevated TSH levels in childhood obesity. J Clin Res Pediatr Endocrinol 2014;6(2):100–4.

[71] Unuvar T, Anık A, Catlı G, et al. Isolated hyperthyrotropinemia in childhood obesity and its relation with metabolic parameters. J Endocrinol Invest 2014;37(9):799–804.

[72] Biondi B. Thyroid and obesity: an intriguing relationship. J Clin Endocrinol Metab 2010;95(8):3614–7.
[73] Reinehr T. Thyroid function in the nutritionally obese child and adolescent. Curr Opin Pediatr 2011;23(4):415–20.
[74] Ortiga-Carvalho TM, Oliveira KJ, Soares BA, et al. The role of leptin in the regulation of TSH secretion in the fed state: in vivo and in vitro studies. J Endocrinol 2002;174(1): 121–5.
[75] Catli G, Kir M, Anik A, et al. The effect of L-thyroxine treatment on left ventricular functions in children with subclinical hypothyroidism. Arch Dis Child 2015;100(2):130–7.
[76] Cerbone M, Capalbo D, Wasniewska M, et al. Cardiovascular risk factors in children with long-standing untreated idiopathic subclinical hypothyroidism. J Clin Endocrinol Metab 2014;99(8):2697–703.
[77] Garin MC, Arnold AM, Lee JS, et al. Subclinical hypothyroidism, weight change, and body composition in the elderly: the Cardiovascular Health Study. J Clin Endocrinol Metab 2014;99(4):1220–6.
[78] Hyland KA, Arnold AM, Lee JS, et al. Persistent subclinical hypothyroidism and cardiovascular risk in the elderly: the cardiovascular health study. J Clin Endocrinol Metab 2013;98(2):533–40.
[79] Kim TH, Choi HS, Bae JC, et al. Subclinical hypothyroidism in addition to common risk scores for prediction of cardiovascular disease: a 10-year community-based cohort study. Eur J Endocrinol 2014;171(5):649–57.
[80] Pasqualetti G, Tognini S, Polini A, et al. Is subclinical hypothyroidism a cardiovascular risk factor in the elderly? J Clin Endocrinol Metab 2013;98(6):2256–66.
[81] Gopalakrishnan S, Chugh PK, Chhillar M, et al. Goitrous autoimmune thyroiditis in a pediatric population: a longitudinal study. Pediatr 2008;122(3):e670–4.
[82] Lazar L, Frumkin RB, Battat E, et al. Natural history of thyroid function tests over 5 years in a large pediatric cohort. J Clin Endocrinol Metab 2009;94(5):1678–82.
[83] Moore DC. Natural course of 'subclinical' hypothyroidism in childhood and adolescence. Arch Pediatr Adolesc Med 1996;150(3):293.
[84] Radetti G, Gottardi E, Bona G, et al. The natural history of euthyroid Hashimoto's thyroiditis in children. J Pediatr 2006;149(6):827–32.
[85] Wasniewska M, Salerno M, Cassio A, et al. Prospective evaluation of the natural course of idiopathic subclinical hypothyroidism in childhood and adolescence. Eur J Endocrinol 2008;160(3):417–21.
[86] Zois C, Stavrou I, Svarna E, et al. Natural course of autoimmune thyroiditis after elimination of iodine deficiency in northwestern Greece. Thyroid 2006;16(3):289–93.
[87] De Luca F, Corica D, Pitrolo E, et al. Idiopathic and mild subclinical hypothyroidism in childhood: clinical management. Minerva Pediatr 2014;66(1):63–8.
[88] Fatourechi V. Subclinical hypothyroidism: an update for primary care physicians. Mayo Clin Proc 2009;84(1):65–71.
[89] Jaruratanasirikul S, Leethanaporn K, Khuntigij P, et al. The clinical course of Hashimoto's thyroiditis in children and adolescents: 6 years longitudinal follow-up. J Pediatr Endocrinol Metab 2001;14(2):177–84.
[90] Casey BM. Subclinical hypothyroidism and pregnancy. Obstet Gynecol Surv 2006;61(6): 415–20 [quiz: 423].
[91] Haddow JE, Palomaki GE, Allan WC, et al. Maternal thyroid deficiency during pregnancy and subsequent neuropsychological development of the child. N Engl J Med 1999;341(8):549–55.
[92] Fardella CE, Gloger S. Neurobehavioral and psychological changes induced by hyperthyroidism: diagnostic and therapeutic implications. Expert Rev Neurother 2002;2(5): 709–16.

[93] Loomba-Albrecht LA, Bremer AA, Styne DM, et al. High frequency of cardiac and behavioral complaints as presenting symptoms of hyperthyroidism in children. J Pediatr Endocrinol Metab 2011;24(3-4):209-13.

[94] Hazen EP, Sherry NA, Parangi S, et al. Case records of the Massachusetts General Hospital. Case 10-2015. A 15-year-old girl with Graves' disease and psychotic symptoms. N Engl J Med 2015;372(13):1250-8.

[95] Sohal APS, Dasarathi M, Lodh R, et al. Speech and language delay in two children: an unusual presentation of hyperthyroidism. J Pediatr Endocrinol Metab 2013;26(11-12): 1171-4.

[96] Tamagno G, Celik Y, Simó R, et al. Encephalopathy associated with autoimmune thyroid disease in patients with Graves' disease: clinical manifestations, follow-up, and outcomes. BMC Neurol 2010;10(1):27.

[97] New Members. Nav Eng J 2005;117(3):11-2.

[98] Baba M, Terada A, Hishida R, et al. Persistent hemichorea associated with thyrotoxicosis. Intern Med 1992;31(9):1144-6.

[99] Javaid A, Hilton DD. Persistent chorea as a manifestation of thyrotoxicosis. Postgrad Med J 1988;64(756):789-90.

[100] Pozzan GB, Battistella PA, Rigon F, et al. Hyperthyroid-induced chorea in an adolescent girl. Brain Dev 1992;14(2):126-7.

[101] Ristic AJ, Svetel M, Dragasević N, et al. Bilateral chorea-ballism associated with hyperthyroidism. Mov Disord 2004;19(8):982-3.

[102] Fidler SM, O'Rourke RA, Buchsbaum HW. Choreoathetosis as a manifestation of thyrotoxicosis. Neurology 1971;21(1):55-7.

[103] Fischbeck KH, Layzer RB. Paroxysmal choreoathetosis associated with thyrotoxicosis. Ann Neurol 1979;6(5):453-4.

[104] Loh L-M, Hum AY, Teoh HL, et al. Graves' disease associated with spasmodic truncal flexion. Parkinsonism Relat Disord 2005;11(2):117-9.

[105] Åberg HE, Herbai GL, Westerberg C-E. Recurrent and reversible cerebellar ataxia with concomitant episodes of hyperthyroidism. Acta Med Scand 2009;199(1-6):331-4.

[106] Seeherunvong T, Diamantopoulos S, Berkovitz GD. A nine year old girl with thyrotoxicosis, ataxia, and chorea. Brain Dev 2007;29(10):660-1.

[107] Mitchell RS, Yager JY, Marks SD. Childhood onset demyelination and graves' disease: shared antigen or autoimmune clustering? J Pediatr Endocrinol Metab 2007;20(11): 1233-6.

[108] Vergely N, Garnier P, Guy C, et al. Seizure during Graves' disease. Epileptic Disord 2009;11(2):136-7.

[109] Lin CS, Garnier P, Guy C, et al. Thyrotoxicosis accompanied with periodic seizure attacks a case report and review of literature. Zhonghua Yi Xue Za Zhi (Taipei) 1992;50(4): 335-7.

[110] Kelley DE. Thyrotoxic periodic paralysis. Report of 10 cases and review of electromyographic findings. Arch Intern Med 1989;149(11):2597-600.

[111] Ober KP. Thyrotoxic periodic paralysis in the United States: report of 7 cases and review of the literature. Medicine 1992;71(3):109-20.

[112] Kung AWC. Thyrotoxic periodic paralysis: a diagnostic challenge. J Clin Endocrinol Metab 2006;91(7):2490-5.

[113] Cassio A, Corrias A, Gualandi S, et al. Influence of gender and pubertal stage at diagnosis on growth outcome in childhood thyrotoxicosis: results of a collaborative study. Clin Endocrinol 2006;64(1):53-7.

[114] Bossowski AT, Reddy V, Perry LA, et al. Clinical and endocrine features and long-term outcome of Graves' disease in early childhood. J Endocrinol Invest 2007;30(5):388-92.

[115] Koutras DA. Disturbances of menstruation in thyroid disease. Ann N Y Acad Sci 1997;816:280-4.

[116] Numbenjapon N, Costin G, Gilsanz V, et al. Low cortical bone density measured by computed tomography in children and adolescents with untreated hyperthyroidism. J Pediatr 2007;150(5):527–30.

[117] Numbenjapon N, Costin G, Pitukcheewanont P. Normalization of cortical bone density in children and adolescents with hyperthyroidism treated with antithyroid medication. Osteoporos Int 2011;23(9):2277–82.

[118] Crocker MK, Kaplowitz P. Treatment of paediatric hyperthyroidism but not hypothyroidism has a significant effect on weight. Clin Endocrinol 2010;73(6):752–9.

[119] Dale J, Daykin J, Holder R, et al. Weight gain following treatment of hyperthyroidism. Clin Endocrinol 2001;55(2):233–9.

[120] van Veenendaal NR, Rivkees SA. Treatment of pediatric Graves' disease is associated with excessive weight gain. J Clin Endocrinol Metab 2011;96(10):3257–63.

[121] Klein I, Ojamaa K. Thyroid hormone and the cardiovascular system: from theory to practice. J Clin Endocrinol Metab 1994;78(5):1026–7.

[122] Gurdogan M, Ari H, Tenekecioğlu E, et al. Predictors of atrial fibrillation recurrence in hyperthyroid and euthyroid patients. Arq Bras Cardiol 2016;106(2):84–91.

[123] Channick BJ, Adlin EV, Marks AD, et al. Hyperthyroidism and mitral-valve prolapse. N Engl J Med 1981;305(9):497–500.

Advances in Pediatrics 63 (2016) 227–254

ADVANCES IN PEDIATRICS

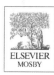

Advances in Pediatric Pharmacology, Therapeutics, and Toxicology

Laura A. Wang, MIPH[a],
Michael Cohen-Wolkowiez, MD, PhD[a,b,*],
Daniel Gonzalez, PharmD, PhD[c]

[a]Duke Clinical Research Institute, Duke University Medical Center, 2400 Pratt Street, Durham, NC 27705, USA; [b]Department of Pediatrics, Children's Health Center, College of Medicine, Duke University, T901, Durham, NC 27705, USA; [c]Division of Pharmacotherapy and Experimental Therapeutics, UNC Eshelman School of Pharmacy, University of North Carolina at Chapel Hill, 301 Pharmacy Lane, CB #7569, Chapel Hill, NC 27599, USA

Keywords

• Pediatrics • Pharmacology • Pharmacokinetics • Toxicology

Key points

• Pediatric research continues to expand in both the United States and in Europe as a result of ongoing efforts to promote pediatric drug development and labeling.

• Areas in major need of drug development including rare and ultra rare diseases have seen new advancements. However, drug development for other populations such as neonates continues to experience limited progress.

• Despite the progress made in 2014 and 2015 much work remains, including gathering more data on medications that are currently available and developing new, safe, and effective therapies for pediatric patients.

D. Gonzalez is funded by K23HD083465 from the National Institute for Child Health and Human Development (NICHD) and by the nonprofit Thrasher Research Fund (www.thrasherresearch.org). M. Cohen-Wolkowiez receives support for research from the National Institutes of Health (NIH) (1R01-HD076676-01A1), the National Center for Advancing Translational Sciences of the NIH (UL1TR001117), the National Institute of Allergy and Infectious Diseases (NIAID) (HHSN272201500006I and HHSN272201300017I), the NICHD (HHSN275201000003I), the Food and Drug Administration (1U01FD004858-01), the Biomedical Advanced Research and Development Authority (HHSO100201300009C), and the nonprofit Thrasher Research Fund (www.thrasherresearch.org) and from industry for drug development in adults and children (www.dcri.duke.edu/research/coi.jsp).

*Corresponding author. Duke Clinical Research Institute, PO Box 17969, Durham, NC 27715. E-mail address: michael.cohenwolkowiez@duke.edu

0065-3101/16/$ – see front matter
http://dx.doi.org/10.1016/j.yapd.2016.04.015

INTRODUCTION

Over the past 2 years there have been numerous advancements in drug development for pediatric patients. In 2014 and 2015, the Food and Drug Administration (FDA) approved more than 70 product label changes related to pediatric populations (Table 1), resulting in more than 530 overall since the enactment of the Best Pharmaceuticals for Children Act in 2002 and the Pediatric Research Equity Act in 2003 [1]. There were more than 10 approvals of new drugs specifically for the treatment of pediatric indications in the past 2 years, including several for rare or ultrarare diseases, which reflects the major advancements that have occurred for drug development for these populations. In the European Union, there have been more than 30 new authorizations by the European Medicines Agency (EMA) for medications for use in pediatric populations. Additionally, the Paediatric Committee of the EMA has approved more than 135 new pediatric investigation plans for new studies [2,3]. The greatest numbers of pediatric investigation plans are in the areas of endocrinology and infectious disease, with 20 and 19, respectively, followed by oncology and gastroenterology. Furthermore, there have been many contributions by investigator-initiated studies that have led to a greater understanding of the use and effects of medications prescribed to children. Even though it has been recognized that there is a major need for drug development for neonates, these is still a lack of information on the safety and efficacy of drugs that are used in this population [4].

Given the numerous advancements over the past 2 years, the goal of this article is to highlight specific developments in pediatric pharmacology, toxicology, and therapeutics from January 2014 through October 2015. The updates were extracted from the FDA Pediatric Labeling Information Database, EMA Public Assessment Reports database, EMA Opinions and Decisions on Paediatric Investigation Plans database, clinicaltrials.gov, PubMed, and Embase. Articles were selected to identify important developments within various therapeutic areas.

ANESTHESIA

Sedation

Dexmedetomidine is a selective α_2-agonist that acts centrally in the brainstem to inhibit norepinephrine release, which results in sedative and anesthetic effects without causing respiratory depression [5]. It is currently FDA approved for use in adult patients for up to 24 hours while intubated and on mechanical ventilation in the intensive care setting but has been used off-label in pediatric patients as an adjunct to sedation regimens and is increasingly used as a primary sedative agent [6].

Given the lack of data surrounding dexmedetomidine usage in neonates, a phase 2/3, open-label study was performed with the goal of characterizing the safety, efficacy, and pharmacokinetic (PK) properties of dexmedetomidine in preterm and term neonates between 28 weeks and 44 weeks of gestational age [7]. The neonates were divided into 2 groups, with group 1 including preterm neonates born at 28 weeks' to 35 weeks' gestational age and group 2 including term neonates born at 36 weeks' to 44 weeks' gestational age. The investigators found that 90% of patients did not require midazolam for added sedation while receiving dexmedetomidine infusion. In regard to PK parameters, the neonates born between 28 weeks and 35 weeks seemed to have a lower weight-adjusted plasma clearance (0.3 L/h/kg vs 0.9 L/h/kg) and a prolonged terminal elimination half-life (7.6 hours vs 3.2 hours) compared with neonates born between 36 weeks and 44 weeks There were no serious adverse events related to dexmedetomidine usage and none that led to discontinuation of sedation; 56 adverse events were reported in 26 patients (26/42, 62%), with 11 (11/18, 61%) in group 1 and 15 (15/24, 63%) in group 2. Three patients (3/42, 7%) reported 4 adverse events related to dexmedetomidine, including hypertension, hypotension, and agitation. Overall, the investigators concluded that the PK of dexmedetomidine is different in neonates compared with older children and adults, indicating lower doses may be required for the same level of sedation and to limit potential adverse effects [7].

A majority of pediatric data for dexmedetomidine come from studies examining usage for less than 72 hours [8]. As such, the safety of dexmedetomidine during long-term use was studied in a group of 98 patients under 21 years of age who received 0.2 μg/kg/h to 0.7 μg/kg/h for greater than 72 hours. The median (range) age of the cohort was 3.8 years (0.04–17) and duration of dexmedetomidine use was 141 hours (72–2472). There was a statistically significant reduction in both heart rate and systolic blood pressure (BP) from baseline after initiation of sedation and a decreased need for opioids and benzodiazepines. After cessation of the infusion, however, there was a significant increase in heart rate and both systolic and diastolic BP; 21% of patients required either a new antihypertensive agent or the addition of clonidine for the treatment of rebound tachycardia and hypertension. Other withdrawal effects included agitation tremors and decreased sleep [8]. Overall, the investigators concluded that longer-term dexmedetomidine administration in the intensive care setting is safe and effective. Prominent withdrawal symptoms, however, may occur and patients should be monitored for tachycardia and hypertension on discontinuation of the medication.

Pain management

In August of 2015, the FDA approved controlled-release oxycodone hydrochloride (Oxycontin) for use in patients 11 years and older with pain and who are opioid tolerant and receiving a minimum daily dose of 20 mg of oxycodone. This approval was based on an open-label clinical trial of 155 opioid-tolerant pediatric patients with moderate to severe chronic pain. Mean (range) duration of therapy was 20.7 days (1–43) and daily dose was 33.30 mg/d (20–140) [9]. More than 50% of patients experienced any adverse event, with the most frequently reported vomiting, nausea, headache, fever, and constipation. Pain was assessed using a revised FACES Pain Rating Scale, which was scored by the patient during screening, after the first dose, and twice daily (morning and evening) at the time of each dose. The mean (SD) score at baseline was 4.44

Table 1
Select drug label changes made by US Food and Drug Administration in 2014 and 2015

Generic name	Trade name	Indication studied	Summary of label change(s)
Abacavir sulfate and lamivudine	Epzicom	HIV-1 infection	Expanded indication from adults to pediatric patients weighing at least 25 kg
Acyclovir/hydrocortisone	Xerese	Treatment of recurrent herpes labialis	Expanded indication to include pediatric patients ≥ 6 y of age
Amphetamine	Dyanavel XR	ADHD	Safety and efficacy established in patients 6–17 y of age
Aripiprazole	Abilify	Maintenance treatment of irritability associated with autistic disorder	Effectiveness was not established in a 12-wk clinical trial in 85 pediatric patients 6–17 y of age
Aprepitant	Emend	Prevention of nausea and vomiting associated with highly and moderately emetogenic cancer chemotherapy	Indicated for patients 12 y of age and older and patients <12 y who weigh at least 30 kg
Asenapine	Saphris	Treatment of schizophrenia and acute manic or mixed episodes associated with bipolar I disorder	Safety and effectiveness established in by placebo-controlled, double-blind trial of 403 patients 10–17 y of age
Atazanavir	Reyataz	Treatment of HIV-1 infection	Oral powder approved for use in pediatric patients at least 3 mo and weighing between 10 and $\leq$25 kg, and was then expanded to patients 3 mo and older weighing 5 to <10 kg and to those weighing >25 kg
Beclomethasone dipropionate	QNASL	Treatment of nasal symptoms associated with seasonal allergic rhinitis and perennial allergic rhinitis	Expanded indication to pediatric patients $\geq$4 y
Bortezomib	Velcade	Relapsed ALL and lymphoblastic lymphoma	Effectiveness in pediatric patients with relapsed pre-B ALL has not been established
Calcipotriene/ betamethasone dipropionate	Taclonex	Treatment of psoriasis vulgaris	Expanded indication to patients 12–17 y of age

Generic	Brand	Indication	Details
Cysteamine bitartrate	Procysbi	Treatment of nephropathic cystinosis	Expanded indication to pediatric patients down to 2 y
Darbepoetin alfa	Aranesp	Initial treatment of anemia in pediatric patients with chronic kidney disease	Indication expanded to include patients from 1–18 y of age
Duloxetine hydrochloride	Cymbalta	Treatment of generalized anxiety disorder	Safety and effectiveness established in 10-wk, placebo-controlled trial of 272 patients with generalized anxiety disorder 7–17 y of age
Entecavir	Baraclude	Treatment of chronic hepatitis B virus infection	Approved for use in pediatric patients ≥ 2 y
Erlotinib	Tarceva	Treatment of recurrent or refractory ependymoma	Safety and effectiveness not established in pediatric patients based on an open-label, multicenter trial with 25 patients (median age 14 y, range 3–20 y)
Finafloxacin	Xtoro	Treatment of acute otitis externa	Safety and effectiveness established in patients ≥ 1 y by 2 randomized multicenter placebo-controlled trials of 1234 patients
Fluticasone furoate	Arnuity ellipta	Maintenance treatment of asthma as prophylactic therapy	Approved for use in patients ≥ 12 y
Fluticasone proprionate	Cutivate	Treatment of atopic dermatitis	Indication expanded to patients ≥ 3 mo of age
Lamivudine and raltegravir	Dutrebis	Treatment of HIV-1 infection	Indicated in pediatric patients 6–16 y of age weighing at least 30 kg
Lamotrigine	Lamictal	Maintenance treatment of bipolar disorder	Safety and effectiveness were not established for patients 10–17 y of age based on a double-blind placebo controlled trial in 301 patients
Levalbuterol	Xopenex inhalation solution	Treatment of asthma or reactive airway disease	Effectiveness was not established a trial in 291 patients from 2–5 y of age and another trial in 88 patients from birth to <2 y of age
Levetiracetam	Keppra	Treatment of POSs, PGTCs, myoclonic seizures	Safety and effectiveness established for adjunctive treatment of POS in patients 1 mo to 16 y, PGTC in patients 6–16 y, and myoclonic seizures in patients 12–16 y
Levetiracetam	Keppra XR	Adjunctive therapy in the treatment of POSs	Safety and effectiveness established in patients ≥ 12 y

(continued on next page)

Table 1
(continued)

Generic name	Trade name	Indication studied	Summary of label change(s)
Memantine hydrochloride	Namenda XR	Treatment of autism spectrum disorders	Safety and effectiveness not established in 2 12-wk controlled trials of 578 patients 6–12 y of age
Meropenem	Merrem IV	Treatment of complicated intra-abdominal infections	Expanded indication to pediatric patients <3 mo of age
Mesalamine	Asacol	Maintenance of remission of mildly to moderately active ulcerative colitis	Safety and effectiveness have not been established in pediatric patients
Mesalamine	Delzicol	Treatment of mild to moderately active ulcerative colitis	Expanded indication to patients 5 y and older
Methylphenidate hydrochloride	Aptensio XR	Treatment of ADHD	Safety and effectiveness established in patients 6–17 y of age
Mometasone furoate	Asmanex HFA	Maintenance of asthma as prophylactic therapy	Approved for use in children ≥12 y
Naftifine hydrochloride	Naftin	Treatment of interdigital tinea pedis	Expanded indication to include pediatric patients 12–18 y
Olopatadine hydrochloride	Pazeo	Treatment of ocular itching associated with allergic conjunctivitis	Safety and effectiveness established in patients ≥2 y
Omalizumab	Xolair	Treatment of chronic idiopathic urticarial	Approved for treatment of chronic idiopathic urticarial in children ≥12 y who remain symptomatic despite H1 antihistamine treatment
Oxycodone hydrochloride	Oxycontin extended-release tablets	Management of pain severe enough to require daily, around-the-clock, long-term opioid treatment	Safety and efficacy established in patients 11–16 y of age
Palonosetron hydrochloride	Aloxi	Prevention of chemotherapy-induced nausea and vomiting and postoperative nausea and vomiting	Approved for use in pediatric patients 1 mo to ≤17 y

Drug	Indication	Labeling
Perampanel (Fycompa)	Treatment of PGTCs	Safety and efficacy established in patients ≥12 y of age in a randomized, double-blind, placebo-controlled multicenter trial with 11 patients
Rifapentine (Priftin)	Treatment of latent tuberculosis infection caused by Mycobacterium tuberculosis in combination with isoniazid	Safety and effectiveness established in pediatric patients 2–17 y of age
Rilpivirine (Edurant)	HIV-1 infection in treatment-naïve patients	Expanded indication from adults to pediatric patients 12–18 y of age
Rufinamide (Banzel)	Adjunct treatment of seizures associated with Lennox-Gastaut syndrome	Indication expanded to patients ≥1 y of age
Sapropterin dihydrochloride (Kuvan)	Treatment to reduce blood phenylalanine levels in patients with hyperphenylalaninemia due to tetrahydrobiopterin-responsive phenylketonuria	Expanded indication to include 1 mo to 4 y
Selegiline (Emsam)	Treatment of MDD	Effectiveness was not established in a multicenter randomized, double-blind, placebo-controlled, flexible-dose trial in 308 adolescents 12–17 y
Spinosad (Natroba)	Treatment of head lice infestation	Indication expanded to patients ≥6 mo of age
Tiotropium bromide (Spiriva Respimat Inhalation Spray)	Long-term maintenance treatment of asthma	Safety and efficacy established in patients 12–17 y of age
Topiramate (Topamax)	Prophylaxis of migraine headache	Approved for use in children ≥12 y
Valganciclovir (Valcyte)	Prevention of CMV disease in heart transplant patients	Indication expanded to patients 1–4 mo of age
Zolmitriptan (Zomig Nasal Spray)	Acute treatment of migraine with or without aura	Efficacy established in patients 12–17 y of age

Data from The FDA Pediatric Labeling Information Database. Available at: http://www.accessdata.fda.gov/scripts/sda/sdNavigation.cfm?sd=labelingdatabase. Accessed November 20, 2015.

(3.250) compared with the morning 3.13 (2.569) and evening 3.42 (2.974) of the fourth week. As such, the trial concluded that controlled-release oxycodone is safe and effective at controlling pain in this opioid-tolerant pediatric population.

CARDIOLOGY

Pulmonary hypertension

Sildenafil is a phosphodiesterase type-5 inhibitor that lowers pulmonary vascular resistance and is used in patients with single-ventricle heart defects [10]. Because children with single-ventricle heart defects have altered hepatic physiology that might influence drug metabolism, a study was conducted to determine the effect of elevated hepatic pressure on the PKs of sildenafil in this population [11]. A population PK model was developed for 20 children with a median (range) age of 3.2 years (0.8–5.3) receiving single-dose intravenous sildenafil during cardiac catheterization. The analysis showed that increased hepatic pressure affected the clearance of desmethyl-sildenafil, the active metabolite, but not of sildenafil. An increase of hepatic pressure from 4 mm Hg to 18 mm Hg was predicted to decrease desmethyl-sildenafil clearance by approximately 7-fold. Additionally, predicted drug exposure increased in subjects with hepatic pressures greater than or equal to 10 mm Hg compared with less than 10 mm Hg by approximately 1.5-fold (median area under the concentration vs time curve, 533 µg/h/L vs 792 µg/h/L). As such, the investigators concluded that hepatic pressure should be considered when prescribing sildenafil for children with single-ventricle defects [11].

The randomized, double-blind, placebo-controlled trial, Sildenafil in Treatment-Naïve Children, Aged 1–17 years, With Pulmonary Arterial Hypertension (STARTS)-1, was designed to evaluate the safety and efficacy of sildenafil citrate in children and adolescents. The study found that exercise capacity and hemodynamics improved in patients receiving medium and high doses of sildenafil, and preliminary data published for STARTS-2, a trial examining long-term greater than 2-year treatment, showed increased mortality at higher doses [12]. This resulted in statements issued by both the FDA and EMA in 2012 that warned against off-label use of the medication [13,14]. The FDA released an updated safety communication in 2014 advising against the chronic use of sildenafil in children [15]. Data from STARTS-2 were fully published in 2014 and showed that even though children randomized to higher doses of sildenafil had an unexplained increase in mortality, all dosage groups showed favorable survival for children with pulmonary arterial hypertension [16]. Estimated Kaplan-Meier survival rates were 94%, 93%, and 88% for low-dose, medium-dose, and high-dose groups, respectively. Within the study groups, 87%, 89%, and 80%, respectively, were shown to be alive after 3 years from the start of treatment. Hazard ratios for mortality were 3.95 (95% CI, 1.46–10.65) for high-dose versus low-dose groups and 1.92 (95% CI, 0.65–5.65) for medium-dose versus low-dose groups. The investigators noted, however, that multiple analyses raised uncertainty regarding the survival and dose relationship.

Hypertension

Losartan is an angiotensin II receptor blocker that is used as an antihypertensive therapy in adults and children over 6 years of age. Losartan has been shown to reduce BP in a dose-dependent manner in children between the ages of 6 and 16 [17]. A 12-week randomized, open-label, dose-ranging study with a 2-year extension was conducted to assess safety and efficacy of losartan in a group of 101 children 6 months to 6 years of age with hypertension [18]. Patients were randomized to receive either 0.1 mg/kg/d (low dose), 0.3 mg/kg/d (medium dose), or 0.7 mg/kg/d (high dose). The dosage was titrated to the next dose level at 3 weeks, 6 weeks, and 9 weeks up to 1.4 mg/kg/d up to 100 mg/d if adequate BP control was not achieved. Over the course of the study, losartan was well tolerated and the incidence of adverse events was low and comparable between the groups. The investigators concluded that children between 6 months and 6 years of age taking losartan, 0.1 to 0.7 mg/kg/d, had significantly lower systolic and diastolic BP, although there was no dose-response relationship [18].

Lisinopril is a long-acting angiotensin-converting enzyme inhibitor that prevents the conversion of angiotensin I to angiotensin II in the renin-angiotensin-aldosterone system to lower BP. It is FDA approved for the treatment of essential hypertension in adult and pediatric patients over 6 years of age. In adult kidney transplant patients, lisinopril has been shown to prolong allograft survival by affecting intraglomerular hemodynamics and reducing the activity of profibrotic and inflammatory mediators [19]. To understand the effects of lisinopril on pediatric kidney transplant patients, a trial was conducted to determine the PK, pharmacodynamic, and safety profile of lisinopril in this population [20]; 22 patients between the ages of 7 and 17 were divided into 2 groups based on prior lisinopril exposure (lisinopril naïve vs lisinopril per standard of care). Patients in the lisinopril naïve group received a once-daily dose of 0.1 mg/kg (low), 0.2 mg/kg (medium), or 0.4 mg/kg (high) whereas the standard-of-care patients received doses of the medication as part of their ongoing care. Lisinopril was generally well tolerated and was associated with lowering of BP at approved pediatric dosages. The investigators found that the PK of lisinopril in patients with a kidney transplant was comparable to previous children who had not undergone a kidney transplant. Clearance was not affected by age after scaling allometrically for size across the age range studied. Additionally, clearance was proportional to dose and increased in proportion to estimated glomerular filtration rate. As such, it is recommended that pediatric kidney transplant patients receive the currently approved pediatric dose with consideration for estimated glomerular filtration rate [20].

DERMATOLOGY

Atopic dermatitis

In 2014, the American Academy of Pediatrics released updated recommendations regarding management and treatment of atopic dermatitis due to an increasing incidence nationwide. New data suggest that atopic dermatitis results from primary abnormalities of the skin barrier, which has placed a new focus on the importance of a skin-directed management approach [21]. These recommendations emphasize maintenance skin care, such as the use of daily moisturizers, in addition to the use of topical corticosteroids for active disease.

Topical calcineurin inhibitors, including tacrolimus and pimecrolimus, are FDA approved as second-line treatments for mild to severe atopic dermatitis in children over 2 years of age. Tacrolimus and pimecrolimus show comparable efficacy and safety and are suitable and cost-effective alternatives to topical corticosteroids, although the uncertain risk for malignancy should be considered [22–24]. Topical calcineurin inhibitors are also commonly prescribed off-label to infants and young children because compliance to topical steroids can be poor due to parental concerns regarding side effects [25]. A 5-year phase 3 study in 2418 infants found that pimecrolimus had similar efficacy to topical corticosteroids [26]. Additionally, the data suggest that long-term management of mild to moderate atopic dermatitis in infants with either pimecrolimus or topical corticosteroids was safe and without any effect on the immune system. As such, both are reasonable first-line treatment options.

GASTROENTEROLOGY
Inflammatory bowel disease: ulcerative colitis and Crohn disease
Pediatric inflammatory bowel disease is characterized by chronic, recurrent inflammation of the gastrointestinal tract and includes 2 subcategories, Crohn disease and ulcerative colitis. Patients with ulcerative colitis experience inflammation isolated to the mucosa that most commonly occurs in the colon and rectum. Pediatric patients with ulcerative colitis tend to experience a more severe form of the disease that evolves rapidly with a higher prevalence of pancolitis (70%–90%) than in adults [27,28].

Mesalamine is a 5-aminosalicylate that is used for the management of ulcerative colitis in both adults and pediatric populations [29,30]. Two pediatric label changes were made for mesalamine in the past 2 years [1]. Delayed-release oral mesalamine capsule (Delzicol) is now approved for the treatment of mild to moderate ulcerative colitis in pediatric patients 5 years of age and older, which was based on data from studies in 82 patients 5 years to 17 years of age [31]. The second label change was for another mesalamine delayed-release formulation (Asacol), which was originally approved for the treatment of mild to moderate ulcerative colitis in patients 5 years and older in 2012 based on a 6-week trial period. The label change includes the statement that efficacy was not demonstrated for the maintenance of remission of mild to moderate ulcerative colitis in this same age group [32]. This was based on a 26-week trial of 2 dosage levels in 39 patients age 5 to 17.

Crohn disease is another form of inflammatory bowel disease that is characterized by transmural inflammation of the gastrointestinal mucosa leading to the formation skip lesions. Similar to ulcerative colitis, studies have shown that the onset of Crohn disease is typically more severe in younger patients [27]. Adalimumab (Humira) is an anti–tumor necrosis factor antibody that functions as an immunosuppressing agent and is approved for the induction and maintenance of clinical remission of moderate to severe Crohn disease in adults. In 2014, the FDA expanded the age range for use in pediatric patients 6 years and older as a treatment option when other treatments, including infliximab, have failed. The approval for pediatric use was based on the results of a phase 3 double-blind, randomized trial in 192 patients, which showed that adalimumab was able to induce and maintain remission in patients 6 years to 17 years of age with moderate to severe Crohn disease with a comparable safety profile to that of adult patients [33].

Constipation

Functional constipation is associated with infrequent or painful defecation, fecal incontinence, and abdominal pain and is a common problem in childhood that often starts during the first year of life [34]. The European Society for Paediatric Gastroenterology, Hepatology, and Nutrition and the North American Society for Pediatric Gastroenterology, Hepatology, and Nutrition released updated consensus guidelines in 2014 for the evaluation and treatment of functional constipation in infants and children [35]. The updated guidelines recommend polyethylene glycol (PEG) with or without electrolytes orally, 1 g/kg/d to 1.5 g/kg/d, for 3 to 6 days as first-line treatment of children presenting with fecal impaction. PEG is further recommended as a maintenance treatment at a starting dosage of 0.4 g/kg/d, which should be adjusted with clinical response. Lactulose is recommended if PEG is not available, although recent studies have shown that lactulose is not as effective as PEG in the treatment of chronic constipation is children 1 year to 3 years of age [36]. Maintenance treatment should continue for up to 2 months or until all symptoms have resolved for 1 month. The updates do not recommend the routine use of lubiprostone, linaclotide, or prucalopride because there have been no randomized trials published establishing their safety and efficacy in children. Lubiprostone was evaluated, however, in an open-label study in 109 patients between the ages of 3 and 17 and was found efficacious and well tolerated. Patients on lubiprostone experienced a significant increase in the number of spontaneous bowel movements per week compared with the group receiving placebo (3.1 vs 1.5, $P<.0001$). The most common adverse events included nausea, vomiting, diarrhea, abdominal pain, and headache [37].

Gastroesophageal reflux disease

Gastroesophageal reflux disease (GERD) is characterized by the regurgitation of gastric acid into the esophagus. GERD in infancy is generally self-limiting and improves with age whereas older children who develop GERD along with other medical comorbidities tend to experience a more prolonged disease course [38,39]. Rabeprazole (Aciphex), a proton pump inhibitor, was approved for the treatment of GERD in adolescents 12 years to 17 years of age in 2008 [1]. The age range for rabeprazole was expanded to include children 1 year of age and older in 2013 [40]. A follow-up study was conducted to evaluate the maintenance of efficacy and safety in children between the ages of 1 year and 11 years who had received 12 weeks of treatment and were maintained on the same dose for an additional 24 weeks. Subjects were originally random-ized into 2 groups during the treatment phase to receive either 0.5 mg/kg or 1.0 mg/kg of rabeprazole. Children who weighed 6 kg to 14.9 kg received up to 5 mg/d to 10 mg/d and children greater than or equal to 15 kg received 10 mg/d to 20 mg/d. The primary study outcome was evaluated with esopha-gogastroduodenoscopy and histology; 64 patients who achieved healing during the 12-week treatment phase were enrolled in the 24-week maintenance phase. The overall healing rate was 90%, with 100% of children in the low-weight group reporting maintained healing compared with 89% (10 mg) and 85% (20 mg) in the high-weight group [41].

GENETIC AND METABOLIC DISEASES

Significant advancements have been made in the treatment of rare genetic and metabolic diseases. A milestone for pediatric rare disease drug legislation occurred in 2012 with passage of the Creating Hope Act (CHA) as part of FDA Safety and Innovation Act. The CHA focuses on the use of priority re-view vouchers as a market incentive for companies to develop drugs for rare pediatric diseases. Since the enactment of the CHA, 4 priority review vouchers were issued with the approval of new entities for rare or ultrarare pediatric dis-eases. Additionally, as part of a requirement under a provision of FDA Safety and Innovation Act, a public meeting was held in 2014 to discuss ways to encourage and accelerate the development of new therapies for children with rare diseases. This culminated in the release of a new strategic plan on accelerating the development of therapies for pediatric rare diseases by the FDA [42].

In February 2014, elosulfase alfa (Vimizim) became the first FDA-approved treatment of Morquio A syndrome for patients 5 years and older [43]. Muco-polysaccharidosis type IV A, also known as Morquio A syndrome, is a rare autosomal recessive lysosomal storage disorder caused by a deficiency in N-acetylgalactosamine sulfate sulfatase (GALNS), leading to the accumulation of keratin sulfate and chondroitin-6-sulfate. Morquio A syndrome is clinically characterized by severe skeletal deformities as well a constellation of other developmental abnormalities, including corneal opacities, hepatosplenomegaly, and structural heart disease. In March 2015, cholic acid (Cholbam) was approved for the treatment of patients with bile acid synthesis disorders as well as patients with Zellweger spectrum peroxisomal disorders [44]. These disorders are characterized by reduced bile flow, steatorrhea, and malabsorp-tion of fatty acids and fat-soluble vitamins, leading to liver disease and growth abnormalities over time. For patients with bile acid synthesis disorders, a single-arm trial following more than 50 patients over 18 years showed im-provements in baseline liver function and weight gain over time [45]. Lastly, uridine triacetate (Xuriden) was approved by the FDA in September 2015 for the treatment of hereditary orotic aciduria, an extremely rare autosomal recessive metabolic disorder, which is thought to affect fewer than 20 people worldwide [46,47].

INFECTIOUS DISEASE
Pharmacokinetics
Several advancements have been made in characterizing the PK properties of anti-infective agents in pediatric populations (Table 2).

Pneumonia
Community-acquired pneumonia is a major cause of hospitalization of children in the United States [48]. It is most commonly caused by *Streptococcus pneumonia* but due to uncertainty of the causative organism and susceptibility patterns in

Table 2
Pediatric antimicrobial pharmacokinetic studies published in 2014 and 2015

Drug name	Patient population	Pharmacokinetic analysis approach	Dosing modifications recommended for studied population (yes/no)
Antimicrobials			
Ampicillin [94]	Neonates	Population	Yes
Azithromycin/ chloroquine [95]	Children and adults	Population	Yes
Ciprofloxacin [96]	Neonates and infants	Population	Yes
Clindamycin [97]	Neonates, infants, children, adolescents	Population	Yes
Piperacillin/ tazobactam [98]	Children	Population	Yes
Piperacillin/ tazobactam [99]	Infants	Population	Yes
Teicoplanin [100]	Children	Population	No
Teicoplanin [101]	Children, adolescents	Population	Yes
Antifungals			
Fluconazole [102]	Children	Population	Yes
Micafungin [103]	Children, adolescents	Noncompartmental	No
Micafungin [104]	Children, adolescents	Population	Yes
Antivirals			
Acyclovir [105]	Infants	Population	Yes
Fosamprenavir/ ritonavir [106]	Children, adolescents	Noncompartmental	No
Fosamprenavir/ ritonavir [107]	Infants, children	Noncompartmental	No
Lopinavir/ritonavir [108]	Infants, children	Noncompartmental	No
Nevirapine [109]	Children, adolescents	Noncompartmental	No
Raltegravir [110]	Neonates	Noncompartmental	No
Raltegravir [111]	Children, adolescents	Noncompartmental	No
Raltegravir [112]	Infants, children, adolescents	Population	No
Vancomycin [113]	Infants, children, adolescents	Compartmental	No
Zidovudine [114]	Children	Noncompartmental	No
Antiparasitic			
Benznidazole [115]	Children	Population	Yes

the clinical setting, patients are frequently prescribed broad-spectrum antibiotics as empirical therapy [49]. The Pediatric Infectious Disease Society and the Infectious Diseases of Society of America published guidelines in 2011 for the treatment of uncomplicated community-acquired pneumonia in pediatric patients and recommended the empiric use of narrow-spectrum coverage with agents, such as ampicillin or penicillin G [50]. A multicenter retrospective cohort study was conducted to compare the effectiveness of empiric treatment with narrow-spectrum versus broad-spectrum therapy [51]. Children between the ages of 2 months and 18 years (n = 492) who had been discharged with a diagnosis of community-acquired pneumonia and received either narrow-spectrum or broad-spectrum therapy in the first 2 days of hospitalization were included in the study. Narrow coverage was defined as amoxicillin, ampicillin, penicillin, or amoxicillin/clavulanic acid and broad coverage was defined as a second-generation or third-generation cephalosporin or fluoroquinolones. The study found that patients on narrow-spectrum therapy had a 10-hour shorter length of hospitalization ($P = .4$) with no other significant differences in outcomes. As such, the investigators concluded that both narrow-spectrum and broad-spectrum coverage are associated with similar outcomes [51]. Similarly, a prospective randomized study in 58 children between 3 months and 15 years of age found that penicillin G was as safe and effective as cefuroxime for the treatment of community-acquired pneumonia [52].

Hepatitis B
Entecavir (Baraclude) is a reverse transcriptase inhibitor that was approved for the treatment of chronic hepatitis B in adult patients in 2004. In 2014, the FDA expanded the indication age range to include pediatric patients 2 years of age and older. This was based on 2 clinical trials in pediatric patients ages between 2 years and 18 years with hepatitis B envelope antigen–positive chronic hepatitis B infection and compensated liver disease [53].

HIV
Significant progress has been made over the past decade in decreasing the incidence of HIV in pediatric populations. In 2014, Joint United Nations Programme on HIV/AIDS (UNAIDS) reported a 60% reduction in the number of new infections in children under 15 years of age between 2001 and 2013, from 500,000 to approximately 200,000 cases. Pediatric HIV/AIDS is currently estimated to affect 3.2 million children worldwide, which is approximately 9% of the global HIV/AIDS population [54]. In the past 2 years, there have been multiple FDA labeling changes for HIV drugs for use in pediatric populations. Atazanavir (Reyataz), which was previously available as a capsule for patients 6 years and older, became available in a new dosage form as an oral powder for patients greater than 3 months of age and weighing at least 5 kg. Abacavir (Ziagen) and lamivudine (Epivir) both underwent label revisions to provide new information on once-daily dosing for pediatric patients 3 months and older. A label change for combined lopinavir-ritonavir (Kaletra) recommended that the drug be administered twice daily and not once daily in pediatric patients.

Combination lamivudine-raltegravir tablets (Dutrebis) were approved for the treatment of HIV infection in adult and pediatric patients over 6 years of age and weighing at least 30 kg [55]. The indication for rilpirivone (Edurant) and the combination medication abacavir sulfate-lamivudine (Epzicom) was expanded from adults to include pediatric patients.

During the initiation of antiretroviral therapy (ART), both CD4 percentage (CD4%) and age are important factors [56,57]. Investigators of the Pediatric AIDS Clinical Trials 390/Paediatric European Network for Treatment of AIDS 9 (PENPACT-1) quantified the impacts of ART initiation at different ages and CD4% on CD4% recovery after 4 years in pediatric patients 0 to 17 years of age [58]. Overall, 72% of 162 vertically infected, immunosuppressed children recovered to normal CD4% within 4 years of ART initiation. Those who had mild or advanced immunosuppression as defined by World Health Organization criteria were more likely to recover to normal CD4% compared with those who were considered severely immunosuppressed at baseline. Additionally, for each 5-year increase in baseline age, the proportion of children achieving recovery declined by 19%. The study concluded that combining baseline CD4% and age effects resulted in greater than 90% recovery after 4 years when ART was initiated with mild immunosuppression at any age or with advanced immunosuppression less than 3 years of age [58].

Congenital cytomegalovirus

Congenital cytomegalovirus (CMV) infection is a leading cause of sensorineural hearing loss in infants and children [59]. Approximately 10% to 15% of infants with congenital CMV infection are symptomatic at birth, and up to 20% of all infected children develop long-term sequelae, including cognitive impairment and sensorineural hearing loss [60]. Neonates with symptomatic congenital CMV involving the central nervous system can be treated with 6 weeks of intravenous ganciclovir, or oral valganciclovir, which has been shown to improve outcomes at 6 months of life [61]. A randomized, placebo-controlled trial of valganciclovir therapy in neonates with symptomatic congenital CMV was conducted to compare 6 months versus 6 weeks of therapy [62]; 96 neonates with gestational age greater than or equal to 32 weeks and postnatal age less than or equal to 30 days and who weighed at least 1800 g were randomized to receive oral valganciclovir at a dose of 16 mg/kg twice daily for either 6 weeks (followed by 4.5 months of placebo) or 6 months. Brainstem auditory evoked response was assessed at baseline and performed in combination with visual-reinforcement audiometry to assess hearing at 6 months, 12 months, and 24 months. Additionally, the Bayley-III scale to assess infant and toddler development was administered at 12 months and 24 months. The results of the 6-month hearing assessment were similar between the 2 groups. Hearing, however, was more likely to be improved or to remain the same at 12 months in the 6-month group compared with the 6-week group (73% vs 57%, $P = .01$). The benefit in the 6-month group was maintained at 24 months (77% vs 64%, $P = .04$). Additionally, patients in the 6-month group had better neurodevelopmental scores on the Bayley-III. Overall, the investigators concluded that treating neonates with symptomatic CMV for 6 months did not improve hearing in the short term but was associated with improved outcomes in the long term [62].

Pneumococcal disease

Premature infants, in particular those less than 32 weeks' gestational age, are at increased risk for invasive pneumococcal disease due to factors, such as an reduced maternal-fetal transfer of pneumococcal antibodies and immature immune system [63,64]. Despite this increased risk for infection, vaccination of preterm infants is often delayed [65]. A clinical trial was conducted to evaluate the immune response and safety profile of the 13-valent pneumococcal conjugate vaccine (PCV13) in preterm infants compared with term infants on the same vaccination schedule [66]; 200 healthy infants (preterm, n = 100, and term, n = 100) between 42 and 98 days postnatal age were enrolled in a phase 4, open-label, multicenter parallel-group study. Infants received PCV13 at 2 months, 3 months, 4 months (infant series), and 12 months of age (toddler dose), along with other routine vaccinations. The primary study objective was to evaluate the immune response 1 month after administration of the infant series and 1 month after the toddler dose. The secondary objective was to measure the safety profile based on incidence of local reactions, systemic events, and adverse events. Most subjects in the study achieved an immunoglobulin G (IgG) concentration greater than or equal to 0.35 μg/mL for all serotypes, with greater than 85% after completing the infant series and greater than 97% after the toddler dose. Preterm infants were found to have an overall lower IgG geometric mean concentration compared with term infants. The geometric mean, however, increased at similar amounts for both groups after the toddler dose at 12 months, and the difference in IgG response between the 2 groups almost disappeared. The vaccination was tolerated well regardless of gestational age. The investigators concluded that a majority of subjects in both groups were able to exceed the World Health Organization threshold of protection and functional antibody response after the infant series [66].

NEUROLOGY

Migraines

Triptans are vascular 5-hydroxytryptamine 1 receptor agonists that cause vasoconstriction and are an option for migraine treatment and prophylaxis in adult and pediatric populations. Prior to 2014, only 2 triptans were FDA approved for use in pediatric populations: almotriptan for use in adolescents (12–17 years) and rizatriptan (6 years and older) [1]. Over the past 2 years, 2 additional triptans have been approved for the acute treatment of migraines in adolescent patients 12 years to 17 years of age. The first is zolmitriptan (Zomig), which was approved in 2014 based on a randomized, double-blind, placebo-controlled trial of 310 patients with an established diagnosis of migraine for at least 1 year with a typical untreated migraine attack lasting 3 hours or more. Two hours after the initiation of treatment, 30% of patients who had received 5 mg of zolmitriptan reported no more headache pain compared with 17% in the placebo group [67].

Sumatriptan in combination with naproxen (Treximet) was also approved in 2014. In terms of efficacy, 3 different doses of sumatriptan/naproxen were found to be superior to placebo at reducing headache severity from moderate or severe pain to no pain at 2 hours' postdose (10/60 mg, 30/180 mg, and 85/500 mg vs placebo, 29%, 27%, 24% vs 10%, $P<0.1$) [68].

Topiramate (Topamax) is an antiepileptic medication that is also used for migraine treatment and prophylaxis. In pediatric populations, it is approved for the treatment of partial-onset seizures (POSs) or primary generalized tonic-clonic seizures (PGTCs) both as a monotherapy or adjunctive treatment. In 2014, topiramate was also approved for migraine prophylaxis in adolescent patients 12 years to 17 years of age [69].

Seizures

Benzodiazepines are considered a first-line therapy for the treatment of status epilepticus (SE) in pediatric patients [70]. Diazepam is currently FDA approved for the treatment of SE in pediatric patients whereas lorazepam is not. Previous studies have suggested, however, that lorazepam may have potential advantages compared with diazepam, such as improved effectiveness in terminating convulsions, a longer duration of action, and a lower incidence of respiratory depression [71,72]. A study was conducted to determine if lorazepam has better efficacy and safety than diazepam for the treatment of pediatric SE [73]; 273 patients between 3 months and 18 years of age presenting with convulsive SE to 11 US academic pediatric emergency departments were enrolled and randomized to receive 0.1 mg/kg of lorazepam or 0.2 mg/kg of diazepam. The primary efficacy outcome was cessation of convulsions by 10 minutes without additional recurrence within 30 minutes, which occurred in 72.1% of patients in the diazepam group and 72.9% of patients in the lorazepam group with an absolute efficacy difference of 0.8% (95% CI, −11.4%–9.8%). For the primary safety outcome, 16.0% of patients in the diazepam group and 17.6% of patients in the lorazepam group required mechanical ventilation, resulting in an absolute efficacy difference of 1.6% (95% CI, −9.9% to 6.8%). There were no statistically significant differences in secondary outcomes between the 2 groups. As such, the investigators concluded that lorazepam for the treatment of SE in pediatric patients did not have improved efficacy or safety over diazepam [73].

ONCOLOGY

Two label changes were made for oncology drugs in the past 2 years [1]. For erlotinib (Tarceva), which is used in the treatment of refractory or recurrent ependymoma, the label change includes a statement that safety and effectiveness have not been established in pediatric patients. This is based on a phase 2 study in 25 pediatric patients which was terminated prematurely for lack of efficacy [74]. For bortezomib (Velcade), a drug used in the treatment of relapsed acute lymphoblastic leukemia (ALL) and lymphoblastic lymphoma, the label change states that the effectiveness in pediatric patients with relapsed pre-B ALL has not been established.

Dinutuximab (Unituxin) became the third novel agent approved for the treatment of a pediatric cancer in the past 25 years [75]. Dinutuximab is a monoclonal antibody targeting GD2, a glycolipid that promotes cell growth in neuroblastoma. It is approved for the treatment of high-risk neuroblastoma in combination with isotretinoin, interleukin 2, and granulocyte-macrophage colony-stimulating factor in patients who have shown some response to first-line therapy but require further treatment. The approval was based on a phase 3 study in 226 patients who had already completed multidrug chemotherapy, surgery, radiation therapy, and stem cell transplant [76].

PULMONARY AND ALLERGY
Asthma
There were multiple label changes for antiasthmatic therapies in 2014 and 2015. Mometasone furoate (Asmanex HFA) and fluticasone furoate (Arnuity Ellipta), which are used as maintenance treatment and prophylactic therapy, have both been approved for use in patients 12 years and older. For levalbuterol (Xopenex Inhalation Solution) used to treat reactive airway disease or asthma, the first label change stated that efficacy was not established in pediatric patients from 0 to 5 years of age. This was later updated to state that levalbuterol was not indicated for pediatric patients less than 4 years of age. A placebo-controlled clinical trial found no statistical difference in the primary efficacy endpoint and an increased incidence of adverse events in the study group compared with the placebo group [77].

Terbutaline is a β_2-receptor agonist that is administered intravenously to patients who do not improve on initial treatments for severe acute asthma. A retrospective chart review of 120 subjects admitted to the pediatric ICU for severe asthma and receiving treatment with terbutaline was conducted to determine if earlier terbutaline administration was associated with improved outcomes [78]. Of the patients who had received terbutaline for a significantly shorter amount of time (0.69 hours $\pm$ 1.38 hours vs 2.91 hours $\pm$ 2.47 hours, $P<.001$), 60% of patients required mechanical ventilation compared with 27% of patients who had received terbutaline sooner. The study suggests that earlier administration of terbutaline may be beneficial in patients with severe acute asthma and decrease the incidence of respiratory failure [78].

Allergic rhinitis
Drug label changes were made for 4 drugs indicated for the treatment of allergic rhinitis. The indication for omalizumab (Xolair), originally approved in 2003 for asthma, was expanded to include the treatment of chronic idiopathic urticarial in patients 12 years and older. The approved age range for ciclesonide (Zetonna) for the treatment of perennial allergic rhinitis was expanded from 12 years and older to include patients 6 years to 11 years of

age. Use of beclomethasone diproprionate (QNASL) for the treatment of nasal symptoms associated with seasonal and perennial allergic rhinitis was expanded to include patients 4 years and older. Finally, the age category for azelastine indicated for the treatment of seasonal allergic rhinitis was expanded to include patients as young as 6 months of age. Two new approvals were made for the treatment of allergic rhinitis associated with grass pollen allergies. The first was a combination allergen extract of Sweet Vernal, Orchard, Perennial Rye, Timothy, and Kentucky Blue Grass Mixed Pollens (Oralair), which was the first approved sublingual alternative to allergy shots [79]. The approval was based on studies conducted in the United States and Europe in 2500 patients from the ages of 10 years through 65 years. Patients taking the extract experienced a 16% to 30% reduction in symptoms compared with those who received the placebo [80]. The second approval was for another allergen extract of Timothy Grass Pollen (Grastek) in patients 5 years to 65 years of age, which showed a similar reduction in symptoms in a trial in 1501 patients [81].

Intranasal corticosteroids are frequently prescribed for the control of symptoms associated with allergic rhinitis. Triamcinolone acetonide aqueous nasal spray (Nasacort) has been approved in the United States for more than a decade for treating symptoms related to perennial and seasonal allergic rhinitis in both adults and children 2 years and older [1]. Previous studies have yielded varying results regarding the potential systemic effects of intranasal corticosteroid, such as growth retardation. The first randomized controlled trial based on FDA guidelines to assess the long-term effect of intranasal triamcinolone acetonide examined the difference in the growth velocity of children between 3 years and 9 years of age who were treated for 12 months [82]. The randomized, double-blind, placebo-controlled, parallel-group multicenter study was composed of a 4-month to 6-month screening period followed by a 12-month treatment phase and a 2-month post-treatment follow-up. After screening and baseline visits, the patients were stratified by age group (3–5 years vs 6–9 years) and gender and were randomized to receive either 110 µg of intranasal triamcinolone acetonide or placebo for 12 months. The investigators found that triamcinolone acetonide had a small, statistically significant effect on growth velocity (-0.45 cm/y, 95% CI, $-.78$–0.11; $P = .01$). During the follow-up period, however, the growth velocity in the triamcinolone acetonide increased to approach the baseline growth velocity [82].

Cystic fibrosis

Ivacaftor, which was originally approved for the treatment of patients with the *G551D* cystic fibrosis transmembrane conductance regulator gene mutation in children 6 years and older, has been approved by the FDA for use in children over 2 years of age [1]. Additionally, the combination lumacaftor-ivacaftor was approved for the treatment of patients 12 years and older who are homozygous for the *F508del* mutation based on 2 phase 3 randomized trials (TRAFFIC and TRANSPORT) totaling 1108 patients [83]. The groups receiving different daily doses of lumacaftor-ivacaftor for 24 weeks showed improvement in predicted forced expiratory volume in 1 second (FEV_1). The mean (95% CI) absolute improvement in percentage of predicted FEV_1 for 600 mg/d lumacaftor-ivacaftor was 2.6% (1.2–4.1) and 400 mg every 12 hours was 3.0% (1.6–4.4) over the placebo group ($P<.001$). Additionally, patients experienced an increase in body mass index and a reduced frequency of pulmonary exacerbations [83]. Lumacaftor-ivacaftir combination treatment was well tolerated with the incidence of adverse events similar between the groups.

PSYCHIATRY

Five label changes were made for psychiatric drugs between 2014 and 2015 [1]. First, asenapine (Saphris) is now approved for the treatment of acute manic or mixed episodes associated with bipolar I disorder in patients between 10 years and 17 years of age. Safety and efficacy were established in a phase 1 study in 403 patients. Asenapine was not shown effective in the treatment of schizophrenia in adolescents ages 12 years to 17 years [84]. Second, a 24-week open-label safety study for escitalopram oxalate (Lexapro) did not identify any new safety concerns in 118 children 7 years to 11 years of age with major depressive disorder (MDD). The label change states that escitalopram oxalate is safe and well tolerated in this population even though efficacy was not established. Third, selegiline (Emsam) also used for the treatment of MDD failed to demonstrate efficacy in adolescents 12 years to 17 years of age based on a phase 4 study in 306 patients. Additionally, selegiline is contraindicated in children under 12 years of age due to increased risk of hypertensive crisis compared with adults and adolescents. Fourth, safety and efficacy for lamotrigine (Lamictal) used in the maintenance of bipolar disorder was not established for patients 10 years to 17 years of age. Lastly, a study of duloxetine hydrochloride (Cymbalta) in 272 patients for the treatment of generalized anxiety disorder established safety and efficacy in children 7 years to 17 years.

Advances in pharmacotherapies for attention-deficit/hyperactivity disorder (ADHD) are covered in this issue (See Leung AKC, Hon KL: Attention-Deficit Hyperactivity Disorder, in this issue).

RHEUMATOLOGY
Juvenile idiopathic arthritis

Juvenile idiopathic arthritis (JIA) is the most common rheumatic disease of childhood and is composed of several subgroups of autoimmune diseases depending on onset and disease course [85]. Polyarticular JIA is characterized by the involvement of greater than or equal to 5 joints within 6 months of the onset of illness. Adalimumab is an anti–tumor necrosis factor antibody that is approved for the treatment of moderate to severe polyarticular JIA in patients greater than or equal to 4 years of age [1]. A phase 3, open-label, multicenter trial was conducted to determine the safety, efficacy, and PK profile of adalimumab in children between the ages of 2 years and 4 years with moderate to severe polyarticular JIA [86]. Each patient received 24 mg/m^2 of adalimumab subcutaneously every other week for a minimum of 24 weeks and was allowed to continue concomitant treatments, including methotrexate, nonsteroidal anti-inflammatory drugs, or low-dose steroids. The study followed 32 patients with a mean (SD) age of 3.0 (0.72) years and duration of polyarticular JIA of 12 (9.3) months. Patients received a mean duration (SD) of 515 (245) days of adalimumab exposure; 90.6% of patients reported at least 1 adverse event, with infections and worsening of JIA the most frequent. Adalimumab was associated with sustained improvement of core JIA disease parameters as defined by the American College of Rheumatology pediatric score for up to 96 weeks. Mean steady state concentrations were within the range observed in older populations of children between ages 14 and 17 [87]. Overall, the investigators concluded that adalimumab therapy with or without concomitant methotrexate was well tolerated and effective for the treatment of moderate to severe polyarticular JIA in this population [86].

Systemic JIA is another subgroup of childhood arthritis with onset of disease that is characterized by high fever, rash, hepatosplenomegaly, lymphadenopathy, anemia, and occasionally macrophage activation syndrome [88]. Patients may also experience poor long-term outcomes, such as growth failure, musculoskeletal deformities, and osteoporosis [89]. Rilonacept is an inhibitor of interleukin-1, which is a mediator in the inflammatory cascade that contributes to the pathogenesis of systemic JIA. It is currently only FDA approved for the treatment of cryopyrin-associated periodic syndromes in adults and children 12 years and older [90]. The Randomized Placebo Phase Study of Rilonacept in the Treatment of Systemic Juvenile Idiopathic Arthritis (RAPPORT) trial was conducted to determine the safety and efficacy of rilonacept in the treatment of systemic JIA [91]; 71 children between the ages of 18 months and 19 years were randomized to receive either 24 weeks of rilonacept treatment or 4 weeks of placebo followed by 20 weeks of treatment. At week 4, 57% of the patients receiving rilonacept had a response compared with 27% of patients receiving the placebo ($P = .016$). The most common adverse events were the exacerbation of systemic JIA and elevated transaminase levels. A PK analysis conducted as part of this study found that rilonacept clearance increased with increasing body weight and age and decreased with increasing serum albumin levels. Overall, it was observed that the range of exposure after a loading dose of 4.4 mg/kg followed by 2.2 mg/kg weekly maintenance doses used in the RAPPORT trial were comparable to values observed in adult populations [92].

SYMPTOMATIC CARE

Clonidine is an α_2-adrenergic agonist that is used in conjunction with morphine for the treatment of withdrawal in neonatal abstinence syndrome (NAS). To determine whether single-agent clonidine treatment is as effective as morphine in the treatment of NAS, a pilot randomized double-blind single-center study was conducted [93]. A total of 31 infants greater than or equal to 35 weeks' gestational age were enrolled in the study and randomized to receive morphine (0.4 mg/kg/d) or clonidine (5 µg/kg/d) divided into 8 doses. Neurobehavioral performance was assessed using the NICU Network Neurobehavioral Scale (NNNS) 1 week and 2 weeks to 4 weeks after start of treatment. The Bayley-III and Preschool Language Scale, Fourth Edition, were administered at 1-year adjusted age. The study found that duration of treatment of infants on morphine (n = 15) was significantly longer compared with clonidine (n = 16). Additionally, NNNS scores improved with clonidine but not morphine and 1-year motor, cognitive, and language scores did not differ between the 2 groups. The investigators concluded that clonidine single-agent therapy is as effective as morphine used for the treatment of NAS [93]. Because this was a small pilot study, a large randomized multicenter trial is necessary.

SUMMARY

There has been major progress in the development of drugs for pediatric patients over the past 2 years. The top areas under investigation included infectious disease, in particular antivirals, and antiallergy and antiasthma medications. Other areas of progress included anti-inflammatory medications used in the treatment of gastrointestinal disease and antiepileptics for pediatric seizures. Additionally, there has been a recent surge in the development of medications for the treatment of rare diseases that affect pediatric populations, specifically inherited metabolic disorders.

References

[1] U.S. Food and Drug Administration. Pediatric labeling information database. Available at: http://www.accessdata.fda.gov/scripts/sda/sdNavigation.cfm?sd=labelingdatabase. Accessed November 20, 2015.
[2] European Medicines Agency. Opinions and decisions on paediatric investigation plans. Available at: http://www.ema.europa.eu/ema/index.jsp?curl=pages/medicines/landing/pip_search.jsp. Accessed November 15, 2015.
[3] European Medicines Agency. Public assessment reports. Available at: http://www.ema.europa.eu/ema/index.jsp?curl=pages/medicines/landing/epar_search.jsp&mid=WC0b01ac058001d125. Accessed November 15, 2015.
[4] Laughon MM, Avant D, Tripathi N, et al. Drug labeling and exposure in neonates. JAMA Pediatr 2014;168(2):130–6.
[5] Tan JA, Ho KM. Use of dexmedetomidine as a sedative and analgesic agent in critically ill adult patients: a meta-analysis. Intensive Care Med 2010;36(6):926–39.
[6] Tobias JD. Dexmedetomidine: applications in pediatric critical care and pediatric anesthesiology. Pediatr Crit Care Med 2007;8(2):115–31.
[7] Chrysostomou C, Schulman SR, Herrera Castellanos M, et al. A phase II/III, multicenter, safety, efficacy, and pharmacokinetic study of dexmedetomidine in preterm and term neonates. J Pediatr 2014;164(2):276–82.e1–e3.
[8] Whalen LD, Di Gennaro JL, Irby GA, et al. Long-term dexmedetomidine use and safety profile among critically ill children and neonates. Pediatr Crit Care Med 2014;15(8):706–14.
[9] Oxycontin extended release tablets [package insert]. Purdue Pharma LP. Available at: http://www.accessdata.fda.gov/drugsatfda_docs/label/2015/022272s027lbl.pdf. Accessed November 6, 2015.
[10] Reinhardt Z, Uzun O, Bhole V, et al. Sildenafil in the management of the failing Fontan circulation. Cardiol Young 2010;20(5):522–5.
[11] Hill KD, Sampson MR, Li JS, et al. Pharmacokinetics of intravenous sildenafil in children with palliated single ventricle heart defects: effect of elevated hepatic pressures. Cardiol Young 2016;26(2):354–62.

[12] Barst RJ, Ivy DD, Gaitan G, et al. A randomized, double-blind, placebo-controlled, dose-ranging study of oral sildenafil citrate in treatment-naive children with pulmonary arterial hypertension. Circulation 2012;125(2):324–34.

[13] U.S. Food and Drug Administration: FDA drug safety communication: FDA recommends against use of Revatio (sildenafil) in children with pulmonary hypertension. 2012. Available at: http://www.fda.gov/Drugs/DrugSafety/ucm317123.htm. Accessed November 1, 2015.

[14] European Medicines Agency: Revatio: Summary of product characteristics. Available at: http://www.ema.europa.eu/docs/en_GB/document_library/EPAR_-_Product_Information/human/000638/WC500055840.pdf. Accessed October 10, 2015.

[15] U.S. Food and Drug Administration: FDA clarifies Warning about Pediatric Use of Revatio (sildenafil) for Pulmonary Arterial Hypertension. 2014. Available at: http://www.fda.gov/Drugs/DrugSafety/ucm390876.htm. Accessed November 1, 2015.

[16] Barst RJ, Beghetti M, Pulido T, et al. STARTS-2: long-term survival with oral sildenafil monotherapy in treatment-naive pediatric pulmonary arterial hypertension. Circulation 2014;129(19):1914–23.

[17] Shahinfar S, Cano F, Soffer BA, et al. A double-blind, dose-response study of losartan in hypertensive children. Am J Hypertens 2005;18(2 Pt 1):183–90.

[18] Webb NJ, Wells TG, Shahinfar S, et al. A randomized, open-label, dose-response study of losartan in hypertensive children. Clin J Am Soc Nephrol 2014;9(8):1441–8.

[19] Inigo P, Campistol JM, Lario S, et al. Effects of losartan and amlodipine on intrarenal hemodynamics and TGF-beta(1) plasma levels in a crossover trial in renal transplant recipients. J Am Soc Nephrol 2001;12(4):822–7.

[20] Trachtman H, Frymoyer A, Lewandowski A, et al. Pharmacokinetics, pharmacodynamics, and safety of lisinopril in pediatric kidney transplant patients: implications for starting dose selection. Clin Pharmacol Ther 2015;98(1):25–33.

[21] Tollefson MM, Bruckner AL, Section On Dermatology. Atopic dermatitis: skin-directed management. Pediatrics 2014;134(6):e1735–44.

[22] Legendre L, Barnetche T, Mazereeuw-Hautier J, et al. Risk of lymphoma in patients with atopic dermatitis and the role of topical treatment: a systematic review and meta-analysis. J Am Acad Dermatol 2015;72(6):992–1002.

[23] Chia BK, Tey HL. Systematic review on the efficacy, safety, and cost-effectiveness of topical calcineurin inhibitors in atopic dermatitis. Dermatitis 2015;26(3):122–32.

[24] Huang X, Xu B. Efficacy and safety of tacrolimus versus pimecrolimus for the treatment of atopic dermatitis in children: a network meta-analysis. Dermatology 2015;231(1):41–9.

[25] Charman CR, Morris AD, Williams HC. Topical corticosteroid phobia in patients with atopic eczema. Br J Dermatol 2000;142(5):931–6.

[26] Sigurgeirsson B, Boznanski A, Todd G, et al. Safety and efficacy of pimecrolimus in atopic dermatitis: a 5-year randomized trial. Pediatrics 2015;135(4):597–606.

[27] Abraham BP, Mehta S, El-Serag HB. Natural history of pediatric-onset inflammatory bowel disease: a systematic review. J Clin Gastroenterol 2012;46(7):581–9.

[28] Gower-Rousseau C, Dauchet L, Vernier-Massouille G, et al. The natural history of pediatric ulcerative colitis: a population-based cohort study. Am J Gastroenterol 2009;104(8): 2080–8.

[29] Aloi M, Nuti F, Stronati L, et al. Advances in the medical management of paediatric IBD. Nat Rev Gastroenterol Hepatol 2014;11(2):99–108.

[30] Turner D, Levine A, Escher JC, et al. Management of pediatric ulcerative colitis: joint ECCO and ESPGHAN evidence-based consensus guidelines. J Pediatr Gastroenterol Nutr 2012;55(3):340–61.

[31] Delzicol [package insert]. Warner Chilcott. Available at: http://www.accessdata.fda.gov/drugsatfda_docs/label/2015/204412s006lbl.pdf. Accessed October 17, 2015.

[32] Asacol [package insert]. Warner Chilcott. Available at: http://www.accessdata.fda.gov/drugsatfda_docs/label/2015/019651s025lbl.pdf. Accessed October 17, 2015.

[33] Hyams JS, Griffiths A, Markowitz J, et al. Safety and efficacy of adalimumab for moderate to severe Crohn's disease in children. Gastroenterology 2012;143(2):365–74.e2.

[34] Loening-Baucke V. Constipation in early childhood: patient characteristics, treatment, and longterm follow up. Gut 1993;34(10):1400–4.

[35] Tabbers MM, DiLorenzo C, Berger MY, et al. Evaluation and treatment of functional constipation in infants and children: evidence-based recommendations from ESPGHAN and NASPGHAN. J Pediatr Gastroenterol Nutr 2014;58(2):258–74.

[36] Treepongkaruna S, Simakachorn N, Pienvichit P, et al. A randomised, double-blind study of polyethylene glycol 4000 and lactulose in the treatment of constipation in children. BMC Pediatr 2014;14:153.

[37] Hyman PE, Di Lorenzo C, Prestridge LL, et al. Lubiprostone for the treatment of functional constipation in children. J Pediatr Gastroenterol Nutr 2014;58(3):283–91.

[38] Tighe M, Afzal NA, Bevan A, et al. Pharmacological treatment of children with gastro-oesophageal reflux. Cochrane Database Syst Rev 2014;(11):CD008550.

[39] Nelson SP, Chen EH, Syniar GM, et al. One-year follow-up of symptoms of gastroesophageal reflux during infancy. Pediatric Practice Research Group. Pediatrics 1998;102(6):E67.

[40] Haddad I, Kierkus J, Tron E, et al. Efficacy and safety of rabeprazole in children (1-11 years) with gastroesophageal reflux disease. J Pediatr Gastroenterol Nutr 2013;57(6):798–807.

[41] Haddad I, Kierkus J, Tron E, et al. Maintenance of efficacy and safety of rabeprazole in children with endoscopically proven GERD. J Pediatr Gastroenterol Nutr 2014;58(4):510–7.

[42] United States Department of Health and Human Services, Food and Drug Administration: Report: Complex Issues in Developing Drugs and Biological Products for Rare Diseases and Accelerating the Development of Therapies for Pediatric Rare Diseases Including Strategic Plan: Accelerating the Development of Therapies for Pediatric Rare Diseases. 2014. Available at: http://www.fda.gov/downloads/RegulatoryInformation/Legislation/SignificantAmendmentstotheFDCAct/FDASIA/UCM404104.pdf. Accessed November 1, 2015.

[43] Sanford M, Lo JH. Elosulfase alfa: first global approval. Drugs 2014;74(6):713–8.

[44] U.S. Food and Drug Administration: FDA approves Cholbam to treat rare bile acid synthesis disorders. 2015. Available at: http://www.fda.gov/NewsEvents/Newsroom/PressAnnouncements/ucm438572.htm. Accessed October 26, 2015.

[45] Cholbam [package insert]. Asklepion Pharmaceuticals LLC. Available at: http://www.accessdata.fda.gov/drugsatfda_docs/label/2015/205750s000lbl.pdf. Accessed October 20, 2015.

[46] U.S. Food and Drug Administration: FDA approves new orphan drug to treat rare autosomal recessive disorder. 2015. Available at: http://www.fda.gov/NewsEvents/Newsroom/PressAnnouncements/ucm457867.htm. Accessed October 15, 2015.

[47] Xuriden [package insert]. Wellstat Therapeutics Corporation. Available at: http://www.xuriden.com/FPI.pdf. Accessed October 4, 2015.

[48] Lee GE, Lorch SA, Sheffler-Collins S, et al. National hospitalization trends for pediatric pneumonia and associated complications. Pediatrics 2010;126(2):204–13.

[49] Ambroggio L, Tabb LP, O'Meara T, et al. Influence of antibiotic susceptibility patterns on empiric antibiotic prescribing for children hospitalized with community-acquired pneumonia. Pediatr Infect Dis J 2012;31(4):331–6.

[50] Bradley JS, Byington CL, Shah SS, et al. The management of community-acquired pneumonia in infants and children older than 3 months of age: clinical practice guidelines by the Pediatric Infectious Diseases Society and the Infectious Diseases Society of America. Clin Infect Dis 2011;53(7):e25–76.

[51] Queen MA, Myers AL, Hall M, et al. Comparative effectiveness of empiric antibiotics for community-acquired pneumonia. Pediatrics 2014;133(1):e23–9.

[52] Amarilyo G, Glatstein M, Alper A, et al. IV Penicillin G is as effective as IV cefuroxime in treating community-acquired pneumonia in children. Am J Ther 2014;21(2):81–4.

[53] Baraclude [package insert]. Bristol-Meyers Squibb. Available at: http://www.accessdata.fda.gov/drugsatfda_docs/label/2014/021797s018021798s019lbl.pdf. Accessed November, 7, 2015.

[54] Joint United Nations Programme on HIV and AIDS (UNAIDS): Gap Report. 2014. Available at: http://www.unaids.org/sites/default/files/media_asset/UNAIDS_Gap_report_en.pdf. Accessed October 23, 2015.

[55] Dutrebis [package insert]. Merck Sharp & Dohme Corp. Available at: http://www.accessdata.fda.gov/drugsatfda_docs/label/2015/206510lbl.pdf. Accessed October 18, 2015.

[56] HIV Paediatric Prognostic Markers Collaborative Study. Predictive value of absolute CD4 cell count for disease progression in untreated HIV-1-infected children. AIDS 2006;20(9): 1289–94.

[57] Puthanakit T, Saphonn V, Ananworanich J, et al. Early versus deferred antiretroviral therapy for children older than 1 year infected with HIV (PREDICT): a multicentre, randomised, open-label trial. Lancet Infect Dis 2012;12(12):933–41.

[58] Yin DE, Warshaw MG, Miller WC, et al. Using CD4 percentage and age to optimize pediatric antiretroviral therapy initiation. Pediatrics 2014;134(4):e1104–16.

[59] Fowler KB, Boppana SB. Congenital cytomegalovirus (CMV) infection and hearing deficit. J Clin Virol 2006;35(2):226–31.

[60] Dollard SC, Grosse SD, Ross DS. New estimates of the prevalence of neurological and sensory sequelae and mortality associated with congenital cytomegalovirus infection. Rev Med Virol 2007;17(5):355–63.

[61] Kimberlin DW, Lin CY, Sanchez PJ, et al. Effect of ganciclovir therapy on hearing in symptomatic congenital cytomegalovirus disease involving the central nervous system: a randomized, controlled trial. J Pediatr 2003;143(1):16–25.

[62] Kimberlin DW, Jester PM, Sanchez PJ, et al. Valganciclovir for symptomatic congenital cytomegalovirus disease. N Engl J Med 2015;372(10):933–43.

[63] Okoko BJ, Wesumperuma LH, Hart AC. Materno-foetal transfer of H. influenzae and pneumococcal antibodies is influenced by prematurity and low birth weight: implications for conjugate vaccine trials. Vaccine 2001;20(5–6):647–50.

[64] Omenaca F, Garcia-Sicilia J, Boceta R, et al. Antibody persistence and booster vaccination during the second and fifth years of life in a cohort of children who were born prematurely. Pediatr Infect Dis J 2007;26(9):824–9.

[65] Gagneur A, Pinquier D, Quach C. Immunization of preterm infants. Hum Vaccin Immunother 2015;11(11):2556–63.

[66] Martinon-Torres F, Czajka H, Center KJ, et al. 13-valent pneumococcal conjugate vaccine (PCV13) in preterm versus term infants. Pediatrics 2015;135(4):e876–86.

[67] Zomig nasal spray [package insert]. AstraZeneca. Available at: http://www.accessdata.fda.gov/drugsatfda_docs/label/2015/021450s008lbl.pdf. Accessed November 10, 2015.

[68] Treximet [package insert]. Pernix Therapeutics. Available at: http://www.accessdata.fda.gov/drugsatfda_docs/label/2015/021926s011s012lbl.pdf. Accessed November 10, 2015.

[69] Topamax [package insert]. Janssen. Available at: http://www.accessdata.fda.gov/drugsatfda_docs/label/2014/020505s052, 020844s043lbl.pdf. Accessed November 10, 2015.

[70] Alford EL, Wheless JW, Phelps SJ. Treatment of Generalized Convulsive Status Epilepticus in Pediatric Patients. J Pediatr Pharmacol Ther 2015;20(4):260–89.

[71] Leppik IE, Derivan AT, Homan RW, et al. Double-blind study of lorazepam and diazepam in status epilepticus. JAMA 1983;249(11):1452–4.

[72] Chiulli DA, Terndrup TE, Kanter RK. The influence of diazepam or lorazepam on the frequency of endotracheal intubation in childhood status epilepticus. J Emerg Med 1991;9(1–2):13–7.

[73] Chamberlain JM, Okada P, Holsti M, et al. Lorazepam vs diazepam for pediatric status epilepticus: a randomized clinical trial. JAMA 2014;311(16):1652–60.

[74] Astellas Pharma Inc (OSI Pharmaceuticals): Single-agent Erlotinib in Patients Previously Treated Oral Etoposide in Protocol OSI-774-205- Study Terminated. Available at: https://clinicaltrials.gov/ct2/show/NCT01247922?term=erlotinib&rank=1. Accessed November 20, 2015.

[75] Dhillon S. Dinutuximab: first global approval. Drugs 2015;75(8):923–7.

[76] Yu AL, Gilman AL, Ozkaynak MF, et al. Anti-GD2 antibody with GM-CSF, interleukin-2, and isotretinoin for neuroblastoma. N Engl J Med 2010;363(14):1324–34.

[77] Xopenex inhalation solution [package insert]. Oak Pharmaceuticals. Available at: http://www.respistory.com/aa/ast/XOPENEX-HFA-Prescribing-Information.pdf. Accessed November 20, 2015.

[78] Doymaz S, Schneider J, Sagy M. Early administration of terbutaline in severe pediatric asthma may reduce incidence of acute respiratory failure. Ann Allergy Asthma Immunol 2014;112(3):207–10.

[79] U.S. Food and Drug Administration: FDA approves first sublingual allergen extract for the treatement of certain grass pollen allergies. 2014. Available at: http://www.fda.gov/newsevents/newsroom/pressannouncements/ucm391458.htm. Accessed October 30, 2015.

[80] Stallergenes SA: Oralair [package insert]. Available at: http://www.fda.gov/downloads/BiologicsBloodVaccines/Allergenics/UCM391580.pdf. Accessed November 12, 2015.

[81] Maloney J, Bernstein DI, Nelson H, et al. Efficacy and safety of grass sublingual immunotherapy tablet, MK-7243: a large randomized controlled trial. Ann Allergy Asthma Immunol 2014;112(2):146–53.e2.

[82] Skoner DP, Berger WE, Gawchik SM, et al. Intranasal triamcinolone and growth velocity. Pediatrics 2015;135(2):e348–56.

[83] Wainwright CE, Elborn JS, Ramsey BW, et al. Lumacaftor-Ivacaftor in Patients with Cystic Fibrosis Homozygous for Phe508del CFTR. N Engl J Med 2015;373(3):220–31.

[84] Saphris [package insert]. Forest. Available at: http://pi.actavis.com/data_stream.asp?product_group=1908&p=pi&language=E. Accessed November 15, 2015.

[85] Prakken B, Albani S, Martini A. Juvenile idiopathic arthritis. Lancet 2011;377(9783): 2138–49.

[86] Kingsbury DJ, Bader-Meunier B, Patel G, et al. Safety, effectiveness, and pharmacokinetics of adalimumab in children with polyarticular juvenile idiopathic arthritis aged 2 to 4 years. Clin Rheumatol 2014;33(10):1433–41.

[87] Lovell DJ, Ruperto N, Goodman S, et al. Adalimumab with or without methotrexate in juvenile rheumatoid arthritis. N Engl J Med 2008;359(8):810–20.

[88] Grom AA, Passo M. Macrophage activation syndrome in systemic juvenile rheumatoid arthritis. J Pediatr 1996;129(5):630–2.

[89] Woo P. Systemic juvenile idiopathic arthritis: diagnosis, management, and outcome. Nat Clin Pract Rheumatol 2006;2(1):28–34.

[90] Acralyst [package insert]. Regeneron Pharmaceuticals Inc. Available at: http://www.regeneron.com/Arcalyst/Arcalyst_FPI.pdf. Accessed October 19, 2015.

[91] Ilowite NT, Prather K, Lokhnygina Y, et al. Randomized, double-blind, placebo-controlled trial of the efficacy and safety of rilonacept in the treatment of systemic juvenile idiopathic arthritis. Arthritis Rheumatol 2014;66(9):2570–9.

[92] Autmizguine J, Cohen-Wolkowiez M, Ilowite N, et al. Rilonacept pharmacokinetics in children with systemic juvenile idiopathic arthritis. J Clin Pharmacol 2015;55(1):39–44.

[93] Bada HS, Sithisarn T, Gibson J, et al. Morphine versus clonidine for neonatal abstinence syndrome. Pediatrics 2015;135(2):e383–91.

[94] Tremoulet A, Le J, Poindexter B, et al. Characterization of the population pharmacokinetics of ampicillin in neonates using an opportunistic study design. Antimicrob Agents Chemother 2014;58(6):3013–20.

[95] Zhao Q, Tensfeldt TG, Chandra R, et al. Population pharmacokinetics of azithromycin and chloroquine in healthy adults and paediatric malaria subjects following oral administration of fixed-dose azithromycin and chloroquine combination tablets. Malar J 2014;13:36.

[96] Zhao W, Hill H, Le Guellec C, et al. Population pharmacokinetics of ciprofloxacin in neonates and young infants less than three months of age. Antimicrob Agents Chemother 2014;58(11):6572–80.

[97] Gonzalez D, Melloni C, Yogev R, et al. Use of opportunistic clinical data and a population pharmacokinetic model to support dosing of clindamycin for premature infants to adolescents. Clin Pharmacol Ther 2014;96(4):429–37.

[98] Cies JJ, Jain J, Kuti JL. Population pharmacokinetics of the piperacillin component of piperacillin/tazobactam in pediatric oncology patients with fever and neutropenia. Pediatr Blood Cancer 2015;62(3):477–82.

[99] Cohen-Wolkowiez M, Watt KM, Zhou C, et al. Developmental pharmacokinetics of piperacillin and tazobactam using plasma and dried blood spots from infants. Antimicrob Agents Chemother 2014;58(5):2856–65.

[100] Ramos-Martin V, Paulus S, Siner S, et al. Population pharmacokinetics of teicoplanin in children. Antimicrob Agents Chemother 2014;58(11):6920–7.

[101] Zhao W, Zhang D, Storme T, et al. Population pharmacokinetics and dosing optimization of teicoplanin in children with malignant haematological disease. Br J Clin Pharmacol 2015;80(5):1197–207.

[102] Watt KM, Gonzalez D, Benjamin DK Jr, et al. Fluconazole population pharmacokinetics and dosing for prevention and treatment of invasive Candidiasis in children supported with extracorporeal membrane oxygenation. Antimicrob Agents Chemother 2015;59(7):3935–43.

[103] Albano E, Azie N, Roy M, et al. Pharmacokinetic and safety profiles of repeated-dose prophylactic micafungin in children and adolescents undergoing hematopoietic stem cell transplantation. J Pediatr Hematol Oncol 2015;37(1):e45–50.

[104] Hope WW, Kaibara A, Roy M, et al. Population pharmacokinetics of micafungin and its metabolites M1 and M5 in children and adolescents. Antimicrob Agents Chemother 2015;59(2):905–13.

[105] Sampson MR, Bloom BT, Lenfestey RW, et al. Population pharmacokinetics of intravenous acyclovir in preterm and term infants. Pediatr Infect Dis J 2014;33(1):42–9.

[106] Fortuny C, Duiculescu D, Cheng K, et al. Pharmacokinetics and 48-week safety and antiviral activity of fosamprenavir-containing regimens in HIV-infected 2- to 18-year-old children. Pediatr Infect Dis J 2014;33(1):50–6.

[107] Cotton M, Cassim H, Pavia-Ruz N, et al. Pharmacokinetics, safety and antiviral activity of fosamprenavir/ritonavir-containing regimens in HIV-infected children aged 4 weeks to 2 years-48-week study data. Pediatr Infect Dis J 2014;33(1):57–62.

[108] Musiime V, Fillekes Q, Kekitiinwa A, et al. The pharmacokinetics and acceptability of lopinavir/ritonavir minitab sprinkles, tablets, and syrups in african HIV-infected children. J Acquir Immune Defic Syndr 2014;66(2):148–54.

[109] Giaquinto C, Anabwani G, Feiterna-Sperling C, et al. Steady-state pharmacokinetics of nevirapine extended-release tablets in HIV-infected children and adolescents: an open-label, multiple-dose, cross-over study. Pediatr Infect Dis J 2014;33(7):e173–9.

[110] Clarke DF, Acosta EP, Rizk ML, et al. Raltegravir pharmacokinetics in neonates following maternal dosing. J Acquir Immune Defic Syndr 2014;67(3):310–5.

[111] Nachman S, Zheng N, Acosta EP, et al. Pharmacokinetics, safety, and 48-week efficacy of oral raltegravir in HIV-1-infected children aged 2 through 18 years. Clin Infect Dis 2014;58(3):413–22.

[112] Rizk ML, Du L, Bennetto-Hood C, et al. Population pharmacokinetic analysis of raltegravir pediatric formulations in HIV-infected children 4 weeks to 18 years of age. J Clin Pharmacol 2015;55(7):748–56.

[113] Autmizguine J, Moran C, Gonzalez D, et al. Vancomycin cerebrospinal fluid pharmacokinetics in children with cerebral ventricular shunt infections. Pediatr Infect Dis J 2014;33(10):e270–2.

[114] Fillekes Q, Kendall L, Kitaka S, et al. Pharmacokinetics of zidovudine dosed twice daily according to World Health Organization weight bands in Ugandan HIV-infected children. Pediatr Infect Dis J 2014;33(5):495–8.

[115] Altcheh J, Moscatelli G, Mastrantonio G, et al. Population pharmacokinetic study of benznidazole in pediatric Chagas disease suggests efficacy despite lower plasma concentrations than in adults. PLoS Negl Trop Dis 2014;8(5):e2907.

Advances in Pediatrics 63 (2016) 255–280

ADVANCES IN PEDIATRICS

Attention-Deficit/ Hyperactivity Disorder

Alexander K.C. Leung, MBBS, FRCPC, FRCP (UK & Irel), FRCPCH, FAAP[a],*, Kam Lun Hon, MD, FAAP, FCCM[b]

[a]Department of Paediatrics, Alberta Children's Hospital, University of Calgary, #200, 233–16th Avenue North West, Calgary, Alberta T2M 0H5, Canada; [b]Department of Paediatrics, Chinese University of Hong Kong, 6/F, Clinical Sciences Building, Prince of Wales Hospital, Shatin, Hong Kong, China

Keywords
- Attention-deficit • Hyperactivity • Stimulants • Atomoxetine
- α_2-Adrenergic agonists • Educational intervention • Behavioral intervention

Key points

- Attention-deficit/hyperactivity disorder (ADHD) is the most common behavioral and neurodevelopment disorder, affecting 5% to 7% of school-aged children.
- The disorder is characterized by developmentally inappropriate levels of hyperactivity, impulsivity, and inattention.
- The most current and widely used criteria for diagnosis of ADHD are listed in the *Diagnostic and Statistical Manual of Mental Disorders* (Fifth Edition) (*DSM-5*).
- To arrive at a diagnosis, children should have 6 or more symptoms of the disorder that have persisted for at least 6 months in 2 or more settings to a degree that is maladaptive and inconsistent with developmental level and that impairs social, academic, or occupational functioning.
- People 17 years or older should have at least 5 symptoms. Symptoms must be present prior to age 12 years.

INTRODUCTION

ADHD is characterized by an age-inappropriate level of inattention, hyperactivity, and impulsivity, all of which affect behavioral, emotional, cognitive, academic, and social functions [1,2]. ADHD is the most common behavioral and neurodevelopment disorder of children [3].

This article has been published in part in *Common Problems in Ambulatory Care Pediatrics: Specific Clinical Problems*, volume 2, with permission from Nova Science Publishers, Inc.

Corresponding author. E-mail address: aleung@ucalgary.ca

0065-3101/16/$ – see front matter
http://dx.doi.org/10.1016/j.yapd.2016.04.017

PREVALENCE

The reported prevalence of the disorder ranges from 3% to 11% in school-aged children [4–6]. The wide variation in prevalence results from several factors, including diagnostic criteria used, age and gender of study populations, and geographic areas [1,7]. A meta-analysis of 102 studies (n = 171,756) published in 2007 yielded a pooled prevalence of 5.3% (95% CI, 5.0–5.6) in subjects up to 18 years of age [8]. Most studies were conducted in school-aged children. In a recent meta-analysis of 175 studies, the estimated overall worldwide pooled prevalence was 7.2% (95% CI, 6.7–7.8) [9]. The prevalence is expected to rise further with the adoption of the diagnostic criteria listed in the *DSM-5* [10]. The present consensus is that ADHD occurs in 5% to 7% of school-aged children worldwide [4,10]. ADHD is more commonly diagnosed in white children than in black and Hispanic children [11,12]. The condition is least common in Asian children [11]. The prevalence decreases with age; the disorder persists into adulthood in approximately 40% of affected children [13]. The male-to-female ratio is approximately 3 to 4:1 in epidemiologic surveys and 6:1 in clinic samples [11,14,15]. Girls with ADHD may be less likely to be seen in clinics [16]. Data from the Centers for Disease Control and Prevention show that most children with ADHD have mild (46.7%) or moderate (39.5%) problems [17]. Only less than 14% of affected children have severe ADHD [17].

ETIOPATHOGENESIS

The etiology is multifactorial in most cases and involves complex interactions between susceptible genes and environmental factors [1]. This may explain why some children are susceptible to environmental risks whereas others are somewhat resilient. Children with relatives with the disorder are at high risk for ADHD, suggesting a genetic etiology. The concordance rate is up to 92% for monozygotic twins and 33% for dizygotic twins [18]. The heritability is approximately 76% [7]. Approximately 30% of first-degree relatives of ADHD children are affected [3]. Adoption studies have found increased rates of ADHD in the first-degree biological relatives of nonadopted probands with ADHD compared with the first-degree adopted relatives of adopted probands with ADHD and the first-degree relatives of nonadopted, non-ADHD control probands [19]. Furthermore, adoptive relatives of children with ADHD perform better in measures of attention than biological relatives of children with ADHD [20].

Several candidate genes show statistically significant evidence of association with ADHD based on the pooled odds ratio (1.18–1.46) across studies, namely, dopamine D_2 receptor, dopamine D_4 receptor, and dopamine D_5 receptor genes (*DRD2, DRD4,* and *DRD5*); dopamine transporter-1 gene (*DAT1*); dopamine ß-hydroxylase gene (*DBH*); serotonin transporter genes (*SLC6A3* and *SLC6A4*); serotonin 1B receptor gene (*HTR1B*); glutamate receptor metaboropic genes (*GRM1, GRM5, GRM7,* and *GRM8*); and synaptosomal-associated protein 25 gene (*SNAP-25*) [21–23]. It has been suggested that regions 16p13 and 17p11 likely harbor these genes. An additional support for a genetic contribution to

ADHD is provided by a case-control study of 366 children with ADHD and 1047 controls [24]. In that study, 57 large, rare copy number variants were identified in children with ADHD and 78 in controls (15.6% vs 7.5%). Copy number variants refer to submicroscopic chromosomal structural abnormalities, which can be either duplications or deletions [25]. Although the effects of each gene marker are too small to be of clinical utility, multiple genes, each with a small effect, may together mediate genetic vulnerability [26].

The neurotransmitters mainly implicated are dopamine and norepinephrine [7]. In a meta-analysis of 210 studies (71 studies on the main metabolites and metabolic enzymes of monoaminergic neurotransmission pathway), significantly increased norepinephrine, decreased 3-methoxy-4-hydroxyphenylethylene glycol, decreased monoamine oxidase, and decreased phenylethylamine were found in ADHD subjects compared with controls [27]. The investigators suggested that the biochemical changes resulted from a compensatory response to hyponoradrenergic synaptic activity in ADHD.

A genetic imbalance of catecholamines metabolism in the cerebral cortex seems to play an important role in the pathogenesis of ADHD as evidenced by structural and functional brain imaging and the response to drugs with noradrenergic and dopamine activity [4,28–30]. Decreased activity of serotonin may also be responsible because serotonin is a modulator for dopamine [31]. Reduced dopamine activity has been found in prefrontal-striatal-thalamo-cortical and cerebellar circuits [32–34].

A recent study shows that children with ADHD have lower serum levels of oxytocin compared with neurotypical controls [35]. It has been suggested that decreased levels of oxytocin may play a role in the pathophysiology of ADHD [35]. Another recent study shows that the serum levels of neopterin are significantly higher in ADHD individuals than in controls [36]. Because neopterin is a good indicator of cellular immunity, cellular immunity may have a role in the etiopathogenesis of ADHD [36].

Quantitative EEGs have shown increased theta and decreased alpha or beta activities in some children with ADHD (discussed later) [37]. Neuroimaging studies have identified a delay in cortical maturation and several morphologic abnormalities in the brains (especially the prefrontal areas) of children with ADHD (discussed later) [22,30,38,39].

Factors affecting brain development during prenatal and early postnatal life may play a secondary role [40]. Factors reported associated with ADHD, but not necessarily causal, include unplanned pregnancy, maternal alcoholism, maternal tobacco smoking, maternal use of medication, maternal stress/anxiety, maternal malnutrition, prenatal exposure to neurotoxins (eg, mercury, lead, polychlorinated biphenyls, and hexachlorobenzene), maternal illnesses (eg, infection, diabetes mellitus, preeclampsia, anemia, and trauma), maternal obesity, protracted/complicated delivery, prematurity, low birth weight, intrauterine growth retardation, firstborn, and perinatal complications (eg, hypoxia, trauma, and infection) [41–49]. Television or video game overexposure has also been identified as a risk factor [50].

Postnatal exposure to some environmental toxicants, in particular, tobacco, organophosphate pesticides, polychlorinated biphenyl, and lead, is a recognized risk factor for ADHD [46,47,51].

Low socioeconomic status is a strong risk factor for ADHD [48,49,52]. In a systematic review of 42 studies, 35 studies found a significant univariate association between socioeconomic disadvantage and ADHD [52]. Meta-analyses of dimensions of socioeconomic status and their association with ADHD indicated that children in families of low socioeconomic status were on average 1.85 to 2.21 times more likely to have ADHD than their peers in families of high socioeconomic status.

Dietary factors do not seem to play a role in a majority of children with ADHD [1]. Controlled studies failed to show the effect of food additives (artificial color, artificial flavors, and preservatives) on ADHD [53]. Nevertheless, a small subgroup of children may be sensitive to food additives (especially food coloring) and preservatives and respond adversely to additives and preservatives administered as a challenge [54,55]. The Food Advisory Committee of the US Food and Drug Administration opines that the existing literature does not support a causality between consumption of color additives and ADHD [56]. Some parents of children with ADHD report a worsening of symptoms after excessive ingestion of candy or diet soda. Meta-analyses, however, failed to find an association between intake of sugar or aspartame and ADHD [53,57,58]. Although studies have shown that the behavior of children with ADHD improved during the elimination phase of the oligoallergenic (hypoallergenic/elimination) diet, the behavior also improved during the placebo phase or when the oligoallergenic diet was compared with a placebo diet [59–61]. The current consensus is that food sensitivity has little, if any, role to play in the pathogenesis of ADHD [1,4]. It has been shown that some children with ADHD have significantly lower plasma and blood levels of polyunsaturated fatty acids (omega-3 and omega-6 fatty acids) [62]. The literature today does not indicate causality [63]. A Cochrane systematic review shows little evidence that polyunsaturated fatty acids supplementation provides any benefit for the symptoms of ADHD [62]. Studies examining serum iron and ferritin levels in children with ADHD have yielded conflicting results [64–66]. A preliminary study suggests that lower iron stores in toddlerhood may be a predictor for poor sensitivity to later stimulant use [67]. Further studies are warranted to confirm or refute an association between iron deficiency and ADHD [1]. Studies examining serum zinc levels in children with ADHD also have yielded conflicting results [68–70]. More large-scale, well-designed controlled studies are needed to prove or disprove an association between zinc deficiency and ADHD.

CLINICAL FEATURES AND DIAGNOSIS

ADHD is characterized by developmentally inappropriate levels of hyperactivity, impulsivity, and inattention; such symptoms interfere with, or reduce the quality of, social, academic, or occupational functioning [1]. The presenting symptoms vary with age. Typically, hyperactive and impulsive symptoms are observed when a child is 4 years old and peak in severity when the child is 7 to 8 years old [71]. On the other hand, inattentive symptoms may not be apparent until a child is 8 to 9 years of age [71].

The most widely used criteria for diagnosis of ADHD are listed in the *DSM-5* [10]. The *DSM-5* differentiates 3 presentations of ADHD: the predominantly inattentive, the predominantly hyperactive/impulsive, and a combined presentation [10]. The combined presentation is the most commonly represented subgroup, followed by the inattentive presentation and the hyperactive/impulsive presentation [1]. To meet the criteria for ADHD, children should have 6 or more symptoms of the disorder that have persisted for at least 6 months in 2 or more settings to a degree that is maladaptive and inconsistent with developmental level and that interferes with, or reduces the quality of, social, academic, or occupational functioning. People 17 years and older should have at least 5 symptoms. The 9 symptoms of inattentive presentations are (1) often fails to give close attention to details or makes careless mistakes in school work, work, or other activities; (2) often has difficulty sustaining attention in tasks or play activities; (3) often does not seem to listen when spoken to directly; (4) often does not follow through on instructions and fails to finish school work, chores, or duties in the workplace; (5) often has difficulty organizing tasks and activities; (6) often avoids, dislikes, or is reluctant to engage in tasks that require sustained mental effort (such as school work or homework); (7) often loses things necessary for tasks or activities (eg, school assignments, pencils, books, tools, or toys); (8) often easily distracted by extraneous stimuli; and (9) often is forgetful in daily activities [10]. The 9 symptoms of hyperactive/impulsive presentations are (1) often fidgets with or taps hands or feet or squirms in seat; (2) often leaves seat in classroom or in other situations in which remaining seated is expected; (3) often runs about or climbs excessively in situations in which it is inappropriate (in adolescents or adults, may be limited to subjective feelings of restlessness); (4) often has difficulty playing or engaging in leisure activities quietly; (5) is often "on the go" or often acts as if "driven by a motor"; (6) often talks excessively; (7) often blurts out answers before questions have been completed; (8) often has difficulty awaiting turn; and (9) often interrupts or intrudes on others (eg, butts into conversations, games, or activities) [10]. The combined inattentive and hyperactivity/impulsive presentation describes an individual who has the required number of symptoms from both presentations. Additional required diagnostic criteria for ADHD in the *DSM-5* include (1) the symptoms are not solely a manifestation of oppositional behavior, defiance, hostility, or failure to understand tasks or instructions; (2) several symptoms were present prior to age 12 years; (3) several symptoms are present in 2 or more settings (eg, at home, school, or work; with friends or relatives; and in other activities); (4) there is clear evidence that the symptoms interfere with, or reduce the quality of, social, academic, or occupational functioning; and (5) the symptoms do not occur exclusively during the course of schizophrenia or another psychotic disorder and are not better explained by another mental disorder (eg, mood disorder, dissociate disorder, personality disorder, substance intoxication, or withdrawn) [10].

A diagnosis of ADHD is essentially a clinical one, based on history from the parents, review of the school record, and direct assessment of a child. ADHD may be mild, moderate, or severe, depending on how many symptoms a person has and how those symptoms make daily life difficult [10]. Severity is specified in terms of number of symptoms in excess of those required to make a diagnosis. ADHD is considered mild if there are few, if any, symptoms in excess of those required to make the diagnosis are present and symptoms result in no more than minor impairments in social or occupational functioning [10]. ADHD is considered severe if there are many symptoms in excess of those required to make the diagnosis or several symptoms that are particularly severe are present or the symptoms result in marked impairments in social or occupational functioning [10]. ADHD is considered moderate if symptoms or functional impairment between mild and severe are present. Pervasive development disorders, such as autism spectrum disorder, is no longer an exclusion criterion for a diagnosis of ADHD [10].

Diagnosis can be difficult in preschoolers. Preschoolers with ADHD often present with hyperactivity, oppositional noncompliant behaviors, temper tantrums, and aggression. Young children should, therefore, undergo a comprehensive assessment to evaluate for alternative diagnosis before receiving an ADHD diagnosis [72].

DIFFERENTIAL DIAGNOSIS
There are many developmental, behavioral, and medical conditions that may mimic ADHD (Box 1) [3,40]. Some of these conditions may coexist with ADHD. In early childhood, it may be difficult to distinguish symptoms of ADHD from age-appropriate behaviors in active children [3].

COMORBIDITY
Epidemiologic studies have documented high rates of concurrent psychiatric and learning disorders among individuals with ADHD [3,23,73]. Approximately 60% of children with ADHD have an oppositional defiant disorder, 50% have a mood disorder, 33% have anxiety disorders (eg, generalized anxiety disorder, separation anxiety, and panic disorder), 30% have language or learning problems (eg, dyslexia or dyspraxia), 26% have conduct disorders, 20% have autism spectrum disorder, and 18% have depressive disorders [3,23,40,73–75]. Emotional lability occurs in 38% to 75% of children with ADHD [76]. Approximately 7% of children with ADHD have tics or, rarely, Tourette syndrome [18,23]. Somatic symptoms, poor motor coordination, nocturnal enuresis, binge-eating disorder, and sleeping problems are reported more often in children with ADHD than in children without the disorder [73,74,77–79].

Many children with ADHD experience academic failure, school suspensions/expulsions, peer rejection, bullying at school, adult disapproval, and loss of

Box 1: Differential diagnosis of attention-deficit/hyperactivity disorder

1. Variant of normal/environmental factors
    A. Age-appropriate overactivity
    B. Ineffective discipline
    C. Inappropriate school placement
    D. Child abuse/neglect
    E. Stressful home environment
2. Developmental/sensory problems
    A. Mental retardation
    B. Learning disability
    C. Speech/language disability
    D. Auditory/visual deficit
3. Behavioral/psychological/psychiatric problems
    A. Conduct disorder
    B. Oppositional defiant disorder
    C. Anxiety disorder
    D. Mood disorder
    E. Obsessive-compulsive disorder
    F. Personality disorder
    G. Pervasive development disorder
    H. Autism spectrum disorders
    I. Obsessive-compulsive disorder
    J. Posttraumatic stress disorder
    K. Adjustment disorder
4. Medical problems
    A. Absence seizures
    B. Endocrine disorders (thyrotoxicosis, hypothyroidism, and uncontrolled diabetes mellitus)
    C. Chronic illness
5. Drugs
    A. Drug effect (eg, albuterol, anticonvulsants, or antihistamines)
    B. Substance abuse
6. Sleep deprivation

Modified from Leung AK. Attention deficit hyperactivity disorder. In: Leung AK, editor. Common problems in ambulatory care pediatrics: specific clinical problems, vol. 2. New York: Nova Science Publishers, Inc; 2011. p. 59; with permission from Nova Science Publishers, Inc.

self-esteem [73,78,80]. Compared with their peers, they are approximately 3 times more likely to repeat a grade, 15 times more likely to receive special education services, and less than half as likely to graduate from high school [81–83]. Chronic academic or social failure may result in loss of motivation and learned helplessness [3]. Children with ADHD are at increased risk for child abuse and accidental injuries [73,78,84]. Adolescents and adults with ADHD are at an increased risk for cigarette smoking, alcohol use, substance abuse, depression, anxiety, bipolar disorder, antisocial behavior, and suicidal tendency [23,74,78,85,86]. They are also more likely to be involved in motor vehicle collisions [3,84].

CLINICAL EVALUATION

History

Physicians must rely on parents/caregivers, teachers, and other important adults in a child's life to provide diagnostic evidence of ADHD, because symptoms may be minimal or absent in a 1-to-1 situation, such as an office visit [3]. Review of information about a child's school performance, attention span, distractibility, activity level, behavioral problems, and peer relationships from multiple observers across home and community settings is of utmost importance. It is important that the teachers who provide the information should have regular contact with a child for a minimum of 4 months [71]. Many standardized parent-teacher questionnaires are available for obtaining the required information, such as the Conners Comprehensive Behavior Rating Scales; Conners' Teacher Rating Scale–Revised; Conners' Parent Rating Scale–Revised; ADHD Rating Scale–IV (parent and teacher versions); Child Behavior Checklist; Edelbrock Child Attention/Activity Profile; Conners Abbreviated Teacher Rating Scale; ANSER teacher questionnaire; ADD-H Comprehensive Teacher's Rating Scale; Academic Performance Rating Scale; Swanson, Nolan and Pelham Questionnaire, revised (SNAP-IV-R); and Attention Deficit Disorders Evaluation Scale [1,40,87]. Most of these rating scales are based on the 18 symptoms listed in the *DSM-5* and include a Likert scale scoring system for frequency of symptoms from 0 to 3 (0 = never, 1 = occasionally, 2 = often, and 3 = very often) [3]. These rating scales are helpful in documenting the individual profile of ADHD symptoms as well as assessing the response to treatment [23]. None of these scales should be used, however, in isolation to make or refute a diagnosis.

Although the Preschool Age Psychiatric Assessment has been found useful for preschoolers referred for assessment of ADHD [88], only the Conners Comprehensive Behavior Rating Scales and ADHD Rating Scale–IV Preschool Version have been validated in preschool-aged children [71,89]. ADHD cannot be reliably diagnosed in children under the age of 4 years [90]. The use of validated behavioral rating scales can improve diagnostic confidence [90].

A comprehensive history should be obtained including details of a mother's pregnancy, prenatal exposure to alcohol and tobacco, labor, delivery, perinatal complications, and past health (in particular, heart disease). A child's developmental milestones, speech and language function, early temperament, and daily activities should be reviewed. The medical history, including child's age at onset of ADHD, a review of current symptoms and their severity, and medication use, should be thoroughly documented. A history of appetite disturbance, pica, enuresis, encopresis, and sleep disorder should be sought [79]. Social and family history taking should include inquiry into possible emotional stressors on the child, such as domestic disharmony, financial difficulties, the impact of the disorder on the family, and parental attitude and expectations toward the problem [1]. The presence of ADHD, specific learning disabilities, conduct or anxiety disorders, psychiatric disturbances, and cardiac disorder in other family members is also of relevance. Physicians should also evaluate for the presence of comorbidities and other possible conditions that may mimic or coexist with ADHD [90].

Physical examination

Most children with ADHD have no abnormalities on physical examination, but a thorough examination should be performed to rule out neurologic disorders, cardiac disorders, dysmorphic features, visual and hearing impairment, and other disorders that may mimic ADHD [2]. Children with ADHD have a higher incidence of soft neurologic signs (eg, mixed laterality, clumsiness, and dysdiadochokinesia) than in the general population [1]. Tests of intelligence (eg, Wechsler Intelligence Scale for Children) and educational achievement (eg, Woodcock-Johnson Psycho-Educational Battery–Revised) help rule out intellectual deficits and determine the possibility of learning disabilities [3].

LABORATORY EVALUATION

Laboratory tests, such as complete blood cell count, serum blood level, thyroid function tests, and ECG, are not usually indicated unless indicated by history and physical finding in the clinical evaluation [91]. Electroencephalography (EEG) has, historically, played a focal role in the assessment of neural function in children with ADHD [92]. Quantitative EEG has shown increased theta and decreased alpha or beta activities in some children with ADHD [31]. Many affected children, however, have normal EEGs [93]. A 2013 meta-analysis of 9 controlled studies (n = 1253) focusing on theta-to-beta ratio in individuals aged 6 to 18 years found significant heterogeneity and concluded that EEG profiles (especially an increased theta-to beta-ratio) cannot be used to reliably diagnose ADHD [94]. In spite of the controversy, the Food and Drug Administration approved the use of the Neuropsychiatric EEG-Based Assessment Aid (NEBA) system for diagnosis of ADHD [95]. Suffice to say, NEBA should not be used as a stand-alone tool. Rather, it should be used in conjunction with current gold standard ADHD assessment measures, including clinician direct assessment of the child, and use of diagnostic tools, such as standardized parent-teacher questionnaires. Recently, Saad and colleagues [96] proposed that a personalized theta-to beta-cutpoint, or transition frequency, is a better frame of reference for the measurement of theta-to-beta ratio, which is regarded as a biomarker of ADHD. The transition frequency is the point at which resting and event-related EEG spectra intersect.

Structural MRI studies have demonstrated a slight decrease in size of the corpus callosum, basal ganglia (putamen, globus pallidus, and caudate nucleus), cerebral cortex (in particular, prefrontal cortex and anterior cingulate cortex), white matter tracks, and vermis of the cerebellum and in increased gray matter in the posterior temporal and inferior parietal cortices in some patients with ADHD [22,30,39,97]. Preliminary studies using functional MRI have shown that children with ADHD have reduced blood flow in the basal ganglia, ventral prefrontal cortex, anterior cingulated gyrus, and frontostriatal networks as well as abnormalities in inter-regional connectivity [28,29]. Diffusion tensor imaging studies have shown white matter abnormalities within the limbic network in some patients with ADHD [32,34]. These systems have been implicated in the pathophysiology of ADHD. PET has found disruption of dopamine reward pathway, abnormal dopamine transporter binding, and abnormal dopamine receptor binding in patients with ADHD [97–99]. There are no published PET studies, however, that assess the functioning of neuroepinephrine, serotonin, and other neurotransmitter systems. Currently, neuroimaging technologies lack adequate specificity and sensitivity and their findings are inconsistent [99,100]. Therefore, despite the promise of neuroimaging markers, their clinical utility in the ADHD population remains limited [97].

MANAGEMENT

The goal of treatment is to improve core symptoms of attention, hyperactivity, and impulsivity, improve school performance, optimize functional performance, and remove behavioral obstacles [90]. Treatment should be multimodal and include pharmacologic, educational, and behavioral interventions, alone or in combination, and should be individualized for optimal results. It has been shown that combination therapy with medications and behavior/psychological therapy is superior to behavior/psychological therapy alone [101]. With exceptions, pharmacologic intervention is not recommended for children younger than 6 years of age [34]. Behavioral interventions should be the primary treatment of children with ADHD in this age group [101,102]. Pharmacologic intervention may be considered for preschool children (aged 4–5 years) who have moderate-to-severe functional impairment and who have failed to respond to behavioral interventions [102,103]. Also, it is important to treat comorbid conditions, treatment of which may influence the treatment outcome for ADHD [101,104,105].

Pharmacologic intervention

Currently, the most commonly used medications are stimulants, 1 selective norepinephrine reuptake inhibitor (atomoxetine), and 2 α_2-adrenergic agonists (discussed later) [106]. Ideally, medications should be given every day. Drug holidays on weekends and during school vacations are not usually recommended because drug holidays may destabilize control of a patient's behavior [1,75]. In addition, many learning opportunities occur on nonschool days. Furthermore, learning is enhanced in a child with ADHD where attentiveness is controlled with medication. Pharmacologic intervention should be continued as long as it provides clear benefit without causing significant adverse effects. Some patients require treatment throughout adolescence and adulthood. Periodic discontinuation for a brief period is often used to reaffirm the need for continuing drug therapy [3]. Children with ADHD should be monitored regularly for compliance, response to treatment, and adverse events. Studies have shown that treatment with ADHD drugs may reduce the negative impact of children and improve the long-term outcomes for some ADHD individuals, although not usually back to their normal levels [107].

Stimulants

Many well-designed, placebo-controlled studies have demonstrated beyond doubt that the use of stimulant medications is the most effective intervention for school-aged children with ADHD [40,106]. The American Academy of Pediatrics recommends stimulants as the first line of treatment of ADHD, particularly when no comorbidity is present [108]. Stimulant medications have been shown to induce short-term enhancement of behavioral, academic, and social functioning in the vast majority of children treated. This in turn leads to positive lasting effects on self-esteem, parental child relationships, and peer relationships. Stimulant medications increase the activity of norepinephrine and dopamine in the prefrontal cortex, increase the activity of the extracellular concentrations of norepinephrine and dopamine at the neuronal synapse, increase the release of catecholamines from the presynaptic neurons, block reuptake of catecholamines into the presynaptic neuron, and inhibit monoamine oxidase [109,110]. The available catecholamines, acting as neurotransmitters, stimulate the reticular activating system, limbic system, and other areas of the brain that control attention, arousal, and the inhibitory process.

Stimulants are available in short-acting, intermediate-acting, and long-acting (LA) formulations. The most commonly used short-acting stimulants include methylphenidate (Ritalin and Methylin), dexmethylphenidate (Focalin), dextroamphetamine (Dexedrine, Zenzedi, and ProCentra), and amphetamine/dextroamphetamine (Adderall). Typically, short-acting stimulants have onset of action within 60 minutes and duration of action up to 5 hours [111]. Coadministration of amphetamines with acidic foods decreases the absorption of amphetamines [7]. This interaction does not occur with methylphenidate [7]. Short-acting stimulants must be taken 2 to 3 times a day if full-day coverage is desired [103,111]. The need for frequent dosing can lead to problems with adherence and inconvenient timing of dosing [103]. On the other hand, short-acting methylphenidate is the medication of choice for treatment of ADHD in preschool children [112].

Examples of intermediate-acting methylphenidate include Ritalin sustained release (SR), Metadate extended release (ER), and Methylin ER in the form of SR tablets. Ritalin SR and Metadate ER deliver methylphenidate via a single-pulsed wax matrix [113]. Methylin ER uses a dual-acting hydrophilic polymer-release technology, which controls the release of methylphenidate by diffusion and erosion [113]. Because these intermediate-acting agents have a duration of action of 6 to 8 hours, they can be administered once a day, although most patients may require twice-daily dosing for symptom control throughout the school day and after school [113].

LA and SR preparations of stimulants are generally preferred because they are given once a day, thereby eliminating the need for dosing in school or after school [114]. These preparations could also eliminate the embarrassment and inconvenience that a child may have, which, in turn, may improve compliance [40]. Examples of LA methylphenidate include osmotic release tablets (Concerta), SR bead-filled capsules (eg, Ritalin LA, Metadate CD, and Biphentin), oral suspension (Quillivant XR), and transdermal patch (Daytrana) [40,115,116]. Oral suspension and bead-filled capsules are particularly useful for patients who cannot swallow pills. Bead preparations can be sprinkled into soft foods. Transdermal patch should be considered for patients who cannot take oral medications [111]. Dexmethylphenidate XR (Focalin XR) is marketed as an SR bead-filled capsule, the content of which can be sprinkled into soft foods for children who have difficulty swallowing pills. Examples of LA amphetamines include dextroamphetamine SR (Dexedrine Spansule) and lisdexamfetamine (Vyvanse). For children who have difficulty swallowing pills, the SR capsule of dextroamphetamine SR can be sprinkled into soft foods whereas the capsule of lisdexamfetamine can be opened and mixed with water for immediate use. Amphetamine/dextroamphetamine ER (Adderall XR) contains 25% each of dextroamphetamine saccharate, amphetamine aspartate, dextroamphetamine sulfate, and amphetamine sulfate. Typically, LA stimulants have onset of action within 60 minutes and duration of action up to 12 hours [111]. Many of the LA stimulants (eg, methylphenidate LA, methylphenidate CD, dextroamphetamine SR, and amphetamine/dextroamphetamine ER) have some of the active ingredients in immediate-release beads and the remaining in enteric-coated delayed release beads that begin to release active ingredients hours later [117]. Lisdexamfetamine is a prodrug that is converted to dextroamphetamine and L-lysine in the blood stream with an effect over 10 hours [111].

Unlike most other medications in pediatric use, dosages of stimulants are not weight dependent [3,118]. Doses should begin in the low end of the range and titrate upward every 3 to 7 days until an effective response is obtained or significant side effects are noted [1,112]. In general, most side effects are dose dependent and diminish or resolve with reduction in dosage or with passage of time [3]. The frequency of most side effects is similar with methylphenidate and amphetamines [111]. In general, stimulants are safe with mild, reversible side effects [111]. The most common side effects are insomnia, loss of appetite, weight loss, jitteriness, and rebound moodiness [1,111]. Melatonin is effective in treating sleep problems in children with ADHD [119]. A Cochrane systematic review of 8 randomized trials found that stimulants did not worsen tics in most individuals with tics; nevertheless, they might exacerbate tics in individual cases [120]. At higher doses, some children may experience headache and abdominal pain [1]. Other side effects include motor tics, dry mouth, dizziness, drowsiness, constipation, euphoria, dysphoria, irritability, agitation, anxiety, hallucinations, mania, social withdrawal, nightmares, and medication rebound [103,120–122]. Priapism, peripheral vasculopathy, depression, suicidal ideation, and sudden unexpected death are rare [90,123,124]. Patients treated with transdermal patch may develop contact sensitization and chemical leukoderma if the patch is worn in the same location every day [11]. Transient growth delay may occur with prolonged stimulant treatment [1,125]. Ultimate adult height, however, is often unaffected [1,126]. Although stimulant medication may cause small increases in mean heart rate and mean blood pressure, large cohort studies have not shown an increased risk of cardiovascular adverse events compared with the general pediatric population [91,127]. The present consensus is that stimulant therapy can be initiated if there is no evidence of cardiac disease based on a comprehensive history and physical examination. On the other hand, stimulant medications should not be used in children with previous sensitivity to stimulants, cardiovascular disease, severe arrhythmia, moderate to severe hypertension, hyperthyroidism, anxiety, agitated states, angle-closure glaucoma, Tourette syndrome, or concurrent use of monoamine oxidase inhibitors [1,7,111,128]. A 2013 meta-analysis of 15 longitudinal studies (n = 2565) suggests that treatment of ADHD with stimulant medication does not increase the risk of later substance use disorders [129]. Treatment with stimulant medication may reduce the risk of developing substance use disorders [130]. The present consensus is that children with ADHD are at increased risk for substance use disorders based on the diagnosis, not their treatment with stimulants [131]. The available literature suggests that the consistent misuse and diversion of stimulants is occurring in adolescents and young adults often in the context of enhancing academic performance [114,132].

The response rate for any single stimulant medication is approximately 80% [1]. It is recommended that if a child has adverse effects or does not respond to 1 stimulant medication, another 2 should be tried [1]. Up to 95% of children with ADHD respond to at least 1 stimulant medication without major side effects [18,90]. Lack of response to treatment should lead clinicians to assess the accuracy of the diagnosis and the possibility of undiagnosed coexisting conditions. The most frequent causes of treatment failure are noncompliance, over-reporting of adverse effects by medication-weary parents, inappropriate or unrealistic expectations for mediation response, and attempting to treat symptoms other than the cores symptoms of ADHD [1,133]. Noncompliance may result from dosing inconvenience, social stigma associated with ADHD medication, psychological side effects, and perceived inadequate medication effectiveness [1,134,135]. Several factors may affect response to treatment, namely, intelligence quotient of the affected child, severity of ADHD, parental depression, genetic polymorphisms, and the presence of a comorbid anxiety disorder [131].

Atomoxetine

Atomoxetine (Strattera), a nonstimulant, is a selective norepinephrine reuptake inhibitor with high specificity for the presynaptic norepinephrine transporter and minimal affinity for other neurotransmitter transporters or receptors [115,136]. Dosing of atomoxetine is weight based [112]. Treatment may be initiated with 0.5 mg/kg/d, which may be increased gradually to 1.4 mg/kg/d if necessary (maximum 100 mg/d) [112,136]. Unlike stimulants, the initial onset of action may take 1 to 4 weeks but may require 12 weeks for the full effect to be achieved [137,138]. Responders usually show some changes within 2 weeks [14]. Before initiating treatment, it is important that a physician sets appropriate expectations for the patient and family with regard to the likelihood of a gradual response, which often builds over time [138]. Atomoxetine must be given every day without drug holiday [89]. Adverse effects include loss of appetite, nausea, vomiting, dyspepsia, abdominal pain, headache, dizziness, irritability, fatigue, and sedation. Rarely, priapism, erectile and ejaculatory dysfunction, dysmenorrhea, lowering of seizure threshold, increased risk of liver toxicity, depression, sudden death in patients with significant cardiac disease, and increased risk of suicidal ideation may occur [15,40,75,103,139]. On the other hand, atomoxetine does not cause insomnia or motor tics [1,120]. Also, nonstimulants are less likely to be associated with drug abuse and diversion than stimulants [115].

Head-to-head comparisons of the efficacy of atomoxetine with that of stimulants have shown a greater treatment effect of the stimulants [140,141]. Atomoxetine is recommended if a patient is unresponsive to or unable to tolerate treatment with stimulants [40,115]. Atomoxetine is preferred if there is a strong family preference for a nonstimulant medication, if a patient has an active substance abuse problem, comorbid anxiety, or tic, or if a patient is at risk for stimulant diversion or performance enhancement use [1,74,90,103]. Contraindications to atomoxetine include sensitivity to the medication, concurrent use or use within 14 days of the administration of a monoamine oxidase inhibitor, severe cardiovascular disorder, pheochromocytoma, and glaucoma [111].

α_2-Adrenergic agonists

α_2-Adrenergic agonists, such as ER clonidine (Kapvay) and guanfacine (Intuniv), are less efficacious than stimulants; they have been found beneficial in approximately 50% of patients with ADHD [1,111,142]. Clonidine ER and guanfacine ER may take up to 2 weeks for initial response and up to 4 weeks for full therapeutic effect [89,103]. The initial dose of clonidine ER is 0.1 mg/d, which may be increased if necessary by 0.1 mg weekly (maximum 0.4 mg/d) [112]. The initial dose of guanfacine ER is 1 mg/d, which may be increased if necessary by 1 mg weekly (maximum 4 mg/d) [112]. Compared with clonidine ER, guanfacine ER has a longer half-life [90]. As such, clonidine ER should be administered twice a day whereas guanfacine ER is administered once daily [111,143]. Because guanfacine is metabolized predominately by CYP3A4, dosage should be reduced in patients taking CYP3A4 inhibitors, such as ketoconazole [7,144].

α_2-Adrenergic agonists are usually reserved for those who respond poorly or are intolerant to stimulants or atomoxetine or when there is coexisting significant insomnia, conduct disorder, oppositional defiant disorder, or tic disorder [7,111,142,143]. More commonly, they can be used as adjuncts to stimulant medication in patients who have shown partial response to stimulant medications but are unable to tolerate them at higher doses [103]. α_2-Adrenergic agonists have positive effects on the reduction of impulsivity and hyperactivity but do not have much effect on inattention [1,7,120]. Side effects of clonidine ER include drowsiness, sedation, somnolence, trouble sleeping, fatigue, headache, xerostomia, nausea, abdominal pain, constipation, depression, bradycardia, hypotension, prolonged QT interval, allergic reaction, chest pain, and seizures [26,145,146]. Side effects of guanfacine ER include drowsiness, sedation, somnolence, headache, fatigue, nightmares, dizziness, xerostomia, abdominal pain, bradycardia, hypotension, prolonged QT interval, allergic reaction, and mood changes [26,145–147]. Compared with clonidine ER, guanfacine ER has fewer sedative and hypotensive effects [90].

Antidepressants
Antidepressants have been used off label in the treatment of patients with ADHD who do not benefit or do not tolerate stimulant medications, atomoxetine, and α_2-adrenergic agonists [108,112]. Tricyclic antidepressants, such as desipramine (Norpramin), imipramine (Tofranil and Impril), and nortriptyline (Pamelor and Apo-Nortriptyline), inhibit reuptake of norepinephrine and serotonin [11]. These agents can produce improvement in more than 70% of children with ADHD, although they are not as effective as stimulants [1,145]. Although these medications work fairly well for the improvement of mood, impulsivity, and tolerance of frustration, they work less well for inattention [142]. They are particularly useful for those individuals with concomitant depression, anxiety, conduct disorder, or tic disorder [1]. Side effects include dry mouth, blurred vision, constipation, urinary retention, dizziness, sedation, fatigue, nervousness, loss of appetite (desipramine), increased weight gain (nortriptyline), mild increase in diastolic pressure, mild tachycardia, cardiac arrhythmias, lowering of seizure threshold, suicidal tendency, and discontinuation syndrome consisting of nausea, vomiting, headache, hyperthermia, and irritability [1,112,136,148]. Rarely, bone marrow suppression may occur [112]. The use of tricyclic antidepressants has sharply declined in recent years due to concerns of cardiac toxicity [7]. A cardiac evaluation should be performed before tricyclic antidepressants are administered [111,112].

Bupropion (Aplenzin and Wellbutrin), a moncyclic phenylaminoketone that blocks the reuptake of norepinephrine and dopamine, has more stimulant effect than tricyclic antidepressants [149,150]. The medication has been used in the treatment of depressive disorder and nicotine dependence. Randomized controlled trials of bupropion have shown its efficacy in individuals with ADHD [149–151]. It is of modest efficacy in decreasing hyperactivity and aggressive behavior [111]. Bupropion has a safety profile comparable with methylphenidate [112,150,151]. Side effects include anorexia, bulimia, irritability, insomnia, tics, suicidal ideation, and lowering of seizure threshold [103,111]. Bupropion is an inhibitor of CYP2D6, so dosage adjustment may be necessary for drugs metabolized by this enzyme if taken together with bupropion [152].

Educational intervention

Most children with ADHD do best in small, orderly, structured classrooms where there is a minimum of extraneous distraction and stimulation. Small-group or individualized teaching is very helpful. The classroom seating arrangement should facilitate close supervision of a child with ADHD [118]. Teachers should be sympathetic, understanding, and tolerant and adjust their expectations and the work assignments to the short attention span of a child with ADHD. Frequent reminders may be necessary and should be given tactfully to avoid embarrassing a child. A child's strengths and interests should always be encouraged and accomplishments recognized to build a positive self-image and to enhance self-esteem [117]. Studies have shown that educational interventions delivered in school settings lead to improvement in both symptomatic and academic outcomes [16]. The use of a daily report card can enhance teacher-parent collaboration and facilitate communication between home and school by encouraging parental reinforcement at home for behavior observed during the school hours [74,75]. The use of periodic follow-up ADHD rating scales can be helpful in tracking school progress [103].

Behavioral intervention

Behavioral modification may enhance the therapeutic outcome [153]. Parents should be advised to keep goals realistic and attainable. In general, good behavior or fulfillment of a contract should be reinforced with rewards (eg, a smile, verbal praise, special attention, physical affection, extra privileges, and material benefits), which should immediately follow the positive behavior [1]. Undesirable behavior should be discouraged with mild punishment (eg, verbal disapproval, temporary isolation [time-off], or temporary removal of a privilege). If punishment is required, it should be immediate and inevitable. Because the inability to modify behavior based on previous experience is a particular problem for many children with ADHD, however, punishment should be used only cautiously and with moderation. There is no role for corporal punishment. Parents should be counseled to establish realistic expectations for their child. Household routines should be predictable. Rules should be simple, clear, and as few as possible. Excessive fatigue and overstimulation should be avoided. Checklists prepared for a child may help a child remember articles and assignments.

A meta-analysis of 5 randomized controlled trials (n = 284) evaluating the effectiveness of parental training in children with ADHD showed that parent training was effective in the reduction of parental stress, enhancement of parental stress, and improvement of the child's behavior [154]. It is recommended that psychoeducation be provided to parents and teachers who have to look after children with ADHD [16]. Teachers who have received training about ADHD can provide behavioral intervention in the classroom to help children with ADHD [16]. Parents and teachers who attend more training sessions see greater improvements in the child's behavior.

The Multimodal Treatment Study of Children with ADHD showed that medication was superior to behavioral therapy for reducing the core symptoms of ADHD; the combination of medical and behavioral therapy was not significantly more effective than medication alone for these symptoms [155]. Secondary analyses showed that, compared with medication alone, combined therapy resulted in greater improvements in academic performance and reduction in conduct problems, higher levels of parental satisfaction, and the use of lower doses of stimulant medication [156]. Combined therapy was also superior for treating children of lower socioeconomic status and those with coexisting anxiety [156]. A recent systematic review supports efficacy of behavioral interventions for patients with ADHD [157]. Behavioral interventions may result in decreased negative and increased positive parenting and decreased comorbid conduct problems [157].

Family therapy

Family therapy may be necessary to relieve parents' guilt, frustration, and exhaustion, and to help siblings cope with the jealousy that often results when extra attention is devoted to a child with ADHD [1]. Family therapy should be considered if severe disruption in relationships within the family is evident.

Psychotherapy

Children with ADHD who have significant conduct disorder, antisocial behavior, aggressiveness, depression, or anxiety may benefit from psychotherapy.

Dietary intervention

Various dietary measures have been proposed for treating individuals with ADHD. These include elimination of salicylates, artificial coloring, artificial flavoring, and antioxidant preservatives (ie, the Feingold diet), restriction of sugar intake, oligoallergenic diet, polyunsaturated fatty acid supplementation, iron supplementation, and megavitamin therapy [1]. To date, controlled studies have not substantiated the efficacy of most of these treatments [62,63]. Preliminary studies have shown that omega-3 supplementation and restriction of artificial coloring may be effective [158,159]. These studies have been criticized for their small sample sizes and inclusion often restricted to families where parents have reported an adverse link between food and their child's behavior [74]. At present, most authorities believe that dietary manipulations are not indicated in most children with ADHD [1,4,63,101,108,160]. Nevertheless, if a parent notes that a specific food seems to increase the symptoms of ADHD, the food should be excluded from the diet. Iron supplement should be given to children with low serum iron or ferritin and those with iron deficiency anemia [161].

PROGNOSIS

Prospective follow-up studies have found that approximately 40% of individuals who had ADHD as children continued to exhibit symptoms by late teens and meet the *DSM* criteria for diagnosis [13]. With increasing age, hyperactivity tends to decrease [1,43]. Hyperactive symptoms are barely noticeable by adolescence, although patients may feel restless or unable to settle down [71]. On the other hand, inattention, impulsivity, disorganization, and relationship difficulties often persist [1,43,101]. Affected individuals are at risk of antisocial behavior, poor academic attainment, substance abuse, poor workplace performance, impaired executive functions, pathologic gambling, Internet addiction, communication disorders, depression, anxiety disorders, marital disharmony, and unemployment [7,85,101,162,163]. ADHD is associated with significantly increased mortality rates. Premature deaths may be attributed to violence/ aggression/fighting, risky behavior, traffic accidents, substance abuse, poor health, criminality, and suicidal tendency [78,164,165]. Comorbid oppositional defiant disorder and conduct disorder increase the risk of premature death further [164]. Factors that may predict the persistence of ADHD into adulthood include severity of symptoms, comorbidity, low IQ of the child, family history of ADHD, and family adversity [1,102]. Conversely, favorable outcome may result from early diagnosis, appropriate therapy, and support both from home and school [33].

References

[1] Leung AK. Attention-deficit hyperactivity disorder. In: Leung AK, editor. Common problems in ambulatory pediatrics: specific clinical problems, vol. 2. New York: Nova Science Publishers, Inc; 2011. p. 55–66.

[2] Leung AK, Lemay JF. How to treat patients with ADHD. Can J Diagn 2002;19(9):97–110.

[3] Leung AK, Lemay JF. Attention deficit hyperactivity disorder: an update. Adv Ther 2003;20: 305–18.

[4] Krull KR. Attention deficit hyperactivity disorder in children and adolescents: epidemiology and pathogenesis. In: Post TW, editor. Waltham (MA): UpToDate; Accessed September 14, 2015.

[5] Perou R, Bitsko RH, Blumber SJ, et al, Center for Disease Control and Prevention. Mental health surveillance among children - United States, 2005-2011. MMWR Surveill Summ 2013;62(Suppl 2):1035.

[6] Visser SN, Danielson ML, Bitsko RH, et al. Trends in the parent-report of health care provider-diagnosed and medicated attention-deficit/hyperactivity disorder: United States, 2003-2011. J Am Acad Child Adolesc Psychiatry 2014;53:34–46.

[7] Bokor G, Anderson PD. Attention-deficit/hyperactivity disorder. J Pharm Pract 2014;27: 336–49.

[8] Polanczyk G, de Lima MS, Horta BL, et al. The worldwide prevalence of ADHD: a systematic review and metaregression analysis. Am J Psychiatry 2007;164:942–8.

[9] Thomas R, Sanders S, Doust J, et al. Prevalence of attention-deficit/hyperactivity disorder: a systematic review and meta-analysis. Pediatrics 2015;135:e994–1001.

[10] American Psychiatric Association. Attention-deficit/hyperactivity disorder. In: Diagnostic and statistical manual of mental disorders. 5th edition. Arlington (VA): American Psychiatric Association; 2013. p. 59–65.

[11] Getahun D, Jacobsen SJ, Fassett MJ, et al. Recent trends in childhood attention-deficit/ hyperactivity disorder. JAMA Pediatr 2013;167:282–8.

[12] Miller TW, Nigg JT, Miller RL. Attention deficit hyperactivity disorder in African American children: what can be concluded from the past ten years? Clin Psychol Rev 2009;29: 77–86.

[13] Biederman J, Mick E, Faraone SV, et al. Age-dependent decline of symptoms of attention deficit hyperactivity disorder: impact of remission definition and symptom type. Am J Psychiatry 2000;157:816–8.

[14] Jamdar S, Sathyamoorthy BT. Management of attention-deficit/hyperactivity disorder. Br J Hosp Med 2007;68:360–6.

[15] Keen D, Hadjikoumi I. ADHD in children and adolescents. Clin Evid 2011;02:312.

[16] Richardson M, Moore DA, Gwernan-Jones R, et al. Non-pharmacological interventions for attention-deficit/hyperactivity disorder (ADHD) delivered in school settings: systematic reviews of quantitative and qualitative research. Health Technol Assess 2015;19(45):1–470.

[17] Centers for Disease Control and Prevention. Increasing prevalence of parent-reported attention-deficit/hyperactivity disorder among children - United States, 2003 and 2007. MMWR Morb Mortal Wkly Rep 2010;59:439–43.

[18] Goldman LS, Genel M, Bezman RJ, et al. Diagnosis and treatment of attention-deficit/ hyperactivity disorder in children and adolescents. JAMA 1998;279:1100–7.

[19] Sprich S, Biederman J, Crawford MH, et al. Adoptive and biological families of children and adolescents with ADHD. J Am Acad Child Adolesc Psychiatry 2000;39:1432–7.

[20] Alberts-Corush J, Firestone P, Goodman JT. Attention and impulsivity characteristics of the biological and adoptive parents of hyperactive and normal control children. Am J Orthop 1986;56:413–23.

[21] Elia J, Glessner JT, Wang K, et al. Genome-wide copy number variation study associates metabotropic glutamate receptor gene networks with attention deficit hyperactivity disorder. Nat Genet 2012;44:78–84.

[22] Schubiner H, Katragadda S. Overview of epidemiology, clinical features, genetics, and prognosis of adolescent attention-deficit/hyperactivity disorder. Adolesc Med 2008;19: 209–15.

[23] Spencer TJ, Biederman J, Mick E. Attention-deficit/hyperactivity disorder: diagnosis, lifespan, comorbidities, and neurobiology. J Pediatr Psychol 2007;32:631–42.

[24] Williams NM, Zaharieva I, Martin A, et al. Rare chromosomal deletions and duplications in attention-deficit hyperactivity disorder: a genome-wide analysis. Lancet 2010;376:1401–8.

[25] Golmirzaei J, Namazi S, Amiri S, et al. Evaluation of attention-deficit hyperactivity disorder risk factors. Int J Pediatr 2013;2013:953103.

[26] Feldman HM, Reiff MI. Attention deficit-hyperactivity disorder in children and adolescents. N Engl J Med 2014;370:838–46.

[27] Scassellati C, Bonvicini C, Faraone SV, et al. Biomarkers and attention-deficit/ hyperactivity disorder: a systematic review and meta-analysis. J Am Acad Child Adolesc Psychiatry 2012;51:1003–19.

[28] Cubillo A, Halari R, Ecker C, et al. Reduced activation and inter-regional functional connectivity of fronto-striatal networks in adults with childhood attention-deficit hyperactivity disorder (ADHD) and persisting symptoms during tasks of motor inhibition and cognitive switching. J Psychiatr Res 2010;44:629–39.

[29] DePue BE, Burgess GC, Willcutt EG, et al. Inhibitory control of memory retrieval and motor processing associated with the right lateral prefrontal cortex: evidence from deficits in individuals with ADHD. Neuropsychologia 2000;48:3909–17.

[30] Seidman LJ, Valera EM, Makris N, et al. Dorsolateral prefrontal and anterior cingulate cortex volumetric abnormalities in adults with attention-deficit/hyperactivity disorder identified by magnetic resonance imaging. Biol Psychiatry 2006;60:1071–80.

[31] Oades RD. Dopamine-serotonin interaction in attention-deficit hyperactivity disorder. Prog Brain Res 2008;172:543–65.

[32] Chen L, Huang X, Lei D, et al. Microstructural abnormalities of the brain white matter in attention-deficit/hyperactivity disorder. J Psychiatry Neurosci 2015;40:280–7.

[33] Kulkarni M. Attention deficit hyperactivity disorder. Indian J Pediatr 2015;82:267–71.

[34] Lawrence KE, Levitt JG, Loo SK, et al. White matter microstructure in subjects with attention-deficit/hyperactivity disorder and their siblings. J Am Acad Child Adolesc Psychiatry 2013;54:431–40.

[35] Sasaki T, Hashimoto K, Oda Y, et al. Decreased levels of serum oxytocin in pediatric patients with attention-deficit/hyperactivity disorder. Psychiatry Res 2015;228:746–51.

[36] Ceylan MF, Uneri OS, Guney E, et al. Increase levels of serum neopterin in attention-deficit hyperactivity disorder (ADHD). J Neuroimmunol 2014;273:111–4.

[37] Shi T, Li X, Zhao N, et al. EEG characteristics and visual cognitive function of children with Attention deficit hyperactivity disorder (ADHD). Brain Dev 2012;34:806–11.

[38] Gornick MC, Addington A, Shaw P, et al. Association of the dopamine receptor D4 (DRD4) gene 7-repeat allele with children with attention-deficit/hyperactivity disorder (ADHD): an update. Am J Med Genet B Neuropsychiatr Genet 2007;144B(3):379–82.

[39] Shaw P, Eckstrand K, Sharp W, et al. Attention-deficit/hyperactivity disorder is characterized by a delay in cortical maturation. Proc Natl Acad Sci U S A 2007;104:19649–54.

[40] Pliszka SR, AACAP Work Group on Quality Issues. Practice parameter for the assessment and treatment of children and adolescents with attention-deficit/hyperactivity disorder. J Am Acad Child Adolesc Psychiatry 2007;46:894–921.

[41] Chang Z, Lichtenstein P, D'Onofrio BM, et al. Maternal age at childbirth and risk for ADHD in offspring: a population-based cohort study. Int J Epidemiol 2014;43:1815–24.

[42] Curran EA, O'Neill SM, Cryan JF, et al. Research review: Birth by caesarean section and development of autism spectrum disorder and attention-deficit/hyperactivity disorder: a systematic review and meta-analysis. J Child Psychol Psychiatry 2015;56:500–8.

[43] French WP. Assessment and treatment of attention-deficit/hyperactivity disorder: part 1. Pediatr Ann 2015;44:114–20.

[44] Mann JR, McDermott S. Are maternal genitourinary infection and pre-clampsia associated with ADHD in school-aged child ren? J Atten Disord 2011;15:667–73.

[45] Mill J, Petronis A. Pre- and peri-natal environmental risks for attention-deficit hyperactivity disorder (ADHD): the potential role of epigenetic processes in mediating susceptibility. J Child Psychol Psychiatry 2008;49:1020–30.

[46] Lanphear BP. Attention deficit hyperactivity disorder. A preventable epidemic? Arch Pediatr Adolesc Med 2012;166:1182–4.

[47] Nigg J. Environment, developmental origins, and attention-deficit/hyperactivity disorder. Arch Pediatr Adolesc Med 2012;166:387–8.

[48] Nomura Y, Marks DJ, Grossman B, et al. Exposure to gestational diabetes mellitus and low socioeconomic status: effects on neurocognitive developments and risks of attention-deficit/hyperactivity disorder in offspring. Arch Pediatr Adolesc Med 2012;166:337–43.

[49] Schmitt J, Romanos M. Prenatal and perinatal risk factors for attention-deficit/hyperactivity disorder. Arch Pediatr Adolesc Med 2012;166:1074–5.

[50] Swing EL, Gentile DA, Anderson CA, et al. Television and video game exposure and the development of attention problems. Pediatrics 2010;126:214–21.

[51] Bouchard MF, Bellinger DC, Wright RO, et al. Attention-deficit/hyperactivity disorder and urinary metabolites of organophosphate pesticides. Pediatrics 2010;125:e1270–7.

[52] Russell AE, Ford T, Williams R, et al. The association between socioeconomic disadvantage and attention-deficit/hyperactivity disorder (ADHD): a systematic review. Child Psychiatry Hum Dev 2015. [Epub ahead of print].

[53] Millicap JG, Yee MM. The diet factor in attention-deficit/hyperactivity disorder. Pediatrics 2012;139:330–7.

[54] Harley JP, Matthews CG, Eichman P. Synthetic food colors and hyperactivity in children: a double-blind challenge experiment. Pediatrics 1978;62:975–83.

[55] Weiss B. Synthetic food colors and neurobehavioral hazards: the view from environmental health research. Environ Health Perspect 2012;120:1–5.

[56] Quick Minutes: food advisory committee meeting March 30-31, 2011. Available at: http://www.fda.gov/AdvisoryCommittees/CommitteesMeetingMaterials/FoodAdvisoryCommittee/ucm250901.htm. Accessed August 25, 2015.
[57] Rojas NL, Chan E. Old and new controversies in the alternative treatment of attention-deficit hyperactivity disorder. Ment Retard Dev Disabil Res Rev 2005;11:116–30.
[58] Wolraich ML, McGuinn L, Doffing M. Treatment of attention deficit hyperactivity disorder in children and adolescents: safety considerations. Drug Saf 2007;30:17–26.
[59] Carter CM, Urbanowicz M, Hemsley R, et al. Effects of a few food diet in attention deficit disorder. Arch Dis Child 1993;69:564–8.
[60] Egger J, Stolla A, McEwen LM. Controlled trial of hyposensitisation in children with food-induced hyperkinetic syndrome. Lancet 1992;339:1150–3.
[61] Schmidt MH, Mocks P, Lay B, et al. Does oligoantigenic diet influence hyperactive/conduct-disordered children - a controlled trial. Eur Child Adolesc Psychiatry 1997;6:88–95.
[62] Gillies D, Sinn JK, Lad SS, et al. Polyunsaturated fatty acids (PUFU) for attention deficit hyperactivity disorder (ADHD) in children and adolescents. Cochrane Database Syst Rev 2012;(7):CD007986.
[63] Rajyaguru P, Cooper M. Role of dietary supplementation in attention-deficit hyperactivity disorder. Br J Psychiatry 2013;202:398–9.
[64] Bener A, Kamal M, Bener H, et al. Higher prevalence of iron deficiency as strong predictor of attention deficit hyperactivity disorder in children. Ann Med Health Sci Res 2014;4(Suppl 3):S291–7.
[65] Donfrancesco R, Parisi P, Vanacore N, et al. Iron in ADHD: time to move beyond serum ferritin levels. J Atten Disord 2013;17:347–57.
[66] Oner P, Oner O, Azik FM, et al. Ferritin and hyperactivity ratings in attention deficit hyperactivity disorder. Pediatr Int 2012;54:688–92.
[67] Turner CA, Xie D, Zimmerman BM, et al. Iron status in toddlerhood predicts sensitivity to psychostimulants in children. J Atten Disord 2012;16:295–303.
[68] Arnold LE, Disilvestro RA, Bozzolo D, et al. Zinc for attention-deficit/hyperactivity disorder: placebo-controlled double-blind pilot trial alone and combined with amphetamine. J Child Adolesc Psychopharmacol 2011;21:1–19.
[69] Ghanizadeh A, Berk M. Zinc for treating children and adolescents with attention-deficit hyperactivity disorder: a systematic review of randomized controlled clinical trials. Eur J Clin Nutr 2013;67:122–4.
[70] Oner O, Oner P, Bozkurt OH, et al. Effects of zinc and ferritin levels on parent and teacher reported symptom scores in attention deficit hyperactivity disorder. Child Psychiatry Hum Dev 2010;41:441–7.
[71] Krull KR. Attention deficit hyperactivity disorder in children and adolescents: clinical features and evaluation. In: Post TW, editor. Waltham (MA): UpToDate; Accessed September 14, 2015.
[72] Law EC, Sideridis GD, Prock LA, et al. Attention-deficit/hyperactivity disorder in young children: predictors of diagnostic stability. Pediatrics 2014;133:659–67.
[73] Daley D. Attention-deficit hyperactivity disorder: a review of the literature. Child Care Health Dev 2006;32:193–204.
[74] Tarver J, Daley D, Sayal K. Attention-deficit hyperactivity disorder (ADHD): an updated review of the essential facts. Child Care Health Dev 2014;40:762–74.
[75] Verkuijl N, Perkins M, Fazel M. Childhood attention-deficit/hyperactivity disorder. BMJ 2015;350:h2168.
[76] Childress AC, Sallee FR. Emotional lability in patients with attention-deficit/hyperactivity disorder: impact of pharmacotherapy. CNS Drugs 2015; http://dx.doi.org/10.1007/s40263-015-0264-9.
[77] Leung AK. Nocturnal enuresis. In: Bope ET, Kellerman RD, editors. Conn's current therapy. Philadelphia: Elsevier; 2015. p. 1122–4.

[78] Reinhardt MC, Reinhardt CAU. Attention deficit-hyperactivity disorder, comorbidities, and risk situations. J Pediatr (Rio J) 2013;89:124–30.

[79] Robson WL, Jackson HP, Blackhurst D, et al. Enuresis in children with attention-deficit hyperactivity disorder. South Med J 1997;90:503–5.

[80] Sciberras E, Ohan J, Anderson V. Bulling and peer victimisation in adolescent girls with attention-deficit/hyperactivity disorder. Child Psychiatry Hum Dev 2012;43:254–70.

[81] Baweja R, Mattison RE, Waxmonsky JG. Impact of attention-deficit hyperactivity disorder on school performance: what are the effects of medication? Paediatr Drugs 2015;17(6): 459–77.

[82] Galera C, Melchior M, Chastang JF, et al. Childhood and adolescent hyperactivity-inattention symptoms and academic achievement 8 years later: the GAZEL YOUTH study. Psychol Med 2009;39:1895–906.

[83] Kent KM, Pelham WE Jr, Molina SS, et al. The academic experience of male high school students with ADHD. J Abnorm Child Psychol 2011;39:451–62.

[84] Dalsgaard S, Leckman JF, Mortensen PB, et al. Effect of drugs on the risk of i njuries in children with attention-deficit hyperactivity disorder: a prospective cohort study. Lancet Psychiatry 2015;2:702–9.

[85] Thapar A, Cooper M, Jefferies R, et al. What causes attention deficit hyperactivity disorder? Arch Dis Child 2012;97:260–5.

[86] Young J. Common comorbidities seen in adolescents with attention-deficit/hyperactivity disorder. Adolesc Med 2008;19:216–28.

[87] Alda JA, Serrano-Troncoso E. Attention-deficit hyperactivity disorder: agreement between clinical impression and the SNAP-IV screening tool. Actas Esp Psiquiatr 2013;41:76–83.

[88] Greenhill LL, Posner K, Vaughan BS, et al. Attention deficit hyperactivity disorder in preschool children. Child Adolesc Psychiatr Clin N Am 2008;17:347–66.

[89] Subcommittee on Attention-Deficit/Hyperactivity Disorder, Steering Committee on Quality Improvement and Management, Wolraich M, Brown L, Brown RT, et al. ADHD: clinical practice guideline for the diagnosis, evaluation, and treatment of attention-deficit/hyperactivity disorder in children and adolescents. Pediatrics 2011;128:1007–22.

[90] Felt BT, Biermann B, Christner JG. Diagnosis and management of ADHD in children. Am Fam Physician 2014;90:456–64.

[91] Berger S. Cardiac evaluation of patients receiving pharmacology for attention deficit hyperactivity disorder. In: Post TW, editor. Waltham (MA): UpToDate; Accessed September 14, 2015.

[92] Lenartowicz A, Loo SK. Use of EEG to diagnose ADHD. Curr Psychiatry Rep 2014;16:498.

[93] Fayyazi A, Khajeh A. Does electroencephalography contribute to examining children with attention deficit hyperactivity disorder? Iran J Child Neurol 2014;8:65–7.

[94] Arns M, Conners CK, Kraemer HC. A decade of EEG theta/beta ratio research in ADHD: a meta-analysis. J Atten Disord 2013;17:374–83.

[95] Food and Drug Administration. De novo classification request for neuropsychiatric EEG-based assessment aid for ADHD (NEBA) system. K112711. 2013. Available at: http://www.accessdata.fda.gov/cdrh_docs/reviews/K112711.pdf.

[96] Saad JF, Kohn MR, Clarke S, et al. Is the theta/beta EEG marker for ADHD inherently flawed? J Atten Disord 2015 [pii: 1087054715578270].

[97] Cortese S, Castellanos FX. Neuroimaging of attention-deficit/hyperactivity disorder: current neuroscience-informed perspectives for clinicians. Curr Psychiatry Rep 2012;14: 568–78.

[98] Jucaite A, Fernell E, Halldin C, et al. Reduced midbrain dopamine transporter binding in male adolescents with attention-deficit/hyperactivity disorder: association between striatal dopamine markers and motor hyperactivity. Biol Psychiatry 2005;57:229–38.

[99] Weyandt L, Swentosky A, Gudmundsdottir BG. Neuroimaging and ADHD: fMRI, PET, DTI findings, and methodological limitations. Dev Neuropsychol 2013;38:211–25.

[100] Arnsten AFT, Berridge CW, McCracken JT. The neurobiological basis of attention-deficit/ hyperactivity disorder. Prim Psychiatry 2009;16:47–54.

[101] Krull KR. Attention deficit hyperactivity disorder in children and adolescents: overview of treatment and prognosis. In: Post TW, editor. Waltham (MA): UpToDate; Accessed September 14, 2015.

[102] Kaplan G, Adesman A. Clinical diagnosis and management of attention-deficit hyperactivity disorder in preschool children. Curr Opin Pediatr 2011;23:684–92.

[103] French WP. Assessment and treatment of attention-deficit/hyperactivity disorder: part 2. Pediatr Ann 2015;44:160–8.

[104] Connor DF. Pharmacological management of pediatric patients with comorbid attention-deficit hyperactivity disorder oppositional defiant disorder. Pediatr Drugs 2015; http:// dx.doi.org/10.1007/s40272-015-0143-3.

[105] Pringsheim T, Hirsch L, Gardner D, et al. The pharmacological management of oppositional behaviour, conduct problems, and aggression in children and adolescents with attention-deficit hyperactivity disorder, oppositional defiant disorder, and conduct disorder: a systematic review and meta-analysis. Part 2: antipsychotics and traditional mood stabilizers. Can J Psychiatry 2005;60:52–61.

[106] Pringsheim T, Hirsch L, Gardner D, et al. The pharmacological management of oppositional behaviour, conduct problems, and aggression in children and adolescents with attention-deficit hyperactivity disorder, oppositional defiant disorder, and conduct disorder: a systematic review and meta-analysis. Part 1: psychostimulants, alpha-2 agonists, and atomoxetine. Can J Psychiatry 2005;60:42–51.

[107] Shaw M, Hodgkins P, Caci H, et al. A systematic review and analysis of long-term outcomes in attention deficit hyperactivity disorder: effect of treatment and nontreatment. BMC Med 2012;10:99.

[108] American Academy of Pediatrics, Committee on Quality Improvement, Subcommittee on Attention-Deficit/Hyperactivity Disorder. Clinical practice guidelines: treatment of the school-aged child with attention deficit/hyperactivity disorder. Pediatrics 2001;108: 1033–44.

[109] Devilbiss DM, Berridge CW. Cognition-enhancing doses of methylphenidate preferentially increase prefrontal cortical neuronal responsiveness. Biol Psychiatry 2008;64: 626–35.

[110] Wilens TE. Effects of methylphenidate on the catecholaminergic system in attention-deficit/ hyperactivity disorder. J Clin Psychopharmacol 2008;28:S46–53.

[111] Krull KR. Pharmacology of drugs used to treat attention deficit hyperactivity disorder in children and adolescents. In: Post TW, editor. Waltham (MA): UpToDate; Accessed September 14, 2015.

[112] Warikoo N, Faraone SV. Background, clinical features and treatment of attention deficit hyperactivity disorder in children. Expert Opin Pharmacother 2013;14:1885–906.

[113] Sugrue D, Bogner R, Ehret MJ. Methylphenidate and dexmethylphenidate formulations for children with attention-deficit/hyperactivity disorder. Am J Health Syst Pharm 2014;71: 1163–70.

[114] Wilens T, Adler LA, Adams J, et al. Misuse and diversion of stimulants prescribed for ADHD: a systematic review of the literature. J Am Acad Child Adolesc Psychiatry 2008;47:21–31.

[115] Findling RL. Evolution of the treatment of attention-deficit/hyperactivity disorder in children: a review. Clin Ther 2008;30:942–57.

[116] Katzman MA, Sternat T. A review of OROS methylphenidate (Concerta(®)) in the treatment of attention-deficit/hyperactivity disorder. CNS Drugs 2014;28:1005–33.

[117] McCough JJ, Biederman J, Greenhill LL, et al. Pharmacokinetics of SL1381 (Adderall XR), an extended-release formulation of Adderall. J Am Acad Child Adolesc Psychiatry 2003;42:684–91.

[118] Rappley MD. Attention deficit-hyperactivity disorder. N Engl J Med 2005;352:165–73.

[119] Herman JH. Attention deficit/hyperactivity disorder and sleep in children. Sleep Med Clin 2015;10:143–9.

[120] Pringsheim T, Steeves T. Pharmacological treatment for Attention Deficit Hyperactivity Disorder (ADHD) in children with comorbid tic disorders. Cochrane Database Syst Rev 2011;(4):CD007990.

[121] Mosholder AD, Gelperin K, Hammad TA, et al. Hallucinations and other psychotic symptoms associated with the use of attention-deficit/hyperactivity disorder drugs in children. Pediatrics 2009;123:611–6.

[122] Ross RG. Psychotic and manic-like symptoms during stimulant treatment of attention deficit hyperactivity disorder. Am J Psychiatry 2006;163:1149–52.

[123] Cakin-Memik N, Yildiz O, Sismanlar SG, et al. Priapism associated with methylphenidate: a case report. Turk J Pediatr 2010;52:430–4.

[124] Yu ZJ, Parker-Kotler C, Tran K, et al. Peripheral vasculopathy associated with psychostimulant treatment in children with attention-deficit/hyperactivity disorder. Curr Psychiatry Rep 2010;12:111–5.

[125] Charach A, Figuerosa M, Chen S, et al. Stimulant treatment over 5 years: effect on growth. J Am Acad Child Adolesc Psychiatry 2006;45:415–21.

[126] Harstad EB, Weaver AL, Katusic SK. ADHD, stimulant treatment, and growth: a longitudinal study. Pediatrics 2014;134:e935–44.

[127] Hammerness PG, Karampahtsis C, Babalola R, et al. Attention-deficit/hyperactivity disorder treatment: what are the long-term cardiovascular risks? Expert Opin Drug Saf 2015;14:543–51.

[128] Kaplan G, Newcorn JH. Pharmacotherapy for child and adolescent attention-deficit hyperactivity disorder. Pediatr Clin North Am 2011;58:99–120.

[129] Humphreys KL, Eng T, Lee SS. Stimulant medication and substance use outcomes: a meta-analysis. JAMA Psychiatry 2013;70:740–9.

[130] Harstad EB, Levy S, Committee on substance abuse. Attention-deficit/hyperactivity disorder and substance abuse. Pediatrics 2014;134:e293–301.

[131] Kiely B, Adesman A. What we do not know about ADHD… yet. Curr Opin Pediatr 2015;27:395–404.

[132] Advokat C, Scheithauer M. Attention-deficit hyperactivity disorder (ADHD) stimulant medications as cognitive enhancers. Front Neurosci 2013;7:82.

[133] Obioha O, Adesman A. Pearls, perils, and pitfalls in the assessment and treatment of attention-deficit/hyperactivity disorder in adolescents. Curr Opin Pediatr 2014;26:119–29.

[134] Gajria K, Lu M, Sikirica V, et al. Adherence, persistence, and medication discontinuation in patients with attention-deficit/hyperactivity disorder - a systematic literature review. Neuropsychiatr Treat 2014;10:1543–69.

[135] Toomey SL, Sox CM, Rusinak D, et al. Why do children with ADHD discontinue their medication? Clin Pediatr 2012;51:763–9.

[136] Pierce K. Treatment of attention-deficit/hyperactivity disorder. Pediatr Ann 2011;40:556–62.

[137] Bushe CJ, Savill NC. Systematic review of atomoxetine data in childhood and adolescent attention-deficit hyperactivity disorder 2009-2011: focus on clinical efficacy and safety. J Psychopharmacol 2014;28:204–11.

[138] Savill NC, Buitelaar JK, Anand E, et al. The efficacy of atomoxetine for the treatment of children and adolescents with attention-deficit/hyperactivity disorder: a comprehensive review of over a decade of clinical research. CNS Drugs 2015;29:131–51.

[139] Bangs ME, Jin L, Zhang S, et al. Hepatic events associated with atomoxetine treatment for attention-deficit hyperactivity disorder. Drug Saf 2008;31:345–54.

[140] Dittman RW, Cardo E, Nagy P, et al. Efficacy and safety of lisdexamfetamine dimesylate and atomoxetine in the treatment of attention-deficit/hyperactivity disorder: a

head-to-head randomized, double-blind, phase IIIb study. CNS Drugs 2013;27: 1082–92.

[141] Hanwella R, Senanayake M, De Silva V. Comparative efficacy and acceptability of methylphenidate and atomoxetine in treatment of attention-deficit hyperactivity disorder in children and adolescents: a meta-analysis. BMC Psychiatry 2011;11:176.

[142] Hunt RD, Paguin A, Payton K. An update on assessment and treatment of complex attention-deficit hyperactivity disorder. Pediatr Ann 2001;30:162–72.

[143] Cutler AJ, Brams M, Bukstein O, et al. Response/remission with guanfacine extended-release and psychostimulants in children and adolescents with attention-deficit/hyperactivity disorder. J Am Acad Child Adolesc Psychiatry 2014;53:1092–101.

[144] Cruz MP. Guanfacine extended-release tablets (Intuniv), a non-stimulant selective alpha(2A)-adrenergic receptor agonist for attention-deficit/hyperactivity disorder. P T 2010;35:448–51.

[145] Daley KC. Update on attention-deficit/hyperactivity disorder. Curr Opin Pediatr 2004;16: 217–26.

[146] Scahill L. Alpha-2 adrenergic agonists in children with inattention, hyperactivity and impulsiveness. CNS Drugs 2009;23(Suppl 1):43–9.

[147] Rizzo R, Martino D. Guanfacine for the treatment of attention-deficit hyperactivity disorder in children and adolescents. Expert Rev Neurother 2015;15:347–54.

[148] Otasowie J, Castells X, Ehimare UP, et al. Tricyclic antidepressants for attention deficit hyperactivity disorder (ADHD) in children and adolescents. Cochrane Database Syst Rev 2014;(9):CD006997.

[149] Connors CK, Casat CD, Gualtieri CT, et al. Bupropion hydrochloride in attention deficit disorder with hyperactivity. J Am Acad Child Adolesc Psychiatry 1996;35:1314–21.

[150] Maneeton N, Maneeton B, Intaprasert S, et al. A systematic review of randomized controlled trials of bupropion versus methylphenidate in the treatment of attention-deficit hyperactivity disorder. Neuropsychiatr Dis Treat 2014;10:1439–49.

[151] Jafarinia M, Mohammadi MR, Modabbernia A, et al. Bupropion versus methylphenidate in the treatment of children with attention-deficit/hyperactivity disorder: randomized double-blind study. Hum Psychopharmacol 2012;27:411–8.

[152] Foley KF, DeSanty KP, Kast RE. Bupropion: pharmacology and therapeutic applications. Expert Rev Neurother 2006;6:1249–65.

[153] Antshel KM, Barkley R. Psychosocial interventions in attention deficit hyperactivity disorder. Child Adolesc Psychiatr Clin N Am 2008;12:421–37.

[154] Zwi M, Jones H, Thorgaard C, et al. Parent training interventions for Attention Deficit Hyperactivity Disorder (ADHD) in children aged 5 to 18 years. Cochrane Database Syst Rev 2011;(12):CD003018.

[155] The MTA Cooperative Group. A 14-month randomized clinical trial of treatment strategies for attention-deficit/hyperactivity disorder. Arch Gen Psychiatry 1999;56:1073–86.

[156] Moderators and mediators of treatment response for children with attention-deficit/hyperactivity disorder: the Multimodal Treatment of children with attention-deficit/hyperactivity disorder. Arch Gen Psychiatry 1999;56:1088–96.

[157] Daley D, van der Oord S, Ferrin M, et al. Behavioral interventions in attention-deficit hyperactivity disorder: a meta-analysis of randomized controlled trials across multiple outcome domains. J Am Acad Adolesc Psychiatry 2014;53:835–47.

[158] Bloch MH, Qawasmi A. Omega-3 fatty acid supplementation for the treatment of children with attention-deficit/hyperactivity disorder symptomatology: systematic review and meta-analysis. J Am Acad Child Adolesc Psychiatry 2011;50:991–1000.

[159] Nigg J, Lewis K, Edinger T, et al. Meta-analysis of attention-deficit/hyperactivity disorder symptoms, restriction diet, and synthetic food color additives. J Am Acad Child Adolesc Psychiatry 2012;51:86–97.e8.

[160] Sampson HA, Aceves S, Bock SA, et al. Food allergy: a practice parameter update-2014. J Allergy Clin Immunol 2014;134:1016–25.

[161] Leung AK, Chan KW. Iron deficiency anemia. Adv Pediatr 2001;48:385–408.

[162] Davtian M, Reid RC, Fong TW. Investigating facets of personality in adult pathological gamblers with ADHD. Neuropsychiatry 2012;2:163–74.

[163] Lee SS, Humphreys KL, Flory K, et al. Prospective association of childhood attention-deficit/hyperactivity disorder and substance use and abuse/dependence: a meta-analytic review. Clin Psychol Rev 2011;31:328–41.

[164] Dalsgaard S, Ostergaard SD, Leckman JF, et al. Mortality in children, adolescents, and adults with attention-deficit hyperactivity disorder: a nationwide cohort study. Lancet 2015;385:2190–6.

[165] Faraone SV. Attention deficit hyperactivity disorder and premature death. Lancet 2015;385:2132–3.

Advances in Pediatrics 63 (2016) 281–332

ADVANCES IN PEDIATRICS

Updates in Pediatric Rheumatology

Deborah K. McCurdy, MD

Division of Allergy/Immunology/Rheumatology, Department of Pediatrics, David Geffen School of
Medicine, UCLA, 10833 Le Conte Avenue, Los Angeles, CA 90095, USA

Keywords

• Pediatrics • Rheumatology • Autoimmune disease • Biologics • Biomarkers
• Gastrointestinal Microbiome • Bone Health

Key points

• Provide an overview of the current understanding of the pediatric rheumatic diseases with a discussion of the pathogenesis, clinical features and criteria for diagnosis.

• Review the current standards of treatment, including new therapeutic modalities, in the pediatric rheumatic diseases.

• Review the cytokines and intracellular pathways that are involved in inflammation in autoimmune diseases and discuss the subsequent biologic therapies that have been developed to treat the pediatric rheumatic diseases.

• Discuss the gastrointestinal microbiome and its potential role in autoimmune diseases.

• Discuss bone health and Vitamin D in the pediatric rheumatic diseases.

O ver the last decade, the understanding of the genetic and immunologic basis of autoimmune diseases has expanded, resulting in targeted biologic therapies that have changed the prospects of children with rheumatic diseases. Pediatric rheumatologists have witnessed the advent of biologics that have prevented the chronic and crippling changes of arthritis and have allowed children, who would have been in a wheelchair in another era, to engage in school activities, sports, and dance. There is now the promise of enhanced understanding of autoimmune diseases and multiple and better therapies that will improve clinical outcomes to allow most children with rheumatic diseases to live lives more free of pain and with few limitations.

E-mail address: dmccurdy@mednet.ucla.edu

0065-3101/16/$ – see front matter
http://dx.doi.org/10.1016/j.yapd.2016.04.006

Although advances have been made in many areas of autoimmune diseases, 3 major advances are considered in this article: the use of biologic therapies in children with autoimmune diseases, research into the gastrointestinal (GI) microbiome and its role in autoimmune disease, and current understanding of bone health in children with arthritis and chronic autoimmune diseases. Each of these areas promises to improve the quality of life for children with rheumatic diseases.

RHEUMATIC DISEASES

The rheumatic or autoimmune diseases are also called collagen vascular diseases because the connective tissues, made up of collagen proteins, and the vascular system are affected. However, the disorders are caused not by inherent problems in the connective tissue or vascular system but by aberrant acquired immune responses that are associated with anti–self-antibodies and inflammation resulting in damage to the collagen vascular system and other organs in the body. The anti–self-antibodies associated with each disease process help to define the disease and in some cases to determine the degree of disease activity. Significant progress has been made in classifying each disease with criteria for diagnosis, including clinical and laboratory findings. Although there may be significant overlap, most autoimmune diseases can be classified and this helps in choosing the optimal treatment plan.

Juvenile idiopathic arthritis

Chronic arthritis diagnosed in children younger than 16 years of age and persisting for longer than 6 weeks was initially termed juvenile rheumatoid arthritis (JRA) in North America. This classification included 3 main subtypes of arthritis: oligoarticular, polyarticular, and systemic. The classifications were not inclusive or descriptive. For example, young girls with asymmetric arthritis involving fewer than 4 joints and older boys who were human leukocyte antigen (HLA) B27 positive were included in the oligoarticular subtype. There was no inclusion of psoriatic arthritis (PsA), spondyloarthropathies, or inflammatory bowel disease (IBD) associated arthritis [1,2]. In 2011, the International League of Associations for Rheumatology (ILAR) held a conference with the purpose of identifying arthritis disease groups that were homogenous in presentation to facilitate research on cause, pathogenesis, epidemiology, and clinical outcome studies and treatment trials [2–4]. The final proposal changed the name to juvenile idiopathic arthritis (JIA) and included 7 disease categories based on the features present in the first 6 months of illness: systemic arthritis, rheumatoid factor (RF)–positive polyarthritis, RF-negative polyarthritis, oligoarthritis (also termed pauciarticular arthritis and divided into persistent oligoarthritis, in which arthritis remains confined to ≤4 joints throughout the whole disease course, and extended oligoarthritis, in which arthritis extends to >4 joints after the first 6 months of illness), PsA, enthesitis-related arthritis (ERA), and undifferentiated arthritis. There was a suggestion that there should also be a category of antinuclear antibody (ANA)–positive patient groups because the ANA positivity includes a group of children with early onset of disease, strong female predominance, prevalence of asymmetric arthritis, and increased risk for iridocyclitis, and is divided between the oligoarticular and RF-negative polyarticular groups [5]. To date, this criterion has not been added, but it does include another subtype of JIA that potentially should be considered in study design (Table 1).

Biomarkers

Biomarkers promise to provide guidance in therapeutic decisions in the future. The degree of ongoing inflammation can be difficult to determine in arthritis and uveitis with a persistence of low-grade inflammation that is difficult to fully evaluate clinically. JIA activity is associated with activation of granulocytes and macrophages cells. The S100 proteins, calcium-binding proteins (such as calprotectin) that function as proinflammatory alarmins, are derived from phagocytes and are being used as biomarkers [6–8]. Studies have shown that myeloid related proteins, MRP-8/MRP-14 (S100A8/S100A9 heterodimer) and S100A12 can be used to determine disease activity and the risk of relapse as children with JIA and uveitis are tapered off medications [9]. This test can be done by an enzyme-linked immunosorbent assay method (ELISA) and may be incorporated into treatment management. Other biomarkers are being studied to aid in optimizing therapies in children with JIA [9–11].

Clinical features

JIA is the most common of the rheumatic diseases in children and one of the most common chronic diseases in the pediatric population. In the United States, the incidence is estimated at more than 14 patients per 100,000 population and the prevalence 96 patients per 100,000 population [2,11]. At some point during the disease process, arthritis is present. Arthritis is defined as heat, swelling, pain on motion, and/or limitation of motion. It is different from arthralgia, in which there is pain but no clinical findings. One of the most informative clinical symptoms is the presence of morning stiffness and its duration. Children with arthritis also experience gelling or stiffness after a period of inactivity. JIA is a systemic disease and can affect growth and development of the musculoskeletal system, and often other organs.

Oligoarticular juvenile idiopathic arthritis

Oligoarticular JIA is the most common subtype of JIA, affecting more than 50% of children with JIA. It often affects toddlers and young girls (3–5:1 female/male [F/M]) with a peak incidence of between 1 and 3 years of age and is seen most frequently in those of European background, but does occur in all backgrounds [12]. There are 1 to 4 joints involved, with an asymmetric arthritis; for example, 1 knee (the most common joint involved), wrist, ankle, or elbow, and a smaller joint such as one of the proximal interphalangeal (PIP) joints. The hips or shoulders are less commonly involved and usually there is no involvement of the neck or spine. In most children, the arthritis remains in 4 or fewer joints, but in 30% to 40% the arthritis may become extended after

Table 1

Juvenile idiopathic subtypes (ILAR 2011) and clinical features and optimal treatments

JIA subtype	Joints involved	Age at onset (y)	Gender (female/male)	ANA positive (%)	Other organs involved	Differential diagnosis (common)	Therapy	Prognosis
Oligoarticular JIA Persistent	≤4 Asymmetric (eg, knee, PIP)	2–4	3–5:1	30–65	Uveitis, leg length discrepancy	Septic joint, bone tumor	NSAIDs, steroid injection	Joint instability, uveitis
Oligoarticular JIA Extended	≤4 for 6 mo, but then >4 Asymmetric	2–4	3–5:1	30–65	Uveitis, leg length discrepancy	Septic joint, bone tumor	NSAIDs, MTX, biologics; TNF inhibitors	Joint instability, uveitis
Polyarticular JIA RF negative	≥5 May be asymmetric	2–4	3:1	50	Uveitis, joint instability, rheumatoid nodules	Infectious, postinfectious, malignancy, metabolic arthropathy	NSAIDs, MTX, biologics; TNF inhibitors	Joint instability, uveitis
Polyarticular JIA RF positive	≥5 Symmetric Small and large Joints	Adolescents	10:1	20–30	Rheumatoid nodules, vasculitis, multiple organs	Infectious, postinfectious, malignancy, metabolic arthropathy	NSAIDs, MTX, biologics; TNF inhibitors	Joint instability, joint replacements
sJIA	Variable, usually polyarticular	Throughout childhood Peak 1–5	1:1	<5	Multiple organs, MAS	Sepsis, leukemia, malignancy	Steroids, NSAIDs, MTX, biologics; IL-1 inhibitors	Joint instability, organ damage
Psoriatic	Usually ≤4 Asymmetric Dactylitis, involves axial spine	3–11	1:1	20	Skin	Infectious, malignancy	NSAIDs, MTX, biologics; TNF inhibitors	Joint instability, skin, malignancy
ERA	Usually ≤4 Lower extremities Affects the SI and lumbosacral spine	>6	1:7	Negative	Uveitis, posture and gait abnormalities	Infectious, postinfectious, malignancy	NSAIDs, MTX, biologics; TNF inhibitors	Joint instability, uveitis
Undifferentiated (IBD arthropathy)	Peripheral and axial spine	Older children, adolescents	1:1	±	IBD, skin, vasculopathy, other organs	Infectious, malignancy	Treatment for IBD, MTX	Gastrointestinal, vasculitis

6 months of disease and involve $\geq$ 5 joints. Extended oligoarticular JIA is more severe and similar to polyarticular JIA, but continues with asymmetric joint involvement. The chronic arthritis leads to chronic changes in the joint: flexion contractures, joint subluxation, and instability of the joint. A potential result is a limb length discrepancy with the affected limb being longer. Because of the increased blood flow to the affected joints of children with oligoarthritis, the extremity on the affected side may grow more rapidly with bony overgrowth. Untreated, the joint will ultimately fuse, resulting in a shorted limb. Treatment is designed to prevent joint instability and limb length discrepancies.

Anterior uveitis. The ANA is positive in 30% to 65% of children with oligoarticular JIA and is associated with anterior uveitis in 15% to 30%. Anterior uveitis is inflammation of the iris, anterior uveal tract, and adjacent ciliary body. Often there are no symptoms and, to prevent irreversible changes, ophthalmology visits are scheduled routinely. Children with oligoarticular JIA who are ANA positive, 6 years of age or younger, and have had arthritis for less than 4 years are at high risk for uveitis and should be checked by an ophthalmologist every 3 months. If there is no sign of uveitis for more than 4 years, the risk becomes moderate and the ophthalmology appointments can be scheduled every 6 months [12,13]. Usually local steroid eye drops are used to control the disease, but more than 50% of children with uveitis require methotrexate (MTX) and/or a biologic to control the inflammation. Untreated anterior uveitis may lead to glaucoma, cataracts, and blindness.

Differential diagnosis. The differential includes infections and malignancy. A septic joint requires urgent treatments and, if the onset of pain and swelling is sudden, unremitting, and associated with a fever, the joint should be aspirated and cultured. In addition, radiographs should be obtained to evaluate the joint for effusions and chronic changes, as well as to rule out a malignant tumor involving the bone.

Laboratory tests. The complete blood count (CBC) and acute phase reactants are usually normal. The test with the most prognostic significance is the ANA because it is associated with a greater risk for uveitis. The RF is almost always negative. Synovial fluid analysis shows 5000 to 20,000 white blood cells with normal glucose and protein levels.

Treatment and prognosis. Persistent oligoarticular JIA often responds to nonsteroidal antiinflammatory drugs (NSAIDs), but at times may require a joint injection with an intermediate-acting steroid preparation (triamcinolone) to quickly reduce the swelling and prevent damage. If nonresponsive, MTX, a disease-modifying antirheumatic drug (DMARD), is the second line of treatment. With extended oligoarticular disease, biologic treatments may be needed to control the arthritis. Uveitis is initially treated with steroid eye drops (prednisolone acetate), but may require MTX or biologics to control the inflammation. The prognosis with current therapies is positive and few children have permanent joint damage. The major concern is for those with anterior uveitis, which may result in permanent changes and decreased vision. If there is not a good response to the local treatments and MTX within several months, the monoclonal tumor necrosis factor (TNF) alpha inhibitors (adalimumab, infliximab) are now an important component in the treatment of uveitis. Of note, the fusion protein etanercept has been associated with the onset of uveitis and is not used in treatment of uveitis. In cases of severe or unremitting uveitis, the anti-TNF monoclonal, infliximab (Remicade), often offers a rapid decrease in inflammation (although not US Food and Drug Administration [FDA] approved for treatment of JIA in children). Other biologics, such as rituximab, daclizumab, tocilizumab, and abatacept, are being used in those cases refractory to anti–TNF-α therapy, but clinical trials are yet to be done [14].

Polyarticular juvenile idiopathic arthritis

Polyarticular JIA occurs in approximately 20% to 40% of patients with JIA and these children have 5 or more joints affected by arthritis [15]. RF-negative polyarticular JIA is the most common (85%) and often presents in young girls (3:1 F/M) between 2 and 4 years of age. In Canada, there is noted to be a higher incidence in First Nations children, but the RF-negative polyarticular JIA can be seen in all backgrounds. The disease onset is usually insidious, with additional joints affected over time. The arthritis can be asymmetrical, but usually involves both sides of the body. Often the temporomandibular joint is involved and results in micrognathia with pain and difficulty opening the mouth and chewing. The spine is usually not involved until late in the disease, but can result in ankyloses and atlantoaxial subluxation. Unlike oligoarticular JIA, polyarticular and systemic JIA are associated with marked inflammation and a catabolic state, that results in growth failure. In the past, the vertical height was commonly affected and limb length was shortened. In polyarticular and systemic JIA, there is shortening of the affected joints with resultant shortening of the extremities relative to the other side and to the spine, if the disease is active during periods of rapid growth. Approximately 50% are ANA positive and are at increased risk of anterior uveitis (Fig. 1).

RF-positive polyarticular JIA is most common in adolescent girls (10:1 F:M) of all ethnic backgrounds, with symmetric joint disease that involves the small and large joints, much like RA. The RF positivity is associated with more severe joint damage, as it is in RA.

Differential diagnosis. The differential is broad and a diagnosis is made after exclusion of infection, malignancy, and metabolic diseases. Infectious or postinfectious arthritis, as seen with viral infections or acute rheumatic fever, may have polyarticular joint involvement. In arthritis following a streptococcal infection, the arthritis is usually migratory. Malignancies, such as leukemia, may present

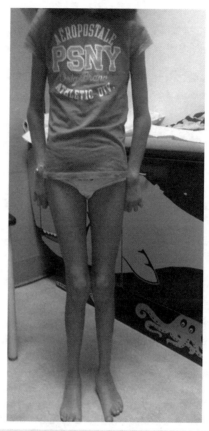

Fig. 1. RF-Negative Polyarticular JIA showing severe arthritis and cachexia when the inflammation is not well controlled. Note the shortened toes on the left foot secondary to arthritis.

with arthritis, but usually the laboratory tests are helpful in making the diagnosis. Metabolic and genetic disease may have associated arthropathies.

Laboratory tests. The CBC often shows anemia, usually the anemia of chronic disease, and may show a slightly increased white blood cell count (WBC). The erythrocyte sedimentation rate (ESR) and C-reactive protein level (CRP) are often increased. The ANA is positive in 50% and in younger children may be associated with anterior uveitis. With active joint inflammation, a cyclic citrullinated peptide antibody test (CCP) helps to assess the degree of inflammation in the joints. The synovial fluid has increased numbers of cells, but usually fewer than 100,000.

Treatment and prognosis. Before 1999, children with polyarticular JIA usually had ongoing inflammation of their joints and required NSAIDs and MTX. Many had hours of morning stiffness and required intensive physical therapy to prevent contractures and atrophy. Despite these treatments, the disease often remained active. Since the advent of biologics, the prognosis has changed markedly. In polyarticular JIA, the biologics that target TNF are effective in most of these patients and the prognosis has been improving over the last decade. Treatment is started early and stratified so that, if there is not an adequate response to NSAIDs and MTX in 1 to 2 months, more aggressive treatment, usually with a TNF inhibitor, is indicated [16–18]. There are many NSAIDs available, but usually naproxen is used first because its safety profile is well known in children and it is taken twice per day rather than requiring dosing 3 to 4 times per day. Depending on the severity of the arthritis, MTX is started concurrently or, if NSAIDs do not control the inflammation, 1 to 2 months later. The dose is usually 10 to 15 mg/m^2 given once per week orally or subcutaneously. If MTX is not tolerated, leflunomide (Arava) may be substituted at the following doses: for patients less than 20 kg, 10 mg every alternate day by mouth; 20 to 40 kg, 10 mg daily by mouth; greater than 40 kg, 20 mg daily by mouth. All of these medications may cause liver toxicity and the liver function tests (LFTs) should be checked every 1 to 3 months. There are other available DMARDs, including sulfasalazine, but these are used less frequently in children. The biologics are discussed separately later.

Systemic juvenile idiopathic arthritis

Systemic-onset JIA (sJIA) is present in 5% to 15% of patients with JIA and presents with high fevers, rashes, lymphadenopathy, hepatosplenomegaly, and arthritis [19]. Although the exact incidence is unknown, in Europe the incidence is estimated at 0.3 to 0.8 per 100,000. There is no clear ethnic predilection. Boys and girls are equally affected and although sJIA can occur throughout childhood, the peak of onset is at 1 to 5 years of age. The acute nature of the clinical presentation and the laboratory features of activation of the innate immune system, with rare autoantibodies and high interleukin (IL)-1 levels, are similar to diseases seen in the autoinflammatory or periodic fever syndromes [20,21]. By definition, the fever must be greater than 39°C and return to less than 37°C between peaks for at least 3 days (called a quotidian fever). During the fever or at times of stress, the patients may have a salmon-colored rash that is usually nonpruritic and evanescent. There may be a Koebner phenomenon (Fig. 2) that appears at the sites of trauma. These rashes may be difficult to see on dark skin tones. Criteria established by ILAR include arthritis and a quotidian fever of ≥2 weeks with 1 or more of the following: rash, lymphadenopathy, hepatosplenomegaly, and/or serositis. Arthritis may not be present at the time of the initial fever and may be delayed for up to 6 months. Usually the arthritis is polyarticular, but it may present in only 1 joint. Other organ systems are frequently involved. The cardiac system is affected and there is often tachycardia and, in up to 30% of children, pericarditis and pericardial effusions. The lymph nodes, liver, and spleen are often enlarged and there may be a mild hepatitis. There may be involvement of the lungs and central nervous system (CNS), but less commonly. One curiosity is that about 50% of children with sJIA go into remission and it is not possible to predict this at onset. In contrast, up to 8% develop macro-phage activation syndrome (MAS), which previously was associated with mor-tality in more than 20% of children. Now, with earlier recognition and more aggressive therapy, mortality has decreased to 8%.

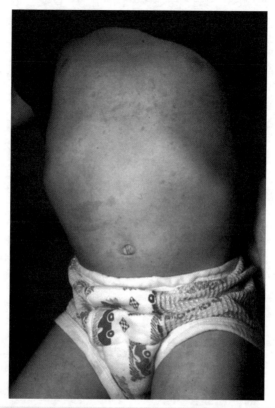

Fig. 2. The rash of systemic JIA with the Koebner phenomenon seen on the abdomen.

Macrophage activation syndrome in systemic juvenile idiopathic arthritis. A frequent complication of sJIA is MAS that occurs as a full-blown picture in about 8% of children; however, a partial picture may be seen much more frequently. MAS may occur in systemic lupus erythematosus (SLE) and other autoimmune diseases, during infections, or with malignancies, but proportionately it is most commonly seen with sJIA. Despite a better understanding of this disease and early recognition and treatment, there is still significant morbidity and mortal-ity in up to 8% of children. MAS has been called a cytokine storm because there are high levels of IL-1, TNF-α, IL-6, and IL-18, and associated activation of T cells and macrophages [20–24]. The picture is similar to that of hemopha-gocytic lymphohistiocytosis (HLH), a genetic defect in perforin or associated genes that causes a defect in cytolytic activity and natural killer (NK) cell function [23–26]. The accumulation of target cells that do not undergo apoptosis because of abnormalities in the perforin pathway fuels inflammation. In 2004, criteria were developed for the diagnosis of HLH and, because MAS is similar, these criteria are helpful. The criteria for HLH established by the International Histiocyte Society include either: (1) a molecular diagnosis of mutations in perforin (PRF1) or mammalian uncoordinated protein (MUNC13-4) or (2) 5 out of the following 8 criteria: persistent fever; spleno-megaly; cytopenias (affecting ≥ 2 of 3 lineages in the peripheral blood); hyper-triglyceridemia and/or hypofibrinogenemia; hemophagocytosis in the bone marrow, spleen, or lymph nodes; serum ferritin level ≥ 500 μg/L; low or ab-sent NK cell activity; and/or increased serum soluble interleukin 2 receptor alpha (sIL2Rα) level [19].

The onset of MAS is sudden and severe and usually occurs early in the dis-ease. The fever that was following a quotidian pattern becomes persistent and is associated with bruising and bleeding, mental status changes (including irritability, seizures, coma), lymphadenopathy, hepatosplenomegaly, and liver dysfunction. There is a precipitous decrease in at least 2 of 3 blood cell lines (leukocytes, erythrocytes, and platelets) and the ESR secondary to hypofibrinogenemia.

Tests that are helpful in the diagnosis of MAS include the CBC, comprehen-sive metabolic panel, ferritin, D dimer, fibrinogen, triglycerides, serum sIL2Rα, cluster differentiation 163 (CD163) (a macrophage that binds hemoglobin-haptoglobin complexes), and NK cell function.

The treatment should be started immediately and should include intrave-nous methylprednisolone pulse therapy (maximum dose of 1 gram) for three 3 days followed by methylprednisolone 2 to 3 mg/kg/d divided every 6 to 8 hours. Often this is not sufficient and cyclosporine A (2–5 mg/kg/d) is started at onset or if there is not a clear response. In a protocol established by the In-ternational Histiocyte Society, etoposide is the next line of therapy and this pro-tocol is followed for primary HLH by most hematologists. Because of the serious side effects of etoposide, most rheumatologists use biologics, including IL-1 inhibitors and TNF-α inhibitors. The IL-1 inhibitors may prove to be the optimal treatment of MAS that does not respond quickly to pulse steroids and cyclosporine therapy. Recent studies show the efficacy of Kineret (Anakinra) or other IL-1 inhibitors or IL-6 inhibitors [27–29].

Differential diagnosis. The differential of sJIA includes systemic infections and malignancies and a full work-up is indicated. At times, steroids are necessary to control the inflammation and a bone marrow test may be indicated to rule out malignancy before starting therapy.

Laboratory tests. There is marked increase in the levels of acute inflammatory markers in sJIA with high white counts with a shift to the left, and high platelet counts, ESR, and CRP levels. The high platelet count helps in differentiating sJIA from leukemia. There is usually profound anemia that seems to be iron deficient, but the bone marrow often shows adequate iron stores that are not being used secondary to inflammation. If a synovial aspiration is done, the cell count is 50,000 to 100,000/µL. Clinicians should be aware that these patients may develop MAS, especially early in the course of the disease. With persistent fevers and rash, the CBC, and liver enzyme, ferritin, and D-dimer levels should be monitored in order to start treatment early if MAS is present.

Treatment and prognosis. Children with sJIA are the least likely to respond to the initial treatment with NSAIDs and MTX alone, although occasionally NSAIDs control the disease manifestations. The current recommendation is to start IL-1 inhibitors early to control the systemic disease. Often children with sJIA do not respond to TNF-α inhibitors. Children with MAS are urgently treated with high-dose steroids (pulse Solu-Medrol 30 mg/kg up to 1000 mg for 3 days) and started on cyclosporine and concurrently started on an IL-1 inhibitor [29] or an IL-6 inhibitor [30]. The prognosis is guarded in many of these children. Although 80% respond favorably to treatment, 20% have ongoing disease and/or develop MAS despite treatment. Despite the recent advances in treatment, these children are still at increased risk for mortality (1% in North America) and for permanent joint damage and increased morbidity/mortality, including cardiac involvement, CNS involvement, and MAS.

Psoriatic arthritis

The criteria for PsA as established by ILAR include psoriasis and 2 of the following: dactylitis (swelling of the entire digit), nail pitting or onycholysis, and/or psoriasis in a first-degree relative [31]. Psoriasis presents in 0.5% to 1% of children and in most the arthritis usually starts later. This type of arthritis, excluding dactylitis, may have a presentation similar to oligoarticular JIA in 68% to 94% of children, but unlike oligoarticular disease can involve the shoulder, hip, spine, sacroiliac joint (SI), and small joints. Treatment is similar to the treatment of JIA, with NSAIDs, MTX, and biologics depending on the severity.

Enthesitis-related arthritis and juvenile ankylosing spondylitis

The ILAR criteria for ERA include arthritis or enthesitis and 2 or more of the following: onset of arthritis in a boy more than 6 years old; SI joint or lumbosacral tenderness, presence of HLA-B27, family history of HLA-B27–associated diseases, and/or acute symptomatic anterior uveitis [32]. To make a diagnosis of JAS, the axial skeleton must also be involved, most often the SI joint, and changes are noted on imaging. The exact incidence and prevalence are unknown, but ERA/JAS is much less common then JIA. ERA is more frequent in boys (1.4–7:1 M:F), but does occur in girls, usually with less severity. The onset is after 6 years of age, but the mean age of onset is 10 to 13 years. The arthritis usually is oligoarticular, involving the lower extremities, including the hip. Tarsitis (inflammation of the tarsal joints) and enthesitis (inflammation at the attachment of ligaments and tendons) is seen in ERA. Involvement of the axial spine usually occurs later in the disease and is associated with HLA-B27 positivity. On forward flexion of the spine, there is decreased forward movement (documented by the Schober test) and flattening of the back. Other organ systems may be involved, most often uveitis in 3% to 7% of children, which, unlike oligoarticular JIA, is associated with redness and pain. The treatment is similar to JIA, but often MTX is not as effective and TNF inhibitors are started earlier or in the place of MTX. The disease course is variable and remissions have been reported in up to 44% of patients. Damage to the hip and SI joints may occur, but often there is less axial involvement than is seen in adult-onset ankylosing spondylitis.

Undifferentiated
Other arthritis and arthropathies are included in this subtype, but the most common are the arthropathies associated with IBD. This arthritis occurs in 7% to 21% of patients with IBD and may follow a polyarticular course, but often also involves the SI and axial skeleton [33]. The arthritis occurs during the course of IBD when the gastrointestinal disease is active. Usually the symptoms improve when the IBD is controlled, but in a small percentage of children the joint pain persists and NSAIDs and MTX are used to control the arthritis.

Outcomes for juvenile idiopathic arthritis
Etanercept was approved for use in children in 1999 and the previous outcome studies are no longer valid. A recent study of 43 children from the Netherlands concluded that 67% of patients who started etanercept had inactive disease and 20% did not require ongoing treatment of arthritis [34]. As new outcomes for patients with JIA are reported, a clearer picture of the future for children with JIA will emerge.

Systemic lupus erythematosus
SLE epitomizes autoimmune disease, because most patients have 6 or more autoantibodies and multiple organ system involvement [35]. Some autoantibodies are associated with disease pathogenesis and disease activity (eg, anti–double-stranded DNA [dsDNA] antibodies and renal involvement), but most autoantibodies are helpful in diagnosis but not clearly associated with pathogenesis or prognosis. The clinical presentation varies from only sun-sensitive rashes and arthritis to severe disease with multiorgan system involvement. In the pediatric and adolescent population with SLE, the presentation and course are often more severe, with renal, CNS, and other organ system involvement. ANAs are present in greater than 90% of patients with SLE, but can also be seen in many other diseases and in normal populations (up to 15%). Other more specific autoantibodies are usually present and, in some cases, help to optimize treatment and aid in prognosis [35–39]. The goal of treatment is to bring the immune system into balance by decreasing the inflammation.

Epidemiology
Incidence and prevalence
Approximately 20% of the cases of SLE are diagnosed in the pediatric population (<19 years old). The incidence is approximately 6 to 18.9 per 100,000 among white girls, 20 to 30 per 100,000 among African Americans girls, and 16 to 36.7 per 100,000 among Puerto Rican girls [35–40].

Ethnic background
In people of Hispanic, African, Native American, and Asian backgrounds, SLE
is not rare, although it is difficult to determine the incidence and prevalence
in children because there have not been extensive studies in the childhood population. However, SLE is present in all ethnic backgrounds, and is seen
throughout the world.

Age and gender
Although SLE may present at any age, most presentations in childhood and
adolescence are around the time of puberty. The F:M ratio varies from 4:1
to 13:1 depending on the ethnicity of the cohort.

Clinical presentation
The criteria for SLE were established by the American College of Rheumatology (ACR) in 1982 and modified in 1997 to include antiphospholipid
(aPL) antibodies [35,38]. There are 11 criteria and 4 of the 11 clinical and
laboratory findings must be present at some point during the disease to establish a diagnosis of SLE. The criteria are approximately 95% specific and sensitive for an SLE diagnosis (Box 1).
   Usually patients present with constitutional symptoms such as fever, fatigue,
and weight loss. Often there is a history of a photosensitive rash and swelling of
the joints. There may also be systemic inflammation with lymphadenopathy
and hepatosplenomegaly. In the pediatric populations, more than 80% have
renal involvement, either at onset or at some point in their disease [35–40].
Any and all organs may be involved. The most commonly involved organ

---

Box 1: SLE criteria for diagnosis (1997); 4 out of 11 required for diagnosis

- Malar rash
- Discoid rash
- Photosensitivity
- Oral ulcers
- Nonerosive arthritis
- Pleuritis or pericarditis
- Renal disorder
- Seizures or psychosis
- Hematologic disorder
- Positive autoantibodies
  - Anti–double-stranded DNA
  - Anti-Smith
  - Antiphospholipid antibody/lupus anticoagulant
- Positive antinuclear antibody

systems include the mucocutaneous, musculoskeletal, hematologic, renal, CNS, cardiac, and pulmonary systems.

The skin is frequently involved and is often a clinical clue to the diagnosis. The malar or butterfly rash is a classic rash seen in SLE and is usually photosensitive, but only 60% of patients have this type of rash at onset. The discoid rash that is deeper and involves the dermis is seen less commonly in the pediatric population, but if present is usually in those of African descent. Oral and nasal ulcers occur in 10% to 30% and Raynaud's in 15% to 20% of patients, but multiple other rashes may be seen less commonly, including vasculitis, bullous lesions, and ischemic lesions. These rashes are not specific for SLE. Arthritis involving the both the small and large joints and myositis or myalgia are often present at onset and during disease flares, but usually respond quickly to treatment. Anemia, thrombocytopenia, and leukopenia may be present in 50% to 75% of patients. Most often, patients have a normochromic, normocytic anemia typical of anemia of chronic disease, but the Coombs test is positive in 30% to 40% of patients and 10% to 15% have significant hemolysis. Thrombocytopenia is present in 15% to 45% of patients and is associated with a poorer prognosis.

Renal involvement is a major concern in the pediatric population, with approximately 50% of patients presenting with lupus nephritis and 80% to 90% developing renal disease during the first few years. The kidney is especially vulnerable to autoimmune diseases. The glomerulus is a filtering unit in which small capillaries form loops in which are housed the mesangial cells. The mesangial cells are monocytes that are important in filtration, regulation of blood flow, structural support, and phagocytosis. In SLE, the mesangial cells are affected by autoantibodies and immune complexes to become activated and proliferate. The World Health Organization classifies lupus nephritis (classes I–VI) based on mesangial proliferation and resultant inflammation and destruction of the glomeruli. Treatment and prognosis are based on the histologic classification and a renal biopsy is imperative to determine the optimal treatment. Mild renal involvement is seen in class I (mesangial involvement with immune deposits) and class II (mesangial involvement with immune deposits and increased cellularity) and both usually respond to treatment used for SLE in general; hydroxychloroquine and/or low-dose steroids. The concern is for class III focal (<50% of the glomeruli with focal involvement within the glomerulus) and class IV diffuse (>50% of glomeruli, with inflammation/ destruction throughout the glomerulus) glomerulonephritis because both can be associated with hypertension, edema, and progression to renal failure. For classes III and IV, treatment with high-dose steroids and immunosuppression is indicated to prevent ongoing damage. Class V membranous glomerulonephritis (subepithelial immune deposits that result in thickening of the basement membrane of the glomerulus) is characterized by proteinuria and a slower progression to renal failure. Class V is also treated with steroid and often immunosuppression is needed. Class VI glomerulonephritis (advanced sclerotic lesions) has irreversible scarring and there is no benefit to immunosuppressive treatment (Box 2). With more aggressive and consistent treatment overall

Box 2: Lupus nephritis: World Health Organization classification

I. Normal

II. Mesangial disease

III. Focal proliferative: less than 50% glomeruli

IV. Diffuse proliferative: greater than 50% glomeruli

V. Membranous-subepithelial immune deposits

VI. Sclerosing

survival for patients with renal involvement has improved, with markedly improved 5-year and 10-year survival rates [35–40].

Neuropsychiatric lupus occurs in 20% to 95% of patients with SLE, depending on the definition used [39]. Often children present with difficulty concentrating and poor school performance and this is now thought to be related to SLE. Lupus headaches are the most frequent clinically documentable presentation and are defined as a migrainelike, unremitting headache requiring narcotic analgesics. If refractory to treatment, lupus headaches may indicate active CNS vasculitis, increased intracranial pressure, or cerebral vein thrombosis. Thrombotic events are often associated with aPL antibodies and a full work-up with urgent imaging, including MRI, magnetic resonance angiography (MRA), and magnetic resonance venography (MRV) are indicated if thrombosis is suspected (Fig. 3). In these cases, MRI with contrast and MRA and/or MRV help to show whether there has been bleeding or an ischemic event or whether there is demyelination or CNS vasculitis. The MRI/MRA may be normal in antibody-mediated cerebritis, but the cerebrospinal fluid (CSF) shows an increase in immunoglobulin (Ig) G synthesis. These patients may present with psychosis (30%–50%), seizures, movement disorders, cognitive impairment, and coma (Table 2).

Cardiac involvement is seen in 15% to 25% of patients, with symptoms including tachycardia, arrhythmias, and chest pain, but electrocardiogram changes occur in up to 68% who may be asymptomatic. The pericardium is most commonly involved with pericardial effusions. The myocardium and valves can also be affected and sterile verrucous vegetations or Libman-Sacks endocarditis may impair valvular function. With chronic inflammation there is an increased risk of premature arthrosclerosis and one of the highest mortalities in young adults with SLE is from myocardial infarction. The lungs may be involved in 25% to 75% of patients and pleuritis is the most common manifestation, often associated with pleural effusions. Because of the disease and medications, opportunistic infections are concerning and often present as a pneumonia. Infection remains the leading cause of mortality in patients with SLE. Imaging studies, especially high-resolution chest computed tomography (CT) and pulmonary function tests (PFTs) are indicated if pulmonary disease is suspected. Other organ systems, such as the GI tract, ocular involvement, and thyroiditis are seen fairly commonly.

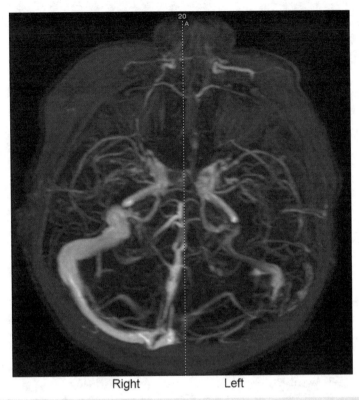

Right   Left

Fig. 3. MRV image of venous thrombosis: hypoplastic left transverse, sigmoid, and anterior superior sagittal sinus. Decreased flow through left transverse and sigmoid sinuses and left jugular. Partial thrombosis/hypoplastic vessels with focal narrowing of the superior sagittal sinus just above the torcula.

Antiphospholipid syndrome

The antiphospholipid syndrome (APS) is an acquired autoimmune prothrombotic state associated with aPL antibodies and beta-2 glycoprotein I (β_2GPI, apolipoprotein H) antibodies. aPL antibodies are directed against phospholipids that are found in cell membranes throughout the body and, as such, are composed of many different antibodies with different epitopes. The most common aPL antibodies are the anticardiolipin antibodies (aCL) and the lupus anticoagulant (LAC). The term lupus anticoagulant is a misnomer and the condition is so called because the phospholipid-dependent partial thromboplastin time (PTT) cascade is prolonged in the presence of aPL antibodies. In contrast, the affected patients are at risk of a thrombotic event because the aPL antibodies bind to the epithelial membranes of blood vessels and activate clotting mechanisms. aPL antibodies alone may be associated with infection, malignancies, or autoimmune states, but are usually benign and transient. There is a risk of thrombosis when the

Table 2
Neuropsychiatric Lupus (NP-Lupus) Laboratory Test and Imaging

NP-Lupus	Labs May Show	CT	MRI	MRA	Angio	LP
Cerebral Hemorrhage	Thrombocytopenia Antibodies to clotting factors	Positive for bleed	Positive for bleed	May show vasculitis	May show vasculitis	Protein: high May have autoantibodies
Cerebral Stroke	Anti-phospholipid Ab	Positive for ischemic changes	Positive for ischemic changes	May show vasculitis	May show vasculitis	Protein: high May have autoantibodies
CNS Vasculitis	May have autoantibodies Labs may be normal	Often appears Normal	Often appears Normal	May show vasculitis	Standard for CNS vasculitis	Protein: high May have autoantibodies
Demyelination	May have autoantibodies Labs may be normal	Often appears Normal	Positive with contrast	Usually normal	Usually normal	Protein: high MBP Oligoclonal bands IgG synthesis: high
Cognitive Dysfunction/ Psychosis	Usually has autoantibodies Labs may be normal	Often appears Normal	May appear Normal	Usually Normal	Usually Normal	Protein: normal or high IgG synthesis Anti-ribosomal P antibodies

Table 3
Biologics Used in Pediatric Rheumatic Diseases

Target	TNF Inhibitors			IL-1 Inhibitors			IL-6	Decreased T Cell Activation	B cell	Decreased B Cell Activation	Th 17 Cells	JAK
Name	Etaner-cept[1]	Adalim-umab[2]	Infli-ximab[3]	Anakinra	Rilona-cept[1]	Canakin-umab[2]	Tociliz-umab[2]	Abata-cept[1]	Ritu-ximab[3]	Belim-umab[2]	Ustekin-umab[2]	Tofaciti-nib
Brand Name	Enbrel	Humira	Remicade	Kineret	Arcalyst	Ilaris	Actemra	Orencia	Rituxan	Benlysta	Stelara	Xeljanz
Approved (Children)	1999 >2yo	2004 >4 yo	NA	2012 Infants	2008 >12yo	2009 >2yo	2011 >2yo	2008 6y or older	NA	NA	NA	NA
Dose	0.8 mg/kg q week SQ	15-30 kg 20 mg q 2 week SQ >30 kg 40 mg q 2 week SQ	6-10 mg/kg q 2 weeks x 2 then q month IV	1 mg/kg q day SQ (higher doses may be required)	4.4 mg/kg SQ loading then 2.3 mg/kg q week (max 160mg)	4 mg/kg q 4 weeks SQ	>2yo <30kg 10-12 mg/kg q 2-4 weeks IV >30kg 8 mg/kg q 2 weeks IV	<75 kg 10 mg/kg q 2 weeks x3 then q 4 weeks IV	375 mg/M_2 q 1 week x 4 or 750 mg/M_2 q 2 weeks x 2 IV	10 mg/kg q 2 weeks x3 then q 4 weeks IV	45 mg q 4 week x1 then q 12 weeks SQ	5 mg po BID
Used to Treat	JIA (oligo-ex, poly), PsA, ERA, JAS	JIA (oligo-ex, poly), PsA, ERA, JAS, Uveitis	JIA (oligo-ex, poly), PsA, ERA, JAS, Uveitis, Vasculitis (Takayasu)	JIA (systemic), periodic fevers	JIA (systemic), periodic fevers, Gout	JIA (systemic), periodic fevers	JIA (poly, systemic)	JIA (oligo-ex, poly), Uveitis, Arthritis of SLE, MCTD	SLE, ITP, Evan's, CAPS, Vasculitis (GPA, MPA), JIA (RF+poly)	SLE	PsA, Crohn's	JIA (oligo- ex, poly), ERA/JAS
Toxicity	Inf. reaction, infections, TB, fungal, MS, lymphoma, possibly uveitis	Inf. reaction, infections, TB, fungal, MS, lymphoma	Inf. reaction, infections, TB, fungal, MS, lymphoma	Inj. site reaction, infection, high LFTs	Inf. reaction, infections, infection, high LFTs, lipids	Inf. reaction, infections, infection, high LFTs, neutropenia	Inf./hypersensitivity reactions, infection, TB, malignancy, MS, high lipids, GI perforation	Inf. reaction, infections	Inf. reaction, infections, progressive multifocal encephalopathy (JC polyoma virus)	Inf. reaction, infection	Inf. reaction, infections, infection, high LFTs	Infection, high LFTs Avoid with liver disease

Used with Other Drugs	MTX 10-15 mg/M$_2$ q week po or SQ	MTX 10-15 mg/M$_2$ q week po or SQ	MTX 10-15 mg/M$_2$ q week po or SQ	Cyclosporin 2.5-5 mg/kg/d	MTX 10-15 mg/M$_2$ q week po or SQ	MTX 10-15 mg/M$_2$ q week po or SQ	MTX 10-15 mg/M$_2$ q week po or SQ	Other immune-suppressives	Other immune-suppressives	Other immune-suppressives	MTX 10-15 mg/M$_2$ q week po or SQ

These are the most commonly used biologics as of this date, however, many more are being developed.

The brand name is the name used in the US.

Name: 1. -cept (fusion protein), 2. -umab (humanized monoclonal antibody). 3. -ximab (chimeric monoclonal antibody).

Anakinra: A recombinant form of IL-1 Ra.

Abatacept: CTLA$_4$ binds CD80/86 preventing the binding of CD28 to CD80/86.

Belimumab: Anti-Blys monoclonal antibody

Approved: The date given is the FDA approval in children. Although all are not FDA approved in children, these biologics prove to be optimal in certain cases. Those "Not Approved" (NA) are as of 2015.

Dose: The usual doses, but each may be dosed differently or in higher doses with very active disease

Used to Treat: The uses are expanding and each biologic may have additional uses
Oligoarticular (oligo)
Extended polyarticular (Ex poly)

Toxicity: Only the common ones are listed. Please see the package insert for full information
Injection (Inj)
Infusion (Inf)

Used with other drugs: The use of combined therapies increases the effectiveness in decreasing inflammation. With arthritis, methotrexate (MTX) is often used in combined therapies, however if not tolerated leflunomide (Arava) may be used at <20 kg, 10 mg/q alternate day po, 20-40 kg 10 mg /day po, >40 20 mg/day po. In children with SLE, hydroxychloroquine (Plaquenil) and other immunosuppressives are used in combination. In children with Crohn's medications are combined to control bowel inflammation.

aPL antibodies are found in high titers of IgG or IgM subtypes, are LAC positive, and are associated with anti-β_2GPI. These prothrombotic antibodies persist and are present when retested in 12 weeks. β_2GPI is a positively charged polypeptide that is made by hepatocytes and endothelial cells. The function is not fully elucidated, but it may play a role in preventing clotting on the endothelial surface. Once bound to the negatively charged aPL antibodies, however, β_2GP1 is associated with a pathologic state in which the risk of thrombosis is the greatest. It is estimated that the incidence of APS is 5 per 100,000 and the prevalence is 40 to 50 per 100,000 [41,42]. APS can occur as a primary disease without an associated autoimmune disease, but is most often found in patients with SLE. In children with SLE, aCL, β_2GPI, and LA are found in 44%, 40% and 22% respectively. Children may present with arterial, venous, or small vessel thromboses. Only 16% to 36% of children with aPL antibodies are at risk of having a thrombotic event, but those with LAC positivity have a 28-fold increased risk of a thrombotic event. The most frequent thrombotic event is a deep vein thrombosis followed by cerebral sinus vein thrombosis, portal vein thrombosis, thromboses in the deep veins of the upper extremities, and superficial vein thromboses. Thrombocytopenia and hemolytic anemia may also be secondary to aCL binding to the red cell and platelet membranes. Thrombotic thrombocytopenic purpura and hemolytic uremic syndrome are often complicated by aCLs, although their role is unclear. Treatment in asymptomatic children with SLE may include monitoring the levels of aPL yearly. Some clinicians start hydroxychloroquine (Plaquenil), which has been shown to decrease erythrocyte aggregation on the endothelium. Low-dose aspirin is often used as an anticoagulant, but its efficacy is in question. In cases in which anticoagulation is clearly needed, warfarin (Coumadin), low-molecular-weight heparin (Lovenox), or other anticoagulants are used, often for 6 months or longer. Catastrophic APS (CAPS) is of particular concern because this is a life-threatening disease process in which 3 or more organ systems develop small vessel occlusions within 1 week in association with aPL. Children with CAPS often present with adult respiratory distress syndrome, hypertension, renal failure, and multiple other organ system involvement requiring intensive care therapies. Immediate and aggressive therapy, including anticoagulation, plasmapheresis, and corticosteroids is necessary to reverse the thrombotic storm, but the mortality is still reported at 40% to 50%. In this patient population, lifelong anticoagulant therapy is indicated.

Differential diagnosis
The differential is extensive and, because the presentation of SLE is so variable, infections, malignancy, and other autoimmune diseases must be considered. The criteria for diagnosis are helpful in determining the diagnosis, as are low complement levels (C_3, C_4). Low complement levels lead to poor opsonization of organisms and infection, including opportunistic infections, are a great risk.

Laboratory tests
Autoantibodies are the hallmark of SLE and a positive ANA is found in virtually all of the patients, but is not specific or necessarily associated with

disease manifestations [36–40]. The autoantibodies target intracellular molecules: histone, nonhistone, RNA-binding, cytoplasmic, and nuclear proteins that are thought to be externalized in blebs during apoptosis/necrosis. Anti-DNA antibodies are the most commonly seen (65%–95%) and are associated with disease activity, especially with active renal disease. Anti-Ro and La antibodies (27%–33%) are seen less frequently, but are associated with skin disease and neonatal lupus. Anticardiolipin antibodies (19%–87%) and the LAC (10%–62%) make up the aPL and are associated with an increased risk of thrombosis especially when found in combination with β_2GPI. There is often involvement of the hematologic system, as discussed earlier. The acute phase reactants are often at increased levels and may remain so throughout the course of the disease. One of the most helpful tests to determine disease activity is the measurement of C_3 and C_4 complements. With the binding of antibodies to self-proteins and immune complexes, the complement levels are depleted, and the lower the complement level, the more active the lupus disease process.

Treatment and prognosis
Organ damage can occur early in the disease so it is important to confirm the diagnosis and start treatments as soon as possible [36,39–42]. With mild disease involving primarily musculoskeletal and/or cutaneous symptoms, the child is treated with NSAIDs and antimalarials (hydroxychloroquine 6.5 mg/kg/d; ophthalmology visits every 6–12 months for toxicity). In cases that do not respond, the anti-BLyS monoclonal antibody belimumab (Benlysta) may be useful in treating skin disease and musculoskeletal manifestations [43,44]. Because the disease may progress, it is important to monitor the course routinely. Most often children with SLE present with renal or other organ system involvement and more than 90% require the use of corticosteroids at some point. The kidney is frequently involved in children with SLE and prognosis often depends on the degree of renal involvement and the response to treatment. Patients with class III to IV disease require early and aggressive treatment with an induction and maintenance phase. In the pediatric population, a combination of high-dose glucocorticoids and cyclophosphamide is often required. Pulse methylprednisolone (15–30 mg/kg; maximum 1000 mg) is given intravenously for 3 days, if there is no concern for infection and if the child is not hypertensive. Otherwise, intravenous (IV) methylprednisolone or oral prednisone/prednisolone is started at 2 mg/kg/d in divided doses. Following the methylprednisolone pulse, oral prednisone/prednisolone (1–2 mg/kg/d) is used and slowly tapered once the symptoms and laboratory values improve. Corticosteroids are given in conjunction with an immunosuppression. If the renal biopsy shows very active disease, IV cyclophosphamide administered as monthly pulses (500–1000 mg/m^2) is used in children. The side effects are considerable, including GI disturbances, bone marrow suppression, hemorrhagic cystitis, and gonadal suppression. For this reason, some centers use azathioprine (Imuran 1–2.5 mg/kg/d PO or mycophenolate mofetil (MMF; 600 mg/m^2 PO twice a day) as an induction therapy. Maintenance

therapy is most often with hydroxychloroquine, low-dose steroids, and MMF. Children with class V glomerulonephritis may not require such aggressive treatment, depending on the response to early therapy. Patients with involvement of the CNS often require similar therapy but also benefit from plasmapheresis with 5 to 10 plasma exchanges and rituximab, a humanized monoclonal anti-CD20 antibody that depletes B cells. There are no randomized control trials for the use of rituximab, but often it seems to be useful in cytopenias, APS, and antibody-driven disease. Aspirin or other anticoagulants are used in patients with APS to prevent thrombotic events. Aspirin is thought to be of questionable benefit if there is concern about a procoagulant state and warfarin or the newer anticoagulants are used in children who have had a thrombotic event. Children who have had CAPS are on lifelong anticoagulation. Statins may be useful in adolescents, especially in those with abnormal fasting lipid levels. All the treatments have adverse effects. For example, ibuprofen has been associated with aseptic meningitis in patients with SLE. Corticosteroids must be used judiciously because of the known adverse effects of weight gain, poor skin healing, and osteoporosis, but additionally because approximately 10% of patients with SLE develop avascular necrosis that is associated with steroid use. The risk of infection is always high in patients with SLE and especially so for those requiring immunosuppression. Children and adolescents with SLE should be counselled on diet and physical activity. Monitoring of the fasting lipid levels, supplementation with calcium and vitamin D, and a program of exercise to maintain good bone health are essential. Survival rates have improved markedly with 5-year and 10-year survival rates greater than 95% and 92%, respectively, among pediatric patients, but the prognosis is still guarded for children with SLE, especially as they enter adulthood. Atherosclerosis generally begins in adolescence and is worse in children with SLE because of the inflammation of the disease and the treatments. The risk of myocardial infarction or stroke is 6 to 9 times greater in women with SLE across all ages compared with controls. In the first 2 years, mortality is often associated with infections and severe disease: pancreatitis, pulmonary hemorrhage, thromboembolic disease, and active neuropsychiatric disease. Five years or more after diagnosis, causes of mortality include complications of end-stage renal disease, atherosclerosis, suicide, and less commonly active SLE or infection.

Inflammatory myopathies

Chronic inflammatory myopathies are rare in children, but the most common is juvenile dermatomyositis (JDM) characterized by a vasculopathy and inflammation of muscles, primarily the striated muscles, and skin [45–48]. As with most autoimmune diseases, JDM is thought to be an interplay between genetics and environmental stimuli. Genetic risk factors are being studied and in about half of the patients there is a family history of autoimmune disease. A viral illness may precede the onset of JDM and Coxsackie virus, influenza, group A *Streptococcus*, toxoplasmosis, parvovirus, hepatitis B, *Borrelia*, and leishmania have been associated with disease onset. On muscle or skin biopsy, an angiopathy is noted with an infiltration of plasmacytoid dendritic cells, helper T cells, and B cells around the muscle capillary and endothelium that leads to vascular damage and ischemia of the skin or muscle fibers. The striated muscles are predominately involved, but there can be involvement of the GI and cardiac muscles. Polymyositis is very rare in children, but tends to be severe and difficult to treat. It is not associated with a rash and the disorder is mediated by cytotoxic T cells that destroy muscle fibers.

Epidemiology

Incidence and prevalence

The incidence of JDM is calculated at 3.2 per million children. The prevalence is not known.

Ethnic background

There is no clear ethnic predilection.

Age and gender

The age range at onset of JDM is 5 to 14 years, with a peak at 7.6 years. Adults may also present with dermatomyositis between 45 and 64 years of age and the presentation may be associated with malignancy, but the association with malignancy is rare in JDM. JDM is more frequent in female patients, with an overall F/M ratio of 1.7:1, but may be as high as 2.7:1 [45].

Clinical presentation

The criteria for diagnosis of JDM include symmetric proximal muscle weakness, characteristic cutaneous changes including a heliotrope rash (over the eyelids associated with periorbital edema) and Gottron papules, increased muscle enzyme levels (creatine kinase [CK], aspartate transaminase [AST], alanine aminotransferase ALT, lactate dehydrogenase [LDH], and aldolase), and an electromyogram with myopathy and denervation with a diagnostic confirmation by muscle biopsy [45–48].

The presentation is often an insidious progression over 3 to 6 months with malaise, low-grade fevers, and fatigue. More than 75% of these children have the classic rashes and this may be the initial presentation. There may also be inflammation and erythema of the periungual skin and capillary nail bed with ulceration. Muscle pain or tenderness occurs in 25% to 75% and there is proximal muscle weakness of the neck and abdominal muscles, limb girdle, and lower extremities. On examination, these children are unable to sit up from the supine position without rolling over and using their arms to push them into a sitting position, to rise from sitting to standing, to squat or sit on the floor, and get up without help. On getting up from the floor, the Gowers sign is often present and on walking there may be a truncal sway and a positive Trendelenburg, indicating weakness of the hip muscles. Other musculature may be involved, including the pharyngeal, hypopharyngeal, and palatal muscles, causing dysphonia, aspiration, and/or respiratory distress. It is important to evaluate this urgently with a barium swallow and PFTs and to protect the airway. Often the joints are involved with arthritis and arthralgia. The muscle of the GI tract may be involved, with small ulcerations causing microperforations throughout the bowel. This picture presents with progressive abdominal pain, melena, and hematemesis, or an ileus. Imaging studies may show free intraperitoneal air but, because the perforations are multiple and small, often no free air is noted. This condition is a medical emergency and children should be treated for sepsis and evaluated for possible surgical intervention. Cardiac involvement is rare, but may be life threatening. Myocarditis, conduction defects, and first-degree heart block can be seen and prompt a complete cardiac work-up before any surgeries. The disease presents with an active vasculopathy but, as the disease is treated and the inflammation abates, there may be healing with the laying down of calcinosis in 12% to 43% of patients. Calcification may occur in the skin, muscle belly, or diffusely and is problematic because of recurrent skin ulcerations, limitation of motion, and increased infection rates caused by poor skin integrity. Treatment of calcinosis is difficult and the condition may require surgical removal in some instances.

Laboratory studies
Laboratory studies, including the CBC and inflammatory markers (ESR and CRP), may show normal or slightly increased levels. Levels of the sarcoplasmic muscle enzymes, AST, CK, LDH, and aldolase are increased and contribute to making the diagnosis, and are useful to monitor the effectiveness of therapy. AST and LDH correlate the best with active disease. Usually the CK level is increased, but may fluctuate and is the first to decrease with adequate therapy. The ANA is positive in 10% to 85% of patients and antibodies against small RNA antigens (RNP, Sjogren's Syndrome A/Sjogren's Syndrome B [SSA/SSB]) may be present. Traditional myositis-specific autoantibodies are rare in JDM, although Anti-Jo-1 occurs in 2% to 5% and anti-Mi-2 occurs in 1% to 7% of children. Recently, novel autoantibodies have been associated with JDM and have a predictive value in the disease course. These include: transcription intermediary factor 1 (TIF-1) found in 20–30% of JDM patients and associated with photosensitivity, lipodystrophy and a more chronic course; nuclear matrix protein 2 (NXP2) found in 20–25% of JDM patients and associated with muscle cramps, dysphonia, joint contractures, and possibly with increased risk of calcinosis; and melanoma differentiation- associated protein 5 (MDA5) that is rare in JDM, but is associated with rapidly progressive interstitial lung disease [45]. Some centers offer a myositis panel that includes these autoantibodies. Because of the vasculopathy, the factor VIII–related antigen (von Willebrand factor) may be high in children with active disease. Flow cytometry studies often show increased numbers of CD19+ B cells that play a role in the disease process. MRI, especially the fat-suppressed T2-weighted or short tau inversion recovery sequences, is optimal to show hyperintensity indicating muscle edema.

Treatment and prognosis
Corticosteroids are the initial treatment used for children with JDM [48,49] to decrease the inflammation to improve the skin manifestations and muscle

strength. In addition, corticosteroids used early prevent the chronic inflammation and ischemia that leads to calcinosis. If there is severe inflammation or weakness, a Solu-Medrol pulse (30 mg/kg, maximum 1000 mg, each day for 3 days) or a daily oral prednisone dose of 2 mg/kg is the first line of treatment. JDM may be monocyclic with a good response after the initial treatment. As the strength improves and the muscle enzymes return to normal, steroids are tapered. If the course of JDM is polycyclic (a recurrence after a remission) or chronic (active disease for >2 years) prolonged therapy for more than 2 years is continued. In these cases, if there is an inadequate response or it is not possible to reduce the steroids, MTX (10–15 mg/m^2/wk) is generally the second line of therapy. Hydroxychloroquine (6.5 mg/kg/d) is useful for skin manifestations and can be combined with MTX. Immunosuppressives may be necessary, especially for patients with chronic disease, to treat the vasculopathy of the bowel or other organs. For severe involvement, cyclophosphamide is indicated, but in less severe cases azathioprine or cyclosporine are used [46–50]. More recently, rituximab has been found to reverse severe muscle disease in some studies [50–52]. IL-6 inhibition has proved effective in case reports. Most children with JDM benefit from physical therapy. It is important to protect the skin from ultraviolet (UV) light and tissue injury. Diet and physical activity are important to promote optimal intake of calcium and vitamin D and to prevent osteopenia, muscle atrophy, and contractures. The prognosis is generally good for children with monocyclic and polycyclic disease, but up to 80% may have cutaneous scarring, joint contractures, persistent weakness, muscle dysfunction, and calcinosis.

Scleroderma

Scleroderma is categorized into localized scleroderma (LS) and systemic sclerosis (SS). Both are associated with accumulation of collagen and fibrosis, but the diseases are distinct in that LS is limited to the skin and almost never involves the internal organs, whereas SS has diffuse skin involvement and usually affects multiple internal organs. The pathogenesis is associated with abnormalities of regulation of fibroblasts and production of collagen, and immunologic abnormalities that lead to chronic thickening of the skin and, in SS, other organs.

Localized scleroderma

LS can involve a patch or plaque of skin called morphea or a linear streak of skin. Morphea is divided into circumscribed, usually small patches (superficial or deep), generalized with 2 to 7 plaques, or pansclerotic with circumferential involvement of the limbs. The forms may also be mixed. In children the most common form of scleroderma is morphea and some dermatologists do not think this should be classified as scleroderma when only a small patch of skin is involved. Usually this does not progress and can be monitored or treated locally. The linear form involves the trunk or limb and may cross a joint. If it involves the head and face it is called en coup de sabre, Parry-Romberg syndrome, or progressive hemifacial atrophy [53–56].

Epidemiology

Incidence and prevalence

The prevalence of morphea in children less than 17 years old is estimated to be 50 per 100,000. The incidence of LS approximately is 0.34 to 2.7 per 100,000 [53].

Ethnic background

Linear scleroderma is most often found in children of European background (73%–82%).

Age and gender

Linear scleroderma generally is seen predominantly in the pediatric population, with 67% diagnosed before 18 years of age. Girls are affected slightly more frequently than boys (1.7–3.1:1 F/M).

Clinical manifestations

Morphea, areas of indurated, waxy skin with an ivory center and violaceous halo, is most commonly found on the trunk. The lesions may be small (<1 cm) and are called guttate, or the lesions may be larger and become confluent, called generalized morphea. Deep morphea includes subcutaneous morphea, eosinophilic fasciitis, and morphea profunda, in which the entire skin is thickened and feels bound down. This form is the least common and is considered the most disabling. LS involves streaks of thickened skin and typically involves the upper or lower extremities. The skin can become progressively more indurated and can extend through the dermis, subcutaneous tissue, and muscle to the underlying bone. En coup de sabre involves the scalp and head and is thought to look like the depression caused by a dueling stroke from a sword. The Parry-Romberg syndrome is characterized by a progressive hemifacial atrophy of the skin and tissue beneath. Patients with Parry-Romberg are at risk for dental and ocular abnormalities and may develop a seizure disorder. Although LS involves primarily the skin, some patients develop musculoskeletal complaints.

Laboratory studies

Antinuclear antibodies are present in 23% to 73% of patients, but do not predict the disease course. Antihistone antibodies are detected in 47%, are associated with more extensive localized disease, and may be useful in assessing disease activity.

Treatment and prognosis

Topical therapies are the first line of treatment and include corticosteroid creams, vitamin D creams, tacrolimus, or imiquimod (an immunomodulatory that inhibits the collagen production by fibroblasts). UV phototherapy is sometimes used for superficial lesions. Systemic treatment with MTX is the second line of treatment if the lesions do not resolve or extend further or deeper. If there is an erythematous edge around an extending lesion, some centers start a short course of corticosteroids in combination with MTX. If the lesions do not improve or continue to progress, MMF is useful to inhibit further fibrosis. The difficulty in measuring the lesion size makes it difficult to fully assess response to treatment.

Systemic sclerosis

SS is subdivided by the extent of the skin disease into diffuse cutaneous SS (dSSc) and limited cutaneous SS (lSSc), previously designated as the CREST (calcinosis cutis, Raynaud phenomenon, esophageal dysfunction, sclerodactyly, telangiectasia) syndrome. The systemic form of the disease is rare in children [57].

Epidemiology

Incidence and prevalence

There are worldwide reports of dSSc with an incidence of 0.45 to 1.9 per 100,000 and a prevalence of 24 per 100,000. Children younger than 20 years of age comprise only about 1.2% to 9% of cases.

Ethnic background

Studies suggest that SS is more frequent in African Americans and in Choctaw Native Americans, although it is seen in all ethnic backgrounds.

Age and gender

In children, boys and girls are affected equally, but in adolescents, girls are affected more frequently.

Clinical manifestations

The International Committee on Classification Criteria for Juvenile Systemic Sclerosis developed criteria useful in diagnosis and research [58]. Juvenile SS is defined in children as: age <16 years old and 1 major criterion (presence of skin sclerosis/induration proximal to the metacarpophalangeal or metatarsophalangeal) and at least 2 of the 20 minor criteria that include skin (sclerodactyly, vasculopathy, Raynaud's, nail fold capillary abnormalities, digital tip ulcers), GI (dysphagia, gastroesophageal reflux), renal (renal crisis, arterial hypertension), cardiac (arrhythmias, heart failure), respiratory (pulmonary fibrosis, decreased carbon monoxide diffusion in the lung, pulmonary hypertension), musculoskeletal (tendon friction rubs, arthritis, myositis), neurologic (neuropathy, carpal tunnel syndrome), and autoantibodies (ANA, anticentromere, antitopoisomerase I, antifibrillarin, anti-PM-Scl, antifibrillin, or anti-RNA polymerase I or III). The course is insidious and waxes and wanes, and children and their parents may not notice subtle changes until there is significant impact on function and/or mobility. Usually the child has a history of Raynaud's phenomenon. At the onset, there may be edema of the skin for a few weeks or months and this may offer a window of opportunity for treatment to decrease the inflammation and the resulting fibrosis. Following this the sclerotic phase becomes noticeable, especially over the digits (acrosclerosis, sclerodactyly) and face (circumoral furrowing). In addition, there is atrophy of the skin. Telangiectasia and calcinosis may be seen during this process. Multiple other organ systems are often involved. Arthritis is a symptom in approximately 36% of children, with morning stiffness and pain of the small joints of the hands, knees, and ankles. The cause of the greatest morbidity and mortality is related to involvement of the cardiovascular, pulmonary, renal, and GI systems. The presence of anti–topoisomerase I antibody and rapidly progressing skin involvement are thought to be predictors of renal and cardiac involvement.

Laboratory findings
Often there is an anemia of chronic disease or malnutrition related to poor oral intake and/or absorption. Eosinophilia occurs in approximately 15% of patients. Autoantibodies are present in most patients. There are high titers of ANAs in the speckled pattern in 80% of patients. Antitopoisomerase I (anti–Scl-70) autoantibodies are present in 28% to 34% of patients with dSSc with peripheral vascular disease, digital pitting, pulmonary interstitial fibrosis, renal involvement, and higher mortality. Anticentromere antibodies occurred almost exclusively in patients with lSSc in association with calcinosis and telangiectasias, but are rarely seen in children. Imaging of the chest, especially high-resolution chest CT, helps to monitor pulmonary involvement and PFTs detect interstitial lung disease or signs of pulmonary hypertension.

Treatment and prognosis
The optimal treatment is not yet known for dSSc and lSSc and often patients do not seem to respond to therapies [57]. If there is edema of the skin, some rheumatologists use corticosteroids, but with caution because there is a relationship between the use of high-dose steroids and the development of scleroderma renal crisis. Routinely, MTX or other immunosuppressants are used to treat skin thickening. MMF is proposed to be useful to decrease the laying down of collagen. To treat involvement of the GI tract, GI reflux is treated by H_2 blockers and proton pump inhibitors. Raynaud's and digital ulcers are treated with calcium channel blockers and medications that relax smooth muscles (sildenafil, tadalafil). More recently, iloprost (synthetic analogue of prostacyclin PGI2) is used acutely for severe digital ulcers. Both iloprost and endothelial receptor antagonists (bosentan or macitentan; competitive antagonists of endothelin-1) are useful in pulmonary hypertension to increase vascular dilatation and decrease pulmonary vascular resistance. To decrease inflammation in the lung, cyclophosphamide may be used in severe cases and other immunosuppression (MMF or azathioprine) and hydroxychloroquine in more mild cases. Angiotensin-converting enzyme inhibitors play an important role in preventing a renal crisis. Supportive care is of great importance with attention to skin integrity, joint range of movement, and GI issues with weight loss. The family and child need to be educated as to the disease and its complications, and information for the school and community should be available. Despite all treatment efforts, the prognosis is extremely guarded.

Vasculitis

Vasculitis is an inflammatory process involving the blood vessel wall, and thus any organ system may be involved. Vasculitis may be the primary disease process or complicate an autoimmune disease, infection, or malignancy. In primary vasculitis, the disease is defined by the size of the affected vessels [59–63]. Small vessel disease includes Henoch-Schönlein purpura (HSP), isolated cutaneous leukocytoclastic vasculitis, hypocomplementemic urticarial vasculitis, microscopic polyangiitis, and when associated with granulomas includes granulomatosis with polyarteritis (GPA; formally Wegener), and the Churg-Strauss syndrome (CSS). Medium-sized vessels include polyarteritis nodosa (PAN), cutaneous polyarteritis, and Kawasaki disease (KD). The large vessels are involved in Takayasu arteritis (TA).

Epidemiology

Incidence and prevalence

The incidence of vasculitis is estimated to be 23 per 100,000. HSP and KD are seen most commonly, but the prevalence is difficult to determine because these diseases are self-limited.

Ethnic background

All ethnic backgrounds have been reported to have childhood vasculitis. The incidence of HSP is higher in children of European background, KD is higher in children of Asian background, and Behçet is higher in Turkish children.

Age and gender

For HSP, the peak age is 4 to 6 years and boys are affected more frequently (F:M ratio is 1:2). Most children with KD are less than 5 years old and it occurs more frequently in boys. The mean age for PAN is 9 years and the mean age for GPA is 14 years.

Clinical manifestations

Henoch-Schönlein purpura

The classic picture of HSP is lower-extremity purpura over the legs and buttocks. Arthritis is often seen, can be the presenting feature in about 50% of children, and is present at some point in 75% of children. The arthritis follows an oligoarticular pattern, but self-resolves in 3 to 4 weeks. The GI tract is involved in 50% to 75% of children. Usually the children have a crampy abdominal pain. Most often, this is limited to bowel wall edema, but the course may be complicated by bleeding, intussusception, and in severe cases necrosis of the bowel wall. Proteinuria is present in 20% to 60% and is concerning for renal involvement, but ongoing renal disease is rare and the risk of chronic renal impairment and end-stage renal disease is 2% to 15% and less than 1%, respectively. Occasionally, HSP can be associated with severe edema over the trunk associated with a low albumin level. Rarely there is pulmonary and CNS involvement. The laboratory studies are usually normal, except for occasional increases in the acute phase reactant levels. If there is renal involvement, there may be hematuria or proteinuria. This should be monitored with urine dipstick assessments monthly for 6 months since renal disease may present late and after other clinical symptoms have resolved. The stool should be tested for blood, indicating GI involvement and a need for intervention or therapy. The disease process may recur in up to 33% and the rash often comes in crops made worse by activity. HSP usually self-resolves in less than a month, but may persist for 3 months. Cutaneous leukocytoclastic vasculitis and microscopic polyangiitis are types of hypersensitivity vasculitides that are triggered by infection or drug exposure. The cause is often difficult to determine. The process usually self-resolves in a period of 4 to 8 weeks.

Differential diagnosis. A differential diagnosis includes other diseases associated with purpura, especially infectious causes such as sepsis with diffuse intravascular coagulation. Depending on the symptoms, acute hemorrhagic edema of infancy, immune thrombocytopenic purpura, acute poststreptococcal glomerulonephritis, hemolytic uremic syndrome, and hypersensitivity vasculitis should be considered.

Treatment and prognosis. Most HSP is mild and care is supportive with analgesics and NSAIDs. In children with severe abdominal pain, corticosteroids orally or, if the child is unable to eat, methylprednisolone (1-2 mg.kg per day in divided doses) is used to prevent ongoing GI inflammation. In general, HSP resolves and the outcome is good.

Kawasaki disease

KD is the second most common childhood vasculitis and is of concern because of the possibility of residual cardiac sequelae. The medium-sized blood vessels are involved. The European League Against Rheumatism (EULAR)/Paediatric Rheumatology European Society (PReS) classification criteria for KD are a fever for ≥ 5 days and 4 of the following: bilateral conjunctival injection, mucous membrane changes of the lips and oral cavity, cervical lymphadenopathy, polymorphic exanthem, and rash and/or swelling in the peripheral extremities or perineal area. Fewer than 4 criteria are required if there are fevers and characteristic coronary artery changes.

There are 3 phases in KD: (1) an acute febrile period that lasts up to 14 days, (2) a subacute phase of 2 to 4 weeks, and (3) a convalescent phase that can last months to years. During the first phase, the fever is high ($>38.5°C$) and there are increased concentrations of proinflammatory cytokines, particularly IL-6, IL-1, and TNF-α. During the acute phase, inflammation affecting the heart may include valvulitis, myocarditis, and pericarditis. Coronary dilatation and aneurysms may be detected during the acute phase, but develop during the convalescent phase in up to 20% of children, especially in very young children or if treatment was delayed. There may be multiple organ systems involved, including the GI tract with vomiting, abdominal pain, and hydrops of the gallbladder; the musculoskeletal system with arthritis, and the CNS. Most of the children are very irritable, suggesting an aseptic meningitis and headache.

The laboratory tests show high levels of acute phase reactants, a high WBC with a shift to the left, and high platelet counts. Because of the disturbance of the vessel membranes, the lipid profiles are abnormal and the triglyceride levels are often increased. Antineutrophil cytoplasmic antibodies (ANCAs) may be positive as the disease progresses.

Differential diagnosis. This includes infections, especially viral infections; Epstein-Barr virus, adenovirus, echovirus, measles, toxic shock syndrome, scarlet fever, other autoimmune diseases, and Stevens-Johnson syndrome.

Treatment and prognosis. Early treatment prevents cardiac complications in up to 80% of children. The American Heart Association recommends treatment with high-dose aspirin (80–100 mg/kg/d) and IV immunoglobulin (IVIG; 2 g/kg) within the first 10 days of disease. The aspirin is decreased to an antiplatelet dose of 3 to 5 mg/kg/d after the child is afebrile for 48 hours. If the fever persists or returns, a second course of IVIG is warranted. Infliximab, an anti–TNF-α agent (5 mg/kg), did not prove statistically better than a second IVIG in refractory KD. Because there are high levels of inflammatory cytokines, IL-1 inhibition may prove therapeutic. The ultimate outcome is undetermined to date. Usually children recover from the acute disease, but if there are coronary aneurysms there may be long-term sequelae.

Polyarteritis nodosa

This is an uncommon disease in children, but can be life-threating. The EULAR/PreS formulated criteria for PAN that includes systemic inflammation with evidence of necrotizing vasculitis with abnormalities of medium-sized or small-sized arteries plus 1 of the following: skin involvement (livedo reticularis and infarcts); myalgias; hypertension; peripheral neuropathy; and renal involvement with proteinuria, hematuria, and/or impaired function.

With PAN, there is vascular insufficiency to multiple organ systems. The children tend to be ill with fever, malaise, and weight loss complicated by ischemia to involved organs. Often painful subcutaneous nodules develop along affected vessels and help in the diagnosis. The laboratory tests are consistent with the inflammatory state and the acute phase reactant levels are high with a mild leukocytosis and anemia. The perinuclear antineutrophil cytoplasmic antibody (pANCA) may be positive.

Treatment and prognosis

Corticosteroids are used initially, either oral or IV pulse methylprednisolone. Cyclophosphamide is indicated in severe life-threatening and organ-threatening situations. Plasmapheresis has been shown to be helpful in some cases. Maintenance agents include azathioprine, MTX, IVIG, and MMF. Recent studies suggest that rituximab may treat this disease effectively. The prognosis is guarded because of the severe organ involvement during the acute phase.

Takayasu arteritis
This is a granulomatous vasculitis that affects the large vessels, primarily the aorta and its branches. Criteria include characteristic angiographic abnormalities of the aorta or its main branches and pulmonary arteries plus 1 of the following: abnormal pulses or claudication, blood pressure discrepancy in any limb, bruits, hypertension, and increased acute phase reactant levels. The diagnosis may be difficult to make because the symptoms are usually nonspecific. However, there are clinical clues with absent peripheral pulses, hypertension, CNS symptoms, and claudication. The laboratory tests may be normal, but more often there is increase of the acute phase reactant levels and anemia. Imaging helps to confirm the diagnosis.

Treatment and prognosis
Corticosteroids are the mainstay of treatment and induce remission in up to 60% of patients. Other treatments include azathioprine, cyclophosphamide, and MMF. Of note, infliximab may be beneficial in these patients [59,63]. Some of these children go into remission, but the ultimate prognosis depends on the severity of organ involvement during the acute phase.

Childhood primary central nervous system vasculitis
This may present in children with a fairly acute onset and can include neurologic and/or psychiatric symptoms. Imaging is the mainstay of diagnosis. There are 2 types of childhood primary CNS vasculitis: (1) angiography positive, which is seen on MRA and affects the medium and large vessels; (2) angiography negative, which affects the small vessels. To confirm the diagnosis of small vessel disease, an angiogram or brain biopsy may be required. Of note, the laboratory studies may be normal peripherally with no clues to the extent of the CNS vasculitis. The CSF may show increased protein levels or may be normal. Imaging confirms the diagnosis. Therapy includes corticosteroids, either oral or IV, but most often, cyclophosphamide is necessary to control the vasculits. For maintenance therapy, azathioprine or MMF are used for therapeutic control.

Antineutrophil cytoplasmic antibody vasculitis
There are 3 ANCA-associated vasculitides, with small and medium vessel inflammation: (1) granulomatosis with polyangiitis (GPA; formerly known as Wegener granulomatosis), (2) microscopic polyangiitis (MPA), and (3) Churg-Strauss syndrome (CSS). GPA is a granulomatous, small vessel vasculitis that involves the upper and lower respiratory tracts and the kidneys. MPA is a necrotizing, nongranulomatous, pauci-immune disease that affects the small vessels, usually involving the pulmonary capillaries (capillaritis) with a necrotizing glomerulonephritis. CSS is rare in children, but affects the pulmonary tract in adults with long-standing asthma. The laboratory studies show increased levels of acute phase reactants. Autoantibodies include ANA (20%), RF (50%), and ANCAs. The cytoplasmic antineutrophil cytoplamic antibodies (cANCA) is present in 80% to 90% of patient with GPA. In MPA, and CSS the perinuclear cytoplasmic antibodies (pANCA) are positive in 20% to

40%. The treatments include corticosteroids and cyclophosphamide (oral or IV). Several studies show the efficacy of rituximab in treating GPA and in some centers, this is used as an initial therapy. Despite treatment, there is a high rate of relapse. In milder disease, MTX and corticosteroids are used for induction and MTX may be used for maintenance. In more severe cases, higher doses of steroids and cyclophosphamide are needed. Maintenance therapy includes MTX, MMF, or azathioprine for 18 to 24 months. Studies suggest that infliximab, rituximab, and IVIG (2 g/kg/mo) are options for refractory disease. Depending on the extent of the disease, the prognosis is guarded.

Collaborative efforts

In North America and Europe, pediatric rheumatologists have collaborated to determine clinical presentations, disease course, and optimal treatment algorithms and outcomes. In North America, The Childhood Arthritis and Rheumatology Research Alliance (CARRA) is made up of pediatric rheumatologists from Canada and the United States who study investigator-initiated projects, while the Pediatric Rheumatology Collaborative Study Group (PRCGS), studies industry-initiated clinical trials. The Paediatric Rheumatology International Trials Organization (PRINTO), is a similar European organization. These 3 organizations collaborate and often join in studies to attain statistically significant data to improve the outcomes for children with rheumatic diseases.

BIOLOGICS

Over the last 3 decades, there have been major advances in understanding cytokines and their role in autoimmunity. Cytokines, small proteins that bind to cellular receptors and affect cell signaling, have a profound immunomodulatory role and, when dysregulated, lead to a proinflammatory state and autoimmune disease. There are 7 major cytokine families currently associated with autoimmune diseases: type I/II cytokines, TNF family, IL-1 family, IL-17 cytokines, stem cell factor/receptor tyrosine kinase cytokines, transforming growth factor beta (TGF-β) family cytokines, and chemokines (cytokines that mediate chemoattraction between cells) [64]. Cell signaling is initiated through the binding of the cytokine to its receptor and this in turn activates multiple enzymes that are related to the immune response. This increased understanding of immunoregulation has led to biologic therapies, including monoclonal antibodies, inhibitors of cytokine binding, and enzyme inhibitors, each manufactured to block the binding of the cytokine to the receptor or to interfere with downstream activation induced by cytokine/receptor binding. This recent knowledge has resulted in a plethora of new therapies for autoimmune diseases with the potential for many powerful new immunomodulators that decrease inflammation and prevent the clinical manifestations of autoimmune disease (Table 3).

Nomenclature

Biologics include monoclonal antibodies that when used for therapy have a name ending in -mab. The antibody may be human, with the name ending in -umab, or a mixed human-murine chimeric antibody with the name ending in -ximab. Fusion proteins, containing receptor domains or cell surface markers, end in -cept. The downstream Janus activating kinase (JAK) enzyme inhibitors (Jakanibs) end in -nib. The Jakanibs are not derived from a biological system and thus may be considered DMARDs, but they do target specific molecules, as do biologics.

Adverse events attributed to biologics

Adverse events associated with the use of biologics are important to recognize because some are life threatening. At the site of the injection, some children get injection-site reactions or raised warm erythematous lesions that may be painful or itchy. Minor infections may be associated with an injection-site reaction. The areas may reappear at the time of the next injection and can be concerning to the child and the family. These are the most common side effects. Of far greater concern is the risk of infections, particularly tuberculosis and fungal infections in children on TNF inhibitors [65]. Before starting therapy and yearly, a tuberculosis test should be done and the child must be seen for any prolonged respiratory infection or cough. The risk of malignancy may be greater in children on biologics. The increased risk of lymphomas or skin cancer is being monitored [66]. It is difficult to determine whether the risk is higher in children with JIA, because there is literature that suggests that children with JIA may be at more risk of malignancy then unaffected populations of children. As a precautionary measure the FDA placed a black box warning in 2009 after 48 cases of malignancy were reported, most of them on infliximab for IBD [67]. Concurrent immunosuppressive medications increase the risk and 88% of patients with malignancies were also on azathioprine, 6-mercaptopurine, or MTX. An additional concern regards the development of induced antinuclear and anti-dsDNA antibodies, and other serologic markers of drug-induced lupus, and/or inducing another autoimmune disease [68].

Type I cytokines

Type I cytokines are divided into groups with a common gamma chain, a common beta chain, and a group that binds to glycoprotein 130 (gp 130). Those with a common gamma chain include IL-2, IL-4, IL-7, IL-9, IL-15, and IL-21. Although the functions of each cytokine differ, this group is involved in enhancing cellular immune response and antibody production [69–72]. IL-2 promotes T-cell growth, increases the production of other cytokines, and augments cytolytic activity. There have been at least 2 anti–Il-2 antibodies used in therapy, daclizumab (Zenapax or Zinbryta) and basiliximab (Simulect), and these have shown promise in the treatment of uveitis that does not respond to conventional therapy and in renal transplant rejection [73]. IL-21 promotes differentiation of follicular helper T (TFH) cells and promotes antibody class switching. TFH cells are associated with autoantibody-linked autoimmune diseases, including RA and SLE. Levels of IL-21 are increased in the synovium and serum of patients with RA and increased IL-21 and IL-23 levels are associated with increased disease activity and with more severe radiographic changes in patients with early RA. Monoclonal antibodies to IL-21 decrease disease activation in RA and Crohn's and clinical trials are currently being conducted [74].

The common beta chain cytokines include IL-3, IL-5, and granulocyte-macrophage colony-stimulating factor (GM-CSF). GM-CSF is a proinflammatory growth factor for myeloid cells and is noted to be produced by pathogenic T cells that drive autoimmunity [75]. GM-CSF blockade has been effective for RA in phase II clinical trials using the monoclonal antibody mavrilimumab [76].

IL-6 binds to gp130 and is a proinflammatory cytokine produced by macrophages, endothelial cells, and tissue fibroblasts. IL-6 drives the production of other proinflammatory cytokines such as TNF and IL-1 and all have been associated with the arthritis seen in JIA and RA. Several other clinical features of JIA, including growth retardation and bone osteopenia, have been related to IL-6 effects. Furthermore, studies have shown associations between IL-6 levels and fever spikes, thrombocytosis, and joint involvement [77]. This combination of cytokines also induces the differentiation of type 17 helper T cells, which produces IL-17. IL-17 and TNF act together to promote activation of chondrocytes and fibroblastlike synoviocytes and production of metalloproteinases, which leads to joint destruction in RA.

Tocilizumab (Actemra) is a monoclonal antibody that binds both soluble and membrane-bound IL-6 receptor. In 2011, tocilizumab was approved by the FDA for use in systemic JIA in children ≥ 2 years old [29,78]. The recommended IV dose is 12 mg/kg ($<$30 kg) or 8 mg/kg ($\geq$30 kg) every 2 weeks, but in adults, it is given subcutaneously weekly with good efficacy. Current guidelines recommend it for children with systemic JIA with active systemic features and varying degrees of synovitis with persistent disease activity despite receiving NSAIDs or glucocorticoid monotherapy, MTX, or leflunomide, or a previous biologic [79]. As the efficacy in sJIA was noted, a trial was done in children with polyarticular JIA and more than half improved [80]. Tocilizumab may also be useful in difficult-to-manage myositis. Of note, side effects include infection, neutropenia, transaminitis, and high cholesterol level. It is essential to monitor laboratory tests at each visit. Other humanized monoclonal antibodies to IL-6 RA include sarilumab, sirukumab, and clazakizumab.

Type II cytokines

The type II cytokines include the interferons (INF), type I, II, and III, as a part of a large INF cytokine family. INFs are noted for their ability to decrease viral replication, thereby protecting host cells; however, they have multiple other functions, including activation of NK cells and macrophages, upregulation of antigen presentation through increasing the expression of major histocompatibility complex (MHC) antigens, and generalized activation of the immune system [81,82]. The type I INFs are associated with autoimmunity, including arthritis, SLE, SS, and myositis. There are clinical trials using a monoclonal antibody to INF type I sifalimumab, in SLE and although the disease activity index was unchanged, there was a trend to improved complements and reduction in medications [83].

Jakinibs. Type I and type II cytokines bind to type I and type II cytokine receptors that bind to a kinase family within the cytoplasm, known as the Janus kinases ((JAKs), which include Tyk2, JAK1, JAK2, and JAK3. JAKs are phosphotranferases and catalyze the transfer of phosphate from ATP to various substrates, such as cytokine receptors. This modification allows the recruitment of various signaling molecules, including members of the signal transducer and activator of transcription (STAT) family of DNA binding proteins [84]. By blocking JAK, there is a decrease in multiple cytokines, including IL-2, IL-4, IL-7, IL-9, IL-15, IL-21, IL-6, IL-11, and the INFs [84,85]. Understanding of the JAK pathway has allowed the creation of a unique therapeutic treatment of arthritis and other autoimmune diseases. These treatments are not biologics in the sense that these molecules are not produced by biological processes but function as biologics because they target specific molecules. Usually biologics must be given intravenously or subcutaneously to prevent breakdown of the molecule in the stomach and GI tract, but the jakinibs are oral.

There are now multiple JAK inhibitors. Currently on the market, tofacitinib (Xeljanz) inhibits primarily JAK1 and JAK2. Tofacitinib has been tested in RA, IBD, and psoriasis, as well as in renal transplant rejection and dry eyes. It is effective in patients with RA who have failed classic DMARDs, both as monotherapy and in combination with MTX [86,87]. At present, clinical trials are underway for use in JIA. Other JAK inhibitors inhibit primarily JAK1/JAK2 and include ruxolitinib (Jakafi), which is being used for myelofibrosis but also for autoimmune diseases, and baracitinib (Incyte), which has had promising clinical trials, suggesting it may prove better than MTX for treatment of RA.

Tumor necrosis factor cytokine family

The TNF family is a large family of cytokines that have a similar sequence and structure. Cytokines in this family include TNF-α, TNF-β, CD40L, CD27L, CD30L, fatty acid synthetase ligand (FASL), and many others. TNF is produced by mainly by macrophages but also by other cells of the immune system. Most of the TNF family are found as transmembrane proteins on immune cells that bind their cognate receptors $TNFR_1$, found on the cell surface of many tissues, or $TNFR_2$, found primarily on immune cells. TNF may remain on the cell surface or become soluble and both forms are able to bind to their receptors. Initially TNF-α was discovered through its role in tumor necrosis, but the TNF family has effects on most cells with many varied bioactivities. In general, TNF is a major proinflammatory mediator and may induce apoptosis. As part of the proinflammatory function, TNF-α stimulates IL-1 secretion and induces cell proliferation and differentiation. CD40L is important in B-cell development and activation and CD27L stimulates T-cell activation. Other members of the TNF family are involved in apoptosis and cytotoxic T-cell activation. Once bound, there is a conformational change in the TNF receptor and an inhibitory protein, silencer of death domain (SODD), is dissociated from the death domain and allows the tumor necrosis factor receptor type 1-associated death domain protein (TRADD) to bind and recruit a series of proteins that result in activation of 3 potential pathways: nuclear factor kappa-B (NF-κB), which translocates to the nucleus and is involved in production of proteins that result in cell survival, proliferation, inflammatory response, and antiapoptosis; mitogen-activated protein kinase (MAPK) pathways that activate c-Jun N-terminal kinase (c-JNK), that then translocates to the nucleus and is involved in production of proteins involved in cell differentiation, proliferation, and apoptosis; and induction of the death signal that results in in apoptosis. These pathways provide potential targets for future therapies. TNF-α has been identified as a cytokine with a major role in arthritis and vasculitis [88]. There are thousands of reports of the efficacy of TNF inhibition in arthritis and other proinflammatory states.

Biologic therapies
Tumor necrosis factor inhibitors. Increased levels of TNF have been found in the serum and synovial fluid of children with JIA and TNF has proved to be an effective immunomodulatory target in JIA [89,90]. Etanercept (Enbrel) and adalimumab (Humira) are FDA approved for use in JIA. Current recommendations for treatment of JIA from the ACR, established in 2011 [16], are that patients with arthritis in 4 or fewer joints (persistent oligoarticular JIA, PsA, ERA, and undifferentiated arthritis) start treatment with TNF inhibitors if not controlled by glucocorticoid joint injections and 3 to 6 months of maximum-dose MTX. In patients with arthritis in 5 or more joints (extended oligoarthritis, RF-negative polyarthritis, RF-positive polyarthritis, PsA, ERA, and undifferentiated arthritis) TNF-α inhibitors are recommended if the arthritis is not controlled by maximum-dose MTX. TNF-α inhibitors are recommended for patients with ERA with active disease not controlled by glucocorticoid joint injections and an adequate trial of sulfasalazine. MTX has not proved to be as helpful as the TNF inhibitors in controlling ERA/JAS. The TNF-α inhibitors are now recognized to have therapeutic benefits in several vasculitides. Studies have shown benefits in patients with large vessel vasculitis, both giant cell arteritis and TA, and in those with refractory Behçet disease [91]. Infliximab has been used in small studies in patients with GPA with benefit, but treatment with rituximab may be superior.

Etanercept is a fusion protein of the p75 TNF receptor fused to the Fc region of human IgG$_1$ that binds to TNF-α and TNF-β. By binding to circulating TNF-α and TNF-β, etanercept works as a decoy molecule to prevent TNF interaction with the cell surface receptor and, thus, inhibits downstream activation. In 1999, it became the first biologic agent to be FDA approved for use in children ≥2 years old with moderate to severe polyarticular JIA. In a randomized, double-blind withdrawal study in 69 children with active polyarticular JIA (aged 4–17 years old) without an adequate response to MTX therapy, 74% of patients achieved at least an ACR Pediatric (Pedi) 30 after the initial open-label treatment phase [91]. The ACR Pedi 30 is defined as at least 30% improvement from baseline in 3 of any 6 core criteria, whereas no more than 1 of the remaining criteria can worsen by greater than 30%. The core criteria are (1) physician global assessment of disease activity (scored on a 10-cm visual analog score [VAS]), (2) parent/patient global assessment of overall well-being (scored on a 10-cm VAS), (3) functional ability, (4) number of joints with active arthritis, (5) number of joints with limited range of motion, and (6) ESR. The ACR Pedi 30 is used in many clinical trials [92]. Subsequently, etanercept has been approved for use in children with PsA or ERA. Etanercept is a subcutaneous injection given at a dosage of 0.8 mg/kg/wk or 0.4 mg/kg twice weekly (maximum 50 mg/wk) [93].

Adalimumab (Humira) is a monoclonal IgG_1 antibody that binds both soluble and membrane-bound TNF-α and, thus, has increased efficacy because of both antibody-dependent and complement-dependent cytotoxicity. In 2008, it became FDA approved for use in children ≥ 4 years old with polyarticular JIA. In a randomized, double-blind, placebo-controlled withdrawal study in children with JIA, 83% of patients achieved an ACR Pedi 30 by week 16 on adalimumab [94]. Adalimumab is given subcutaneously, usually every other week, unless the arthritis is very severe. Suggested dosing is 10 mg for children weighing 10 kg to <15 kg, 20 mg for children weighing 15 kg to <30 kg, and 40 mg for children weighing ≥ 30 kg.

Infliximab (Remicade) is a chimeric monoclonal antibody consisting of a mouse Fab fragment antibody and the constant region of human IgG_1 and binds to soluble and membrane-bound TNF-α. It is administered as an intravenous infusion at 3 to 10 mg/kg/mo after giving a loading dose. It is not approved for use in children because a study in 2007 noted no significant difference in achievement of an ACR Pedi 30 by week 14 between patients who received infliximab (3 mg/kg) and placebo [95]. This finding is unfortunate because the study did not have enough patients to reach statistical significance. However, infliximab is of great use in the treatment of severe JIA and uveitis and is used if a child presents with very acute disease or does not respond well to other TNF inhibitors. In uveitis that is refractory to other treatments, infliximab reduces inflammation more rapidly than DMARDs or other biologics. In a systematic review, infliximab and adalimumab provided similar benefits in the treatment of refractory autoimmune uveitis, and both were superior to etanercept, which has been reported to potentially cause uveitis [96,97]. For severe uveitis, higher doses of infliximab (6 to 10 mg/kg) are recommended and at times up to 20 mg/kg have been used in children with refractory uveitis with a good safety profile [98]. Concurrent use of MTX is recommended to prevent the development of human antichimeric antibodies, which seem to correlate with infusion reactions and accelerated drug clearance.

There are multiple TNF inhibitors that are being used with beneficial effects. Certolizumab pegol is a pegylated (conjugated with polyethylene glycol to increase the half-life), monovalent Fab fragment of a humanized monoclonal antibody that binds to TNF-α. Many so-called biosimilars are being produced that inhibit TNF, but they often bind to other epitopes of the molecule, and thus, may provide greater benefit in certain individuals. Golimumab (Simponi) is a humanized monoclonal antibody that is given just once per month.

BlyS inhibitors. B lymphocyte stimulator (BLyS), (also known as B cell–activating factor [BAFF]) is a member of the TNF family, involved in B-cell selection, maturation, and survival. BlyS is produced by immune cells and its production is stimulated by IL-2, TNF-α, and INF. BlyS binds to 3 receptors on B cells: BAFF-receptor 3 (BR3); transmembrane activator, calcium modulator, and cyclophilin ligand interactor (TACI); and B cell–maturation antigen (BCMA). This binding stimulates B-cell maturation and survival from immature B cells to plasma cells. High levels of BlyS are thought to prevent self-tolerance by allowing B cells, that would normally be eliminated because of autoreactivity during the B-cell transition to plasma cells, to survival and produce autoantibodies. Increased BLyS levels have been found in patients with SLE and correlate with SLE disease activity and dsDNA levels [99,100]. Belimumab (Benlysta) is a monoclonal antibody to circulating BlyS that inhibits the binding to the BR3, TACI, and BCMA on B cells to prevent the survival of autoreactive B cells. In initial studies, there was not a marked improvement between patients treated with belimumab and controls, but in a phase II poststudy analysis patients with SLE treated for more than 52 weeks showed improvements compared with control patients with SLE [101,102]. At present belimumab is used for patients with difficult-to-control rashes and arthritis and allows corticosteroids to be tapered. Of note, it takes more than 3 to 6 months to see maximum effects.

Interleukin-1 cytokine family

The IL-1 cytokine family currently includes a group of 11 cytokines, including IL-1α, IL-1β, IL-1Ra and IL-18, IL-36α, IL-36β, and IL-36γ. Most of the cytokines in this family are synthesized as precursor proteins in the cytosol of monocytes and cleaved to a shorter active molecule using the inflammasome/caspase-1–dependent processing system. The mature molecule is then secreted. Once bound to their receptors, members of the IL-1 cytokine family activate signal transduction through myeloid differentiation primary response gene 88 (MYD88) and interleukin-1 receptor-activated protein kinase (IRAK). Ultimately these signaling pathways lead to activation of many transcription factors, such as NF-κB, AP-1, JNK, and p38 MAPK, and result in expression of proinflammatory cytokines, chemokines, and secondary mediators of the inflammatory response. The use of inhibitors to IL-1 has changed the disease course for patients with sJIA, decreasing the fevers, rashes, and joint pain [78]. In many cases, the acute manifestations of MAS are controlled by IL-1 inhibitors and the morbidity and mortality is decreased. There have also been reports of the use of IL-1 inhibition and therapeutic benefits in Behçet and in immune-mediated sensorineural hearing loss [91,103]. There are several IL-1 inhibitors that have transformed the treatment of children with autoinflammatory diseases driven by IL-1 and children with sJIA. The 3 used most often are anakinra (Kineret), rilanocept (Arcalyst), and canakinumab (Ilaris).

Anakinra is a recombinant version of the IL-1 receptor antagonist and competes with IL-1 for receptors on the cell surface to prevent downstream signaling. It is given subcutaneously daily and the suggested dosage is 1 to 2 mg/kg daily (up to 100 mg), but during acute inflammation some clinicians advocate much higher doses to control disease manifestations. Since 2013, anakinra has been recommended as the first line of treatment of sJIA if the systemic features and the arthritis persist despite glucocorticoids, NSAIDs, and/or MTX [104–106]. Of note, anakinra is used to treat MAS and may play a lifesaving role in decreasing the cytokine and macrophage storm [107]. Several studies in JIA have shown anakinra's efficacy. In 2011, a multicenter double-blind study showed that anakinra was effective in decreasing levels of the inflammatory markers CRP and ESR and in decreasing arthritis. However, there was a large dropout rate because of adverse events [104]. In another study in 2011 that used anakinra as the first line of therapy, greater than 90% of patients responded at least partially and 60% went into remission [105]. Younger children were more likely to have only a partial response. These results are encouraging and although the numbers are small, taken together, they confirm the efficacy of anakinra in JIA. The adverse effects are similar to those of most biologics and infection is the biggest concern, but, in addition, the injections are required daily and are painful, making this form of therapy less desirable if another alternative is available.

Rilonacept is a fusion protein made of portions of the IL-1 receptor linked to the Fc portion of human IgG and is effective as a soluble decoy by binding IL-1β and preventing its interaction with cell surface receptors. It is given as a loading subcutaneous dose of 4.4 mg/kg (maximum 320 mg) followed by a weekly maintenance dose of 2.2 mg/kg (maximum 160 mg/wk). There is a study that shows that it is effective in sJIA. During the initial 1-month phase there was not a significant difference between rilonacept and placebo, but the systemic features resolved by 3 months and the prednisone dose was decreased [108]. A study in 2014, in which rilonacept was used before initiating corticosteroids in systemic JIA, showed that 85% of patients improved in systemic and articular symptoms [109]. It is approved for children ≥12 years old in the treatment of cryopyrin-associated periodic syndromes, including familial cold autoinflammatory syndrome and Muckle-Wells syndrome.

Canakinumab is a monoclonal antibody that binds to IL-1β. This once-per-month subcutaneous medication at a dose of 4 to 8 mg/kg (300 mg/mo maximum) is recommended for sJIA with persistent active systemic features and arthritis and for children with autoinflammatory diseases. The efficacy in sJIA was reported in 2012 in a study that showed an 84% response with improvement in arthritis and systemic features [110]. Because of the once-per-month dosing, children are often transitioned to this medication from other IL-1 inhibitors.

Interleukin-17 cytokine family
The IL-17 cytokine family includes IL-17A, IL-17B, IL-17C, IL-17D, IL-25, and IL-17F. Stimulated by IL-23, the cytokines are produced by helper T cells and

are proinflammatory cytokines that, when bound to the IL-17R receptor, induce the production of many other cytokines (IL-6, granulocyte colony-stimulating factor [G-CSF], GM-CSF, IL-1β, TGF-β, TNF-α) and chemokines. IL-17 is commonly associated with the delayed-type hypersensitivity reaction and allergic responses but also with immune/autoimmune diseases. Signal transduction by these receptors is equally diverse and transcription factors such as TNF receptor associated factor (TRAF6), JNK, Erk1/2, p38, AP-1, and NF-κB have been implicated in IL-17–mediated signaling. Recently 2 monoclonal antibodies that decrease IL-17 levels have been approved for moderate to severe plaque psoriasis and PsA. Ustekinumab (Stelera) is a monoclonal antibody that binds to IL-12 and IL-23, preventing their interaction with the IL-12 and IL-23 receptor complexes. IL-23 inhibits Th17 cells and thus IL-17. Ustekinumab was recently approved by the FDA for use in PsA when 43.8% of patients treated achieved ACR20 (RA improved by 20%) at week 24 [111]. A monoclonal antibody to IL-17 receptor A, secukinumab, is now being used for treatment of psoriasis and is being studied for use in PsA [112,113]. Clinical trials are showing superiority to placebo for both the skin and joints. A similar monoclonal anti–IL-17 receptor A antibody, brodalumab is being tested for use in plaque psoriasis [114].

Inhibition of the costimulatory pathway of T cells with antigen-presenting cells

For a T cell to be activated, 2 signals must be presented by the antigen-presenting cell: the MHC combined with the antigen that binds with the T cell receptor and the CD80/CD86 molecule (B7-1/B7-2) that binds to CD28 on the T cell. When these 2 signals interact together, there is costimulation that results in activation of the T cell. To modulate and prevent excessive T-cell stimulation, there is another receptor: the cytotoxic T cell–associated antigen 4 (CTLA-4). This receptor has a higher affinity to bind CD80/CD86. Abatacept (Orencia) takes advantage of this higher affinity and is a fusion protein made up of the Fc region of the IgG1 fused to the extracellular domain of CTLA-4. Abatacept binds to the CD80/CD86 molecule, blocking the second costimulatory signal and preventing T-cell activation. In children who fail TNF-α inhibition, abatacept can prove beneficial. It has been noted to be effective in about 70% of children with JIA, including 39% of TNF-α blockade failures. There were also fewer flares of arthritis once improved compared with placebo-treated children. The safety profile of abatacept is generally good [115].

B-cell–targeted therapy

Rituximab (Rituxan) is a monoclonal antibody against the protein CD20, which is primarily found on the surface of pre-B and mature B cells, resulting in B-cell lysis by antibody-dependent and complement-dependent cytotoxicity and apoptosis. As such, rituximab has proved very effective in non-Hodgkin lymphoma. However, the removal of B cells from the circulation also prevents maturation to plasma cell and antibody production. Decrease in antibody levels, including autoantibodies, is the goal in treatment of active autoimmune disease. Another beneficial effect of rituximab in autoimmune diseases is that

B cells may act as antigen-presenting cells and this mode of T-cell stimulation is markedly decreased after rituximab. In antibody-medicated complications of SLE and in JDM and GPA, rituximab has been lifesaving. The efficacy of rituximab in SLE has not been clearly proven, but there are several studies that show benefit. In a review between 2002 and 2007, case reports of 188 patients with SLE treated with rituximab were identified and 91% showed a significant improvement in 1 or more of the systemic manifestations. Among the 103 patients with lupus nephritis, there was an overall rate of therapeutic response of renal involvement in 91% [116]. Infection was the most frequent adverse event. In a study from 2014, 54 patients with lupus nephritis received cyclophosphamide, MMF, or rituximab and outcomes were compared at 3 and 12 months. Rituximab was as effective as the other 2 treatment arms in this study [117]. These studies are small and larger studies need to be done to prove the efficacy of rituximab in lupus nephritis. The use of rituximab in GPA is now well recognized and it is used early in the disease course to achieve remission and prevent flares [118]. There is a report of treatment with rituximab resulting in clinical improvement in myositis early or later in the disease course [51]. There are now many other monoclonal antibodies against proteins on the B-cell surface that have a similar effect.

DIET, ANTIBIOTICS, THE MICROBIOME, AND AUTOIMMUNITY

Over the last decade, parents of children with autoimmune diseases have expressed increased concern that autoimmune disease is caused by a so-called leaky gut. A *New York Times* article by Susannah Meadows in February 2013 chronicled the history of a young boy diagnosed with JIA and subsequently treated with alternative therapy for a leaky gut. This story was thought by the pediatric rheumatology community to be biased, negating standard therapies and promoting untried alternative medications, but underscored the necessity to study the role of the GI tract in autoimmune disease. In 2015, a study from the United Kingdom noted a link between antibiotic use and a 2-fold increase of JIA. The increased risk depended on the dose of antibiotics and was greatest for antibiotic exposures that occurred within 1 year of diagnosis. The investigators postulated that antibiotics caused an alteration of the intestinal microbiome (microorganisms found in the GI tract), with subsequent immune dysregulation [119].

The role of the GI tract in the pathogenesis of arthritis has clear implications in certain types of arthritis, such as reactive arthritis, ankylosing spondylitis, and IBD-associated arthritis, but is not as clearly associated with other JIA subtypes or other autoimmune diseases [120,121]. A leaky gut or increased intestinal permeability caused by the gut microbiome is increasingly studied for its role in autoimmune disease. The microbiome is now understood to modulate the immune system, either maintaining homeostasis or promoting inflammation when the makeup of the microbiota is imbalanced, termed dysbiosis. Determination of the GI microbiota is complex because many of the bacteria in the GI tract are difficult to culture and it is necessary to do DNA sequencing to adequately identify the microorganisms. The intestinal epithelial and immune cells are in direct contact with the microorganisms and this has epigenetic effects. Through direct contact of bacteria and/or metabolites with the epithelial and immune cells, the Toll-like receptors and nucleotide-binding oligomerization domain isoforms are triggered and activate the innate immune system [122,123]. In addition, the inheritance of certain HLA antigens may bind bacterial proteins and induce an acquired immune response [124]. Studies in RA and SLE suggest that there are increased and conversely diminished microorganisms that, when imbalanced, induce a proinflammatory state [125–129]. Of note, in a study from Finland in 30 children with JIA, certain bacteria, Actinobacteria and Fusobacteria, were found only in patients with JIA and Lentisphaerae only in controls. The investigators concluded that JIA is characterized by a low level of Firmicutes and an abundance of Bacteroidetes, and this resembles what has been found in type 1 diabetes [130]. There is much to learn about the microbiome in autoimmune diseases, but understanding this system may have important ramifications in treating and preventing the disease.

Probiotics are often used by families to provide the so-called good bacteria that help to regulate the immune system. Several studies have reported that probiotic supplementation diminished the disease activity and inflammatory status of patients with RA [130–132]. To date, the role of probiotics in the therapy for autoimmune disease is not clear and this treatment is not routinely advised.

The role of gluten and gluten sensitivity, even without evidence of celiac disease, is also thought to be helpful to control disease symptoms by some families of children with an autoimmune disease. Often both gluten and dairy are eliminated from the diet with reported benefits. Although there is literature on the Internet about avoiding gluten in autoimmune disease, there are no controlled clinical studies that clearly addressed avoiding gluten in patients without documented celiac disease. Gluten may provide the pathway to a different microbiome, but the understanding of the role of gluten in autoimmune disease is, as yet, not known.

Because there is no current cure for autoimmune diseases, parents and patients frequently seek alternative therapies that may have validity once studied, but should not preclude conventional treatments in severe or complicated disease. However, a healthy diet is important, and patients should be counselled on a healthy diet and exercise.

BONE HEALTH IN CHILDREN WITH AUTOIMMUNE DISEASES

Bone health in children with autoimmune diseases is often compromised because of inflammation, loss of muscle strength, and the use of medications, especially glucocorticoids, to control the disease. There is a tight regulation between osteoclasts and osteoblasts in bone remodeling and homeostasis and inflammation can profoundly affect this balance. Osteoclasts are derived from hematopoietic stem cells and stimulated by macrophage colony-stimulating factor and receptor for NF-κB ligand (RANKL) to become multinucleated cells that attach to the bone matrix and dissolve bone through phosphatases, lysosomal enzymes, and integrins [133]. To prevent bone destruction and control remodeling, osteoclast function is regulated by the receptor for NF-κB (RANK)/RANKL/osteoprotegerin (OPG) pathway. OPG is a cytokine receptor produced by osteoblasts (derived from mesenchymal stem cells) that inhibits differentiation of the osteoclast precursors to regulate resorption. Osteoblasts promote bone growth by stimulating matrix mineralization, and production of type I collagen, osteocalcin, fibronectin, alkaline phosphatase, and collagenase. Regulators of bone remodeling include parathyroid hormone (PTH), vitamin D, TGF-β, and RANKL. Osteoblast proliferation, differentiation, and survival are controlled by the Wnt/LRP5/β-catenin pathway. This fine balance is influenced by cytokines. IL-1, IL-6, and TNF are released by osteoblasts to activate osteoclast maturation. As osteoclasts resorb bone, there is release of TGF-β and insulinlike growth factors 1 and 2. The proinflammatory state seen with many of the autoimmune diseases is associated with high levels of TNFα, IL-β, and IL-6, which promote the production of osteoclasts and inhibit differentiation of osteoblast, increasing bone resorption and leading to osteopenia/osteoporosis [134,135].

Studies have shown that to optimize bone strength, weight bearing and muscle movement over the joint are necessary. In children with autoimmune disease, there may be limitations in joint mobility and decreased energy secondary to the high catabolic state that occurs with inflammation [136].

To control the disease, corticosteroids are often started and this leads to an increased risk of osteopenia/osteoporosis. Although mechanisms are not completely worked out, corticosteroids cause a negative calcium balance associated with a decreased intestinal calcium absorption and increased urinary calcium excretion that leads to increased bone resorption compared with bone production. Trabecular bone, which is the major constituent of the vertebral bodies, is disproportionately affected compared with cortical bone. Glucocorticoid therapy is also associated with an increased risk of avascular necrosis of bone, most often the femoral heads, leading to collapse and loss of the normal articular surface, resulting in pain and often the need for hip replacement.

Over the last decade, the role of vitamin D in bone health and the immune system is increasingly recognized [137–146]. Insufficiencies or deficiencies in vitamin D are frequently noted in children. A study in 2010 noted vitamin D deficiency (levels <15 ng/mL) in 9% and vitamin D insufficiency (levels <30 ng/mL) in 15% of children and adolescents in the United States [142]. Vitamin D deficiency was highest in non-Hispanic adolescent girls of African descent (60%) and lowest in boys of European descent (1%). Cholecalciferol (vitamin D_3) is produced by the dermis and epidermis when UVB radiation converts 7-dehydrocholesterolin to cholecalciferol. Ergocalciferol (vitamin D_2) is made in mushrooms and yeast and is used in dietary supplements. Fish oils are also rich in vitamin D. Vitamin D is hydroxylated in the liver to 25-hydroxyvitamin D (25[OH]) or in the kidney to dihydroxyvitamin D (1,25[OH]$_2$D). Because vitamin D 25[OH] is stable for 3 weeks, this is usually the form tested for evaluation of vitamin D status. Vitamin D reacts with the vitamin D receptor (VDR). Vitamin D insufficiency/deficiency causes multiple downstream effects, including decrease in the efficiency of intestinal calcium absorption, which results in a decline in the serum ionized calcium concentration, increased PTH level, and subsequently (through RANK/RANKL) increased production of osteoclasts and lower blood phosphorus levels, and subsequently osteoporosis. Vitamin D is now understood to have effects on more than calcium and bone homeostasis. The VDR is found on immune cells and vitamin D can modulate both the innate and acquired immune systems. A deficiency in vitamin D is associated with increased autoimmunity and there are multiple studies suggesting that vitamin D deficiency is found in active SLE and arthritis and that a deficiency is associated with increased immune activation [137–140]. Polymorphisms in the VDR have been shown to be associated with RA and SLE.

Therefore, it is important that normal vitamin D levels are maintained in children with autoimmune disease, not only for optimal bone health but also to provide a stable immune status and decrease immune activation. Current recommendations in the Endocrine Society Clinical Practice Guide-lines are 400 IU daily in infants and children aged 0 to 1 year, and 600 IU daily in children 1 year old and older [144]. The vitamin D 25[OH] blood level should be maintained consistently > 30 ng/mL, which may require doses up to 1000 IU in children and 2000 IU daily in adults [145]. Replacement doses suggested by an Australian and New Zealand consensus statement for patients who are vitamin D deficient are suggested to be 1000 IU/d for infants less than 1 month old, 1000 to 5000 IU/d for infants 1 to 12 months old, and greater than 5000 IU/d for children greater than 12 months old [146].

With severe osteopenia, children with rheumatologic disorders have been treated with bisphosphonate therapy, including alendronate, pamidronate, and clodronate, and each study showed that there was an increase in the bone mineral density in the spine. However, there are concerns about the use of bisphosphonates in children, including possible permanent effects on bone remodeling, impaired healing of fractures, possible damage to growth plates, and impaired linear growth. A notable adverse effect is osteonecrosis of the jaw.

SUMMARY

The pathway to discovery in the treatment of rheumatic diseases has been laid down by those physician scientists who were able to stand at the bedside and analyze the clinical manifestations and use this knowledge to return to the bench to make inroads into the pathogenesis. For several decades, there were few advances in the treatments of rheumatic diseases, but in the last 3 decades the field has advanced and the prognosis for children with arthritis, lupus, myositis, and the vasculopathies is changed so that most children can be just that: children. Clinicians in pediatric rheumatology have united and there is more collaboration both nationally and internationally with the hope that, in the future, every child with a rheumatic disease will receive optimized therapy with new treatments that take the pain and suffering out of having a rheumatic disease.

References

[1] Petty RE, Southwood TR, Manners P, et al. International League of Associations for Rheumatology classification of juvenile idiopathic arthritis: second revision, Edmonton, 2001. J Rheumatol 2004;31(2):390–2.

[2] Petty RE, Laxer RM, Wedderburn LR. Juvenile idiopathic arthritis. In: Petty RE, Laxer RM, Lindsley CB, et al, editors. Textbook of pediatric rheumatology. 7th edition. Philadelphia: Elsevier; 2016. p. 188–204.

[3] Merino R, de Inocencio J, Garcia-Consuegra J. Evaluation of Revised International League of Associations for Rheumatology Classification Criteria for Juvenile Idiopathic Arthritis in Spanish children (Edmonton 2001). J Rheumatol 2005;32:559–61.

[4] Prakken B, Albani S, Martini A. Juvenile idiopathic arthritis. Lancet 2011;377(9783): 2138–49.

[5] Ravelli A, Varnier GC, Oliveira S, et al. Antinuclear antibody-positive patients should be grouped as a separate category in the classification of juvenile idiopathic arthritis. Arthritis Rheum 2011;63(1):267–75.

[6] Vaos G, Kostakis ID, Zavras N, et al. The role of calprotectin in pediatric disease. Biomed Res Int 2013;2013:542363.

[7] Stoll ML, Patel AS, Punaro M. Fecal calprotectin in children with the enthesitis-related arthritis subtype of juvenile idiopathic arthritis. J Rheumatol 2011;38(10):2274–5.

[8] Moncrieffe H, Ursu S, Holzinger D, et al. A subgroup of juvenile idiopathic arthritis patients who respond well to methotrexate are identified by the serum biomarker MRP8/14 protein. Rheumatology (Oxford) 2013;52:1467–76.

[9] Foell D, Wulffraat N, Wedderburn LR, et al. Methotrexate withdrawal at 6 vs 12 months in juvenile idiopathic arthritis in remission: a randomized clinical trial. JAMA 2010;303: 1266–73.

[10] Hinks A, Moncrieffe H, Martin P, et al. Association of the 5-aminoimidazole-4-carboxamide ribonucleotide transformylase gene with response to methotrexate in juvenile idiopathic arthritis. Ann Rheum Dis 2011;70:1395–400.

[11] Weiss JE, Illowite NT. Juvenile idiopathic arthritis. Pediatr Clin North Am 2005;52(2): 413–42.

[12] Petty RE, Lindsley CB. Oligoarticular juvenile idiopathic arthritis. In: Petty RE, Laxer RM, Lindsley CB, et al, editors. Textbook of pediatric rheumatology. 7th edition. Philadelphia: Elsevier; 2016. p. 229–37.

[13] Angeles-Han ST, Pelajo CF, Vogler LB, et al, CARRA Registry Investigators. Risk markers of juvenile idiopathic arthritis-associated uveitis in the Childhood Arthritis and Rheumatology Research Alliance (CARRA) Registry. J Rheumatol 2013;40(12):2088–96.

[14] Hawkins MJ, Dick AD, Lee RJ, et al. Managing juvenile idiopathic arthritis-associated uveitis. Surv Ophthalmol 2015;15:191–5.

[15] Rosenberg AM, Kiem GO. Polyarticular juvenile idiopathic arthritis. In: Petty RE, Laxer RM, Lindsley CB, et al, editors. Textbook of pediatric rheumatology. 7th edition. Philadelphia: Elsevier; 2016. p. 217–28.

[16] Beukelman T, Patkar NM, Saag KG, et al. 2011 American College of Rheumatology recommendations for the treatment of juvenile idiopathic arthritis: initiation and safety monitoring of therapeutic agents for the treatment of arthritis and systemic features. Arthritis Care Res 2011;63(4):465–82.

[17] Ringold S, Weiss PF, Colbert RA, et al, Juvenile Idiopathic Arthritis Research Committee of the Childhood Arthritis and Rheumatology Research Alliance. Childhood Arthritis and Rheumatology Research Alliance consensus treatment plans for new-onset polyarticular juvenile idiopathic arthritis. Arthritis Care Res (Hoboken) 2014;66(7):1063–72.

[18] Webb K, Wedderburn LR. Advances in the treatment of polyarticular juvenile idiopathic arthritis. Curr Opin Rheumatol 2015;5:505–10.

[19] DeBenedetti F, Schnieder R. Systemic juvenile idiopathic arthritis. In: Petty RE, Laxer RM, Lindsley CB, et al, editors. Textbook of pediatric rheumatology. 7th edition. Philadelphia: Elsevier; 2016. p. 205–16.

[20] Ramanan AV, Grom AA. Does systemic-onset juvenile idiopathic arthritis belong under juvenile idiopathic arthritis? Rheumatology (Oxford) 2005;44:1350–3.

[21] Pascual V, Allantaz F, Arce E, et al. Role of interleukin-1 (IL-1) in the pathogenesis of systemic onset juvenile idiopathic arthritis and clinical response to IL-1 blockade. J Exp Med 2005;201:1479–86.

[22] Ogilvie EM, Khan A, Hubank M, et al. Specific gene expression profiles in systemic juvenile idiopathic arthritis. Arthritis Rheum 2007;56:1954–65.

[23] Minoia F, Davì S, Horne A, et al, Pediatric Rheumatology International Trials Organization, Childhood Arthritis and Rheumatology Research Alliance, Pediatric Rheumatology Collaborative Study Group, Histiocyte Society. Clinical features, treatment, and outcome of macrophage activation syndrome complicating systemic juvenile idiopathic arthritis: a multinational, multicenter study of 362 patients. Arthritis Rheumatol 2014;66(11):3160–9.

[24] Grom AA. NK dysfunction: a common pathway in systemic onset juvenile rheumatoid arthritis, macrophage activation syndrome and hemophagocytic lymphohistiocytosis. Arthritis Rheum 2004;50(3):689–98.

[25] Zhang K, Biroschak J, Glass DN, et al. Macrophage activation syndrome in patients with systemic juvenile idiopathic arthritis is associated with MUNC13-4 polymorphisms. Arthritis Rheum 2008;58(9):2892–6.

[26] Vastert SJ, van Wijk R, D'Urbano LE, et al. Mutations in the perforin gene can be linked to macrophage activation syndrome in patients with systemic onset juvenile idiopathic arthritis. Rheumatology (Oxford) 2010;49(3):441–9.

[27] Verbsky JW, White AJ. Effective use of the recombinant interleukin 1 receptor antagonist anakinra in therapy resistant systemic onset juvenile rheumatoid arthritis. J Rheumatol 2004;31:2071–5.

[28] Irigoyen PI, Olson J, Hom C, et al. Treatment of systemic onset juvenile rheumatoid arthritis with anakinra. Arthritis Rheum 2004;50:S437.

[29] Ruperto N, Brunner HI, Quartier P, et al, for the PRINTO, PRCSG. Two randomized trials of canakinumab in systemic juvenile idiopathic arthritis. N Engl J Med 2012;367(25): 2385–95.

[30] De Benedetti F, Brunner HI, Ruperto N, et al, PRINTO, PRCSG. Randomized trial of tocilizumab in systemic juvenile idiopathic arthritis. N Engl J Med 2012;367(25):2385–95.

[31] Nigrovic PA, Sundel RP. Psoriatic arthritis. In: Petty RE, Laxer RM, Lindsley CB, et al, editors. Textbook of pediatric rheumatology. 7th edition. Philadelphia: Elsevier; 2016. p. 256–67.

[32] Tse SML, Petty RE. Enthesitis related arthritis. In: Petty RE, Laxer RM, Lindsley CB, et al, editors. Textbook of pediatric rheumatology. 7th edition. Philadelphia: Elsevier; 2016. p. 238–55.

[33] Lindsley CB, Laxer RM. Arthropathies of inflammatory bowel disease. In: Petty RE, Laxer RM, Lindsley CB, et al, editors. Textbook of pediatric rheumatology. 7th edition. Philadelphia: Elsevier; 2016. p. 268–73.

[34] Anink J, Prince FHM, Dijkstra M, et al. Long-term quality of life and functional outcome of patients with juvenile idiopathic arthritis in the biologic era: a longitudinal follow-up study in the Dutch Arthritis and Biologicals in Children Register. Rheumatology 2015;54(11):1964–9.

[35] Tan EM, Cohen AS, Fries JF, et al. The 1982 revised criteria for the classification of systemic lupus erythematosus. Arthritis Rheum 1982;25:1271–7.

[36] Klein-Gitelman M, Lane JC. Systemic lupus erythematosus. In: Petty RE, Laxer RM, Lindsley CB, et al, editors. Textbook of pediatric rheumatology. 7th edition. Philadelphia: Elsevier; 2016. p. 285–317.

[37] Cunninghame Graham DS. Genome-wide association studies in systemic lupus erythematosus: a perspective. Arthritis Res Ther 2009;11(4):119.

[38] Hochberg MC. Updating the American College of Rheumatology revised criteria for the classification of systemic lupus erythematosus. Arthritis Rheum 1997;40:1725.

[39] Benseler SM, Silverman ED. Systemic lupus erythematosus. Pediatr Clin North Am 2005;52:443–67.

[40] von Scheven E, Bakkaloglu A. What's new in paediatric SLE? Best Pract Res Clin Rheumatol 2009;23(5):699–708.

[41] Avcin T, O'Neil K. Antiphospholipid syndrome. In: Petty RE, Laxer RM, Lindsley CB, et al, editors. Textbook of pediatric rheumatology. 7th edition. Philadelphia: Elsevier; 2016. p. 318–35.

[42] Mina R, von Scheven E, Ardoin SP, et al, Carra SLE Subcommittee. Consensus treatment plans for induction therapy of newly diagnosed proliferative lupus nephritis in juvenile systemic lupus erythematosus. Arthritis Care Res (Hoboken) 2012;64(3):375–83.

[43] Horowitz DL, Furie R. Belimumab is approved by the FDA: what more do we need to know to optimize decision making? Curr Rheumatol Rep 2012;14(4):318–23.

[44] Furie R, Toder K, Zapantis E. Lessons learned from the clinical trials of novel biologics and small molecules in lupus nephritis. Semin Nephrol 2015;35(5):509–20.

[45] Rider LG, Lindsley CB, Miller FW. Juvenile dermatomyositis. In: Petty RE, Laxer RM, Lindsley CB, et al, editors. Textbook of pediatric rheumatology. 7th edition. Philadelphia: Elsevier; 2016. p. 351–83.

[46] Feldman BM, Rider LG, Reed AM, et al. Juvenile dermatomyositis and other idiopathic inflammatory myopathies of childhood. Lancet 2008;371:2201–12.

[47] Reed AM, McNallan K, Wettstein P, et al. Does HLA-dependent chimerism underlie the pathogenesis of juvenile dermatomyositis? J Immunol 2004;172:5041–6.

[48] Wedderburn LR, Rider LG. Juvenile dermatomyositis: new developments in pathogenesis, assessment and treatment. Best Pract Res Clin Rheumatol 2009;23(5):665–78.

[49] Ruperto N, Pistorio A, Oliveira S, et al. Prednisone versus prednisone plus ciclosporin versus prednisone plus methotrexate in new-onset juvenile dermatomyositis: a randomized trial. Lancet 2015;387(10019):671–8.

[50] Huber AM, Robinson AB, Reed AM, et al, Juvenile Dermatomyositis Subcommittee of the Childhood Arthritis and Rheumatology Research Alliance. Consensus treatments for moderate juvenile dermatomyositis: beyond the first two months. Results of the second Childhood Arthritis and Rheumatology Research Alliance consensus conference. Arthritis Care Res (Hoboken) 2012;64(4):546–53.

[51] Oddis CV, Reed AM, Aggarwal R, et al, RIM Study Group. Rituximab in the treatment of refractory adult and juvenile dermatomyositis and adult polymyositis: a randomized, placebo-phase trial. Arthritis Rheum 2013;65(2):314–24.

[52] Vermaak E, Tansley SL, McHugh NJ. The evidence for immunotherapy in dermatomyositis and polymyositis: a systematic review. Clin Rheumatol 2015;34(12):2089–95.

[53] Li SC, Pope E. Localized scleroderma. In: Petty RE, Laxer RM, Lindsley CB, et al, editors. Textbook of pediatric rheumatology. 7th edition. Philadelphia: Elsevier; 2016. p. 406–17.

[54] Laxer RM, Zulian F. Localized scleroderma. Curr Opin Rheumatol 2006;18(6):606–13.

[55] Christen-Zaech S, Hakim MD, Afsar FS, et al. Pediatric morphea (localized scleroderma): review of 136 patients. J Am Acad Dermatol 2008;59(3):385–96.

[56] Zulian F. Systemic sclerosis and localized scleroderma in childhood. Rheum Dis Clin North Am 2008;34(1):239–55.

[57] Zulian F. Systemic sclerodermas. In: Petty RE, Laxer RM, Lindsley CB, et al, editors. Textbook of pediatric rheumatology. 7th edition. Philadelphia: Elsevier; 2016. p. 384–405.

[58] PRES/ACR/EULAR ad hoc Committee on Classification Criteria for JSSc, Zulian F, Woo P, Athreya BH, et al. The Pediatric Rheumatology European Society/American College of Rheumatology/European League Against Rheumatism provisional classification criteria for juvenile systemic sclerosis. Arthritis Rheum 2007;57:203–12.

[59] Petty RE, Cabral DA. Vasculitis and its classification. In: Petty RE, Laxer RM, Lindsley CB, et al, editors. Textbook of pediatric rheumatology. 7th edition. Philadelphia: Elsevier; 2016. p. 448–51.

[60] Ozen S, Ruperto N, Dillon MJ, et al. EULAR/PReS endorsed consensus criteria for the classification of childhood vasculitides. Ann Rheum Dis 2006;65:936–41.

[61] Ozen S, Pistorio A, Iusan SM, et al. EULAR/PRINTO/PRES criteria for Henoch-Schonlein purpura, childhood polyarteritis nodosa, childhood Wegener granulomatosis and childhood Takayasu arteritis: Ankara 2008. Part II: final classification criteria. Ann Rheum Dis 2010;69:798–806.

[62] Cabral DA, Uribe AG, Benseler S, et al. Classification, presentation, and initial treatment of Wegener's granulomatosis in childhood. Arthritis Rheum 2009;60:3413–24.

[63] Weiss PF. Pediatric vasculitis. Pediatr Clin North Am 2012;59(2):407–23.

[64] O'Shea JJ, Holland SM, Staudt LM. JAKs and STATs in immunity, immunodeficiency, and cancer. N Engl J Med 2013;368:161–70.

[65] Bongartz T, Sutton AJ, Sweeting MJ, et al. Anti-TNF antibody therapy in rheumatoid arthritis and the risk of serious infections and malignancies: systematic review and meta-analysis of rare harmful effects in randomized controlled trials. JAMA 2006;295(19):2275–85.

[66] Beukelman T, Haynes K, Curtis JR, et al. Rates of malignancy associated with juvenile idiopathic arthritis and its treatment. Arthritis Rheum 2012;64(4):1263–71.

[67] Diak P, Siegel J, La Grenade L, et al. Tumor necrosis factor alpha blockers and malignancy in children: forty-eight cases reported to the Food and Drug Administration. Arthritis Rheum 2010;62(8):2517–24.

[68] Atzeni F, Turiel M, Capsoni F, et al. Autoimmunity and anti-TNF-alpha agents. Ann N Y Acad Sci 2005;1051:559–69.

[69] Rochman Y, Spolski R, Leonard WJ. New insights into the regulation of T cells by γc family cytokines. Nat Rev Immunol 2009;9:480–90.

[70] O'Shea JJ, Schwartz DM, Villarino AV, et al. The JAK–STAT pathway: impact on human disease and therapeutic intervention. Annu Rev Med 2015;66:311–28.

[71] Schwartz DM, Bonelli M, Gadina M, et al. Type I/II cytokines, JAKs, and new strategies for treating autoimmune diseases. Nat Rev Rheumatol 2016;12(1):25–36.

[72] McInnes IB, Schett G. Cytokines in the pathogenesis of rheumatoid arthritis. Nat Rev Immunol 2007;7(6):429–42.

[73] Aktas S, Colak T, Baskin E, et al. Comparison of basiliximab and daclizumab with triple immunosuppression in renal transplantation. Transplant Proc 2011;43(2):453–7.

[74] Spolski R, Leonard WJ. Interleukin-21: a double-edged sword with therapeutic potential. Nat Rev Drug Discov 2014;13:379–95.

[75] Papatriantafyllou M. Cytokines: GM-CSF in focus. Nat Rev Immunol 2011;11:370–1.

[76] Burmester GR, Weinblatt ME, McInnes IB, et al. Efficacy and safety of mavrilimumab in subjects with rheumatoid arthritis. Ann Rheum Dis 2013;72:1445–52.

[77] De Benedetti F, Martini A. Is systemic juvenile rheumatoid arthritis an interleukin 6 mediated disease? J Rheumatol 1998;25(2):203–7.

[78] Ringold S, Weiss PF, Beukelman T, et al. 2013 update of the 2011 American College of Rheumatology recommendations for the treatment of juvenile idiopathic arthritis: recommendations for the medical therapy of children with systemic juvenile idiopathic arthritis and tuberculosis screening among children receiving biologic medications. Arthritis Rheum 2013;65(10):2499–512.

[79] Yokota S, Imagawa T, Mori M, et al. Efficacy and safety of tocilizumab in patients with systemic-onset juvenile idiopathic arthritis: a randomized, double-blind, placebo-controlled, withdrawal phase III trial. Lancet 2008;371(9617):998–1006.

[80] Brunner HI, Ruperto N, Zuber Z, et al. Efficacy and safety of tocilizumab in patients with polyarticular-course juvenile idiopathic arthritis: results from a phase 3, randomised, double-blind withdrawal trial. Ann Rheum Dis 2015;74(6):1110–7.

[81] Higgs BW, Liu Z, White B, et al. Patients with systemic lupus erythematosus, myositis, rheumatoid arthritis and scleroderma share activation of a common type I interferon pathway. Ann Rheum Dis 2011;70:2029–36.

[82] Rönnblom L, Eloranta ML. The interferon signature in autoimmune diseases. Curr Opin Rheumatol 2013;25(2):248–53.

[83] Petri M, Wallace DJ, Spindler A, et al. Sifalimumab, a human anti-interferon-α monoclonal antibody, in systemic lupus erythematosus: a phase I randomized, controlled, dose-escalation study. Arthritis Rheum 2013;65(4):1011–21.

[84] O'Sullivan LA, Liongue C, Lewis RS, et al. Cytokine receptor signaling through the Jak-Stat-Socs pathway in disease. Mol Immunol 2007;44(2):497–506.

[85] Haan C, Kreis S, Margue C, et al. Jaks and cytokine receptors—an intimate relationship. Biochem Pharmacol 2006;72(11):1538–46.

[86] LaBranche TP, Jesson MI, Radi ZA, et al. JAK inhibition with tofacitinib suppresses arthritic joint structural damage through decreased RANKL production. Arthritis Rheum 2012;64(11):3531–42.

[87] Fleischmann R, Kremer J, Cush J, et al. Placebo-controlled trial of tofacitinib monotherapy in rheumatoid arthritis. N Engl J Med 2012;367(6):495–507.

[88] McInnes IB, Schett G. The pathogenesis of rheumatoid arthritis. N Engl J Med 2011;365:2205–19.

[89] Zeggini E, Thomson W, Kwiatkowski D, et al. Linkage and association studies of single-nucleotide polymorphism-tagged tumor necrosis factor haplotypes in juvenile oligoarthritis. Arthritis Rheum 2002;46(12):3304–11.

[90] Lovell DJ, Giannini EH, Reiff A, et al. Etanercept in children with polyarticular juvenile rheumatoid arthritis. Pediatric Rheumatology Collaborative Study Group. N Engl J Med 2000;342(11):763–9.

[91] Pazzola G, Muratore F, Popitone N, et al. Biologics in vasculitides: where do we stand, where do we go now? Presse Med 2015;44:e231–9.

[92] Giannini EH, Ruperto N, Ravelli A, et al. Preliminary definition of improvement in juvenile arthritis. Arthritis Rheum 1997;40:1202–9.

[93] Horneff G, Ebert A, Fitter S, et al. Safety and efficacy of once weekly etanercept 0.8 mg/kg in a multicentre 12 week trial in active polyarticular course juvenile idiopathic arthritis. Rheumatology (Oxford) 2009;48(8):916–9.

[94] Lovell DJ, Ruperto N, Goodman S, et al. Adalimumab with or without methotrexate in juvenile rheumatoid arthritis. N Engl J Med 2008;359(8):810–20.

[95] Ruperto N, Lovell DJ, Cuttica R, et al. A randomized, placebo-controlled trial of infliximab plus methotrexate for the treatment of polyarticular-course juvenile rheumatoid arthritis. Arthritis Rheum 2007;56(9):3096–106.

[96] Pasadhika S, Suhler EB, Cunningham ET. Use of biologic agents in the treatment of uveitis—review. Curr Opin Ophthalmol 2007;18(6):481–6.

[97] Simonini G, Druce K, Cimaz R, et al. Current evidence of anti-tumor necrosis factor α treatment efficacy in childhood chronic uveitis: a systematic review and meta-analysis approach of individual drugs. Arthritis Care Res (Hoboken) 2014;66(7):1073–84.

[98] Tambralli A, Beukelman T, Weiser P, et al. High doses of infliximab in the management of juvenile idiopathic arthritis. J Rheumatol 2013;40(10):1749–55.

[99] Stohl W, Metyas S, Tan SM, et al. B Lymphocyte stimulator overexpression in patients with systemic lupus erythematosus. Arthritis Rheum 2003;12:3475–86.

[100] Petri M, Stohl W, Chatham W, et al. Association of plasma b lymphocyte stimulator levels and disease activity in systemic lupus erythematosus. Arthritis Rheum 2008;58:2453–9.

[101] Stohl W, Scholz JL, Cancro MP. Targeting BLyS in rheumatic disease: the sometimes-bumpy road from bench to bedside. Curr Opin Rheum 2011;23:305–10.

[102] Wallace D, Navarra S, Houssiau F, et al. Safety profile of belimumab in patients with active systemic lupus erythematosus: pooled phase 2/3 data. Ann Rheum Dis 2011;70(Suppl 3):318.

[103] Vambutas A, Lesser M, Mullooly V, et al. Early efficacy trial of anakinra in corticosteroid-resistant autoimmune inner ear disease. J Clin Invest 2014;124(9):4115–22.

[104] Zeft A, Hollister R, LaFleur B, et al. Anakinra for systemic juvenile arthritis: the Rocky Mountain experience. J Clin Rheumatol 2009;15(4):161–4.
[105] Quartier P, Allantaz F, Cimaz R, et al. A multicentre, randomised, double-blind, placebo-controlled trial with the interleukin-1 receptor antagonist anakinra in patients with systemic-onset juvenile idiopathic arthritis (ANAJIS trial). Ann Rheum Dis 2011;70(5):747–54.
[106] Nigrovic PA, Mannion M, Prince FH, et al. Anakinra as first-line disease modifying therapy in systemic juvenile idiopathic arthritis: report of forty-six patients from an international multicenter series. Arthritis Rheum 2011;63(2):545–55.
[107] Ravelli A, Grom AA, Behrens EM, et al. Macrophage activation syndrome as part of systemic juvenile idiopathic arthritis: diagnosis, genetics, pathophysiology and treatment. Genes Immun 2012;13:289–98.
[108] Lovell DJ, Giannini EH, Reiff AO, et al. Long-term safety and efficacy of rilonacept in patients with systemic juvenile idiopathic arthritis (sJIA). Arthritis Rheum 2013;65(9):2486–96.
[109] Vastert SJ, de Jager W, Noordman BJ, et al. Effectiveness of first-line treatment with recombinant interleukin-1 receptor antagonist in steroid-naive patients with new-onset systemic juvenile idiopathic arthritis: results of a prospective cohort study. Arthritis Rheum 2014;66(4):1034–43.
[110] Ruperto N, Brunner HI, Quartier P, et al, for the PRINTO and PRCSG. Two Randomized Trials of Canakinumab in Systemic Juvenile Idiopathic Arthritis. N Engl J Med 2012;367:2396–406.
[111] Ritchlin C, Rahman P, Kavanaugh A, et al. Efficacy and safety of the anti-IL-12/23 p40 monoclonal antibody, ustekinumab, in patients with active psoriatic arthritis despite conventional non-biological and biological anti-tumour necrosis factor therapy: 6-month and 1-year results of the phase 3, multicentre, double-blind, placebo-controlled, randomised PSUMMIT 2 trial. Ann Rheum Dis 2014;73(6):990–9.
[112] McInnes IB, Mease PJ, Kirkham B, et al. Secukinumab, a human anti-interleukin-17A monoclonal antibody, in patients with psoriatic arthritis (FUTURE 2): a randomised, double-blind, placebo-controlled, phase 3 trial. Lancet 2015;386:1137.
[113] Mease PJ, McInnes IB, Kirkham B, et al. Secukinumab inhibition of interleukin-17A in patients with psoriatic arthritis. N Engl J Med 2015;373:1329.
[114] Lebwohl M, Strober B, Menter A, et al. Phase 3 studies comparing brodalumab with ustekinumab in psoriasis. N Engl J Med 2015;373:1318.
[115] Goldzweig O, Hashkes PJ. Abatacept in the treatment of polyarticular JIA: development, clinical utility, and place in therapy. Drug Des Devel Ther 2011;5:61–70.
[116] Ramos-Casals M, Sotos MI, Cuadrado MI, et al. Rituximab in systemic lupus erythematosus: a systematic review of off-label use in 188 cases. Lupus 2009;18(9):767–76.
[117] Moroni G, Raffiotta F, Trezzi B, et al. Rituximab vs mycophenolate and vs cyclophosphamide pulses for induction therapy of active lupus nephritis: a clinical observational study. Rheumatology 2014;53(9):1570–7.
[118] Charles P, Neel A, Tieulie N, et al, on behalf of the French Vasculitis Study Group. Rituximab for induction and maintenance treatment of ANCA-associated vasculitides: a multicentre retrospective study on 80 patients. Rheumatology 2014;53(3):532–9.
[119] Horton DB, Scott FI, Haynes K, et al. Antibiotic exposure and juvenile idiopathic arthritis: a case-control study. Pediatrics 2015;136:e333.
[120] Klareskog L, Padyukov L, Lorentzen J, et al. Mechanisms of disease: genetic susceptibility and environmental triggers in the development of rheumatoid arthritis. Nat Clin Pract Rheumatol 2006;2(8):425–33.
[121] Catrina AI, Deane KD, Scher JU. Gene, environment, microbiome and mucosal immune tolerance in rheumatoid arthritis. Rheumatology (Oxford) 2014;55(3):391–402.
[122] McClure R, Massari P. TLR-dependent human mucosal epithelial cell responses to microbial pathogens. Front Immunol 2014; http://dx.doi.org/10.3389/fimmu.2014.00386.
[123] Leifera CA, McConkey C, Li S, et al. Linking genetic variation in human Toll-like receptor 5 genes to the gut microbiome's potential to cause inflammation. Immunol Lett 2014;162(2):3–9.

[124] Sparks JA, Costenbader KH. Genetics, environment, and gene-environment interactions in the development of systemic rheumatic diseases. Rheum Dis Clin North Am 2014;40(4):637–57.

[125] McLean MH, Dieguez D Jr, Miller LM, et al. Does the microbiota play a role in the pathogenesis of autoimmune diseases? Gut 2015;64(2):332–41.

[126] Scher JU, Abramson SB. The microbiome and rheumatoid arthritis. Nat Rev Rheumatol 2011;7:569–78.

[127] Mu Q, Zhang H, Luo XM. SLE: another autoimmune disorder influenced by microbes and diet? Front Immunol 2015; http://dx.doi.org/10.3389/fimmu.2015.00608.

[128] Taneja V. Arthritis susceptibility and the gut microbiome. FEBS Lett 2014;588(22): 4244–9, Elsevier.

[129] Proal AD, Albert PJ, Marchall TG. The human microbiome and autoimmunity. Curr Opin Rheumatol 2013;25(2):234–40.

[130] Tejesvi MV, Arvonen M, Kangas SM, et al. Faecal microbiome in new-onset juvenile idiopathic arthritis. Eur J Clin Microbiol Infect Dis 2015;35(3):363–70.

[131] Vaghef-Mehrabany E, Alipour B, Homayouni-Rad A, et al. Probiotic supplementation improves inflammatory status in patients with rheumatoid arthritis. Nutrition 2014;30(4):430–5.

[132] Mandel DR, Eichas K, Holmes J. *Bacillus coagulans*: a viable adjunct therapy for relieving symptoms of rheumatoid arthritis according to a randomized, controlled trial. BMC Complement Altern Med 2010;10:1.

[133] Teitlebaum SL. Osteoclasts: what do they do and how do they do it? Am J Pathol 2007;170(2):427–35.

[134] Clements TL, Rosen CJ. The insulin like growth factor system and bone. Insulin-like growth factors. Austin (TX): Landes Bioscience; 2003.

[135] Kogianni G, Noble BS. The biology of osteocytes. Curr Osteoporos Rep 2007;5(2):81–6.

[136] Cimaz R, Ward L. The impact of rheumatic disease and their treatment on bone strength and development in childhood. In: Textbook of pediatric rheumatology. Philadelphia: Elsevier; 2016.

[137] Aranow C. Vitamin D and the immune system. J Investig Med 2011;59(6):881–6.

[138] Dusso AS, Brown AJ, Slatopolsky E. Vitamin D. Am J Physiol Ren Physiol 2005;289(1): F8–28.

[139] Ritterhouse LL, Crowe SR, Niewold TB, et al. Vitamin D deficiency is associated with an increased autoimmune response in healthy individuals and in patients with systemic lupus erythematosus. Ann Rheum Dis 2011;70:1560–74.

[140] Robinson AB, Tangpricha V, Yow E, et al, APPLE Investigators. Vitamin D deficiency is common and associated with increased C-reactive protein in children and young adults with lupus: an Atherosclerosis Prevention in Pediatric Lupus Erythematosus substudy. Lupus Sci Med 2014;1(1):e000011.

[141] Lee YH, Bae SC, Choi SJ, et al. Associations between vitamin D receptor a meta-analysis. Mol Biol Rep 2011;38:3643–51.

[142] Melamed ML, Kumar J. Low levels of 25-hydroxyvitamin D in the pediatric populations: prevalence and clinical outcomes. Ped Health 2010;4(1):89–97.

[143] Holick MF. Sunlight and vitamin D for bone health and prevention of autoimmune diseases, cancers, and cardiovascular disease. Am J Clin Nutr 2004;80(6 Suppl.):1678S–88S.

[144] Holick MF, Binkley NC, Bischoff-Ferrari HA, et al. Evaluation, treatment, and prevention of vitamin D deficiency: an Endocrine Society clinical practice guideline. J Clin Endocrinol Metab 2011;96(7):1911–30.

[145] Misra M, Pacaud D, Petryk A, et al. Vitamin D deficiency in children and its management: review of current knowledge and recommendations. Pediatrics 2008;122(2):398–417.

[146] Munns C, Zacharin MR, Rodda CP, et al. Prevention and treatment of infant and childhood vitamin D deficiency in Australia and New Zealand: a consensus statement. Med J Aust 2006;185(5):268–72.

Advances in Pediatrics 63 (2016) 333–355

ADVANCES IN PEDIATRICS

Advances in Autism—2016

Edward Goldson, MD

Department of Pediatrics, Children's Hospital Colorado, University of Colorado School of Medicine, 13123 East 16th Avenue, Aurora, CO 80045, USA

Keywords

- Autism • Kanner • Asperger • Early start Denver model (ESDM)
- Applied behavioral analysis (ABA) • Defensor tension imaging (DTI) • Lovaas

Key points

- To have some understanding of the history of autism.
- To review the changes in the DSM-5 and to understand they include the key diagnostic features of an autism spectrum disorder.
- To learn about newer central nervous system imaging technique - diffusion tensor imaging - and its implications for acquiring a greater understanding of the neurophysiology of autism.
- To review a current researched behavioral technique for the treatment/management of children on the autism spectrum.

INTRODUCTION

Autism, or autism spectrum disorder (ASD) as it is now termed, continues to be a topic of interest, research, controversy, political debate, and discussion about the use of economic, medical, and psychological resources. Once considered a rare disorder affecting approximately 4 to 5 in 10,000 children [1], it is now considered a common disorder. Two to 3 years ago, the incidence of autism was estimated to be 1 in 68 children [2,3]. The most recent numbers from the Centers for Disease Control and Prevention are that 1 in 45 children meet the criteria for an ASD [4]. This number is a far cry from the 5 in 10,000 estimate and continues to generate much heated discussion. Despite the impact ASD has had on our medical, social, and political lives and the controversy it has engendered, we, as a community of professionals and lay persons, still do not have the kind of understanding for ASD as we have for

Disclosure Statement: The author has no conflicts of interest.

E-mail address: edward.Goldson@childrenscolorado.org

0065-3101/16/$ – see front matter
http://dx.doi.org/10.1016/j.yapd.2016.04.014

other medical conditions. The purpose of this article is to provide an update on the new taxonomy of ASD, to describe some of the new neuroimaging and evaluation techniques now available to researchers and clinicians, and to discuss some of the newer behavioral techniques involved in the treatment of children with ASD.

HISTORICAL OVERVIEW

Leo Kanner, a child psychiatrist working in Baltimore, is considered to have first described autism and is certainly the first to publish his findings in English, in 1943 [5]. He described 11 children between the ages of 2 and 11 years of age (8 boys) with behavioral and neurologic challenges that he designated as having "Autistic Disturbances of Affective Contact." Kanner noted these children had a fundamental disorder, which "is the children's *inability to relate themselves* in the ordinary way to people and situations from the beginning of life" [5] (p242). He observed these children demonstrated 3 behavioral patterns: (1) extreme autistic aloneness. The child "...whenever possible disregards, ignores, shuts anything that comes to the child from the outside"; (2) delayed echolalia. They could say words and had amazing memories, but the ability to use this language pragmatically was almost nonexistent; (3) "The child's behavior is governed by an *anxiously obsessive desire for the maintenance of sameness*"–resistance to change. In addition, these children had relatively large heads, and one had epilepsy. More concisely and with more precision, Kanner articulated the following behavioral characteristics of the child with autism: (1) a failure to develop relationships with other people before 30 months of age; (2) problems of development of normal language; and (3) ritualistic and obsessional behaviors ("insistence on sameness") [4].

Of interest historically and conceptually is the work of Hans Asperger, an Austrian pediatrician, working in Vienna in the 1930s. He also recognized a group similar to the one described by Kanner, but perhaps functioning at a higher level and somewhat older, but with a wide range of cognitive skills. Noteworthy is that Kanner and Asperger viewed these patients differently. Kanner considered autism as rare and having very distinctive behaviors that he gleaned from evaluating young children. Asperger's experience was with patients of a broader age range. He conceived of the disorder as being a spectrum of individuals with profound intellectual disabilities and behavioral challenges to children with extraordinary capabilities. He worked at the University of Vienna along with other clinicians at the *Heilpädagogik Station* (therapeutic education) established by Erwin Lazar in 1911. Asperger published, in German, descriptions of his patients, his impressions of their behavior, and the strategies designed to meet their needs, which were also articulated through the philosophy of the clinic. Unfortunately, because of World War II, this information did not reach beyond the German-controlled world. It should be noted that during this period, Asperger worked in an Austria that was strongly influenced by the eugenics movement, which was very much in vogue and sought to "improve the human stock." Eugenics was also taken on by the Nazis during this time when the Nazis were embarking on their goal to rid German-occupied territories (and ultimately all of Europe) of individuals who had some form of illness or disability and were not in keeping with the ideal of the "Aryan race." In 1938, Asperger gave the first public talk on autism in history when he spoke to a group of Nazis because he knew they were targeting his patients—children we would now consider to fall on the autism spectrum—to be removed from the community because of their disabilities. Recognizing this philosophic and political thrust, Asperger worked hard to convince the Nazis that his patients had skills that would benefit the Nazi agenda. It appears, however, that he was not entirely convincing, and government agents made several visits to the *Heilpädagogik Station* to arrest Asperger and to ship off his patients. Fortunately, Asperger was saved by one of the officers who thought he was good at what he did and respected him, and so, Asperger survived the war [1]. It is unclear what happened to his patients.

Both Kanner and Asperger were astute physicians and drew on a highly capable, sophisticated group of clinicians around them. What is of interest and importance is that they were exposed to different populations of children and so arrived at different perceptions of causation and treatment. We have more access to Kanner's work because it took place in the United States and by the fact that during this period there was little interaction between Austria and the United States because of the Nazi control of Austria and later World War II.

Many thought the behaviors described by Kanner and Asperger were new phenomena of the modern world. Kanner did not. He was, among other things, a scholar of medieval history and found references describing patients similar to his young charges in the older literature. These children were portrayed as agents of evil who were influenced by horrible forces [1]. Silberman cites the eighteenth century Swiss poet Gottfried Keller in a description of a 7-year-old girl with behaviors described by both Kanner and Asperger in a later century. The poet reports the physician had nothing to offer her, so she was turned over to a minister whose cruel (from our perspective) ministrations and "treatments" ultimately led to her death [1] (pp178–179). Thus, it would seem what Kanner and Asperger and our contemporaries were describing was not a new disease but one that has existed for centuries under different names.

As mentioned previously, one of the striking differences in the formulation of autism was that Kanner conceived of it as rare, occurring in very young children he observed who had very distinctive challenging behaviors. Asperger's experience was with a much broader age range. He conceived the disorder as being a spectrum that included individuals with profound intellectual disabilities and behavioral challenges to children with extraordinary capabilities. Asperger, rather than wanting to cure these children, wanted to identify and celebrate what skills they had and help them find their place in the world as happy, productive human beings. Kanner saw these young patients as being terribly ill and a drain on their parents and society. He saw them as a rare group of individuals with a distinct set of behavioral characteristics. With time, he also came to see them as the product of toxic environments contributed to by their parents. Thus emerged the false idea of the "refrigerator mother" later further perpetrated by Bruno Bettelheim, leading to some very aversive "therapeutic" interventions at the Orthogenic Clinic in Chicago. Blaming parents for children with psychiatric conditions was a societal norm from the 1940s to the 1970s, that is, the concept of the schizophrenogenic mother. Both men saw this disorder as a psychiatric disorder, although Kanner had an inkling there was a strong neurologic component. Asperger had a sense there was a strong genetic component contributing to his charges' challenges.

Asperger, on the other hand, following Lazar's lead, did not see these individuals as "patients" but as bakers, barbers, musicians, academics, and engineers. In the *Heilpädagogik Station*, by taking a multidisciplinary approach, he sought to help each child to attain his or her potential. In addition, he saw them as falling on a spectrum that he called "an autism continuum," each with unique traits. The clinic sought to be a microcosm of a more humane society rather than a place to treat psychological problems. Lazar created an environment, which Asperger later elaborated upon and expanded, where children could learn to interact with others in a context of respect and appreciation. The curriculum included the study and participation in music, literature, nature, art, athletics, and speech therapy [1] (pp84–85). The program developed was individualized and based on a method of intense observation of the child in all aspects of her or his life: in class, at play, at the dinner table as well as based on the results of a battery of tests. In addition, Asperger would spend considerable time just being with the children: talking, reading, and playing with them. As Oliver Sachs in his book, *An Anthropologist on Mars* [6], states:

> No two people with autism are the same: its precise form or expression is different in every case. Moreover, there may be a most intricate (and potentially creative) interaction between the autistic traits and the other qualities of the individual. So, while a single glance may suffice for clinical diagnosis, if we hope to understand the autistic individual, nothing less than a total biography will do.

During the early years with Asperger describing the children he encountered in Vienna and Kanner in the United States involved in the same process, the question of childhood schizophrenia emerged. A group of children similar to those observed by Kanner and Asperger had been described by a Russian psychiatrist, Grunia Sukhareva. These individuals had similar traits as those with schizophrenia, but in contrast to adult schizophrenics, these children improved, whereas at that time, adults did not. Sukhareva proposed the term schizophrenoid personality disorder, but was uncertain as to whether it had any relationship to adult schizophrenia, as it was then understood. In retrospect, it appears that many children diagnosed with childhood schizophrenia may indeed really have been children who were autistic and who Asperger might have considered to be classified on the *autism continuum*. Suffice it to say, this led to much discussion and controversy among workers in the field. However, in the end, it has been agreed on that childhood schizophrenia and ASD are distinct and different entities and identified as such in 1980 in the Diagnostic and Statistical Manual of Mental Disorders (DSM)-III.

What has emerged from these many years of work, disagreement, personality conflicts, egos, as well as a variety of interpretations along with extraordinary clinical insights and creative thinking has been a constellation of behaviors associated with a clinical picture now called ASD and which is now accepted as being a neurologic disorder. Jean Aicardi, the French neurologist, described this neurodevelopmental entity as follows:

> Autism is a … behavioral symptom constellation signaling underlying nervous system dysfunction

> —Aicardi, 1998 [7]

From what has been observed and what is understood physiologically about autism, this is a reasonable characterization of ASD. The clinical picture of this disorder has been further characterized as describing individuals with deficits in language and social relationships in the presence of restrictive, repetitive, and stereotyped behaviors, interests, and activities. This characterization is also the way Kanner first described his young patients. The question then raised is, what behaviors reflect these descriptions? Solomon [8] describes the core issue in ASD as follows: "Intellectual ability is not part of autism per se; the syndrome is rooted in a disruption of social function." He also identified the characteristic symptoms, but noted that not every individual with autism will have all of these traits. At the same time, these are the symptoms one will generally find among children falling on the autism spectrum:

Lack of or delay in speech
Poor nonverbal communication
Repetitive movement, including flapping arms and other self-stimulating behavior
Minimal eye contact
Diminished interest in friendships
Lack of spontaneous or imaginative play
Compromised empathy, insight, and sociability
Diminished capacity for emotional reciprocity
Rigidity
Highly focused interests
A fascination with objects, such as spinning wheels and sparkling things
Concrete thinking
Difficulty understanding metaphor, humor, irony, and sarcasm
Can be obsessive, have stereotyped behavior
Attachments formed to random objects
Tendency to arrange toys by color and size rather than playing with them
Engagement in self-injurious behavior, including hand biting and head-banging
Have sensory motor deficits
Many do not point to things but have to lead someone to what they wish
Some have echolalia
Diction may lack intonation
Food rituals and limited diet

Sensory processing challenges, such as being sensitive to crowds, touch, clothing
  tags
Some may appear normal after birth but then regress between 16 and 20 months
Some may have extreme symptoms, such as smearing feces, not sleeping for
  prolonged periods of time, having a very high energy level, having an inability
  to connect to another human, and having a propensity for random acts of
  violence

The author also adds these children are usually "predictably unpredictable."

One final comment needs to be inserted here and was noted previously. There was a strong feeling first with Kanner and then Bruno Bettelheim and others that it was the parents, particularly mothers, who were the cause of autism: toxic parenting. This formulation led to cruel treatment of these struggling children and their families and set back clinical care and research for many years. It has finally been dispensed with. The clearest formulation is the one put forth by Aicardi that autism is a neurologic disorder that is influenced by genetics and the environment but not by "refrigerator" mothers. Eventually, parents became strong advocates for their children, founding organizations and striving to obtain effective therapies and community inclusion.

REVISED DIAGNOSTIC CRITERIA FOR AUTISM

Much of the debate about autism has revolved around the criteria by which a diagnosis of ASD is made; this is the focus of this section of the article. Among the recent changes, or advances, in autism has been the appearance in the DSM-5 of the revision of the diagnostic criteria. After much storm and debate, autism is now more firmly established as a neurodevelopmental disorder. There is strong evidence that there is a powerful genetic component to the disorder, yet it is acknowledged that environmental factors may also play an important role in causing autism or at least contributing to its presence. To date, there is no specific gene or genes associated with an ASD, although there are many candidate genes. It is also known that there is a strong association with other genetic disorders, such as the fragile X syndrome, tuberous sclerosis, Down syndrome, and others. In addition, there appears to be an association with extremely low birth weight and infection as well as paternal age. The core deficits that mark the diagnosis of an ASD are (1) impairment in social interaction; (2) impairment in communication; and (3) the presence of restricted repetitive and stereotyped behaviors/interest/activities. The question then emerged as how best to consistently diagnose an ASD. Bernard Rimland, a psychologist with a child with ASD, had some checklists that were helpful. However, it was not until 1980 when Eric Schopler at the University of North Carolina and colleagues introduced the Childhood Autism Rating Scale and when the DSM-III was published that the autism triad was first really articulated [9]. This work then anticipated the framing of the autism spectrum model introduced in the DSM-III-R published in 1987 [10]. The release in 1988 of the movie *Rain Man* resulted in increased public awareness about autism. About 6 months later, Rutter and Wing led an international team that developed a comprehensive tool–Autism Diagnostic Observation Schedule–for the evaluation of children ages 5 to 8 years of age with problems with communication, social interaction, and play. This work was later published by Lord and colleagues [11] in 1989. These criteria were then included in the DSM-IV in 1994 [12] and were considered the gold standard of autism assessment [1] (pp395–396). In the DSM-IV, autism was grouped under the umbrella of Pervasive Developmental Disorders (PDD). The groupings included (1) autistic disorder, which includes the symptoms described later with or without intellectual impairment; (2) Asperger syndrome, which is characterized by intellectually intact children who had impaired social interactions, restricted interests, and repetitive behaviors. These children achieved their developmental milestones as did typical children and had reasonable adaptive skills. They have at times been referred to as "Little Professors" because they have strong language skills, can integrate complex ideas, and focus on areas of interest. Also included under this umbrella is Pervasive Developmental Disorder Not Otherwise Specified (PDD-NOS). In addition, the DSM-IV included Disintegrative Disorder of Childhood and Rett syndrome, now known to be caused by a defective regulatory MECP2 gene. Nearly all cases of Rett syndrome, which usually affect women, are caused by a mutation in the methyl CpG binding protein 2, or *MECP2* gene. In 1999, scientists identified the gene that is thought to control the functions of many other genes. Although it is difficult to truly assess cognitive function in individuals with Rett syndrome, many think that in association with well-described stereotypic behaviors and a neurodegenerative course, many of these individuals may also be intellectually impaired, but there is not complete agreement on this issue. As a result of this mutation, Rett syndrome is now placed with syndromes rather than under the PDD umbrella; this is also done with the fragile X syndrome, although it also has a strong association with ASD. Disintegrative Disorder of Childhood is considered to be a very rare neurologic disorder. For the purposes of this discussion, the diagnostic criteria for autistic disorders in the DSM-IV are presented in later discussion and do not include the specific criteria for Asperger syndrome or PDD-NOS.

Consider next the DSM-IV criteria for autism and attend to the differences and their possible significance.

"The essential features of Autistic Disorder are the presence of markedly abnormal or impaired development in social interaction and communication, and a markedly restricted repertoire of activity and interest. The manifestations of this disorder vary greatly depending on the developmental level and chronological age of the individual. Autistic Disorder is sometimes referred to as "Early Infantile Autism, Childhood Autism, or Kanner's Autism" (page 70; DSM-IV). It is no longer considered a form of schizophrenia.

The DSM-IV was published in 1994 and was revised in 2000 [13]. The text revision is significant in that it corrected an error in the original DSM-IV, where it was stated that PDD-NOS could be diagnosed if an individual had severe and pervasive impairment in the development of reciprocal social interaction or verbal and nonverbal communication or when stereotyped behavior, interests, and activities were present. That is to say, only 1 of the 3 of the triad need to be present. The revised version corrected this and stated that 2 of 3 of the triad had to be present.

About every 10 years, the DSM is totally reviewed, leading to reformulations and, in some cases, deletions of entities or the addition of newly recognized disorders. The process of achieving this goal is very involved and can be time consuming and at times controversial. The rewriting of the autism criteria was very complicated, and there are ongoing ripple effects. The DSM is considered the gold standard for the diagnostic criteria for autism. Furthermore, the measurement tools in the evaluation of children suspected of falling on the autism spectrum reflect the characteristics of the disorder as articulated in the DSM. However, along with the clinical aspects of diagnosis, this document also had political and social repercussions. Value judgments about the children and their families were made by clinicians and the public in general. Many parents viewed their child with Asperger syndrome as not being "autistic," and by implication "better" than children with ASD. In some school districts, services were not provided for children with the "diagnosis" of Asperger syndrome. Families developed support groups for children with Asperger syndrome and saw their children as being separate, or different, from children with the diagnosis of autism. There were controversies among the experts as to the nosology of autism: what is included under ASD and what is not and what it should be called. One of the critical realities in the diagnosis of an ASD is that, to date, there are no specific biological markers and the diagnosis is based on formal and informal observation of behavior, not on radiographic or biochemical findings. It is a clinical diagnosis with all of the challenges involved in such diagnoses. As such, this is a challenge for most psychiatric disorders, yet changes and new conceptualizations for these entities seem to be more accepted and seem to be less controversial. The nature of the history of autism being viewed initially as a psychiatric disorder caused by the mother and then becoming recognized as a neurodevelopmental disorder was a major paradigm shift. The way children with these symptoms were perceived varied among the professionals like the differences in perceptions noted between Kanner and Asperger. Among other issues, Asperger's work was not recognized (and perhaps ignored) outside of Europe until the 1970s. Among the confounding factors for this was the fact that Asperger's work was published in German during World War II and so was not easily available to the non-German-speaking scientific community.

The nature of the revision in the DSM-5 [14] of the criteria for what was called in the DSM-IV PDD led to much controversy among the specialists. These controversies also became known by the families of children with autism. As discussed later, all of the subcategories (Asperger, PDD-NOS) were discarded and replaced in the DSM-5 with the term ASD. Among the greatest concerns of professionals and the public was that with the new formulations many children, particularly those previously diagnosed with PDD-NOS under the DSM-IV criteria, would not be identified and diagnosed, and so not receive the supports they needed. Studies determined to assess the validity of these concerns in field studies demonstrated that with the new criteria, this was not the case, and the new formulation was valid [15,16]. It is hoped that these findings should alleviate the concerns about identification. However, among many families, there is an investment in the fact that the child has Asperger or PDD-NOS because many feel their child does not have autism. Thus, specific interest groups have emerged that involve only children with Asperger; they single out members of this group and perceive them as different from other individuals who fall on the autism spectrum. At the same time, what has emerged, even before DSM-5, are many self-advocacy groups such as Autism Speaks, Autistic Self-Advocacy Network, and others that have worked to support and advocate for all individuals with an ASD at local, state, and national levels.

The new criteria are really not terribly new in that they cover the deficits in language as well as social relatedness, but combine them into one category. The second category is the stereotypic behaviors. This new formulation of the criteria was done based on extensive research and seemed to reflect the current understanding of the disorder. In addition, this formulation eliminated redundancies and overlap between the social interaction and communication criteria. A big change in the DSM-5 criteria is the inclusion of hyperactivity or hypoactivity to sensory input or unusual interest in sensory aspects of the environment. This inclusion highlights the increased incidence of sensory difficulties in children with ASD. In addition, what the new criteria create and articulate is the concept of a spectrum (which is what Asperger described when he coined the phrase "autism continuum"). With respect to the extent of involvement and treatment, the concept of categories of needs is very consistent with the idea of a spectrum and speaks to the breadth and range of the clinical picture. There are 3 levels of complexity noted in the DSM-5 that apply to language and social needs and to the stereotypic, repetitive behaviors. A child identified as being at level 1 requires some supports. A child at level 2 is considered to require substantial supports in all arenas, and one at level 3 requires very substantial supports. These levels of need identify how involved the child is. However, the author suggests there is also a built-in sense that the extent of involvement may change, acknowledging fluidity of the disorder even within the setting of the core deficits. A child with ASD is one who presents with a clinical picture characterized by deficits in language and social relationships with or without intellectual disability and also includes the presence of stereotypic repetitive behaviors and thus meets the criteria for an ASD. This reframing of the criteria and the clear articulation that autism is a spectrum disorder and that it needs to be conceptualized as such is what the author would consider one of the advances in autism. The new classification is broader, allows for flexibility, and realistically describes the child and the range of challenges these children may have. The child and his or her challenges become the focus of the assessment. One is not treating a diagnosis but a child. As in the

DSM-IV criteria, a child with chromosomal or other established syndromes is excluded, although we are aware that some conditions, such as the fragile X syndrome, Down syndrome, very low birth weight, and neurologic conditions, such as Rett syndrome, have a strong association with ASD. The hope is that this classification will help to identify more children on the autism spectrum and lead to their receiving appropriate supports and follow-up. Moreover, this formulation very much reflects Asperger's broad view of the disorder rather than Kanner's narrow one. It is worthwhile to acknowledge that in the 1930s Asperger was far ahead of his time and was a strong advocate for children who viewed their world through somewhat different prisms, yet had the capability of becoming productive participants in their communities.

CENTRAL NERVOUS SYSTEM STRUCTURAL FINDINGS ASSOCIATED WITH CHILDREN MEETING THE CRITERIA FOR AN AUTISM SPECTRUM DISORDER

One of the challenges in the diagnosis of psychiatric disorders is that there are few specific biological markers associated with observed behavioral abnormality. The paucity of specific biological markers is also true for neurodevelopmental disorders, such as ASD. Thus, there has been a long and intense search for anatomic variations or abnormalities of central nervous system structures among individuals with ASD. The purpose of this section is to describe a relatively new technique that is enabling scientists to visualize and analyze the structure and function of the microstructures of brain, particularly the white matter (WM). It was noted years ago in neuropathologic studies that there were abnormal changes in the limbic system, including the amygdala and hippocampus. The amygdala is critical for social perception such as recognizing faces and facial expressions, forming associations between specific stimuli, reward value, recognizing the affective significance of stimuli, and perceiving body movements including gaze direction and cross-modal association. The hippocampal system is important for memory function. In addition to the limbic system, changes were found in the cerebellum [17]. A review of neuroimaging studies on individuals with ASD found no focal lesions in the limbic system. However, studies of the cerebellum found variations in size of the cerebellar vermis, and the entire vermis was smaller than that of controls. However, functional neuroimaging studies revealed, with PET, decreased serotonin synthesis in the frontal cortex and thalamus and increased serotonin synthesis in the dentate nuclei in children with ASD, which is different from that in typical children and adults [18]. In other words, there is no question that there are neuroanatomical differences between children with ASD and those without the disorder. In addition, there were functional differences noted with the PET studies [17]. Furthermore, it is known that individuals with ASD have an uneven cognitive profile. Such individuals have been able to perform simple information-processing tasks at the level of their peers, but are unable to perform higher-order tasks. Thus, although it is important to examine localized differences in the brain, it became apparent that it is important to examine neural networks and how they communicate information with different parts of the brain.

As is so often the case, one needs to await the arrival of new technologies. This is true when ASD is considered as well as other neurodevelopmental disorders that do not have focal abnormalities but rather subtle changes or variations in their structure and function. One new imaging technology is diffusion tensor imaging (DTI). DTI is an MRI noninvasive sensitive technique used to visualize WM pathways in the brain and analyze their microstructure. DTI measures the diffusion, or random motion, of water molecules as a function of direction. The diffusion of water is sensitive to, and influenced by, the spacing, orientation, and density of microstructures that are barriers of brain tissue, such as membranes, cytoskeleton, and myelin. The fibrous tissue of WM bundles restricts the diffusion of water perpendicular to WM tracts more than in the parallel direction. This directional dependence of water diffusion is called diffusion anisotropy. It is known that WM consists of tracts of bundles of nerves that facilitate communication in the brain. Changes to the microstructure properties of the tracts, such as myelination, inflammation, and axonal density, have an effect on diffusion anisotropy and so may reflect differences in the brain's connective properties [19].

Measures generated by DTI (Box 1) include fractional anisotropy (FA), which is a ratio representing the degree to which water diffusion in the brain is greater in one direction than in the other or whether it is equal in all directions. FA is considered to be associated with myelination, axon diameter, fiber density, and fiber coherence, thus being a measure of microstructural integrity [20,21]. High FA values indicate that diffusion is greater in one direction than others and is typically regarded as a property of healthy and mature WM microstructure. Lower FA values indicate less specific directionality and thus less mature WM. In imaging WM, FA increases with maturation, implying nonspecific diffusion because of potentially increased myelination, fiber density, or axonal diameter, that is, more mature fibers. Axial diffusivity (AD) is considered to be related to axonal integrity, and radial diffusivity (RD) changes reflect alterations in myelination [20,22].

Normal WM maturation typically produces increasing FA, decreasing mean diffusivity (MD), and decreasing RD with smaller changes in AD. On the other hand, in WM abnormality, FA is decreased while MD and RD are elevated, which indicates reduced "microstructure integrity." However, in DTI studies

Box 1: Definitions used in diffusion tensor imaging

- Fractional anisotropy (FA) values: orientation-dependent variation of water diffusivity and reflected microstructural properties, such as axon diameter, degree of myelination, fiber packing density, and fiber collimation
- Mean diffusivity (MD): the rate of diffusion averaged over all orientations
- Axial diffusivity (AD): rate of diffusion along the orientation of WM fibers within a tract
- Radial diffusivity (RD): rate of diffusion orthogonal to the fiber orientation

involving children with ASD, it is not always the case because of such factors as heterogeneity of the population, the age of the subject, the presence of different tracts, and methods of obtaining the data.

Travers and colleagues [19] reviewed the English-language DTI research and identified 48 studies. They first reviewed studied group differences in overall WM and differences in the whole brain analysis of children and adults in the ASD group. These individuals had decreased FA and significantly increased MD and RD as compared with the non-ASD groups. The investigators then reviewed the literature on group differences in corpus callosum (CC) WM. The CC WM tracts are part of the largest fiber bundle in the human brain connecting the left and right hemispheres and serves in both the inhibitory and the excitatory modulation of communication between the hemispheres. Among other findings, it was noted that the volume of the CC was less in individuals with ASD as compared with non-ASD subjects. When considering the microstructure of the CC of individuals with ASD, some studies found that the axons of the CC were less myelinated. However, there was considerable heterogeneity in the groups, and it is difficult to draw conclusions as to the significance of these CC findings.

In their review, the investigators found differences in the cingulum bundles, which are the primary intrahemispheric association pathways for the medial cingulate cortex and temporoparietal junction and project to the hippocampus. They found studies where the FA was decreased and/or increased in the WM regions of the anterior cingulum. They also found differences in the arcuate fasciculus/superior fasciculus, which starts in the superior gray matter and extends to the frontal lobe. It has been thought to connect brain areas essential for language understanding and production.

The review from which the above data were gathered is more extensive and detailed and goes beyond the scope of this article. However, the point in looking at some of these data is to emphasize that with new imaging techniques scientists have been able to begin to address important questions about brain structure and function as they relate to ASD. The investigators state:

> From the studies under review, it appears that children (>4 years of age) and young adults with ASD tend to have decreased FA in WM tracts spanning across many regions of the brain. The decrease in FA is often accompanied by an increase in both MD and RD. Additionally, this pattern of decreased FA in ASD may be more applicable to some WM tracts than others, with studies finding the most consistent decrease in FA and ASD in regions such as the CC, cingulum, and WM tracts connecting aspects of the temporal lobe. These white matter tracts have been associated with diverse functions, including motor skill and complex functioning of the temporal lobe [19] (p12).

It should also be noted they caution that in interpreting these data one must take into consideration the measurement models used, the age of the subject, and the individual's cognitive level, among other variables.

In a recent study using DTI it was found that children with ASD had significant differences in the macrostructure and microstructure of the CC. These differences did not involve motor function but rather were associated with sociocognitive deficits [20].

The advent and use of DTI imaging are major advances in the ability to non-invasively measure and evaluate WM in the brain, particularly focusing on the CC, the posterior cingulate cortex, and the limbic portions of the brain. Alterations or differences in these areas are often associated with ASD. This method along with other magnetic imaging modes have opened new areas of research into the function of the brain, which may well provide us with a greater understanding of the underlying mechanisms resulting in ASD. In addition, these findings may offer insights as to what might be effective treatment strategies. These findings and how they may change over time may also be helpful to workers as they evaluate the efficacy, or lack of efficacy, of given therapies.

TREATMENT
Behavioral interventions
For years clinicians have sought to identify successful ways of treating ASD and have begun to identify strategies that appear to be helpful in some cases. However, this is not a new endeavor. In the 1930s, Asperger took over and expanded the *Heilpädagogik Station* (therapeutic education), associated with the University of Vienna. *Heilpädagogik Station* was a clinic dedicated to children whom today would be considered as falling on the autism spectrum and would be "high functioning." As a matter of fact, Asperger coined the term *Autistischen Psychopathen* (*"autistic psychopathy"*), which was then shortened to *"autismus."* At the same time, he noted a continuum of varied symptoms that encompassed social challenges and presented a range of abilities from the most gifted to the most disabled. In other words, "there seemed to be nearly as many varieties of *Autismus* as there were autistic people" [1] (p98). Silberman notes Asperger did not see these individuals as being sick or evil, but rather as engaging the world differently than others. Thus, as Silberman puts it, "The job of the staff of the *Heilpädagogik Station*, as Asperger saw it, was to teach these children how to put their autistic intelligence to work… Instead of treating them as patients, he saw them as indispensable allies in developing methods of pedagogy that would be the most appropriate and effective for them" [1] (p195). The methods used in the clinic were tailored to meet the needs of the children and were imbedded in an integrated program that included music, literature, drama, art, nature study, speech therapy, and athletics.

Unfortunately, over time (as noted above), this approach was replaced by harsher strategies for treatment with no significant improvement. In the 1960s and 1970s, O. Ivar Lovaas, and other investigators, became intrigued by children with autism and sought other strategies to improve their lives. These investigators drew on the concepts of applied behavioral analysis (ABA), in which strategies derived from the principles of behavior are applied systematically to improve socially significant behavior [23]. Experimentation and research are used to identify variables responsible for behavior change. Lovaas was one of the pioneers in applying the strategies derived from behavioral analysis (ABA) to the treatment of children with ASD. Using the ABA model, he and others also sought to establish communicative language [24]. In this context, it is worthwhile to consider Lovaas' conceptualization of autism, which resonates with many of the questions discussed now, some 40 years after he put forth the ABA model. Lovaas notes that "When using such diagnostic label one is typically conceptualizing *autism* as a distinct entity; an underlying process which is seen as the cause of these deviant behaviors" [25] (p111). Lovaas points out that many researchers have focused on one or another underlying process to explain the psychopathology of autism. The author suggests this is Kanner's view, which the author thinks was very different from Asperger's formulation of what has come to be known as ASD. Lovaas goes on to say that, "From a behaviorist viewpoint, it is quite unnecessary to postulate such an underlying *disease* or entity, and indeed it is quite possible that the different autistic behaviors are related to several different kinds of antecedent conditions" [25] (p112). He then says, "In our treatment we have felt that we could develop procedures to help these children overcome their pathological behaviors and develop healthy ones without having to postulate an underlying process such as autism" [25] (p112). Today many continue to conceptualize autism, or ASD, as a single entity. The author suggests that one of the important advances in treatment is the recognition that one is not treating the "disease" per se, but seeking to find ways of helping the child to be more functional and to be able to participate more fully in his or her world while building on existing skills. It should be noted here, and as will be mentioned later, Lovaas' interventions were very intensive and took place over years. At times, he used somewhat aversive methods, such as slapping and the use of mild electric shocking, to get the more difficult children to respond to his therapies. He was criticized for such methods, and these are no longer acceptable or in use. The hope was that with appropriate interventions one could alter the microstructures of the brain associated with the behaviors children with ASD demonstrate.

Lovaas drew on theories of learning behavior. He understood how typical children learn and recognized the challenges children with ASD encountered. Based on his understanding, he turned to behavior modification as a therapeutic intervention. He postulated that one could "...isolate the controlling conditions for each one of their various behaviors... [25] (p112) and treat it. He then comments in the name of efficiency of treatment, "...if we could discover that their various behaviors interacted in the sense that if we changed one behavior, then certain others would change concurrently. But one may also be prepared for the possibility that these behaviors are relatively independent of each other so that as one gains some control over one of them, one does not necessarily gain control over the others" [25] (p112). Central to his thinking was "... that by carefully programming certain environmental consequences, these children could in fact be taught to comply with certain aspects of reality" [25] (p113). He thought that in order to treat children with autism one needed to strengthen positive behaviors by reinforcing them. If they are absent, positive behaviors need to be gradually shaped by rewarding the approximation of the desired behavior with meaningful, positive rewards. If the opposite was the case, then the reward was withheld until the desired behavior was elicited. What Lovaas did was to develop a strategy that has been called Discrete Trial Training (DTT), which was one of other approaches coming out of ABA. DTT isolates the individual skills required and breaks them down into their components, which are then taught individually in "massed trials." First, the child must receive a stimulus, which serves as a cue for the child to respond, and the child must attend to the cue. Second, the child must demonstrate a behavior immediately after the cue. Third, the child must receive a feedback or consequence to her or his response to the cue that indicates that the response was the correct one. Ultimately, it is hoped the child, in response to the stimulus, will demonstrate the desired behavior more quickly, frequently, and consistently and will use the behavior in more of a variety of contexts.

The strategies to accomplish this task involve several steps [23,26]. First, the child's attention must be captured. Second, the sequence of ABC (Antecedent-Behavior-Consequence) must take place. This sequence defines a learning trial. The child has a behavior or is taught a behavior that is a response to some stimulus. "Teaching involves manipulating the antecedent (stimulus) and consequence to either strengthen or weaken the relation between the antecedent and the behavior" [26] (p21). "Increases and decreases in behavior due to the manipulation of the antecedent and consequence are the sine qua non of operant behavioral therapy" [26] (p21). Other components of the process include prompting desired behaviors, managing consequences, fading prompts (systematically decreasing the prompt so that the child responds to the stimulus and not the prompt), shaping behaviors, and chaining behaviors, which means building sequences of behaviors to produce a fluid behavioral response. Finally, there must be a functional analysis of the behavior. This analysis is to evaluate whether a behavior is useful to the child in achieving a goal and is a truly in his or her behavior repertoire as they lead to a reward. This strategy is a first step to understanding what a child's goals are and what skills he or she is currently using to meet these goals. These goals must be determined when looking at what more functional skills are required to be learned in order to meet the desired goal.

Lovaas came to believe that "… much of an autistic child's failure to develop appropriate behavior could be viewed as a function of a more basic failure of his environment to acquire meaning for him…" [25] (p114). In other words, children with autism seemed to learn little by observation and imitation, which are the basic ways typical children acquire knowledge and appropriate behaviors. This deficit in children with ASD is one of the challenges for successful treatment. What essentially needs to take place in order for the autistic child to learn is that the environment and her or his experiences in the environment need to have some meaning for the child. How to accomplish this is the question. Lovaas' answer to that was ABA. However, he also recognized that ABA might well be helpful for children without ASD and should be available to them, as a treatment option.

Lovaas published a paper in 1987 [27] in which he reported on the outcome for children with ASD after a treatment based on the hypothesized method that "construction of a special, intense and comprehensive learning environment for very young autistic children would allow some of them to catch up with their normal peers by first grade" [27] (p4). The therapists identified several behavioral problems, and separate programs were designed to accelerate the development of the desired behavior using the principles of ABA. This intense intervention went on for 40 hours a week for more than 2 years and was carried out by trained student therapists. The parents were also involved in the therapy. If highly aggressive or self-stimulatory behaviors were targeted, they were reduced by ignoring them and providing the child with more socially acceptable behaviors. The converse was also true in that desired behaviors/skills were reinforced with positive consequences. There were 19 subjects in this project. Lovaas reports that 47% of these children achieved normal intellectual function and academic function. Forty percent were mildly developmentally disabled, and 10% were profoundly intellectually disabled. They compared the study group to a matched control group of 40 subjects who did not receive this intensive therapy. Only 2% achieved normal intellectual and academic function, 45% were mildly intellectually disabled, and 53% were severely disabled. Lovaas recognized that many questions were raised by these data. He wondered about the cause or causes for what was defined as autism. He thought that if one were to make a difference in this population that early intervention was critical, that it needed to be provided by highly trained and experienced clinicians, and that each child should have one teacher. He also noted that cost was very high, but it was less expensive than life-long institutionalization.

Over the years, there has been much discussion about Lovaas' model and the amount of time required to effect change. Nevertheless, his work was reported to have success and laid the foundation for the development of other approaches, based on the principles of ABA, but recognizing some of the problems associated with his particular treatment approach. Research in the last few years has drawn on the ABA principles and with expansion and refinement has led to newer educational and therapeutic approaches to working with children with ASD. An excellent review of the different approaches to treatment can be found in the article by Schreibman and colleagues [28]. Other principles contributing to these advances are reviewed.

Schreibman [28,29] noted the more structured approaches such as those used by Lovaas sometimes led to (1) the child not generalizing learned skills across different environments; (2) the presence of escape/avoidance behaviors; (3) a lack of spontaneity; and (4) overdependence on prompts. The identification of these challenges encouraged investigators to focus their attention on improving and expanding the intervention, taking into account both the new research in behavioral principles and an ever-growing understanding of what was known about developmental trajectories and how children learn. In addition, although continuing the emphasis on language development, they began focusing on the early core social and communicative skills that were missing in autism. They came to realize the importance of the affective connection between the child and the therapist, which was one of the major deficits found among children with ASD. Thus, they began incorporating strategies to enhance affective engagement. They came to realize that the highly structured teaching strategies were not entirely meeting the child's needs and that there needed to be a more active collaborative engagement with the child. They recognized that in order to be more successful "...children's learning experiences are strategically designed to actively engage children's attention, help them connect new experiences with existing knowledge, teach within developmental sequences, and, through systematically increasing complexity of the learning experiences, enable them to discover the regularities of the work around them" [28]. In addition, they needed to foster the children's spontaneity and encourage them to contribute to their own learning; this could evolve in the presence of a context of an emotionally supportive and rich environment involving play with objects and with people. The combination of more naturalistic behavioral strategies with an understanding of typical development has led to what are now known as naturalistic developmental behavioral interventions (NDBI) [30]. Many of the earliest interventions in autism now being developed are NDBI. A prime example is the Denver Model (DM) and the Early Start Denver Model (ESDM), which will be explored in more detail in this article. Again, using strategies from ABA but using more naturalistic approaches, the therapists began to use more natural and relevant rewards rather than artificial ones; rewards that the child preferred. Efforts were also made to reinforce approximations and attempts. The environment in which these interactions took place was more naturalistic and developmentally appropriate. Researchers and teachers found the children tended to generalize more and were happiest and more productive doing what they wanted in an environment where they wanted to be. Of note, none of these approaches contradicted ABA criteria. They expanded and refined the clinical approaches and opened areas for research.

Pivotal response training (PRT) is another approach contributing to ABA. Now, with the addition of NDBI, it is thought to be an improvement over DTT. PRT was first introduced in the 1980s by the Koegels [31,32] and Schreibman [29,33]. Workers found improvement in their patients' behavior and function when the treatment took place in a more natural and interactive environment, rather than being always in an adult-directed setting. In addition to the basic principles of ABA, such as reinforcement, prompting, fading, shaking, and chaining, they added motivation and response to multiple cues, self-management, and social initiations. They found with these techniques children were more motivated to perform; their generalization of new skills improved, and they were more responsive and had fewer behavioral issues [33]. With PRT, they found they were able to increase the child's capacity to respond to multiple cues by varying the antecedents, thereby teaching children to express the same behavior to varying stimuli. The strategies involved in PRT differed to some degree from those of traditional ABA. They reflected a greater understanding of how typical children learned and developed and the challenges presented by children with ASD. Thus, first the therapists reinforced the child's attempts at the desired behavior by rewarding even less than desired responses. Second, they alternated requests for new behaviors with requests for already acquired skills. Third, they used reinforcers that were a direct response to the child's behavior. The interaction is child driven rather than being entirely adult driven. For example, if the child is ready to stop, the activity stops. It is not terminated by the adult. Fourth, they fostered taking turns between the therapist and the child, thus including the child as a partner in the interaction, enhancing communication and providing a means of modeling-appropriate behavior that can be imitated and lead to a desired response. Fifth, they always sought to gain the child's attention so that the child understood the task and the stimulus was appropriate. Sixth, they give the child choices in the interaction, thus building the child's motivation and reinforcing the child's spontaneous, self-initiated behavior. Again, this is more child driven as compared with having the interaction always directed by the adult.

There are several programs using ABA, its expansion into the NDBI approach, and including PRT. To review all of these programs is beyond the scope of this article, as was noted above. Thus, for this discussion, the DM and the ESDM are reviewed. It was decided to review ESDM because it uses a curriculum covering all domains of development, is child centered, and aims for a child-positive affect. Moreover, its focus is on teaching communication and is embedded in ongoing social communication and nonverbal communication [26].

The DM is the precursor to ESDM and was developed in the 1980s [34–36]. These researchers understood autism as arising from a primary deficit in social interactions. As a result, the program sought to build relationships with children as a means of enhancing the development of communication. Core features of the program and curriculum included an interdisciplinary team also involving pediatricians. Although the team was involved in reviewing and developing the curriculum, the child had one primary therapist. The DM focused on interpersonal engagement, the development of reciprocal, spontaneous imitation of gestures, facial expressions, and movements. The DM emphasized the development of verbal and nonverbal communication and focused on the cognitive aspects of play as well as partnering with parents. In other words, the curriculum assessed all aspects of the child's development, including play, language, nonverbal communication, and cognition. It was also recognized that many of the children had developmental delays that needed to be addressed as well as medical problems that were barriers to development. Finally, the group came to appreciate the significant difficulties children with ASD had with imitation; this presents a particularly challenging aspect of the disorder because imitation is so much a part of how children learn, thus emphasizing imitation skills was emphasized in the model.

Over time, it became apparent that in order for therapy to be more effective in treating children with ASD, interventions had to start early. This view is held by just about all early intervention programs, no matter what might be the child's challenges, but seemed even more critical for children with an ASD. The ESDM was specifically developed for children with ASD starting at 1 to 3 years and continuing in treatment until ages 4 to 5. As noted above, the ESDM is unique in that it addresses all developmental domains and has a curriculum that is very broad and inclusive and partners strongly with the family. As a matter of fact, the family is coached and becomes one of the major agents for education and change. In addition, the ESDM strongly endorses the concept of NDBI and has made it the mainstay of the environment created in the therapy program. Finally, as an intervention strategy, PRT is the model used. The ESDM takes a developmental view of understanding what underlies the challenges for children with ASD so that perspective is what directs the treatment goals. As in the DM curriculum, a list of specific skills that need to be addressed is sequenced developmentally. The domains that are covered include receptive and expressive communication, joint attention and imitation, social and play skills, cognitive skills, fine and gross motor skills, and self-care skills. Receptive and expressive communication, joint attention, imitation, social development, and play are particular foci of intervention in the ESDM [26]. What is of importance is that the teaching is embedded in play and in the child's day-to-day life experiences. As noted previously, the ESDM brings together strategies drawn from ABA, the DM, and PRT. At the outset of the program, a checklist is developed, and the goals for the child are established. At the end of the 12 weeks, the child is assessed, and new learning objectives put into place. This process is then repeated during the child's therapy.

In 2010, Dawson and colleagues [37] published a paper describing the results of a randomized trial comparing the effect the ESDM and interventions by available community providers. The subjects were 48 children with ASD between 18 and 30 months of age. The ESDM group received 20 hours of ESDM therapy, parent training, and parent delivery of ESDM therapy for 5 or more hours for 2 years or until the subjects were 48 months of age. The other group received yearly assessments with therapies provided in the community. All children received a comprehensive evaluation before starting in the program. Subjects were evaluated at the end of the program by skilled examiners who were naïve to the intervention designated groups. The children in ESDM improved 17.6 points on intelligence testing compared with 7.0 points of improvement in the community group. The ESDM maintained the rate of growth in adaptive behavior comparable to a typical sample of children. The community group showed greater delays in adaptive behavior. Children in ESDM were more likely to change their diagnosis from autism to pervasive developmental disorder. Considering the DSM-5 criteria, which do make this differentiation, it is suggested that the ESDM children required less supports and had overall general improvement in their behavior and general function. The overall conclusion is that the ESDM is a more effective intervention

than what is usually available in the community and that it is extremely important to identify and initiate early interventions for children with an ASD. This
thinking has been percolating in the community for some time, but with
the principles of ABA applied in a naturalistic setting, there is now stronger
evidence, rigorously gathered, to support the need for earlier, more intensive
and sustained interventions for this population of children.

Pharmacologic interventions

One cannot address treatment for children with ASD without mentioning pharmacologic interventions. It is beyond the scope of this article to go into detail,
yet several comments need to be made. First, pharmacologic interventions can
be very helpful, particularly if they are combined with behavioral programs
such as ABA and its various permutations. At the same time, it must be clearly
understood that one is not "treating" the underlying cause for autism, but addressing behaviors associated with autism. Thus, atypical antipsychotics have
been used to help with aggressive, uncontrolled, and psychotic behavior.
Mood stabilizers have been used for mood disorders; stimulants have been
used when there is evidence for attention deficit hyperactivity disorder, and
selective serotonin inhibitors have been used for the treatment of anxiety
and/or depression. These pharmacologic interventions are not used to treat
the core deficits in language development and deficits in social relatedness or
repetitive stereotypic behaviors. The author suggests medications are one
means of helping the child to be more available to his or her environment
and for helping therapists to use behavioral strategies to facilitate growth and
development. Furthermore, the author suggests that whenever it is deemed
necessary to use pharmacologic agents, there must always be a behavioral program in place. It is hoped for most children that behavioral strategies would be
the major intervention, not the use of pharmacologic agents.

DISCUSSION AND SUMMARY

As can be seen, autism, or ASD, has had a convoluted and complicated history
first being noted in the eighteenth century and probably existing long before it
was described in that era. It continues to the present to be a challenging entity
or group of entities. Some often wonder if what Kanner and Asperger
described were in reality different entities. However, that is probably a moot
point at this time because we have clinically identified a constellation of symptoms that are used to evaluate and diagnose individuals as falling on the autism
spectrum. Despite current efforts, we have no definitive biological markers,
although there is some insight as to where in the brain the abnormality resides.
In the author's opinion, the clearest, yet the broadest conception of an ASD
currently is the neurologic framework put forth by Aicardi, noted above.
He proposed that the core mechanism underlying ASD are deficits in communication between the various parts of the brain. Genetic markers are continued
to be pursued, yet we have not been successful in identifying a gene or genes
associated with autism. In addition, many environmental factors have been

considered, but none has been clearly associated with autism. Associations have been identified between the fragile X syndrome and tuberous sclerosis, extremely low birth weight, paternal advanced age, and the clinical characteristics of autism. However, these are only associations. There still are many questions to ask about the epidemiology and abnormality of ASD. One of the questions would be, why do only a portion of children with fragile X or Down syndrome or very low birth weight end up with ASD and others do not? Do these children with genetic disorders have other genetic perturbations leading or contributing to an ASD? What is it about some very low-birth-weight infants that results in them falling on the autism spectrum? The author suggests these, and other, questions about these associations are not trivial. The answers may well become apparent as more is learned about the molecular biology of the brain and tools developed to assess molecular biological mechanisms. In addition, these questions (among others) open up areas for meaningful research into the structure and function of the central nervous system and are not to be discarded as more clinically based research is pursued to answer the autism puzzle. At the same time, it is the author's opinion, and the opinion of others, that resources need to be provided for treatments that have been shown to improve the lives of these children and also resources provided for the research into known treatment of ASD as well as for others that may be developed. Finally, more resources need to be provided for families struggling to access early intervention and ongoing treatment programs where we have begun to be successful in enabling these children to be more functional and involved in the community rather than to be institutionalized at enormous cost to the community and the family.

This article has provided an overview of the salient history of autism. It has addressed the changes in the criteria by which the diagnosis of autism has been made and also discussed new imaging techniques that have the potential to shed more light on neural mechanisms associated with ASD. Finally, a refinement of an established intervention for ASD has been presented along with some of the research attesting to its efficacy. It must be noted that this intervention does not work for all children falling on the autism spectrum and is not the end all in therapy. This article is not meant to be comprehensive. Its purpose was to present the reader with information about some of the changes in the world of autism.

Acknowledgments

Appreciation is extended to Elizabeth Griffith, Terry Katz, and Theresa Schiavone for assistance in the preparation of this article.

References

[1] Silberman S. Neurotribes: the legacy of autism and the future of neurodiversity. New York: Avery; 2015.

[2] American Psychiatric Association. Diagnostic and statistical manual of mental disorders. 5th edition. Washington, DC: American Psychiatric Association; 2013.

[3] Centers for Disease Control and Prevention. Prevalence of autism spectrum disorder among children aged 8 years—autism and developmental disabilities monitoring network, 11 Sites, United States, 2010. MMWR Surveill Summ 2014;63(2):1–21.

[4] Available at: http://www.cdc.gov/nchs/data/nhsr/nhsr087.pdf. Accessed November 13, 2015.

[5] Kanner L. Autistic disturbances of affective contact. The Nervous Child 1943;2:217–50.

[6] Sachs O. An anthropologist on Mars. Knopf; 1995.

[7] Aicardi J. Autism and autistic-like conditions. In: Aiacardi J, editor. Diseases of the nervous system in children. 2nd edition. Cambridge (England): Univfersity Press; 1998. p. 827.

[8] Solomon A. Far from the tree. New York: Scribner; 2012. p. 222.

[9] American Psychiatric Association. Diagnostic and statistical manual of mental disorders, 3rd edition (DSM-III). Washington, DC: American Psychiatric Association; 1980.

[10] American Psychiatric Association. Diagnostic and statistical manual of mental disorders, 3rd edition–revised (DSM-III-R). Washington, DC: American Psychiatric Association; 1987.

[11] Lord C, Rutter M, Goode S, et al. Autism diagnostic observation schedule: a standardized observation of communicative and social behavior. J Autism Dev Disord 1989;19: 185–212.

[12] American Psychiatric Association. Diagnostic and statistical manual of mental disorders, 4th edition (DSM-IV). Washington, DC: American Psychiatric Association; 1994.

[13] American Psychiatric Association. Diagnostic and statistical manual of mental disorders, 4th edition–text revision (DSM-IV). Washington, DC: American Psychiatric Association; 2000. p. 50.

[14] American Psychiatric Association. Diagnostic and statistical manual of mental disorders, 5th edition (DSM-V). Washington, DC: American Psychiatric Association; 2013. p. 50.

[15] Frazier TW, Youngstrom EA, Speer L, et al. Validation of proposed DSM-5 criteria for autism spectrum disorder. J Am Acad Child Adolesc Psychiatry 2012;51:28–40.e3.

[16] Huerta M, Sishop SL, Duncan A, et al. Application of DSM-5 criteria for autism spectrum disorder to three samples of children with DSM-IV diagnoses of pervasive developmental disorder. Am J Psychiatry 2012;169:1056–64.

[17] Goldson E. Autism spectrum disorders. Adv Pediatr 2004;51:63–109.

[18] Flipek PA. Neuroimaging in the developmental disorders: the state of the science. J Child Psychol Psychiatry 1999;40:113–28.

[19] Travers BG, Adluru N, Ennis C, et al. Diffusion tensor imaging in autism spectrum disorder: a review. Autism Res 2012;5(5):289–313.

[20] Hanaie R, Mohri I, Kagitani-Shimono K, et al. Abnormal corpus collosum connectivity, socio-communicative deficits and motor deficits in children autism spectrum disorder: a diffusion tensor imaging study. J Autism Dev Disord 2014;44:2209–20.

[21] Tournier JD, Mori S, Lemmans A. Diffusion tensor imaging and beyond. Magn Reson Med 2011;65:1532–56.

[22] Budde MD, Xie M, Cross AH, et al. Axial diffusivity is the primary correlate of axonal injury in the experimental autoimmune encephalomyelitis spinal cord: a quantitative pixelwise analysis. J Neurosci 2009;29:2805–13.

[23] Cooper JO, Heron TE, Heward WL. Applied behavior analysis. 2nd edition. Upper Saddle River (NJ): Prentice Hall; 2006.

[24] Smith T, Eikeseth S. O.Ivar Lovaas: pioneer of applied behavior analysis and intervention for children with with autism. J Autism Dev Disord 2011;41:375–8.

[25] Lovaas OI, Schreibman L, Koegel RL. A behavior modification approach to the treatment of autistic children. J Autism Child Schizophr 1974;4:111–29.

[26] Rogers SJ, Dawson G. Early start Denver model for young children with autism. New York; London: The Guilford Press; 2010.

[27] Lovaas OI. Behavioral treatment and normal educational intellectual functioning in young autistic children. J Consult Clin Psychol 1987;55:3–9.

[28] Schreibman L, Dawson G, Landa R, et al. Naturalistic developmental behavioral interventions: empirically validated treatments for autism spectrum disorder. J Autism Dev Disord 2015;45(8):2411–28. Available at: Springerlink.com.

[29] Schreibman L. The science and fiction of autism. Cambridge (MA): Harvard University Press; 2005.

[30] Ingersol S, Schreibman L. Teaching reciprocal imitation skills to young children with autism using a naturalistic behavioral approach: effects on language, pretend play, and joint attention. J Autism Dev Disord 2006;36:487–505.

[31] Koegel R, Koegel LK. Generalized responsivity and pivotal behavior. In: Horner RH, Dunlap G, Koegel RL, editors. Generalization and maintenance: lifestyle changes in applied settings. Baltimore (MD): Brookes; 1988. p. 41–66.

[32] Koegel RL, Williams JA. Direct vs. indirect response—reinforcer relationships in teaching autistic children. J Abnorm Child Psychol 1980;8:537–47.

[33] Schreibman L, Koegel R. Training for parents of children with autism: pivotal responses, generalizations, and individualization of interventions. In: Hibbs ED, Jensen PS, editors. Psychosocial treatment for child and adolescent disorders: empirically based strategies for clinical practice. 2nd edition. Washington, DC: American Psychological Assocation; 2005. p. 605–32.

[34] Rogers SJ, Herbison J, Lewis H, et al. An approach for enhancing the symbolic, communicative, and interpersonal functioning of young children with autism and severe emotional handicaps. J Dis Early Childh 1986;10:135–48.

[35] Rogers SJ, Hall T, Osaki D, et al. A comprehensive, integrated, educational approach to young children with autism and their families. In: Harrris SL, Handleman JS, editors. Preschool education programs for children with autism. 2nd edition. Austin (TX): Pro-Ed; 2000. p. 95–134.

[36] Rogers SJ, Lewis H. An effective day treatment model for young children with pervasive developmental disorders. J Am Acad Child Adolesc Psychiatry 1989;28:207–14.

[37] Dawson G, Rogers S, Munson J, et al. Randomized, controlled trial of an intervention for toddlers with autism: the early start Denver model. Pediatrics 2010;125:e17–23.

Advances in Pediatrics 63 (2016) 357–387

ADVANCES IN PEDIATRICS

ELSEVIER
MOSBY

The Center for Human Development in Guatemala
An Innovative Model for Global Population Health

Edwin J. Asturias, MD[a,b], Gretchen Heinrichs, MD, DTMH[a,c],
Gretchen Domek, MD, MPhil[a,b], John Brett, PhD[d],
Elizabeth Shick, DDS, MPH[e],
Maureen Cunningham, MD, MPH[a,b], Sheana Bull, PhD[a],
Marco Celada, MD[a], Lee S. Newman, MD, MA[f],
Liliana Tenney, MPH[f], Lyndsay Krisher, MPH[a],
Claudia Luna-Asturias, MSW[a], Kelly McConnell, MD[a],
Stephen Berman, MD[a,*]

[a]Center for Global Health, Colorado School of Public Health Partners with Children's Hospital Colorado, 13199 E. Montview Boulevard, Campus Box A090, Aurora, CO 80045, USA; [b]Department of Pediatrics, University of Colorado School of Medicine, 13123 E. 16th Avenue, Campus Box B065, Aurora, CO 80045, USA; [c]Department of Obstetrics and Gynecology, University of Colorado School of Medicine, 13001 E. 17th Place, Campus Box C290, Aurora, CO 80045, USA; [d]Department of Anthropology, College of Liberal Arts and Sciences, University of Colorado-Denver, PO Box 173364, Campus Box 103, Denver, CO 80217, USA; [e]School of Dental Medicine, University of Colorado Anschutz Medical Campus, 13065 E. 17th Avenue, Campus Box F833, Aurora, CO 80045, USA; [f]Center for Health, Work & Environment, Colorado School of Public Health, 13001 E. 17th Place, Campus Box B186, Aurora, CO 80045, USA

Keywords
- Population health • Maternal health • Child health • Global health
- Neonatal mortality • Education

Key points
- A private sector/university partnership model can successfully promote population health and sustainable development in impoverished regions of the world.
- This model can leverage the strengths of both the university and private sector.

Continued

*Corresponding author. Center for Global Health, Colorado School of Public Health Partners with Children's Hospital Colorado, 13199 E. Montview Boulevard, Campus Box A090, Aurora, CO 80045. *E-mail address:* stephen.berman@childrenscolorado.org

0065-3101/16/$ – see front matter
http://dx.doi.org/10.1016/j.yapd.2016.04.001

Continued

- This model can successfully integrate service delivery, community development, research, and education.
- This model can provide a community laboratory to evaluate innovative interventions that promote population health.

INTRODUCTION

Population health focuses on the health of a defined population as measured by the health outcomes of groups of individuals and an analysis of how and why these outcomes differ within the population. This approach seeks to understand how these differences are affected by social, economic, cultural, geographic, and genetic factors as well as access to health services. In order to optimize population health, traditional health care delivery systems should integrate and/or coordinate with other systems, such as public health, schools, transportation, water and sanitation, and social services. The population health approach, first implemented in Canada, is now being adapted in many countries, including the United States [1]. Measurement is a critical component of population health. Health care systems need accurate population denominators (population registries) and numerators (patient registries), as well as process and outcome measures that will document progress in improving population health. The project described in this article provides a model for operationalizing a population health approach using a university–private sector–community partnership and the opportunity to evaluate the effectiveness of this integrative approach to achieve significant reductions in morbidity and mortality and promote the sustainable development goals in this extremely poor Guatemalan population. This article describes the population in the region, the structure and governance model of the partnership, and the project's activities that seek to empower the community, transform health, and create opportunity.

THE POPULATION

Guatemala is Central America's most populous country, with 15.4 million people, of whom approximately 40% are of indigenous descent. It is a low-middle income country (LMIC) with a gross domestic product per capita of $3,478 and a human development index of 0.58 in 2012 (an improvement of only 0.1 in the past 2 decades). Guatemala has a national poverty rate exceeding 50% and an extreme poverty rate of 15% [2]. Although 46% of the total population lives in rural areas, 72% of the extremely poor live in those rural areas [2]. Nationally, the child mortality (at 30 per 1000 live births) is the highest in Central America and the third highest in the region. Maternal mortality is also one of the highest in the region. In 2010 the World Health Organization (WHO) estimated a maternal mortality ratio of approximately 120 per 100,000 live births and the more recent World Bank estimates from 2011 to 2015 are around 100 per 100,000 [3,4]. The contraceptive prevalence (at 54%) is one of the lowest in

Latin America [5]. Maternal mortality, child mortality, and malnutrition are higher among rural populations such as those living in the southwest (SW) Trifinio region.

Life is especially difficult in the coastal lowlands of southwestern Guatemala near the border with Chiapas, Mexico. This region is named the SW Trifinio (triangle) for the confluence of the 3 departments (states) of San Marcos, Quetzaltenango, and Retalhuleu (Fig. 1). A few decades ago these cattle and pasturelands were transformed into large agribusiness enterprises to cultivate crops for export (primarily bananas and palm oil), attracting approximately 25,000 people who now live in this area. Given their recent migration and diversity, these aldeas (small communities) lack the community cohesion, shared tradition, and culture of older communities. The region is susceptible to flooding because of its low elevation and close proximity to the Pacayá River, which cannot contain the runoff from Guatemala's high mountains to the northeast. Because most families use pit latrines for waste disposal and shallow wells as their source of water, flooding contaminates the water supply, spreading gastrointestinal disease and promoting mosquito-borne infections. Governmental services are limited, perhaps because of poor coordination among local governments. In 2011, no access to physician care was available in the community and a trip to the nearest city, Coatepeque, to see a doctor took 1 hour and cost more than a month's wages.

THE AGRO-AMERICA–UNIVERSITY PARTNERSHIP

One of the largest employers in the SW Trifinio is Agro-America, a private, family-owned Guatemala agribusiness that operates banana and palm oil plantations in the region. Agro-America has been committed to social investing to improve the human development index of the families and communities in the area. The company has strong social values and pays its workers a living wage above the standard within their industry. In 2011, Agro-America approached the Center for Global Health (CGH) at the Colorado School of Public Health to replace its existing social responsibility program called Mis Mejores Familias, a community educational program developed by the sugar industry. The CGH has a strong track record in global health and is one of 2 WHO Collaborating Maternal and Child Health Centers (not Promoting Family and Child Health) in the Americas. In July of 2011, the CGH, Children's Hospital Colorado (a hospital affiliated with the university), and Agro-America through its foundation Jose Fernando Bolaños Menendez signed a memorandum of understanding to "promote the development of scientific and technical activities, research and projects in the field of public health sciences, that promote the comprehensive improvement of health and human development and mitigate the impact of disasters in the area of influence in Guatemala." The next phase created the governance and legal infrastructure for the project, titled the Center for Human Development (CHD). Agro-America created a new private not-for-profit Guatemalan foundation to run the CHD, called Fundación para la Salud Integral de Guatemaltecos-CU (FSIG; Foundation for Guatemalan Integrated

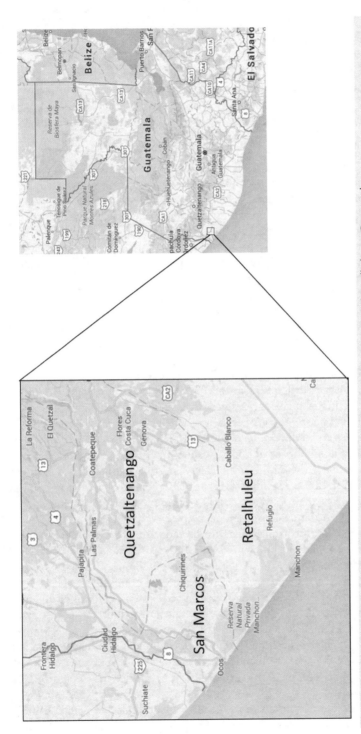

Fig. 1. SW Trifinio at the borders of the departments of San Marcos, Quetzaltenango, and Retalhuleu in Guatemala.

Health–CU). The foundation has 7 members; 4 appointed by Agro-America and 3 appointed by the CGH. The establishment of the foundation for the CHD was critical because the legal department of the university identified obstacles that did not allow the CGH to have university professional staff (faculty) live and work long term in Guatemala. The foundation is responsible for ensuring that all project operations and program activities are in compliance with Guatemalan local laws. It obtains all needed approvals and licenses pertaining to the operation of the clinic, birthing center, laboratory, and pharmacy. It is responsible for the hiring and management of all employees, including managing payroll, benefits, and taxes and maintaining all financial records. The foundation has an executive director, medical director, and chief financial officer. The foundation is also responsible for the approval of and the financial support for hosting volunteer faculty and health care providers who travel to the Guatemala site to work.

Having Agro-America as a partner has many advantages. In addition to its impact on economic opportunity, the project takes advantage of Agro-America's existing infrastructure for human resources, purchasing, information technology, communications, and maintenance. The partnership also benefits from its prior social impact programs and community organizing efforts. Because Agro-America is the major funder, the partnership is able to integrate multiple funding streams and avoid the limitations of funding silos. The CGH, as a hub for the University of Colorado global activities, contributes to the partnership by leveraging expertise from the Schools of Medicine, Nursing, Public Health, Business, Dentistry, Pharmacy, Architecture, and Arts and Sciences. The CGH can create multidisciplinary teams to design and implement the population health strategies. The university also provides clinical support for the project through elective rotations of residents and fellows with faculty oversight.

Public-private partnerships work properly when the following occur: (1) trust and sharing of information between parties, (2) understanding and exploitation of the competencies of each party, and (3) improvement driven by service standards and not by downdriven cost [6–10]. Although the core of the partnership includes a shared commitment to population health and sustainable development, trust is built when each partner recognizes the values and goals of the other. The university must respect and support Ago-America's desire for their efforts and funding to be recognized by the community. The company's goal is to have healthier, more productive employees who will enable the company to become more profitable. The company also benefits in its marketing to existing and potential customers, because buyers are becoming more sophisticated about the ethics of their suppliers and how they address issues of social justice, fairness, and climate change. In contrast, Agro-America must respect and support the university missions in education and research as well as service. Research and educational activities can increase professional resource capacity at the site and provide the expertise needed to develop effective interventions. Funded research grants can also help make the overall project more self-sustaining through indirect cost allocations and recruitment of staff.

Establishing a partnership between a US university and host country corporation is uncommon because universities traditionally partner with host country universities, governmental agencies, or nongovernmental organizations (NGOs) and obtain funding from foundations, United States Agency for International Development (USAID), Centers for Disease Control and Prevention (CDC), National Institutes of Health (NIH), or American multinational corporations. The most obvious reason our model is rare is the difficulty in identifying host country private-sector companies willing to commit to long-term social impact investing in their country's extremely poor communities with a US university partner. If we can document success, the project may stimulate other similar partnerships.

THE STRATEGIC APPROACH TO POPULATION HEALTH

The overall strategic approach for our project is shown in Fig. 2, which displays our vision, mission, community health assessment, and the main domains of the project with their goals, strategies, and outcomes. The domains were identified by a community health assessment and include clinic medical and oral health services with a birthing center, community nursing services, employee health, the environment, economic opportunity, and education. Overarching functions include research, community engagement, and strategic planning/sustainability. This article presents the findings of the community health assessment and the resulting domain and overarching functions' strategies, early outcomes, and challenges.

COMMUNITY HEALTH ASSESSMENT

A community health assessment (CHA) to evaluate the health status and risk determinants of people in the community is the necessary first step in developing a population approach. In September and October 2011, the CGH facilitated home interviews of 287 families using the Mis Mejores Familias homes as index households to conduct the random community sample for those having a child less than 5 years old. This CHA used a cluster sampling technique consistent with the lot quality assurance sampling methodology from the WHO for immunization program evaluation.

The CHA documented that the SW Trifinio aldeas has high levels of food insecurity, maternal depression, maternal morbidity and mortality, neonatal mortality, and child morbidity. Most mothers and children of the aldeas surveyed depended on traditional birth attendants (TBAs) and 1 form of medicine, because there are both financial and access barriers to securing timely formal health care services. Food insecurity was prevalent: of the 287 mothers interviewed, 133 (46.5%) answered that, "Sometimes we have no food to eat" and 30 (10.5%) responded that, "Most of the time we have no food to eat." Seventy percent (n = 201) of participants agreed with the statement, "In the past three months the food we had was not sufficient and we had no money to buy more food." The same proportion (71.5%) reported skipping meals because of insufficient money to buy food, and 148 (51.6%) reported that at

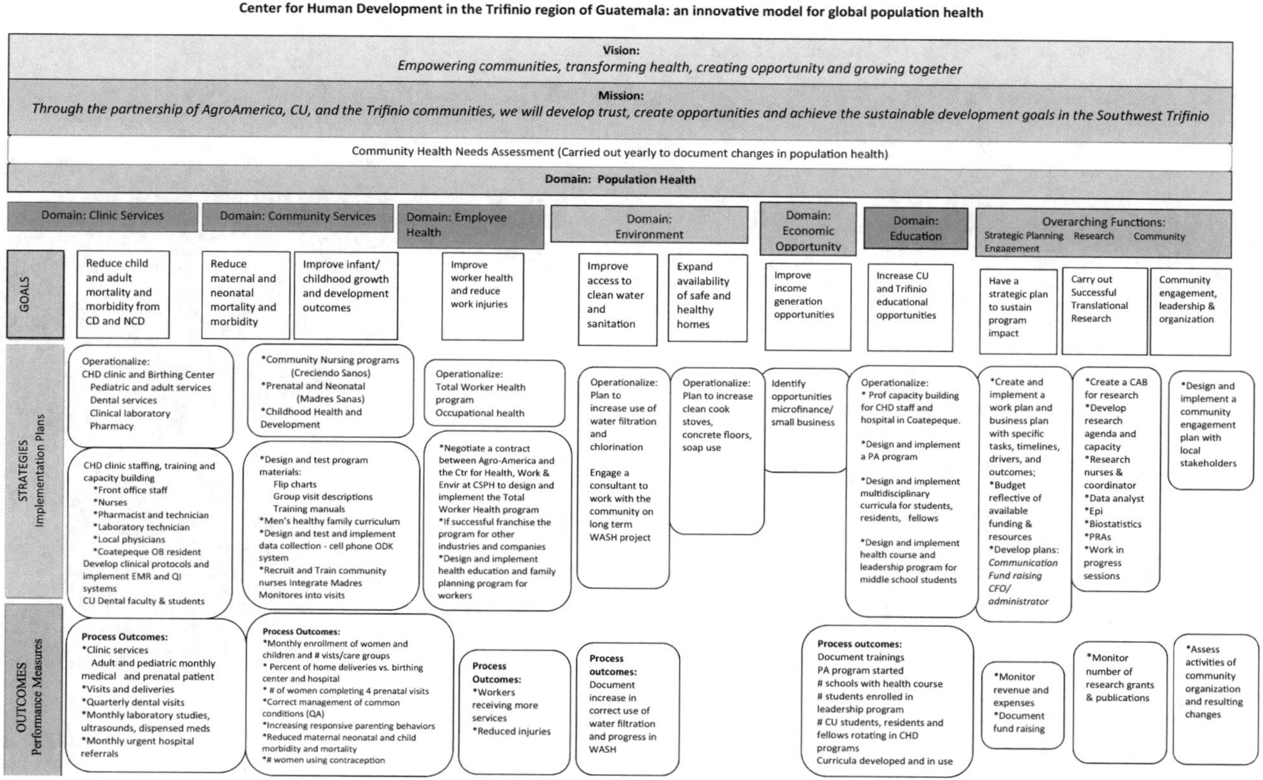

Fig. 2. Strategy map. PA, physician assistant; WASH, water, sanitation, and hygiene.

least 1 member of the family lost weight because of the inability to purchase food. There was a direct relationship between the mother's mental state (level of depression) and food insecurity. Among the 195 mothers with food insecurity, 64 (32.8%) showed signs of significant depression, whereas among the remaining 90 mothers with more food security only 15 (16.6%) showed any depression signs ($P = .003$). Environmental issues related to access to clean water and having appropriate sanitation were serious concerns. Most of the homes (59.6%) used a shallow well as their primary water source and only 25.4% (n = 73) reported access to portable water (aqueducts); 5% used rain or collection tanks and 8% bottled water as their source of drinking water. Covered latrines were the most common means of human waste disposal in 79% of the homes, and 9.8% reported the use of a flushable toilet. Approximately 10% used open latrines or open land or other methods for human waste. Trash was burned on nearby land (n = 190; 66.2%) or buried (n = 43; 15%), and 40 homes (13.9%) reported disposing of waste in the backyard. Only 4.2% used the community waste disposal. Wood stoves were the most common method for cooking (94.1%) (Fig. 3), whereas 5% reported cooking on gas stoves and less than 1% had improved clean-burning stoves. As expected, mothers were poorly educated. Sixty-one of the participants (21.3%) reported not having any formal education and only 52% completed second grade. Despite this, 101 women (35.2%) reported that they could not read and write, noting that the completion of the first or second grade level does not imply freedom from illiteracy. Only 7.5% of mothers had studied beyond the sixth grade.

As part of the survey a modified version of the Edinburgh Post-partum Depression Scale was used, to learn about maternal mental health. The scale used 5 of the 10 original questions to detect maternal depression in the preceding 7 days. Maternal depression was frequently reported. Of the 287 mothers interviewed, 4.2% reported that "they did not see anything good

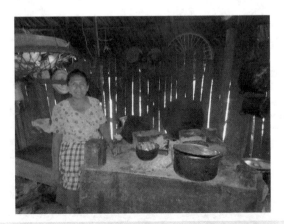

Fig. 3. A wood-fueled cooking stove.

in life and could not smile"; 11.6% reported feeling guilty because their situation was not good, and 9.1% felt very frightened or anxious without reason. In addition, 8.1% were sleepless because of their unhappiness, and 2.5% thought about hurting themselves or preferred to be dead because of their current situation.

Reproductive health problems were clearly identified: 56 (19.5%) of the participants reported 6 or more children, and only 44.9% reported 2 or fewer children. Slightly more than half of the women reported their first pregnancy before the age of 18 years, and 7.8% before the age of 15 years. Sixty-nine percent of the participants reported using TBAs as the primary caregiver for prenatal care and only 9% visited a nurse in the community health center; 12.2% received care from a physician and 6.3% went to a public or private hospital. Consistently, when asked who managed their last delivery, 44.8% reported the use of TBAs, 30% a physician, and 20% received care at the hospitals. Twenty-one percent of the women reported at least 1 abortion or miscarriage, and 30% reported significant complications close to childbirth. Almost 6% of the mothers reported having a stillbirth, which was associated with the lack of adequate prenatal or perinatal care. Having a child die was a frequent occurrence. Forty participants (13.9%) reported having a child die during the first 5 years of life, with more than half of the deaths (55.6%) occurring in the first 2 months of life and 87.3% within the first year of life. Ninety percent of the participating mothers nursed their children for more than 6 months, and 61.7% for more than 12 months. No data were collected about the supplementary feeding practices during the first year of life.

Information on common childhood illness showed that 120 (41.8%) mothers reported diarrhea in the past 2 weeks for at least 1 child less than 5 years of age, and that only 25.7% of children with diarrhea received oral rehydration salts. One in 6 children received antibiotics, 15.6% home remedies, and 12.3% anti-parasitic medications. Similarly, 168 (58.8%) of the mothers reported that at least 1 of their children less than 5 years of age had had a cough in the previous 2 weeks, and 65.2% reported having a cold (upper respiratory infection). Two of every 5 mothers reported at least 1 of their children less than 5 years of age having a fever in the 2 weeks before the survey. The treatment practices included oral rehydration (1.5%), antibiotics (73.8%), and acetaminophen or aspirin (7.5%). If children were ill, 27% visited the community health clinic, 24.9% a nurse, 20.4% a hospital, 13% a family doctor, and only 4.2% sought help directly from the pharmacy clerk. When medications were needed they were obtained at the local pharmacy (43.2%), community health clinic (45.3%), and for a minority in the hospital or physicians. When asked whether the family had sufficient financial resources to purchase the necessary medicines, 252 (88.7%) replied in the negative. When the CHA data were analyzed, plans were made for a community engagement process to share the results and present ideas for possible interventions.

COMMUNITY ENGAGEMENT: A RAPID ANTHROPOLOGIC ASSESSMENT PROCEDURE

After the results of the rapid CHA, it was evident that the next step was to develop an understanding of how the community was organized, its level of function, and how best to develop a partnership with the community to set priorities and build mutual trust. In 2012, the Department of Anthropology at the University of Colorado Denver assembled a team-based qualitative inquiry using triangulation, iterative data collection, and analysis to rapidly understand the situation from the community perspective. The team sought to answer 2 fundamental questions. First, in the absence of functioning state and local government, how do people in these communities organize themselves to meet their basic needs? Second, what is the social and cultural context of health in these communities? During a 2-week period the team conducted 27 formal structured interviews with community leaders and 4 informal interviews with auxiliary nurses. The formal interviews with community leaders included government officials (eg, vice mayors), water managers, disaster preparedness and response officials, Catholic Church workers and evangelical ministers, and participants in the Mis Mejores Familias program [3]. The rapid anthropologic assessment procedure (RAP) produced a visual map of the community leadership and organizational structure and described the areas of dysfunction that made certain groups more vulnerable to social, economic, health, and environmental disturbances. Based on both the CHA and the RAP, 3 major priorities emerged from the communities: (1) access to clean, safe, and sustainable water; (2) access to health care services; and (3) education for children and adolescents. Based on evidence from the CHA and the anthropologic RAP and the expertise of the CGH, the initial focus was to identify interventions that could be rapidly implemented to improve maternal, neonatal, and child health outcomes.

POPULATION HEALTH DOMAINS

The clinic and birthing center: having the facilities needed to provide a medical home.

Clinic services

Establishing a clinic was a high priority for both the community and the Agro-America–University of Colorado partnership. Mr Fernando Bolaños, the founder of Agro-America, dreamed of establishing a clinic for his workers and the community before he died. Therefore, the Bolaños family considered establishing a clinic as a tribute to their late father's memory. A multidisciplinary collaborative process that included Agro-America, its local Guatemalan architect, faculty and students from the College of Architecture and Planning at University of Colorado Denver, and CGH clinical faculty designed the clinical facilities. The facility includes a front check-in area; pediatric, adult, and obstetrics/gynecology examination rooms; a dental room; birthing center; physician workstations; pharmacy; laboratory; and office/conference room space. Architectural plans are shown in Fig. 4 and construction was completed in April

HEALTH CENTER

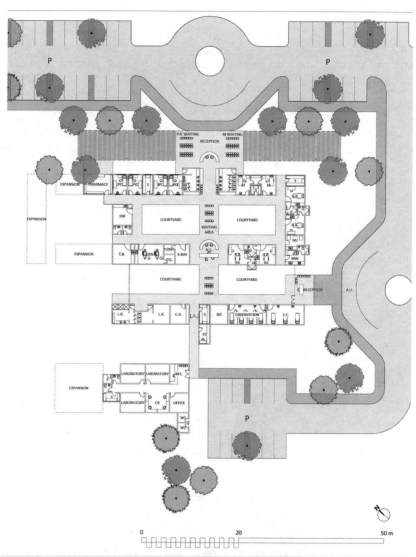

Fig. 4. Clinical facilities floor plan. AU, ambulance unloading area; CA, common area for doctors; CONT, control room; CR, computer room; DENT, dental clinic; DO, doctor office; EC, emergency care; EQ, equipment; IDR, infectious disease room; LR, locker room; M, maternity/women clinic; MW, midwives rest area; NS, nurses station; NU, nursery; P/C, pediatrics/Clinics; P, parking; PC, pediatric clinic; S, storage; ST, sterilization room; T, treatment room; W1, natural waste; W2, medical waste; WS, work station; X, radiography clinic.

2014. The CGH funded the delivery of 2 Project CURE (Commission on Urgent Relief and Equipment) containers that transported donated equipment, furniture, and supplies for the clinic. A server-based electronic medical record, Clinical Fusion, used in school-based clinics in the United States is being implemented and it is close to functional given the remoteness of this site. The clinic started caring for patients on March 14, 2014 (Fig. 5), with staff that included a clerk, 2 nurses, and a laboratory technician. Medical care was provided by University of Colorado pediatric residents and a Guatemalan-American family physician, Dr Marco Celada. As the project became established, the number of students, residents, and faculty traveling to work in Trifinio increased, as shown in Fig. 6. Although the clinic initially focused on children, half of those seeking care were adults with noncommunicable diseases, which provided an opportunity for the pediatric residents to experience family medicine in the global arena, and fostered the need to involve more family and internal medicine residents. One of the principles in establishing this clinic was to avoid competition with the existing, limited public health services (mostly immunizations) staffed with auxiliary nurses. Therefore, the clinic was established as a collaborating second-level facility for outpatient care, safe pregnancy care, and deliveries. The fees were set lower than those of comparable services in Coatepeque, even without considering the saved transportation costs. However, the poverty in the region is so great that any fee may be a significant barrier to seeking care. In trying to balance these concerns, the clinic compromised by setting the cost for employees of Agro-America at $2 and nonemployees at $3. However, mothers and children enrolled in the community outreach maternal and child programs are referred and seen without charge. The laboratory services expanded to include the tests Agro-America required for its employees, as well as routine prenatal testing, Pap smear collection (processing is done by APROFAM), and human immunodeficiency virus and syphilis screening. In addition, the clinic nurses were trained in fetal ultrasonography and the scans were printed so that women could take them to the hospital. A prenatal package with a small monthly payment plan was implemented for visits, laboratory, and ultrasonography costs. The patient volume was initially

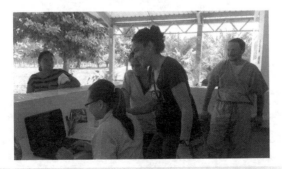

Fig. 5. Checking in the first patient at the clinic.

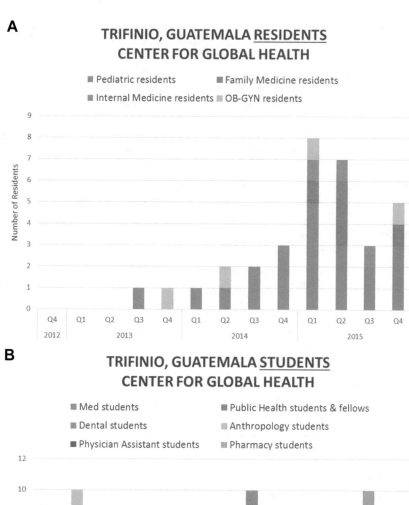

Fig. 6. Residents (A) and students (B) working in the Trifinio 2012 to 2015. OB-GYN, obstetrics/gynecology.

modest but has steadily increased. In the summer of 2015, several positive activities began. The pharmacy became operational; the community nurses began a stronger outreach effort to let families know about the clinic services; clinic leadership met with local leaders regarding clinic offerings; and the clinic's capacity increased as family medicine, internal medicine, and physician assistant rotations began in addition to those of the pediatric residents.

There were several design challenges in building the clinic facilities in an extremely hot climate with torrential rains, annual flooding, and high rates of mosquito-borne illness (dengue and chikungunya). The University of Colorado Denver architecture students came up with several creative ideas about using local materials such as bamboo and river stones enclosed in wire mesh. However, building this way was more expensive than using more traditional cinderblock construction. There were many political problems in obtaining needed licenses and approvals for the clinic, laboratory, and pharmacy operations, which caused delays, and we were under-resourced in terms of on-site management because of financial limitations. After the clinic opening, patient volume was less than expected because there was an initial perception that only corporate employees and their families could receive services at the clinic, as well as confusion as to whether the clinic would see adult patients. We lacked a clear strategy for how to communicate to the community about the clinic services available.

Birthing center
The reasons for excessive maternal mortality and morbidity have traditionally been framed by 3 major delays: (1) delay in recognition that there is a problem, (2) delay in accessing care when the problem has been recognized (financial, physical, transportation barriers), and (3) delay of appropriate care delivery when at the referral facility (caused by supply issues, health worker shortages, or clinical knowledge deficits) [11,12]. Because the CHA found that about half of the pregnant women were delivering at home with a high rate of maternal complications, the project began designing a birthing center based on the midwifery model of care, with TBAs working together with trained delivery nurses within a system of referral and emergency transportation. This approach avoided or ameliorated the traditional 3 delays [13,14]. In April 2012, focused interviews were held with local TBAs to further understand the context in which women receive prenatal care and care during childbirth. Follow-up interviews with the TBAs and a qualitative project collecting birth narratives from community women and TBAs in 2013 increased our understanding of pregnancy behaviors around delivery and common complications. Given this background, the TBAs were recognized as important women of influence in their communities, and we sought to involve them in our ongoing efforts around healthy birth through skills building and clinical team collaboration. This information on pregnancy and delivery complications also helped to design the birthing center and trainings related to healthy pregnancy and childbirth for TBAs, nurses, women, and community members. Protocols and

guidelines were adapted from the university, regional birth centers, and WHO standards to our situation and a training and education program was started for the current TBAs, the skilled birth attendants (SBAs), and the community health nurses (CHNs). Ongoing training in emergency obstetric care has been conducted since July 2013 for TBAs and SBAs. A repetitive curriculum that incorporates the principles of Helping Babies Breathe, Jhpiego's Helping Mother's Survive, and WHO Essential Newborn Care were implemented [15–18]. The curriculum uses simulation and drills to keep practitioners' skills in emergency obstetric management current and promotes team-based practice [19,20]. Evaluations of emergency obstetric skills of CHNs, TBAs, and SBAs are conducted via objective structured clinical examinations at least once per year by faculty visiting the area. Community health and clinic-based nurses were also trained to perform basic ultrasonography scans in pregnancy, identify ultrasonography abnormalities, and to perform pap smears and pelvic examinations. Because access to women's health physicians is severely limited in this area, the task shifting has improved the scope and access to care for the population.

Scheduled to open in May 2016, the birthing center will allow some of the TBAs to shift their patients from home deliveries to the birthing center, providing low-risk patients with the ability to access a culturally appropriate and safer delivery facility closer to their homes, and with assurance that any complicated or high-risk delivery will be referred to the regional hospital in Coatepeque. However, several issues must be resolved for the birthing center to open under the following preestablished guidelines. First, there must be staff to cover 24 hours a day, 7 days a week, with SBAs (physicians, nurses, or trained nurse midwives) who are willing to collaborate with the community TBAs, and there must also be housing accommodation for the staff close to the birthing center. Second, an ambulance with a dedicated, trained driver must be available to transport mothers in labor with complications to a hospital in Coatepeque. An ambulance was purchased and retrofitted but an on-call system for drivers needs to be developed. In addition, an agreement of affiliation with a public hospital in Coatepeque will be established to ensure the proper coordination and referral of patients. Extensive relationship building has already occurred with the obstetrics/gynecology residency program there, to coordinate referrals of outpatient clinical emergencies. Along with the agreement, there is the hope to implement a rotation for local obstetrics/gynecology residents through the birthing center beginning in 2016.

Oral health program
The prevalence of dental problems is very high in the SW Trifinio area. Guatemalan dental professionals can be found in Coatepeque, more than an hour away, but dental care is costly and the lack of transportation limits access to oral health care for most residents. The University of Colorado School of Dental Medicine collaborates with the CGH by funding and providing dental

services at the clinic 3 to 4 times per year. A board-certified pediatric dentist serves as the dental program director at the clinic and has implemented a school-based oral health program (based on WHO guidelines), direct patient care services, and population evaluation. Before opening the dental clinic in June 2014, an oral health needs assessment was performed on schoolchildren attending the Fernando Bolaños Elementary School for the workers' children using previously published experiences [21,22]. A very high incidence of dental disease was noted, with 96% of children having 1 or more decayed teeth. In addition, 44% of children self-reported having dental pain and 20% had visible dental abscesses. An oral health focus group was conducted with the school teachers. The group reported a need for accessible dental care, a high prevalence of toothaches, missing school because of toothaches, facial swelling, and difficulty sleeping at home. A 2-pronged approach to implementing the school-based oral health program was taken: (1) training of the teachers and clinic nurses about oral health and prevention, and (2) a school-based education and brushing program. In June of 2014, 10 teachers and nurses were trained on the causes of dental caries, prevention strategies, and how to identify dental problems and make referrals as needed. In addition, the teachers began a school brushing program, which includes all students keeping a toothbrush at school and brushing their teeth daily. Each time the University of Colorado dental team visits, they hold a school assembly and review oral health via flip chart with all of the children at the school. Also, new toothbrushes and toothpaste are brought to the school to sustain the school brushing program.

Oral health care for workers and the community
The University of Colorado School of Dental Medicine conducts a minimum of 3 dental mission visits per year to provide comprehensive dental care for patients at the clinic. Dental teams consist of School of Dental Medicine faculty, dental students, and volunteer community dentists. Dental services offered include prevention, oral health counseling, and dental treatment, as well as basic fillings and extractions. There have been 4 dental visits since August 2014. Over the course of the first year, the dental team screened 303 school children; had 213 patient visits; and performed 40 preventive visits, 122 fillings, 26 primary tooth crowns, and 274 extractions.

Population evaluation
The initial needs assessment that was performed at the Fernando Bolaños Elementary School in June 2014 was repeated in August 2015. Some students have graduated and new students have been enrolled but the comparisons can be made to show the success of the dental program (Fig. 7). Periodic evaluations will help determine the prospective impact of this program to reduce oral and dental disease in children in the area [23].

The greatest challenge is the lack the funding and resources to use the dental clinic more than 3 to 4 times per year.

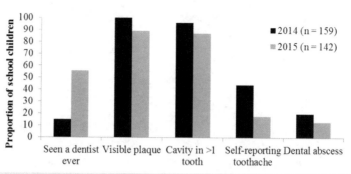

Fig. 7. Impact of a school oral health program at the Fernando Bolaños Elementary School in SW Trifinio in Guatemala.

Community services

The community nursing services program for prenatal care, neonatal home visitation, child visits, and monthly mother-child care group visits, called Creciendo Sanos (Growing Healthy), is a key component of the strategy to reduce maternal, neonatal, and child morbidity and mortality. Both the maternal program component (Madres Sanas [Healthy Mothers]) and child program component (Niños Sanos [Healthy Children]) developed flip charts (with pictures, recognizing the high rates of illiteracy) to deliver educational content to mothers. The front side of the chart has information for the women and the reverse has prompts for the nurses. There are also nurse training manuals for both programs and a manual for the mother-child care group visits. A mobile platform data collection system was established. The community nurses enter data on each visit and care group into a cell phone application that transfers the data to a database using the android-based Open Data Kit (ODK) open source platform. Because ODK is not secure, only the women's project numbers are entered and later matched with the women's names and demographic information stored on a secure platform in REDCap. The data collection system is integral to the community nursing program and allows the assessment of the quality of clinical care delivered; the measurement of key maternal, neonatal, and child health metrics; and evaluation of the programs [24].

Maternal health community nursing programs

Prenatal and delivery care are both critical for maternal and newborn health. Therefore, this maternal community nursing program focuses on improving prenatal care, screening pregnant women for complications, establishing a referral system for high-risk pregnancies, and shifting away from home deliveries. The Madres Sanas program uses a home visiting prenatal and newborn care model with CHNs who deliver 4 prenatal individual or group prenatal care visits, as well as an assessment of the mothers in their immediate postpartum periods. During this visit, CHNs also screen and refer for maternal depression (using the Edinburgh Postnatal Depression Scale). The nurses enter visit data into the prenatal clinical quality improvement database, which allows health information and outcomes on women to be monitored during pregnancy. This monitoring allows for action and/or educational counseling by CHNs for abnormal findings. Based on feedback from mothers participating in this program, the authors developed an Agro-America male worker reproductive education project (piloted in November 2015) on the topics of gender equality, the father's role in a family, and birth spacing methods. The pilot curriculum focuses on the father's role in promoting family health, including the use of birth spacing to encourage optimal health for the child and mother before the next pregnancy, rather than limiting the number of children.

Fig. 8 shows the number of pregnant women registered in the program per month and the number of post-partum visits. Program evaluation occurs in an ongoing manner via the pregnancy and neonatal registry to measure maternal and neonatal mortality and morbidity and the impact of the programs using the following key indicators: number and percentage of women completing 4 prenatal visits during each pregnancy; number and percentage of women less than 19 years old with a pregnancy; number and percentage of women delivering via cesarean; number and percentage of women delivering in a health facility with an SBA; and number and percentage of women choosing a modern form of contraception after delivery.

Pediatric community health nursing program
The Niños Sanos program is an integrated early childhood health and development program that has been specifically designed for the Trifinio population

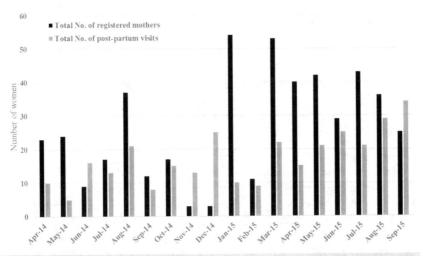

Fig. 8. Number of pregnant women registered by month in the Madres Sanas registry and number of post-partum visits provided. Southwest Trifinio Guatemala 2014 to 2015.

and is based on evidence from the WHO as well as similar programs in other developing regions [25–29]. The importance of integrated interventions to improve early childhood development, health, and nutrition is widely recognized at an international level [30–34]. The first 3 years of a child's life are a critical period for brain growth and development, and this period has significant consequences for long-term functioning. Such interventions have the potential to enhance children's physical growth and socioemotional and cognitive development, as well as the overall economic productivity of a society.

Niños Sanos was informed by 2 initial pilot studies conducted by CGH faculty and medical students from the University of Colorado School of Medicine. An initial early childhood developmental screening study in the Trifinio region in July 2012 found that children had high rates of developmental delays (as defined by the Ages and Stages Questionnaire) and further suggested that families that do not provide adequate cognitive stimulation for their children would benefit from an intervention educating mothers in responsive parenting. Intervention materials integrating ways to promote early childhood development, health, and nutrition were then developed and piloted during a July 2013 study. This study showed that mothers in the Trifinio were able to significantly increase their knowledge about health and development topics following a short interactive flip-chart talk promoting responsive parenting. Mothers further increased their knowledge 1 to 2 weeks after the talk, without any reexposure to the intervention materials, presumably by informal reinforcement with other mothers in the community.

Given the need for an intervention to promote early childhood development and health and the success of early pilot materials in the Trifinio region, Niños Sanos was designed to include an integrated approach to early childhood health and development, combining a series of neonatal home visits, mother-child care groups, and community education sessions to enhance the health and development of children from 0 to 3 years of age. The program starts with 3 neonatal home visits by the CHNs in the first month of life (birth, 2 weeks, and 1 month), based on WHO Essential Newborn Care guidelines, to assess neonates, provide appropriate referrals for sick newborns, and screen for maternal depression (Fig. 9). Small group talks given by the CHNs then occur when the child is 6 months, 12 months, 24 months, and 36 months of age to teach, promote, and reinforce caregiver knowledge of age-appropriate topics, including developmental milestones, good hygiene and hand washing, home management and recognition of common illnesses (including fever, cough, and diarrhea), timely immunizations, safety and injury prevention, and responsive parenting techniques. These visits also include growth monitoring and promotion (with referral for severely malnourished children) and developmental screening. In addition to the community health nurse visits, monthly mother-child interactive care groups start at 2 months of age and continue until the child reaches 3 years (Figs. 10 and 11). These groups use participatory learning to promote cognitive stimulation, provide peer support for the mothers,

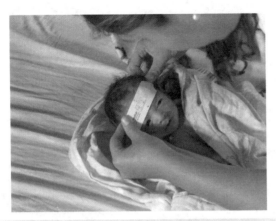

Fig. 9. Neonatal visit with a community nurse during the first week of life.

reinforce caregiver knowledge of health topics, and perform growth monitoring and promotion.

Niños Sanos currently has more than 400 children enrolled. Monthly enrollment is shown in Fig. 12. More than 250 children have received a nurse home visit in the first 2 weeks of life. Program evaluation measuring outcomes and indicators is ongoing. Short-term and midterm goals include increasing identification of sick neonates with referral to the hospital, increasing rates of exclusive breastfeeding before 6 months of age, increasing responsive parenting behaviors (talking, praise, reading, and play), decreasing the incidence of diarrhea, and increasing hand washing with soap. Long-term goals include decreasing neonatal mortality, decreasing infant mortality, decreasing developmental delays, decreasing stunting and the incidence of severe malnutrition,

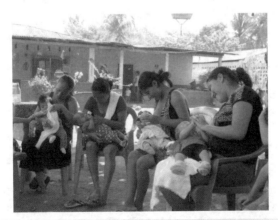

Fig. 10. Mothers using finger puppets to talk with their children in a mother-child care group.

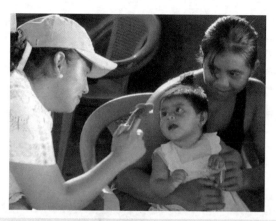

Fig. 11. A community health nurse demonstrates talking to a young child using a finger puppet during a mother-child group visit.

decreasing iron deficiency anemia, and decreasing hospitalizations for pneumonia.

Challenges: community health nursing program

Initially 3 community health technicians and 1 manager were employed to direct the community outreach clinical activities. These technicians had backgrounds in fields outside of medicine (ie, business and social work). Teaching nonclinicians how to diagnose and treat pregnancy, neonatal, and childhood complications was a difficult task. As the program expanded, CHNs who had a more extensive clinical background replaced the community health

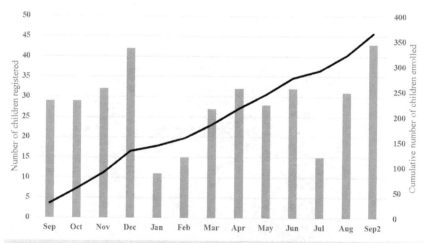

Fig. 12. Total number and cumulative enrollment per month of children less than 1 year of age in the Niños Sanos program at the SW Trifinio, Guatemala 2014 to 2015.

technicians. This change improved the number and quality of patient referrals to the clinical facility and improved the trust of the community. As of February 2015, 6 community nurses and 1 nurse manager had been hired for the maternal and child programs. Transportation for the nurses was another challenge. The usual form of transportation was by motorcycle and the nurses had to carry heavy flip charts, scales, and measuring boards. The center purchased tuk tuks (3-wheeled motorcars) to address this problem (Fig. 13). Finding an appropriate nurse coordinator to supervise the community nurses was difficult but eventually one of the new nurses was promoted and given additional training and ongoing mentoring. In addition, weekly meetings with the community nurses are held via the university's telehealth program, Vidyo, to ensure that program questions and issues are addressed in a timely fashion, and this has improved team morale and communication. An incentive program that rewards both individual effort and team goals has also been developed.

Employee health
Total Worker Health program (adult and occupational health for Agro-America)
CGH and the Center for Health, Work, and Environment of the Colorado School of Public Health have proposed a collaborative project to address total worker health in partnership with Agro-America. Total Worker Health (TWH) is a framework developed by the National Institute for Occupational Safety and Health of the CDC that is designed to integrate occupational safety and health protection with workplace policies, programs, and practices that promote health and prevent disease to advance worker safety, health, and well-being. The project seeks to improve the health, safety, and well-being of Agro-America workers, their families, and the communities in which they do business using the evidence and experience of the Center for Health, Work, and Environment at the University of Colorado [35–37]. The program will incorporate evidence-based guidelines derived from WHO and CDC for the

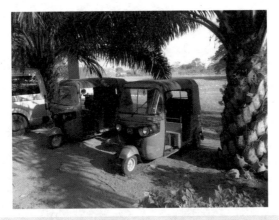

Fig. 13. Tuk tuks; transportation for CHNs.

certification of healthy businesses (Health Links). The goal is to build from the company's strong corporate social responsibility program and the services of the CHD to establish best practices for leading the industry and developing a sustainable model that not only has measurable impact but is scalable to others across industries. Much of what we intend to do has not been tested in LMICs so the experience will provide valuable information about the effectiveness of this approach. Based on an occupational health site visit conducted on June 10, 2015, the following objectives for developing the Agro-America TWH program were determined.

The TWH program will seek to improve the health, safety, and well-being of Agro-America and its workers and consequently improve the health, safety, and well-being of employees and their families. Evidence from similar programs in the United States has shown improvement in worker health and work-related injuries, as well as company performance, via increased employee morale, productivity, employee recruitment and retention, corporate culture, company reputation, and client retention. This program will establish Agro-America as an industry leader and founder of a new global model. To achieve these objectives, focus will be placed on the following 3 main priorities: (1) collect and analyze data to understand the most common work-related injuries and health conditions that have the potential to be addressed through workplace health promotion and health protection activities, (2) identify a multilevel TWH program to address the most urgent needs to improve worker health and safety, and (3) train administrators (managers, supervisors, and foremen) on core skills for supporting TWH on the job.

The TWH program will address the needs of 3 groups. First, the company at large, including key performance indicators to improve worker performance, employee morale, job satisfaction, and contributors to productivity, including retention, reduce absenteeism, and improved return to work, which will position Agro-America to serve as a model for others and to communicate best practices to clients and to the industry. The program will also assist the company in meeting global standards for occupational health and safety and comply with future industry regulations. Second, their employees as administrators (managers, supervisors, foremen), collaborators (field and plant workers), clinicians, community nurses, clinic staff, and office employees will all benefit from having reduced risk for work-related injuries and illnesses. Employee outcomes will include improvement in health risks, overall health, job satisfaction, quicker return to work, and improved quality of life and productivity. In addition, the families of workers and the communities will benefit directly by having access to the clinic, and will therefore have access to new services and better care. They will also benefit indirectly, through the programs that are benefitting employed family members.

Environment: water and sanitation

Agro-America made several attempts to address the clean water issue in the past by providing pumps and pipes to several communities. However, households receiving this water system were either unable or unwilling to pay the small fees needed to maintain the system. As a result, the systems broke down and were abandoned. Agro-America then distributed filters to the homes of employees but in many cases the filters are not being used properly. Given community concerns about the climate and geographic conditions of the area that result in frequent flooding and the recurrent pollution of water sources, the University of Colorado initiated contacts with various NGOs that perform water, sanitation, and hygiene (WASH) projects to conduct a baseline evaluation of needs in the area and propose the development of a water project with 100% coverage in conjunction with communities, local governments, and organizations like Agro-America. Because CGH did not have expertise in this area, several WASH NGOs were consulted and 1 made a site visit. All stressed that a strong community organization would be needed as well as government commitment to a WASH effort. Because we were not able to fund a partner with WASH expertise, the CGH elected to concentrate on the health care priorities first and continue to explore opportunities to make progress on WASH. A program to train local Guatemalan high school students to work on WASH projects in their communities is being explored as part of a leadership program to be started in local schools based on the Reading Village model developed by Larry Dressler in Guatemala.

Economic opportunity

A CU Denver Business School faculty member facilitated a course on entrepreneurship for students to develop a business plan for start-up endeavors at the Trifinio site. The possible endeavors included a transportation company that would serve visitors to the project, a catering service to feed volunteers and visitors, a bakery to make banana bread and muffins, and a company to make sanitary napkins from the banana leaves. Several of these ventures are currently under consideration. The project is creating jobs for local community members in the clinic (clerks, nurses, technicians, drivers, gardeners, maintenance, housekeeping, cooking) and these opportunities will increase as the project expands. Mapping and research projects have provided employment opportunities for many local people. The project is also providing staff with advanced training that will be a valuable asset and result in more opportunities and higher salaries. We also hope to develop additional training programs in laboratory technology and pharmacy, and a physician assistant training program (described later). The TWH program will also generate new positions within Agro-America and, if successfully franchised to other companies, will generate new well-paid employment opportunities for local people.

Education

The project's educational activities have 3 components: (1) CU students, residents, and fellows; (2) Trifinio CHD staff and Coatepeque Hospital staff; and (3) Trifinio secondary and high school students.

CU students, residents, and fellows

The most engaged trainees spending time at the Trifinio site have been pediatric residents and fellows. As of September 2015, 18 pediatric residents participated in rotations at the CHD clinic, and during the 2015 to 2016 academic year, 19 residents elected to take this experience (see Fig. 6). Residents rotating at the site have an on-site Guatemalan physician faculty member and for part of their rotation they also usually have a CGH faculty pediatrician. The residents use a telemedicine system to give case reports to the residency program during noon conference or morning report. This system increases global health exposure to residents not participating and provides the rotating resident with a teaching opportunity. The CGH compiled a handbook for residents and fellows traveling to SW Trifinio. The handbook reviews documentation that residents must provide to the CGH for processing temporary licenses; university requirements for educational travel abroad, including emergency medical and evacuation insurance; and the process for arranging international and in-country travel and accommodation. There is also a structured global health curriculum with appropriate readings and resources.

In 2013, pediatric resident experiences at the CGH SW Trifinio project site catalyzed the creation of a Global Health Track for the University of Colorado pediatric residency program that provides career-focused training and experiences in global health for up to 4 pediatric residents per class. This innovative global health program was designed for those residents who plan to focus their career in global health, or plan to incorporate care of international populations into their practice. Residents in the Global Health Track complete 6 months of global health curriculum throughout the 3-year residency. This curriculum includes 2 months of international experience in Guatemala at the clinic at CHD, a 2-week intensive Global Health and Disasters course (in Denver), experiences in various clinics with global populations, and a continuity clinic at a site with a diverse patient population. Participants also work on a scholarly project that is global health related with mentoring from a faculty member active in global health. The success of the pediatric Global Health Track program and the Trifinio rotations led to having similar rotations for residents in internal medicine, family medicine, obstetrics/gynecology, and occupational and environmental medicine.

Obstetrics and gynecology residents have participated in global health rotations within the site, focusing on specific reproductive health initiatives. One to 2 residents each year have rotated at the site for 2 to 4 weeks at a time, collecting data for research or quality improvement projects. Examples of projects thus far completed include a qualitative family planning needs assessment, a study of the pregnancy database examining factors associated with facility delivery in our population, and a quality improvement project that conducted a needs assessment of the obstetric and neonatal wards at the regional hospital in Coatepeque using a modified WHO hospital survey tool. The findings were reported to the hospital administration. Ongoing women's health projects, including an educational curriculum for the local TBAs, community nursing staff, and a pilot curriculum for male reproductive health education, have been built from the prior resident's findings.

The Physician Assistant (PA) Program in the School of Medicine in collaboration with the CGH has also developed a global health rotation for PA students at the CHD. This rotation includes Spanish language instruction and allows students to gain an understanding of culturally appropriate and interprofessional behaviors under the mentorship of pediatric and family medicine residents and faculty.

Trifinio Center for Human Development staff and Coatepeque Hospital staff

The CGH faculty are providing lectures to the CHD nursing staff and creating a curriculum specific to their role in the community. The lectures are done weekly via telemedicine software and focus on topics such as healthy breastfeeding and childhood illnesses. Faculty from the CGH have also conducted training workshops for the CHD nurses in obstetric emergencies, ultrasonography in pregnancy, and the Helping Babies Breathe program. A group of 10 to 12 TBAs from the community have received specific training in prenatal care practices and normal and emergency delivery skills using the Mama Natalie Birthing Simulator and the Helping Babies Breathe model. CGH faculty have conducted an obstetrics/gynecology residency educational curriculum assessment for the Coatepeque Hospital residency program. The CGH is working with the hospital residency to improve training opportunities via conferences and focused trainings. An external assessment of obstetric services was conducted in February 2015 using a modified WHO Making Pregnancy Safer hospital assessment tool, and the results were presented to the director of obstetric services and head of the hospital.

The CU PA Program is now exploring a partnership with a Guatemalan medical school to establish a joint PA training program at the SW Trifinio site. A needs assessment conducted in 2015 showed that a PA-like professional would be well received by most other health professionals, local leaders, and community members, especially if coming from the community and trained under the US-adapted model.

Southwest Trifinio secondary and high school students

One of the 3 primary concerns surfacing from the CHA and our community engagement activities is school education. A highlighted concern documented by our school survey performed in July of 2015 is the need for a school curriculum on health and sex education. CGH faculty are working with local school officials and community leaders to develop and implement the curriculum in the next school year. CGH faculty are also planning with local leaders a leadership program for 20 high school students that will provide school scholarships and hold biweekly Saturday classes. The students will be trained in basic microbiology and water filtration systems, and will assist families in obtaining and correctly using home water filters. They will also learn about the importance of community organizing and gain leadership skills.

OVERARCHING FUNCTIONS
Research

The CGH established the Translational Global Health Research Initiative (TGHRI) to build the research infrastructure at the SW Trifinio site. The TGHRI was funded by the University of Colorado School of Medicine to enhance the Guatemalan international research facility and to encourage multidisciplinary research within the School of Medicine as well as the schools/colleges of nursing, pharmacy, and dentistry. It offers opportunities for students, residents, fellows, and faculty to investigate the incidence, risk factors, and natural history of communicable and noncommunicable diseases in the Trifinio communities and explore innovative preventive and curative therapies and interventions [38]. Having this infrastructure makes CGH and School of Medicine faculty more competitive in obtaining research funding from international organizations. Faculty at the CGH are now conducting 3 funded research projects totaling $1.37 million: (1) dengue and norovirus disease epidemiology, (2) a randomized clinical trial of a new therapy for acute childhood diarrhea, and (3) a vaccine eHealth trial. A community advisory board has been created to review all proposed research and then assist with community outreach regarding new studies. It is important to properly engage the community in participatory research decision making [38]. Therefore, both a bricks-and-mortar and community engagement foundation are in place to build a significant translational research center at this site.

One of our challenges in designing and building research facilities has been the need to have gasoline-powered generators because interruptions in electrical power occur frequently in the area. However, when power goes off during the night and weekends when the clinic is closed, a system that will automatically supply power to the refrigerators and freezers that store vaccines, medications, and research specimens is needed. Solar power options are currently being explored for the facilities but these can be costly.

Community organizing

The research community advisory board and other community leaders requested that we perform a geographic information system mapping project to identify households and collect census data of the approximately 25,000 people living in the region. This information would help the communities to advocate for government services, assist in disaster preparedness and response, and more adequately plan and implement population health initiatives. This census helps to gain a better understanding of the demographic make-up of the community, including age and gender distribution, number of current and recent pregnancies, and reach of existing services. This project was performed by the CHD with the assistance of faculty from the CGH. Community leaders spoke about the mapping at local meetings and helped to identify local census workers. These workers were employed by FSIG to collect global positioning system coordinates (latitude, longitude, and altitude) of all residences in 13 communities within the catchment area of Trifinio. Leaders from each community accompanied census workers providing the necessary community engagement and receptiveness. More than 95% of the people living in inhabited homes agreed to participate. The census workers did an excellent job and clearly had the trust of the people. We hope to be able to hire them to work on additional community organizing and service projects. Maps will be provided to local community leaders and the local Ministry of Health to improve their capacity to deliver routine services or aid during natural disasters, which are common in the area. The census and mapping was a successful joint project with the community, and meetings are currently underway to consider how communities would like to use the information. One option under discussion is to name roads and footpaths, assign numbers to the houses, and ask Agro-America to fund signage. The mapping is becoming a community organizing and empowerment tool.

Strategic planning and sustainability

The CGH/University of Colorado, Children's Hospital Colorado, and Agro-America all made a long-term commitment to their partnership. Agro-America set aside 10 acres of land where the clinical, research, educational facilities, and volunteer housing would be built. Agro-America assumed responsibility for the construction of the facilities, clinic maintenance, security, information technology management, and transportation within Guatemala. In addition, Agro-America committed a $200,000 per year fund for 5 years to support development, implementation, and evaluation of FSIG programs by the CGH. Once the clinical services became operational, Agro-America agreed to fund 100% of the clinic and community program cost for the first year, 80% the second, and 60% the third. The financial sustainability of these services will require multiple funding streams in addition to Agro-America, including clinical revenue generation (mostly from patients with social security insurance), indirect cost funds from research, and philanthropic funds. It will be important to have a clear development/fund-raising plan in place with both the CU Foundation and Children's Hospital Colorado Foundation.

Strategic planning and sustainability are used to set priorities, focus energy and resources, strengthen operations, and ensure that collaborators and other stakeholders work toward the common goal of population health. The strategic work plan developed by the CGH management committee specifies the goals; strategies to achieve the goals; and the data system to monitor quality and process outcomes. We will follow best practices for dissemination and implementation science whenever we replicate these interventions and take our programs to new communities. Specifically, we will use the RE-AIM (Reach, Efficacy/Effectiveness, Adoption, Implementation and Maintenance) framework for dissemination and translation.

SUMMARY

The CHD project provides an innovative model for how a host country private agribusiness can partner with a US academic center to improve the population health and the human development index of impoverished communities in

Guatemala. Private sector–academic partnerships can combine the private-sector strengths of managerial efficiency, entrepreneurship, and social responsibility with academic strengths of innovation, technical knowledge, and research capacity to alleviate poverty and improve population health [9,10]. Although the first 3 years show great promise, the challenge of sustainability and achieving significant reductions in maternal, neonatal, and child morbidity and mortality are formidable and will only become apparent over the long term. This project provides a community laboratory to attempt innovative and transformative interventions. Those that prove to be successful and financially feasible can be taken to scale. Therefore, maintaining the commitment to our common goal of improving population health and continuing to build respect and trust with the community and between Agro-America and the university over the next decade will be essential to the success of this project.

Acknowledgments

The authors are grateful for the contributions of the following partners and collaborators: Gustavo Bolaños, Fernando Bolaños, and the Jose Fernando Bolaños Menendez Foundation for their vision and support to improve the human development status and the living standards of the communities at the SW Trifinio; Susan Niermeyer, MD, MPH, FAAP, for her work with Helping Babies Breathe training; Michelle Shiver and Molly Terhune for their strategic administrative and planning support at the CGH; Danilo Midence, Raul Barillas, Bernardo Roehrs, Wilson Serrano, and Guillermo A. Bolaños, MD, for their support at the SW Trifinio area; the clinic, research, and community programs personnel who dedicate their efforts to improve the health of these communities; and the community leaders and members who have supported this innovative vision and model of population health.

References

[1] Will BP, Berthelot JM, Nobrega KM, et al. Canada's Population Health Model (POHEM): a tool for performing economic evaluations of cancer control interventions. Eur J Cancer 2001;37(14):1797–804.

[2] USAID. The United States Global Health Strategy. Guatemala (Central America): USAID; 2010.

[3] Available at: http://www.who.int/maternal_child_adolescent/epidemiology/profiles/maternal/gtm. Accessed July 16, 2015.

[4] Available at: http://data.worldbank.org/indicator/SH.STA.MMRT. Accessed July 16, 2015.

[5] Available at: http://data.un.org/Data.aspx?d=SOWC&f=inID%3A34. Accessed July 16, 2015.

[6] Oechler Solana EF. Public private non-for-profit partnerships: delivering public services to developing countries. Proced Eng 2014;78:259–64.

[7] Durand MA, Petticrew M, Goulding L, et al. An evaluation of the Public Health Responsibility Deal: Informants' experiences and views of the development, implementation and achievements of a pledge-based, public-private partnership to improve population health in England. Health Policy 2015;119(11):1506–14.

[8] Huang TTK, Ferris E, Crossley R, et al. A protocol for developing an evaluation framework for an academic and private-sector partnership to assess the impact of major food and

beverage companies' investments in community health in the United States. BMC Obes 2015;2(36):1–7.

[9] Johnston LM, Finegood DT. Cross-sector partnerships and public health: challenges and opportunities for addressing obesity and noncommunicable diseases through engagement with the private sector. Annu Rev Public Health 2015;36:255–71.

[10] Roehrich JK, Lewis MA, George G. Are public-private partnerships a healthy option? A systematic literature review. Soc Sci Med 2014;113:110–9.

[11] Barnes-Josiah D, Myntti C, Augustin A. The "three delays" as a framework for examining maternal mortality in Haiti. Soc Sci Med 1998;46(8):981–93.

[12] Knight HE, Self A, Kennedy SH. Why are women dying when they reach hospital on time? A systematic review of the 'third delay'. PLoS One 2013;8(5):e63846.

[13] Dotta A, Portanova A, Bianchi N, et al. Accreditation of birth centres: advantages for newborns. J Matern Fetal Neonatal Med 2013;26(4):417–8.

[14] Guliani H, Sepehri A, Serieux J. What impact does contact with the prenatal care system have on women's use of facility delivery? Evidence from low-income countries. Soc Sci Med 2012;74(12):1882–90.

[15] Wall SN, Lee AC, Carlo W, et al. Reducing intrapartum-related neonatal deaths in low- and middle-income countries-what works? Semin Perinatol 2010;34(6):395–407.

[16] Niermeyer S. From the Neonatal Resuscitation Program to Helping Babies Breathe: global impact of educational programs in neonatal resuscitation. Semin Fetal Neonatal Med 2015;20(5):300–8.

[17] World Health Organization. Essential newborn care course. Training manual. Geneva (Switzerland): WHO; 2013.

[18] World Health Organization Guidelines review committee. Recommendation on newborn health. Geneva (Switzerland): WHO; 2013.

[19] Nelissen E, Ersdal H, Ostergaard D, et al. Helping mothers survive bleeding after birth: an evaluation of simulation-based training in a low-resource setting. Acta Obstet Gynecol Scand 2014;93(3):287–95.

[20] Nelissen E, Ersdal H, Mduma E, et al. Helping mothers survive bleeding after birth: retention of knowledge, skills, and confidence nine months after obstetric simulation-based training. BMC Pregnancy Childbirth 2015;15:190.

[21] de Souza AL, Leal SC, Bronkhorst EM, et al. Assessing caries status according to the CAST instrument and WHO criterion in epidemiological studies. BMC Oral Health 2014;14:119.

[22] Mtaya M, Astrøm AN, Tsakos G. Applicability of an abbreviated version of the Child-OIDP inventory among primary schoolchildren in Tanzania. Health Qual Life Outcomes 2007;5: 4023.

[23] McMahon AD, Blair Y, McCall DR, et al. Reductions in dental decay in 3-year old children in Greater Glasgow and Clyde: repeated population inspection studies over four years. BMC Oral Health 2011;11:2924.

[24] Rai RK. Tracking women and children in a Continuum of Reproductive, Maternal, Newborn, and Child Healthcare (RMNCH) in India. J Epidemiol Glob Health 2014;4(3):239–43, Goetzel RZ25.

[25] Aboud FE, Singla DR, Nahil MI, et al. Effectiveness of a parenting program in Bangladesh to address early childhood health, growth and development. Soc Sci Med 2013; http://dx. doi.org/10.1016/j.socscimed.2013.06.020.

[26] Baker-Henningham H, Boo FL. Early childhood stimulation interventions in developing countries: a comprehensive literature review. Washington, DC: Institute for the Study of Labor; 2010.

[27] Eshel N, Daelmans B, de Mello MC, et al. Responsive parenting: interventions and outcomes. Bull World Health Organ 2006;84(12):991–8.

[28] Grantham-McGregor SM, Powell CA, Walker SP, et al. Nutritional supplementation, psychosocial stimulation, and mental development of stunted children: the Jamaican Study. Lancet 1991;338(8758):1–5.

[29] WHO. A critical link: interventions for physical growth and psychological development. A review. Geneva (Switzerland): Department of Child and Adolescent Health, World Health Organization; 1999.

[30] Campbell FA, Ramey CT, Pungello EP, et al. Early childhood education: young adult outcomes from the Abecedarian Project. Appl Dev Sci 2002;6:42–57.

[31] Engle PL, Black MM, Behrman JR, et al, International Child Development Steering Group. Strategies to avoid the loss of developmental potential in more than 200 million children in the developing world. Lancet 2007;369(9557):229–42.

[32] Fernald L, Kariger P, Engle P, et al. Examining early child development in low-income countries: a toolkit for the assessment of children in the first five years of life. Washington, DC: World Bank Human Development Group, The World Bank; 2009.

[33] Grantham-McGregor S, Cheung YB, Cueto S, et al, International Child Development Steering Group. Developmental potential in the first 5 years for children in developing countries. Lancet 2007;369(9555):60–70.

[34] Walker SP, Wachs TD, Gardner JM, et al, International Child Development Steering Group. Child development: risk factors for adverse outcomes in developing countries. Lancet 2007;369(9556):145–57.

[35] Tabrizi M, Henke RM, Benevent R, et al. Estimating the return on investment from a health risk management program offered to small Colorado-based employers. J Occup Environ Med 2014;56(5):554–60.

[36] McCoy K, Stinson K, Scott K, et al. Health promotion in small business: a systematic review of factors influencing adoption and effectiveness of worksite wellness programs. J Occup Environ Med 2014;56(6):579–87.

[37] Newman LS, Stinson KE, Metcalf D, et al. Implementation of a worksite wellness program targeting small businesses: the Pinnacol Assurance health risk management study. J Occup Environ Med 2015;57(1):14–21.

[38] Hardy LJ, Bohan KD, Trotter RT. Synthesizing evidence-based strategies and community-engaged research: a model to address the social determinants of health. Public Health Rep 2013;128(Suppl 3):68–76.

Advances in Pediatrics 63 (2016) 389–401

ADVANCES IN PEDIATRICS

ELSEVIER
MOSBY

Better Transportation to Health Care Will Improve Child Health and Lower Costs

Roy Grant, MA*, Grifin Goldsmith, MPH,
Delaney Gracy, MD, MPH, Dennis Johnson, MPS

Children's Health Fund, 215 West 125th Street, Suite 301, New York, NY 10017, USA

Keywords
• Transportation barriers • Access to health care • Vulnerable children

Key points

- Availability of transportation is essential for timely access to health care services.
- Each year, 4% of children nationwide including 9% of children in low income households miss an appointment because transportation was not available.
- Lack of transportation is associated with missed appointments, problems filling prescriptions, poor management of chronic conditions, and preventable emergency room use.
- Our geomapping of 2 southern states shows that the distance from home to a safety net clinic is relatively short, often less than 5 miles.
- There are many effective ways to improve transportation access to health care using existing public transit resources.

INTRODUCTION

Economically vulnerable children experience serious health disparities, including higher incidence of acute and chronic conditions, worse outcomes, higher mortality rates, and difficulty accessing services [1]. Most efforts to improve access focus on ability to pay. The major impact of health reform (the Affordable Care Act of 2010 or "ACA") has been to increase health insurance coverage through commercial insurance exchanges and expanded Medicaid eligibility. Even with insurance coverage, other access barriers remain.

In the first section of this article we review the literature discussing transportation availability as a barrier to child health care access and the clinical benefits

*Corresponding author. *E-mail address*: roygrant.roy@gmail.com

0065-3101/16/$ – see front matter
http://dx.doi.org/10.1016/j.yapd.2016.04.003

and cost savings of providing transportation assistance. We next present a new study demonstrating a 2-stage method to identify and describe geographic areas at risk of transportation-related access barriers. We found that in even the most rural counties, the distance from population centers to safety net health clinics was relatively short, and that most of these counties had limited public transit services. We applied these results to make recommendations intended to alleviate transportation barriers to health care access.

TRANSPORTATION AND HEALTH CARE ACCESS

Transportation disadvantage

In a 2014 report, the Government Accountability Office (GAO) defined "transportation-disadvantaged" populations as those who "cannot provide their own transportation due to age, disability, or income constraints" to access health care or other needed services [2]. This is a very broad definition that does not take into account the mobility options open to people with household income below the poverty level, known disability status, or who are 65 or older. Wallace and colleagues [3] reviewed estimates of the size of the transportation disadvantaged population and found them to range from 528,000 to 15.5 million, depending on definition and data source.

The determination of transit disadvantage is more accurately assessed through personal and community resources: availability of a car or other privately owned vehicle and/or public transportation in the community. By these criteria, transportation barriers are most prominent among low-income populations living in communities with limited public transportation services, such as rural areas, small cities, and increasingly with shifting population demographics, suburban communities [4,5].

Transportation barriers disproportionately affect families with lower income. The percentage of income spent on transportation, including commuting to work, is highest for low-income households. This is notable in all geographic areas, including large cities such as New York and Los Angeles, where housing costs are also very high [6]. People in households with annual incomes less than $25,000 are 7 times less likely to own a vehicle than are those with higher income [7].

Among adults living in rural areas, owning or having access to a car, and having a driver's license, are significantly associated with keeping more medical appointments [8]. An estimated 1.6 million rural households do not own a car [9]. As many as 40% of rural communities do not have any available public transportation services. Of those with transit services, 28% are very limited in coverage. This leaves barely one-third, 32%, having adequate public transportation available [10].

Geographic access and workforce shortages

The extent to which transportation is a potential health care access barrier reflects health geography, where people live relative to where they obtain health care. These spatial relationships may be analyzed using Geographic

Information System (GIS) technology. This methodology has contributed to small area studies that intensively explore health care needs, utilization patterns, and resources within a specific geographic area to identify need for additional health and transit resources [11]. One effective application of GIS in health planning is the measurement of straight-line distances from residential areas mapped by census block groups to health facilities mapped by address [12].

Ascertaining approximate travel distances can facilitate planning to improve transportation resources. This is especially important for low-income communities in which there are often health care workforce shortages. With fewer health professionals in the community, the distance from home to a health care provider may be longer because of their scarcity and distribution [13].

Workforce shortages are reflected in the federal designation of health professional shortage areas (HPSAs). This designation is generally based on a low ratio of providers to population, and is also used for areas with populations demonstrating a high level of need; for example, high poverty rates. People living in a HPSA often have the related problems of poor access to health care and worse health status than people in better resourced communities [14].

Rural communities are disproportionately affected by workforce shortages; 65% of rural counties are federally designated primary care HPSAs [15]. The Health Resources and Services Agency (HRSA) reported that 60 million people live in one of the 6325 federally designated primary medical care HPSAs [16]. Based on Census Bureau demographics, this includes approximately 15 million children.

When an area has a HPSA designation, the health care workforce may be augmented by developing federally qualified health centers (FQHC) and rural health clinics (RHC). These community health centers provide primary and preventive health services, and many also provide mental health and dental care. The federal government provides core funding of these clinics through the HRSA Bureau of Primary Health Care (BPHC). This funding is supplemented by insurance reimbursement for services provided, primarily from Medicaid.

These clinics have become an essential component of the health care safety net for low-income communities. Nationally, community health centers served 23 million predominantly low-income patients in 2014, including one-third of children living in families with incomes below the federal poverty level. Most were covered by public insurance (including 41% on Medicaid or Children's Health Insurance Program) or were uninsured (35%). Nearly half (49%) of community health centers are located in rural areas [17–19].

Transportation and child health access
With 1 child in 5 living in poverty, limited transportation availability has a direct impact on access to child health care. Qualitative studies using parent interview or survey methodologies show this to be a problem especially for low-income and Medicaid populations. Transportation problems affect

adherence with pediatric primary care appointments in urban clinics, accounting for 21% of missed appointments in one study [20,21]. In a 2012 study of children with uncontrolled asthma in rural Arkansas schools, 20% had difficulty accessing asthma care because transportation was not available [22]. In a 2010 study of nonurgent pediatric use at a rural Mississippi hospital emergency room (ER), 10% of parents reported that they were unable to access health care services for the presenting problem before coming to the ER because transportation was not available. The most frequently cited reason for the ER visit was asthma or other upper respiratory concerns [23].

We have previously reported our survey studies designed to assess the extent to which transportation availability is a barrier to child health access. The survey results show that 4% of children in the United States missed at least 1 health care appointment each year because transportation was not available. This included 9% of children with household incomes below $50,000. Parents also reported that nearly one-third (31%) of these children subsequently were seen in a hospital ER for the condition associated with the missed appointment. Based on Census Bureau data, this suggests that more than 750,000 pediatric ER visits could be avoided annually with improved transportation access to primary care sites [4,24].

Distance, transportation, and chronic health conditions

Many studies have explored the relationship of travel distance and transportation availability as factors affecting chronic disease management. Syed and colleagues [25] reviewed 61 peer-reviewed articles and concluded that they provided strong evidence that long distance to a health care site and restricted availability of transportation were associated with missed appointments, difficulty filling prescriptions, compromised management of chronic conditions, and increased ER use. Longer travel distances (typically defined as >10 miles) are associated with worse glycemic management for patients with diabetes [26]; inability to complete radiation therapy for breast cancer [27]; worse outcomes for patients with sickle cell anemia [28]; and inability to maintain life-saving dialysis treatment for patients with end-stage renal disease [29]. Facilitating transportation to primary care improves follow-up for patients seen in emergency settings for acute asthma exacerbations [30]. In a survey of nearly 4000 adults living in rural counties in 8 states, 36% reported transportation problems when keeping medical appointments. Transportation difficulties were associated with not filling prescriptions and not taking prescribed medications [31].

In a 2005 report prepared by Altarum Institute for the Transportation Research Board of the National Academies of Science, Hughes-Cromwick and colleagues [32] assessed the cost of providing transportation services to facilitate access to care relative to the assumed savings attributable to reduced hospital and ER use. After noting that the population that misses health care appointments because of transportation barriers has a higher prevalence of chronic conditions than the general population, the investigators found that transportation services saved more money than they cost for people with asthma, heart disease, and diabetes. Transit services were highly cost-effective for people with end-stage renal disease. Additional savings were attributable to increased access to preventive services, including cancer screening.

Making transportation to health care sites available is essential to bending the cost curve, a major goal of the ACA. Treating and managing chronic conditions represent 85% of the total annual health care expenditures in the United States [33].

Nonemergency medical transportation

Nonemergency medical transportation (NEMT) is a required benefit for patients covered by Medicaid. These services are supposed to be provided for patients who need transportation services to keep medically necessary appointments. Annual expenditures for NEMT represent only 1% of total Medicaid spending nationally. With Medicaid expansion under the ACA, it has been anticipated that there would be a corresponding increase in demand for and delivery of Medicaid NEMT [34].

There is evidence that effective delivery of Medicaid NEMT enhances access to care and improves management of chronic conditions for ambulatory care sensitive conditions (ACSCs), including asthma and diabetes [35,36]. Ambulatory care sensitive conditions are chronic conditions that with proper management in primary care should not require hospitalization or ER use [37].

The requirement to provide NEMT, however, has become optional for states under ACA Medicaid expansion. When officials from Iowa requested a federal waiver from their obligation to provide NEMT to people newly enrolled in Medicaid, it was granted by the federal Centers for Medicaid and Medicare Services (CMS) [38]. Iowa officials subsequently requested an extension of the waiver despite survey findings from their state that showed 20% of new enrollees and 10% of those previously enrolled in Medicaid did not have adequate transportation to keep medical appointments [39].

Following Iowa's example, Medicaid NEMT waivers were requested by and granted for Pennsylvania and Indiana. Arkansas implemented a prior authorization process that did not require a waiver [40]. Requiring authorization before transportation is provided may limit timely access to medically necessary transportation services. These policy decisions to modify the NEMT requirement were contrary to well-established and readily available evidence of the value of transportation for health care access.

In the next section of this article, we present a new study that helps to elucidate the nature of services that would provide effective health-related transportation services in high-risk communities. Based on these results, we offer recommendations for policies to enhance transportation access.

IDENTIFYING RISK FOR TRANSPORTATION BARRIERS TO ACCESS

We previously reported on our preliminary study of risk for transportation barriers that focused on Mississippi because of its high child poverty rate, high percentage of rural counties, and poor child health indicators [24]. In this study, we replicated and expanded on that preliminary study. The goal of the study was to demonstrate a 2-stage method to identify geographic areas at risk of transportation barriers and to generate information that can be used in public health planning to improve health care access. In this replication study, we included a second state, Tennessee, which has demographic and child health indicators closer to those of the United States than does Mississippi, and we conducted additional data analyses. Our updated data included new health center sites developed with expansion funding made available through the ACA.

Methods

Our 2-stage methodology consisted of (1) an objective assessment of each county in the 2 states to identify and describe those at high risk of transportation barriers; and (2) geomapping of each county, locating safety net clinics and population centers to calculate distances between them.

First, we applied the Health Transportation Shortage Index (HTSI) to each county in Mississippi and Tennessee (n = 177) to quantify risk of transportation barriers. The HTSI was developed in 2012 as a tool to assess geographic areas that should be targeted for interventions to improve transportation resources for health care access. It is a validated protocol in which 5 factors associated with transportation barriers to primary care are assessed and scored [4]. The factors, and the data sources we used in this study, were as follows: metro-rural status (assessed by Census Bureau population); poverty rate, which was also a proxy for private vehicle ownership (source: US Department of Agriculture, Economic Research Service); HPSA status (as reported by HRSA); number of safety net clinics (sources: BPHC, state primary care associations, and state departments of health); and availability and type of public transportation (sources: state departments of transportation and the American Public Transportation Association). In addition, we conducted Internet searches for each county to ensure that we identified all relevant resources and to resolve any inconsistencies or ambiguities, especially where multiple data sources were used for the same factor.

We included as safety net clinics FQHCs and RHCs with a bricks-and-mortar ("permanent") street address that were open to the community for primary care. We excluded part-time, special purpose, and special population clinics, such as school-based health centers, health care for the homeless sites, mobile clinic programs, and clinics that only provided mental health or dental services. We included safety net hospitals and state or county department of health centers if they provided primary care services and were open to the community. We refer to these collective resources as "clinics."

Because federal and state governments report relevant data by county, we used the county as the unit of analysis. Data were coded and scored per the HTSI protocol, and the factor scores summed for a total score from 0 to 14. We defined as "high risk" those counties that had a total score indicative of high (fourth quartile) rates of ACSC-related hospital and ER use. In the

HTSI validation study, this was established as a score higher than 7 [4,41]. We conducted comparative analyses among the counties to describe the characteristics of high-risk counties. Data were analyzed in SPSS version 23 (IBM SPSS Statistics, IBM Corporation, Chicago, IL).

In the second stage of this methodology, we used GIS software to map each county in the 2 states. Clinics were mapped by longitude and latitude for street address. Population data by census block groups were obtained from the Census Bureau through the GIS software and mapped. Tables of clinic addresses and census block groups were linked, and the maps were layered. We calculated Euclidian (straight-line) distances in miles from the population-weighted center of each county (a point representative of the place in which the preponderance of the population lives) to the nearest clinic, including a clinic in a contiguous county if it was found to be nearest.

Esri ArcGIS version 10 (Esri, Inc, Redlands, CA) was used for mapping and distance calculations. Data tables were linked in SAS version 8 (SAS Institute, Inc, Cary, NC).

Results

Although there was a significantly higher percentage of high-risk counties in Mississippi than in Tennessee, there were no significant differences in the characteristics of high-risk counties between the states. We therefore conducted our analyses for the 2 states combined. Of the 177 counties in the 2 states, 104 (59%) were identified as having a high risk of transportation barriers to care. These counties were significantly more rural ($P<.01$) and had significantly higher child poverty rates (mean = 36% vs 29%; $P<.01$) than other counties in the states. Although there were significantly more high-risk counties with HPSA designations ($P<.01$), 21% of full-county HPSAs did not score in the high-risk range. At least 1 safety net clinic was present in 88% of high-risk counties.

In the high-risk counties, 76% had demand-response (paratransit) services, where users must call 24 to 72 hours ahead to schedule a pick-up and 17% had partial fixed route services, with designated stops and schedules but services that did not cover the entire county and/or had limited hours and days of operation. Seven percent had no public transit services.

High-risk counties did not differ significantly from the other counties in the states in mean distance from the population center to the nearest safety net clinic (5.4 miles compared with 5.6 miles for the other counties). Fig. 1 presents a map of a high-risk county showing the population-weighted centroid and clinic locations. In 87% of high-risk counties, the straight-line distance was less than 10 miles, and in 95% the distance was less than 15 miles. For many of the high-risk counties with the highest child poverty rates, distances to clinics were within 5 miles, as shown in Fig. 2.

Policy recommendations

This study confirmed that for most high-risk (poor, rural) counties, safety net clinics are well located relative to population centers, distances from most

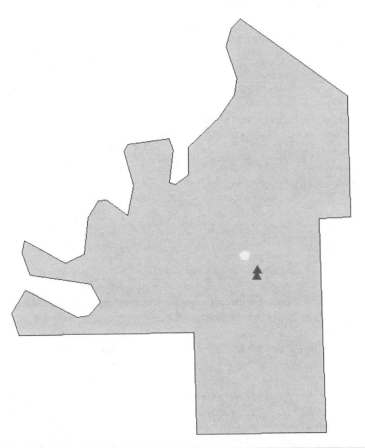

Fig. 1. Coahoma County, MS. Triangles = clinics. Circle = population-weighted centroid.

residences to clinics are relatively short, and at least limited public transportation is available. Based on these findings and a review of effective health-related transportation interventions, we offer the following recommendations to improve transportation access to health care.

Mobility management

A first step in better aligning transit availability with health care access would be commitment to joint transportation planning that includes robust representation from transportation and health sector officials. The benefits of transit services for health care access are well known in the transportation sector [42–44]. Outcomes of this joint planning process could include targeted support for transportation coordinator or mobility manager positions at clinics to ensure that public transit is available for times that appointments are scheduled. Arranging transportation should be considered an integral

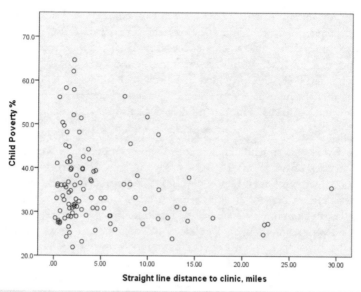

Fig. 2. Distances to clinics are short for high-poverty high-risk counties.

part of care coordination and included in the medical home model as promoted in the ACA and supported in many states with enhanced reimbursement.

Modifying paratransit services

There are effective models to coordinate paratransit services with health clinics. One approach is to incorporate limited fixed-route services in the existing paratransit system, adding scheduled service and routes with stops that incorporate safety net clinics and heavily populated areas. Another approach is to develop contracts between clinics and paratransit providers to use public transportation services for health clinic access. Contracts also may be made between counties or states and paratransit providers [45].

Transportation provided by health clinics

Clinics may directly provide transportation services for their patients independent of public transit. This is an important "enabling" service that many FQHCs provide to improve patient access [46]. One clinic in Mississippi received state funding to expand its health transportation services, and subsequently developed a transportation system that has become a major public transit provider [47]. A more modest approach would be for clinics to purchase a van, hire a driver, and provide transportation from the surrounding residential areas to the clinic, not unlike hotel shuttle services that bring guests from airports. Transportation services may be Medicaid reimbursable as an "other ambulatory service," the same billing category as case management [48].

Strengthening Medicaid nonemergency medical transportation
Despite being required, Medicaid transportation services are inconsistently provided, and millions of patients covered by Medicaid miss medically necessary appointments each year because transportation was not available [3,49]. Effective NEMT services provided in a brokerage model have been found to improve management of chronic conditions and save more money than they cost for adults with diabetes and children with asthma [35,36].

Coordinating transportation resources
The GAO has recommended better coordination among the multiple transportation services provided by the federal government. These services currently are fragmented and inefficiently used. Deploying special purpose vehicles (eg, Head Start vans) for health care and other human service access when idle enhances community mobility with economic benefits and cost savings compared with sole reliance on public transit services. These savings may be reinvested in services to improve community transportation infrastructure [46,50].

Limitations of the study

We did not include primary care providers in private practice in this replication study. In our preliminary study, we included private practitioners identified through multiple data sources including Internet searches for each county. There were 2 or fewer pediatricians in 90% of the high-risk counties, with a somewhat higher number of family practice physicians. The inclusion of private practitioners did not substantially alter distance calculations. Additionally, their availability would have to be established individually based on whether Medicaid, and new Medicaid patients, are accepted. These features could change over time, whereas the availability of fixed site clinics is more likely to remain stable.

For this study, we used data that applied to child health care. We do not, however, consider the results to be specific to pediatrics. Child poverty rates are highly correlated with overall county poverty rates [4]. Virtually all of the clinics we included also provide adult services. Children of course live with adults, their parents, and households without children were included in the census block group data used in the study. The results of this study may therefore be generalized to adult access.

Finally, straight-line distances only approximate actual travel distances. The use of straight-line distance, as noted previously, is generally accepted in GIS studies of geospatial access. This methodology has the advantage of being replicable over time and in diverse geographic areas. Travel distances are influenced by traffic patterns, road conditions, and other factors that vary over time, sometimes in a matter of hours. We believe that straight-line distance calculations are sufficiently accurate to serve as the basis for public health planning. Their replicability makes them an appropriate methodology for future studies of geospatial access to health care.

References

[1] US Department of Health & Human Services (HHS), Agency for Healthcare Research & Quality (AHRQ). National Healthcare Quality and Disparities Report, 2014. 2015. Available at: http://www.ahrq.gov/sites/default/files/wysiwyg/research/findings/nhqrdr/nhqdr14/2014nhqdr.pdf. Accessed December 14, 2015.

[2] U.S. Government Accountability Office (GAO). Transportation disadvantaged populations: nonemergency medical transportation not well coordinated, and additional federal leadership needed. 2014. Available at: http://www.gao.gov/assets/670/667362.pdf. Accessed December 14, 2015.

[3] Wallace R, Hughes-Cromwick P, Mull H, et al. Access to health care and nonemergency medical transportation: two missing links. In: Transportation Research Record: journal of the transportation research board no. 1924. Washington, DC: Transportation Research Board of the National Academies; 2005. p. 76–84.

[4] Grant R, Johnson D, Borders S, et al. The health transportation shortage index: the development and validation of a new tool to identify underserved communities. New York: Children's Health Fund; 2012. Available at: http://issuu.com/childrenshealthfund/docs/chf_htsi-monograph__2_?e=6796486/1866261. Accessed December 14, 2015.

[5] Silver D, Blustein J, Weitzman BC. Transportation to clinic: findings from a pilot clinic-based survey of low-income suburbanites. J Immigr Minor Health 2012;14:350–5.

[6] Roberto E. Commuting to opportunity: the working poor and commuting in the United States. Metropolitan Policy Program at Brookings. Available at: https://web.stanford.edu/group/scspi/_media/pdf/key_issues/transportation_policy.pdf. Accessed December 14, 2015.

[7] United States Department of Transportation. Moving people. Available at: http://www.rita.dot.gov/bts/sites/rita.dot.gov.bts/files/ch2_tsar2012_0.pdf. Accessed December 14, 2015.

[8] Arcury TA, Preisser JS, Gester WM, et al. Access to transportation and health care utilization in a rural region. J Rural Health 2005;21:31–8.

[9] Brown D. Rural transportation at a glance. Agriculture information bulletin # 795. 2005. Available at: http://www.ers.usda.gov/publications/aib795/aib795_lowres.pdf. Accessed December 14, 2015.

[10] TRIP: A national transportation research group. Rural connections: challenges and opportunities in America's Heartland. 2015. Available at: http://www.tripnet.org/docs/Rural_Roads_TRIP_Report_May_2015.pdf. Accessed December 14, 2015.

[11] McLafferty SL. GIS and health care. Annu Rev Public Health 2003;24:25–42.

[12] Higgs G. A literature review of the use of GIS-based measures of access to health care services. Health Serv Outcomes Res Methodol 2004;5:119–39.

[13] McGrail MR, Humphreys JS, Ward B. Accessing doctors at times of need–measuring the distance tolerance of rural residents for health-related travel. BMC Health Serv Res 2015;15:212.

[14] Liu J. Health professional shortage and health status and health care access. J Health Care Poor Underserved 2007;18:590–8.

[15] National Rural Health Association. Health care workforce distribution and shortage issues in rural America. Available at: http://www.ruralhealthweb.org/index.cfm?objectid=3D776162-3048-651A-FEA70F1F09670B0D. Accessed December 14, 2015.

[16] Bureau of Health Workforce. Health resources and services administration (HRSA). U.S. Department of Health & Human Services. Designated health professional shortage areas, statistics as of December 3, 2015. Available at: https://ersrs.hrsa.gov/ReportServer?/HGDW_Reports/BCD_HPSA/BCD_HPSA_SCR50_Smry&rs:Format=PDF (cached). Accessed December 7, 2015.

[17] National Association of Community Health Centers (NACHC). A sketch of community health centers: chartbook, December 2014. Available at: www.nachc.com/client/Chartbook_2014.pdf. Accessed December 14, 2015.

[18] NACHC. The role of health centers in lowering preventable emergency department use. Fact sheet, July 2015. Available at: https://www.nachc.com/client/documents/ED_FS_20151.pdf. Accessed December 14, 2015.

[19] NACHC. Removing barriers to care: community health centers in rural areas. Fact sheet, October 2013. Available at: https://www.nachc.com/client/documents/Rural%20Fact%20Sheet%20-%20November%202011.pdf. Accessed December 14, 2015.

[20] Yang S, Zarr RL, Kass-Hout TA, et al. Transportation barriers to accessing health care for urban children. J Health Care Poor Underserved 2006;17:928–43.

[21] Samuels RC, Ward VL, Melvin P, et al. Missed appointments: factors contributing to high no-show rates in an urban pediatrics primary care clinic. Clin Pediatr (Phila) 2015;54:976–82.

[22] Perry TT, Vargas PA, McCracken A, et al. Underdiagnosed and uncontrolled asthma: findings in rural schoolchildren in the Delta region of Arkansas. Ann Allergy 2008;101:375–81.

[23] Grant R, Ramgoolam A, Betz R, et al. Challenges to accessing pediatric health care in the Mississippi Delta: a survey of emergency department patients seeking non-urgent care. J Prim Care Community Health 2010;1:152–7.

[24] Grant R, Gracy D, Goldsmith G, et al. Transportation barriers to child health care access remain after health reform. JAMA Pediatr 2014;168:386.

[25] Syed ST, Gerber BS, Sharp LK. Traveling towards disease: transportation barriers to health care access. J Community Health 2013;38:976–93.

[26] Zgibor JC, Gieraltowski LB, Talbott EO, et al. The association between driving distance and glycemic control in rural areas. J Diabetes Sci Technol 2011;5:494–500.

[27] Peipins LA, Graham S, Young R, et al. Time and distance barriers to mammography facilities in the Atlanta area. J Community Health 2011;36:675–83.

[28] Liem RL, O'Suoji C, Kingsberry PS, et al. Access to patient-centered medical homes in children with sickle cell disease. Matern Child Health J 2014;18:1854–62.

[29] Cohen SD, Sharma T, Acquaviva K, et al. Social support and chronic kidney disease: an update. Adv Chronic Kidney Dis 2007;14:335–44.

[30] Baren JM, Shofer FS, Ivey B, et al. A randomized, controlled trial of a simple emergency department intervention to improve the rate of primary care follow-up for patients with acute asthma exacerbations. Ann Emerg Med 2001;38:115–22.

[31] Wroth TH, Pathman DE. Primary medication adherence in a rural population: the role of the patient-physician relationship and satisfaction with care. J Am Board Fam Med 2006;19:478–86.

[32] Hughes-Cromwick P, Wallace R, Mull H, et al. Cost benefit analysis of providing non-emergency medical transportation. Washington, DC: Transportation Research Board; The National Academies; 2005 Altarum Institute. Contractor's final report. Available at: http://altarum.org/sites/default/files/uploaded-publication-files/05_project_report_hsd_cost_benefit_analysis.pdf. Accessed December 14, 2015.

[33] Anderson G. Chronic care: making the case for ongoing care. Princeton (NJ): Robert Wood Johnson Foundation and Johns Hopkins Bloomberg School of Public Health; 2010. Available at: http://www.rwjf.org/content/dam/farm/reports/reports/2010/rwjf54583. Accessed December 14, 2015.

[34] Federal Transit Administration, Transportation Cooperative Research Program (TCRP). Research Results Digest 109: impact of the Affordable Care Act on non-emergency medical transportation (NEMT): assessment for transit agencies. Available at: http://onlinepubs.trb.org/onlinepubs/tcrp/tcrp_rrd_109.pdf. Accessed December 14, 2015.

[35] Thomas LV, Wedel KR. Nonemergency medical transportation and health care visits among chronically ill urban and rural Medicaid beneficiaries. Soc Work Public Health 2014;29:629–39.

[36] Kim J, Norton EC, Stearns SC. Transportation brokerage services and Medicaid beneficiaries' access to care. Health Serv Res 2009;44:145–61.

[37] Laditka JN, Laditka SB, Probst JC. Health care access in rural areas: evidence that hospitalization for ambulatory care-sensitive conditions in the United States may increase with the level of rurality. Health Place 2009;15:761–70.

[38] Cross-Call J, Solomon J. Approved demonstrations offer lessons for states seeking to expand Medicaid through waivers. Washington, DC: Center on Budget and Policy Priorities; 2014 Available at: http://www.cbpp.org/cms/?fa=view&id=4190 http://www.cbpp.org/cms/?fa=view&id=4190. Accessed December 14, 2015.

[39] State of Iowa. Iowa Health and Wellness Plan: NEMT Waiver Amendment. 2014. Available at: http://dhs.iowa.gov/sites/default/files/IA_NEMT_WaiverAmendment090414.pdf. Accessed December 14, 2015.

[40] Musumeci M, Rudowitz R. The ACA and Medicaid expansion waivers. Kaiser Family Foundation commission on Medicaid and the uninsured. 2015. Available at: http://files.kff.org/attachment/issue-brief-the-aca-and-medicaid-expansion-waivers. Accessed December 14, 2015.

[41] Borders S. The Children's Health Fund's Health Transportation Shortage Index (HTSI): a new measure of accessability. Grand Valley State University. Available at: http://faculty.gvsu.edu/borderss/HTSI_Final_Draft.pdf. Accessed December 14, 2015.

[42] Ferrell CE. The benefits of transit in the United States: a review and analysis of benefit-cost studies. Mineta Transportation Institute; 2015. Available at: http://transweb.sjsu.edu/PDFs/research/1425-US-transit-benefit-cost-analysis-study.pdf. Accessed December 14, 2015.

[43] National Center for Transit Research (NCTR). Cost-benefit analysis of rural and small urban transit. 2014. Available at: http://www.nctr.usf.edu/wp-content/uploads/2014/07/77060-NCTR-NDSU03.pdf (cached). Accessed December 14, 2015.

[44] Community Transportation Association of America (CTAA). Medicaid expansion and premium assistance: the importance of non-emergency medical transportation (NEMT) to coordinated care for chronically Ill patients. 2014. Available at: http://web1.ctaa.org/webmodules/webarticles/articlefiles/NEMTreportfinal.pdf. Accessed December 14, 2015.

[45] Burkhardt JE, Koffman D, Murray G. Economic benefits of coordinating human service transportation and transit services. TCRP. Available at: http://onlinepubs.trb.org/onlinepubs/tcrp/tcrp_rpt_91.pdf (cached). Accessed December 14, 2015.

[46] Association of Asian Pacific Community Health Organizations (AAPCHO) and NACHC. Highlighting the role of enabling services at community health centers: collecting data to support service expansion & enhanced funding. 2010. Available at: https://www.nachc.com/client/Enabling_Services.pdf. Accessed December 14, 2015.

[47] Aaron E. Henry Community Health Service Center, Inc. Delta Area Rural Transit System (DARTS). Available at: https://www.aehchc.org/darts/. Accessed December 14, 2015.

[48] HRSA. Comparison of the rural health clinic and federally qualified health center programs. 2006. Available at: http://www.hrsa.gov/ruralhealth2/policy/confcall/comparisonguide.pdf. Accessed December 14, 2015.

[49] Cheung PT, Wiler JL, Lowe RA, et al. National study of barriers to timely primary care and emergency department utilization among Medicaid recipients. Ann Emerg Med 2012;60:4–10.

[50] GAO. Fragmentation, overlap, and duplication: an evaluation and management guide. 2015. Available at: www.gao.gov/assets/670/669612.pdf. Accessed December 14, 2015.

Advances in Pediatrics 63 (2016) 403–428

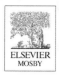

ADVANCES IN PEDIATRICS

ELSEVIER
MOSBY

Toxic Stress in Children and Adolescents

Monica Bucci, MD, Sara Silvério Marques, DrPH, MPH*,
Debora Oh, PhD, MSc, Nadine Burke Harris, MD, MPH

Center for Youth Wellness, 3450 3rd Street, Building 2, Suite 201, San Francisco, CA 94124, USA

Keywords
- Toxic stress • Stress • Adverse childhood experiences • Adversity
- Multisystemic alterations • Chronic disease • Child health • Adolescent health

Key points
- Early life adversity, also referred to as adverse childhood experiences (ACEs), includes stressful or traumatic experiences in childhood and abuse, neglect, and household dysfunction.
- ACEs put children at risk of negative physical, mental, and behavioral health outcomes.
- When a child is exposed to stressors, such as early life adversity, the body's natural stress response can become maladaptive or toxic to the body.
- The toxic stress response results from a disruption of the circuitry between neuroendocrine and immune systems, and it affects multiple biological systems, laying the foundation for long-term health outcomes.

INTRODUCTION

Advances in science have provided evidence of the complex relationship between the social environment, child development, and long-term health outcomes. The medical field, and pediatrics in particular, has become increasingly involved in addressing these complex relationships [1]. Early childhood and adolescence are known to be sensitive periods of development during which biological systems are readily shaped by both positive and negative external influences and experiences [2,3]. Exposure to frequent, prolonged, or intensely negative experiences in childhood (ie, early life adversity) has been associated with long-term negative health outcomes, including ischemic heart disease, cancer, diabetes, asthma, and premature death, among others [1,4–8].

*Corresponding author. *E-mail address*: smarques@centerforyouthwellness.org

0065-3101/16/$ – see front matter
http://dx.doi.org/10.1016/j.yapd.2016.04.002

Investigating the precise biological mechanisms underlying the association between exposure to early life adversity and negative health outcomes is an important emerging field of biomedical research. The current body of data suggests that a maladaptive response to stress during childhood, referred to as a toxic stress response, plays an important role in the pathway from early adversity to disease.

In this article, the authors describe early life adversity and toxic stress, and their implications for pediatric health.

- First, early life adversity and health outcomes are described, including definitions of early life adversity and its prevalence, and associations found between these early experiences and long-term health outcomes.
- Then toxic stress is defined, as part of a continuum of the physiologic stress response and as an important biological pathway linking early life adversity to negative health outcomes. The authors provide an overview of the core anatomic and functional components of the stress response as a foundation for understanding the maladaptive response characteristic of toxic stress. Also presented is evidence of how prolonged exposure to severe or frequent adversity in early life can have an effect on the neuroendocrine immune circuitry that ultimately alters the organism's ability to cease the stress response.
- Finally, the pathogenesis of the toxic stress response is addressed as well as its impact on multiple organ systems, and the risk of negative health outcomes.

EARLY LIFE ADVERSITY AND HEALTH OUTCOMES

Stressful or traumatic events experienced in childhood or adolescence are referred to by many terms, including early life adversity, early life stress, early life trauma, or adverse childhood experiences (ACEs).

In mental and behavioral health, there is an extensive history of studying associations between negative early life experiences and mental and behavioral health outcomes; the Adverse Childhood Experience Study (ACE Study), however, was among the first linking early life adversity and long-term physical health outcomes in a large sample [9]. The categories of adversity used in the ACE Study represent a limited set of risk factors which, although not exhaustive, have become commonly cited as defining categories of adversity in research associating childhood adversity and physical health outcomes. Table 1 exhibits the 3 categories of adversity and definitions used in the ACE Study.

The ACE Study was conducted between 1995 and 1997 at the Kaiser Permanente's Health Appraisal Clinic in San Diego, in collaboration with the Centers for Disease Control and Prevention [9]. The study assessed the associations between ACEs and physical, behavioral, and mental health outcomes. Medical history and data on exposure to ACEs were collected in 2 waves from 18,175 patients of the San Diego clinic (68% overall response rate) [5,9].

In the first wave of the ACE Study, patients were assessed on 2 categories of adversity: abuse and household dysfunction [9]. In the second wave, items on neglect were added [10]. Additional traumatic or stressful experiences with evidence of long-term health impacts include exposure to community violence

Table 1
A adverse childhood experiences, by category

ACE category	Definition
Abuse	• Psychological *Did a parent or other adult in the household ...* ○ Often or very often swear at, insult, or put you down? ○ Often or very often act in a way that made you afraid that you would be physically hurt? • Physical *Did a parent or other adult in the household ...* ○ Often or very often push, grab, shove, or slap you? ○ Often or very often hit you so hard that you had marks or were injured? • Sexual *Did an adult or person at least 5 years older ever ...* ○ Touch or fondle you in a sexual way? ○ Have you touch their body in a sexual way? ○ Attempt oral, anal, or vaginal intercourse with you? ○ Actually have oral, anal, or vaginal intercourse with you?
Neglect	• Emotional *Did you often or very often feel that ...* ○ No one in your family loved you or thought you were important or special? ○ Your family didn't look out for each other, feel close to each other, or support each other? • Physical *Did you often or very often feel that ...* ○ You didn't have enough to eat, had to wear dirty clothes, and had no one to protect you? ○ Your parents were too drunk or high to take care of you or take you to the doctor if you needed it?
Household dysfunction	• Divorce or separation ○ Were your parents ever separated or divorced? • Mother treated violently *Was your mother (or stepmother) ...* ○ Often or very often pushed, grabbed, slapped, or had something thrown at her? ○ Sometimes, often, or very often kicked, bitten, hit with a fist, or hit with something hard? ○ Ever repeatedly hit over at least a few minutes or threatened with, or hurt by, a gun or knife? • Substance abuse ○ Did you live with anyone who was a problem drinker or alcoholic or anyone who used street drugs? • Mental illness ○ Was a household member depressed or mentally ill or attempt suicide? • Criminal behavior in household ○ Did a household member go to prison?

Adapted from Adverse Childhood Experiences Study. Finding your ACE score. Available at: http://www.acestudy.org/yahoo_site_admin/assets/docs/ACE_Calculator-English.127143712.pdf. Accessed May 2, 2016.

[11,12], bullying [13], homelessness [14], parental stress [15], economic hardship [16], and discrimination [17].

Prevalence of early life adversity

Data from the ACE Study indicated that almost two-thirds (63.5%) of adults had at least one ACE, and 12% had 4 or more ACEs [4]. In a more recent, nationally representative sample across 10 states in the United States and the District of Columbia, using data from the Behavioral Risk Factor Surveillance Survey (BRFSS), Gilbert and colleagues [18] also found that approximately two-thirds of adults reported at least one early life adversity. The BRFSS is a cross-sectional population-based telephone survey of noninstitutionalized households. In the BRFSS, early life adversity is defined as abuse (sexual, physical, and emotional) and household dysfunction (having lived with parents/adults who separated/divorced, had a mental illness, abused alcohol, abused drugs, was incarcerated, or was involved in intimate partner violence) experienced before age 18 [18], which is similar to the definition used in the first wave of the ACE Study. Consistent with national data, results from a study using California BRFSS data from 2008, 2009, 2011, and 2013 showed that 61.7% of surveyed adults reported experiencing at least one ACE, and 16.7% reported having experienced 4 or more ACEs [19].

In children, nationally representative studies on ACEs have shown a prevalence of having experienced at least one early life adversity ranging from 33% to nearly 50% of the population [20–22]. Among 701 patients (median age = 7.33 years, SD = 5.47 years) receiving medical services at a community-based primary care clinic in San Francisco, 67.2% of participants had experienced one or more ACE (abuse, neglect, and household dysfunction) and 12% experienced 4 or more ACEs [23]. Among children at high risk for maltreatment, the percentage experiencing at least one early adversity was found to reach as high as 91% [24].

Health outcomes associated with early life adversity

Most studies on early life adversity and health outcomes have been adult retrospective reports of events experienced before age 18 and their adult health outcomes. These studies have been important in identifying associations between early adversity and health outcomes that generally take years to manifest into clinically relevant forms.

Data from the ACE Study suggest a dose-response relationship between the number of ACEs experienced by an individual and negative health outcomes. In comparison with reporting no ACEs, reporting 4 or more ACEs was associated with significantly increased odds of developing 6 of 10 leading causes of death in the United States after adjusting for age, gender, race, and educational attainment: ischemic heart disease (2.20), any cancer (1.90), stroke (2.40), chronic bronchitis or emphysema (3.90), diabetes (1.60), and attempted suicide (12.20) [9,25]. Fig. 1 shows the odds of disease and health risk behavior for those reporting 4 or more ACEs compared with those reporting zero ACEs.

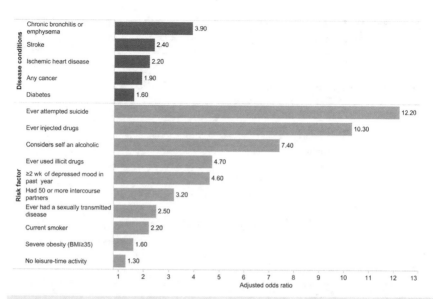

Fig. 1. Odds of outcomes among individuals experiencing 4 or more ACEs. ACEs, adverse childhood experiences; BMI, body mass index. Adjusted for age, gender, race and educational attainment. Referent group 0 ACEs. *Data from* [9]

Additional research on exposure to early life adversity with different populations, including children and adolescents, further supports the conclusion of a relationship between early life adversity and child and adult health outcomes. After 10 years of follow-up, Karlen and colleagues [26] found an association between early life adversity and an increased incidence of childhood illnesses including, dermatitis and eczema, acute upper respiratory illness, otitis media, and viral infections, among others. On the other end of the life span, Brown and colleagues [5] found that people with 6 or more ACEs died nearly 20 years earlier than did those with no ACEs (age 60.6 vs 79.1). Additional findings from various studies on early life adversity and mental, behavioral, and physical health outcomes are summarized in Table 2. In addition to these long-term health consequences, exposure to trauma in childhood has been associated with abnormal development, learning difficulties, and additional pediatric conditions, such as failure to thrive, enuresis, insomnia, and obesity [27].

EARLY LIFE ADVERSITY AND TOXIC STRESS

The etiologic pathways by which the effects of early life adversity becomes embedded in the body and brain of the developing child have yet to be fully understood, but promising research suggests that a dysregulation of the physiologic stress response plays a critical role in the development of negative health outcomes. Although influenced by genetic variability and social and biological protective factors, early life adversity appears to act on the organism as a stressor. Exposure to severe, frequent, and/or prolonged adversity, during

Table 2
Health outcomes associated with early adversity

Outcome	Adults	Children and adolescents
Mental/behavioral health	• Alcoholism • Anxiety • Bipolar disorder • Depression • Difficulty controlling anger • Hallucinations • High stress • Panic reactions • Posttraumatic stress disorder • Smoking • Substance abuse • Suicide	• Bullying • Dating violence • Delinquent behavior • Learning difficulties • Physical fighting • Weapon-carrying
Physical health	• Any cancer • Autoimmune disease • Cardiovascular disease • Chronic lung disease/chronic bronchitis or emphysema • Diabetes • Early death • Fair or poor self-rated health • General poor health • Headaches • Hepatitis or jaundice • Ischemic heart disease • Obesity • Sexual transmitted infections • Sleep disturbances • Skeletal fracture • Stroke	• Acute lower and upper respiratory infections • Adolescent pregnancy • Attention deficit hyperactivity disorder • Asthma • Autism • Conjunctivitis • Dermatitis and eczema • Illness requiring a doctor • Intestinal infectious disease • Lifetime asthma • Otitis media • Overweight or obese • Poor dental health • Poor general health • Pneumonia • Urinary tract infections • Urticaria • Viral infections of unspecified site

Data from Refs. [9,10,20–24,26,125–131].

sensitive periods of development without adequate protective factors in place (eg, supportive caregiving), can cause lasting changes to the stress response regulation. Therefore, toxic stress represents the maladaptive and chronically dysregulated stress response that occurs in relation to prolonged or severe early life adversity [28].

The stress response
The physiologic response to a stressor involves a complex interplay of contextual and biological factors, such as the intensity or severity of the stressor, individual genetic characteristics, gene-environment interactions, family environmental factors, and developmental experiences [29,30]. Protective factors, including biological and social resilience, are also involved in determining how the body responds to environmental stressors [28,29].

The spectrum of the stress response includes positive, tolerable, and toxic stress [1,28], as depicted in Fig. 2. The physiologic response to stress depends on the nature of the stressors and the availability of buffering and coping strategies. Although there is promising evidence from animal studies that the toxic stress response may be mitigated, the extent to which an individual's stress response can move along the continuum is currently unknown [28].

A positive or tolerable stress response is characterized by a return to homeostasis, whereas a toxic stress response may induce lasting changes to the organism. Toxic stress is characterized by prolonged or frequent activation of the stress response that leads to a dysregulation of the neuroendocrine immune circuitry, which produces altered levels of important hormones and neurotransmitters and ultimately changes in brain architecture and multiple organ systems. Because this maladaptive stress response occurs during sensitive periods of development, its effects can become incorporated into long-term regulatory physiologic processes, and subsequently, can increase vulnerability to developmental, biological, mental, and behavioral adverse outcomes, resulting in an increased risk for chronic diseases in adulthood [11].

Anatomy and physiology of the stress response
The stress response has both central and peripheral components. The central components of the stress response include the structures of the central nervous system (CNS): amygdala, hypothalamus, and parts of the brainstem (locus coeruleus in the pons; medulla). The peripheral components of the stress response include the sympatho-adrenomedullary (SAM) axis and the hypothalamic-pituitary-adrenal (HPA) axis. Fig. 3 summarizes the core anatomy of the SAM and HPA axes.

In response to a stressor, the SAM and HPA axes are both activated. The trigger stressor activates the amygdala, which has evolved to detect and signal environmental threats to survival [31]. Activation of the amygdala is modulated by central structures: the hippocampus (important for learning and memory), the prefrontal cortex (implicated in executive functions and cognition), and the locus coeruleus in the pons (responsible for mediating the autonomic effects during stress response) [32]. The complex interplay of the pathways involved in the stress response is highlighted in Fig. 3; key stress-induced hormones are summarized in Table 3.

Activation of the stress response
Sympatho-adrenomedullary axis activation. Once the stimulus is interpreted as a stressor, the SAM axis is activated, releasing catecholamines such as norepinephrine and epinephrine (also known as noradrenaline and adrenaline). The activation of the sympathetic nervous system has both central and peripheral nervous system modulators and operates through a series of interconnected neurons. The locus coeruleus activates the sympathetic neurons in the spinal cord, which are distributed to vessels, major organs, glands, and other parts of the body where they release norepinephrine. Sympathetic neurons also activate the secretion of epinephrine from the adrenal medulla.

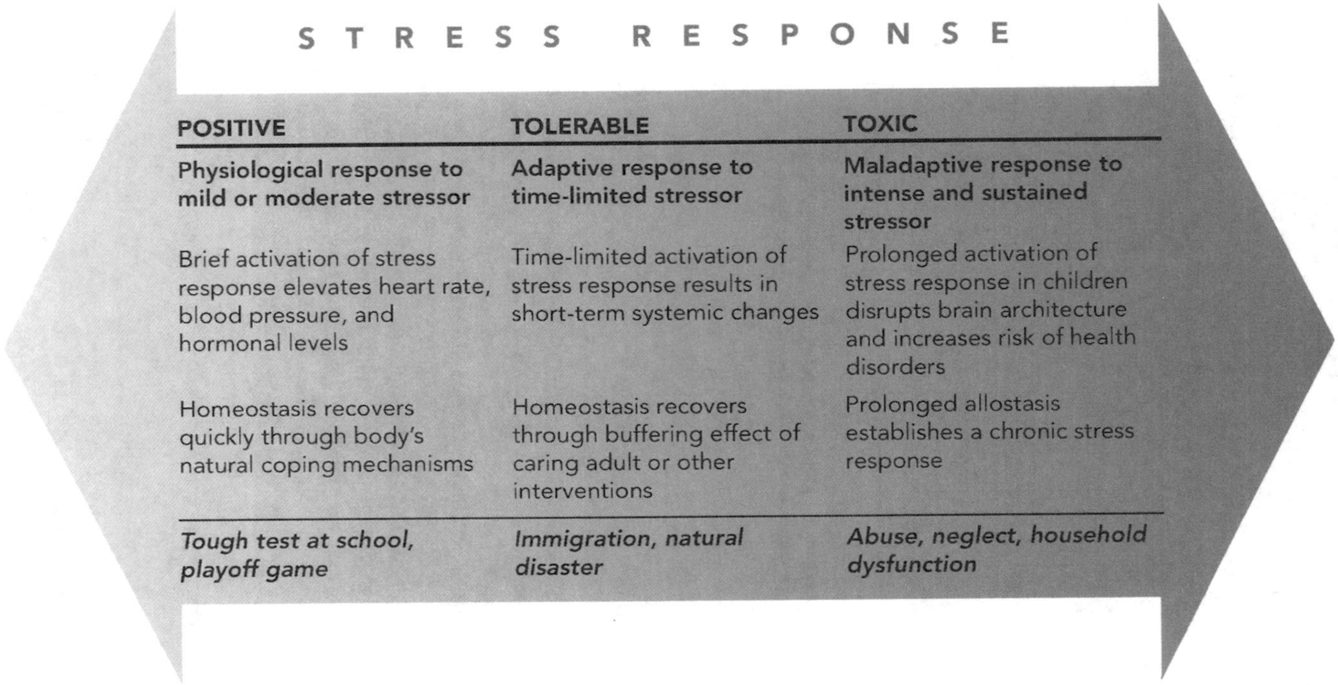

STRESS RESPONSE

POSITIVE	TOLERABLE	TOXIC
Physiological response to mild or moderate stressor	Adaptive response to time-limited stressor	Maladaptive response to intense and sustained stressor
Brief activation of stress response elevates heart rate, blood pressure, and hormonal levels	Time-limited activation of stress response results in short-term systemic changes	Prolonged activation of stress response in children disrupts brain architecture and increases risk of health disorders
Homeostasis recovers quickly through body's natural coping mechanisms	Homeostasis recovers through buffering effect of caring adult or other interventions	Prolonged allostasis establishes a chronic stress response
Tough test at school, playoff game	*Immigration, natural disaster*	*Abuse, neglect, household dysfunction*

Fig. 2. Spectrum of the stress response: positive, tolerable, and toxic.

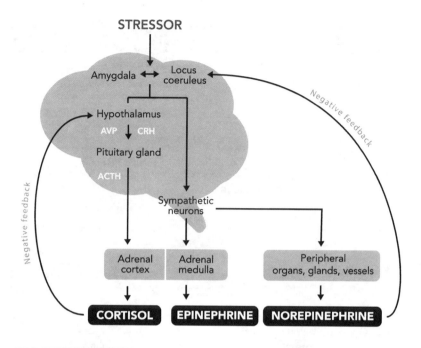

STRESSOR

Fig. 3. Stress response pathway. HPA axis, hypothalamic-pituitary-adrenal axis; SAM axis, sympathoadrenomedullary axis; AVP, arginine vasopressin; CRH, corticotropin-releasing hormone; ACTH, adrenocorticotropin hormone.

Circulating norepinephrine and epinephrine activate the fight-or-flight response to promote redirection and availability of blood, oxygen, and energy to vital organs, through the activation of simultaneous physiologic changes [33,34]. These changes can be described as follows:

- Blood circulation: Constriction of the blood vessels, and increase in the force of cardiac contraction to push blood to the brain, muscles, heart, and other vital

Table 3
Stress-induced hormones

Hormone	Source	Description
CRH	Hypothalamus	Principal regulator of the pituitary-adrenal axis: targets the anterior pituitary
AVP	Hypothalamus and posterior pituitary gland	Targets the anterior pituitary and regulates body's homeostasis
ACTH	Anterior pituitary gland	Targets the adrenal cortex to secrete ACTH
Norepinephrine	Sympathetic neurons in the brain stem (medulla and locus coeruleus)	Activates fight-or-flight response
Epinephrine	Adrenal medulla	Activates fight-or-flight response
Glucocorticoids	Adrenal cortex	Final effectors of the HPA axis. Cortisol is one of the most abundant human glucocorticoids

Abbreviations: ACTH, adrenocorticotropin hormone; AVP, arginine vasopressin; CRH, corticotropin-releasing hormone; HPA axis, hypothalamic-pituitary-adrenal axis.

organs. The effect of these changes is an increase in heart rate, blood pressure, muscle tone, and alertness.

- Respiration: Increase in the respiratory rate and dilation of the small airways in the lungs to increase the intake of oxygen being shunted to the brain and stressed organ systems, where it is most needed.
- Metabolism: Activation of an intermediate metabolic pathway (gluconeogenesis, lipolysis) in order to release stored glucose and fat to be used as an energy source.

Behavioral adaptive changes of the SAM axis activation include the following [35,36]:

- Increased arousal, alertness, and vigilance
- Improved cognition
- Focused attention
- Euphoria
- Enhanced analgesia
- Elevations in body temperature
- Inhibition of vegetative functions (eg, appetite, feeding, digestion, growth, reproduction, and immunity)

Finally, detoxification functions are activated to clear the organism of unnecessary metabolic and catabolic products [35,36].

Hypothalamic-pituitary-adrenal axis activation. In addition to activating the SAM axis in response to a stressor, the amygdala and the locus coeruleus also signal the hypothalamus, inducing activation of the HPA axis [37]. Activation of the HPA axis during exposure to stressors increases the release of corticotropin-releasing hormone (CRH) and arginine vasopressin (AVP) from the hypothalamus to the pituitary gland. In turn, the pituitary gland secretes adrenocorticotropin hormone (ACTH) into the bloodstream. ACTH targets the adrenal cortex, which secretes glucocorticoids. Glucocorticoids are the final effectors of the HPA axis, with cortisol (or hydrocortisone) being the most abundant of the human glucocorticoids [38].

Physiologically normal HPA axis function depends on the balanced activation of two corticosteroid receptors with opposing effects: mineralocorticoid and glucocorticoid receptors [36,39].

- Mineralocorticoid receptors are found in the hypothalamus and regulate blood pressure, the HPA axis circadian rhythm, cerebral glucose availability, and neuronal responsivity, making the organism ready if a fight-or-flight response is needed.
- Glucocorticoid receptors are found in the hypothalamus and anterior pituitary and play an important role in the termination of the stress response through negative feedback inhibition of the secretion of CRH and ACTH. This negative feedback loop serves to limit the duration of the total tissue exposure of the organism to glucocorticoids, minimizing the effects of these hormones on biological systems and shutting down the cascade of effects observed during the response to stress once the organism is no longer exposed to the stressor.

Central nervous system activation. The SAM and HPA axes also interact with other major components of the CNS:

- The reward center (mesocorticolimbic system) is important in cognition and motivation and is a target for substance abuse and drug addiction. This system is composed of dopaminergic neurons of the ventral tegmental area (VTA), involved in anticipatory phenomena and cognitive functions, and is widely implicated in the natural motivational, reinforcement, and reward circuitry of the brain. The VTA contains neurons that project to numerous areas of the brain, including the prefrontal cortex [40–42].
- The emotional center (amygdala-hippocampus complex) is important for memory, decision making, and emotional reactions (especially fear), and it mediates the retrieval and emotional analysis of relevant information of the stressor [40,43].
- The thermoregulatory center increases the core temperature and mediates the pyrogenic effects of proinflammatory cytokines, tumor necrosis factor-α, interleukin (IL)-1, and IL-6 [36].
- The appetite-satiety center in the hypothalamus regulates appetite in response to stress. Acute elevations in CRH concentrations can lead to loss of appetite and anorexia [44,45]. Fasting enhances CRH secretion [44], inhibits the sympathetic nervous system and activates the parasympathetic nervous system [45].

Once the individual is no longer exposed to the stressor, or is in the presence of a supportive caregiver and has effective coping mechanisms that help the body adapt to the stressor, the parasympathetic subdivision of the autonomic nervous system intervenes to withdraw the activation of the SAM axis, while cortisol regulates the activation of the HPA axis through negative feedback inhibition of the secretion of CRH and ACTH [28]. In concert, these processes terminate the stress response and facilitate the return of the body to homeostasis.

Dysregulation of the stress response

The normal physiologic stress response is an adaptive and time-limited process to maintain the homeostasis necessary for survival [46]. Homeostasis is achieved through self-regulating properties that biological systems have in place to maintain the internal stability of key physiologic variables, such as body temperature and energy balance. As part of achieving homeostasis, the organism activates processes that are essential for successful adaptation to prevent an overresponse from both the central and the peripheral components of the stress response. These adaptive processes, known as allostasis, rely on the organism's ability to detect external and internal changes and to activate appropriate adaptive responses [47]. The time-limited nature of the stress response makes its systemic short-term changes tolerable and useful for the healthy development of the child's adaptive stress response [40]. Allostasis becomes adaptive for the organism in the context of coping with a stressful situation. Conversely if the exposure to the stressful situation is intense, chronic, or repeated and occurs during sensitive periods of development and without a buffering factor, it is associated with a prolonged or frequent and dysregulated activation of these allostatic processes [48–50] and can become maladaptive and, over time, toxic.

During a chronic (ie, toxic) stress response, the organism may become unable to regulate the SAM and HPA axes due to a disruption of negative feedback regulation. If the toxic stress response is not buffered, for example, by supporting caregiving and effective coping mechanisms, the organism may fail to regulate the stress response. This dysregulation can lead to a prolonged activation of the SAM and HPA axes and a dysregulation of the release of the stress-induced hormones (eg, cortisol) and catecholamines (eg, epinephrine and norepinephrine). As a result, the circulating stress-induced hormones and catecholamines may become chronically excessive or chronically deficient [35,36,39].

Biological alterations of the stress response

The toxic stress response is particularly concerning for children because the developing brain is highly plastic and influenced by the environment. The dysregulation of the stress response produces significant biological alterations that can damage brain architecture and impact the nervous, endocrine, and immune systems, which are highly integrated biological systems, often referred to as the neuroendocrine immune circuitry [51]. These systems interact reciprocally as the mediators of the toxic stress response. Prolonged or frequent activation of the stress response in early childhood reduces neuronal connections in important areas of the CNS that are key mediators and regulators of the SAM and HPA axes.

Individuals with altered functioning in the nervous, endocrine, and immune systems have been found to be at increased risk for developing chronic disorders [38]. Moreover, epigenetic modifications in childhood play a role in damaging the systems involved in the future response to adversity in adulthood.

Nervous system

In the nervous system, prolonged exposure to early life adversity results in structural and functional alterations in stress-sensitive regions of the brain such as the hippocampus, the amygdala, and the prefrontal cortex [32,52,53]. These regions are thought to play important roles in the regulation of the SAM and HPA axes.

- In the prefrontal cortex, chronic exposure to adversities has been shown to cause reduced prefrontal cortex synaptic plasticity in children and has been associated with selective prefrontal cortex atrophy in adults.
- In the amygdala, chronic exposure to stress has been linked to increased amygdala volume in children and atrophy in adults.
- In the hippocampus, prolonged stress exposure has been associated with reduced hippocampal volume in adults.

Endocrine system

In the endocrine system, prolonged or severe exposure to early life adversity is associated with changes in hormonal levels consistent with chronic activation of the HPA axis: increased CRH levels, lower morning cortisol levels, and elevated afternoon cortisol levels. These changes result in flatter circadian variation and greater daily secretion of cortisol [54], and overall disruption of the feedback inhibition of cortisol on the HPA axis [55,56]. Over time, HPA axis hyperactivity may recede, and in severe cases of prolonged and/or intense toxic stress response, the activity of the HPA axis decreases, to very low or deficient hormonal levels [54].

Immune system

The chronic dysregulation of the HPA axis has profound effects on the immune and inflammatory response, because virtually all the components of the immune response are influenced by glucocorticoids. The neuroendocrine immune circuitry interacts through cytokines, chemical signals that play a key role in regulating both innate and acquired immunity [57] and are essential to development and metabolism of most body tissues and organ systems [58]. The activation of the sympathetic nervous system during a stress response triggers a sustained elevation in the inflammatory response in the organism by inducing the secretion of proinflammatory cytokines in the systemic circulation [59,60]. Proinflammatory cytokines are produced by the immune system to prevent possible infections and are responsible for the activation of complex adaptive response known as sickness behavior, which enhances recovery by conserving energy to combat acute inflammation through the activation of the thermoregulatory and appetite-satiety centers in the brain [61]. Proinflammatory cytokines also interact with the HPA axis during an immune response [62]. They activate the HPA axis to secrete cortisol and, cortisol participates in the negative feedback inhibition to shut down the HPA axis and the inflammatory response, after the threat is removed [62,63].

The prolonged dysregulation observed during a chronic toxic stress response inhibits anti-inflammatory pathways and results in elevation of inflammation levels, such as elevated levels of C-reactive protein (CRP) and proinflammatory cytokines [56,64–66]. In addition, prolonged exposure to stress has been associated with impaired cell-mediated acquired immunity due to the combined effects of glucocorticoid and catecholamine suppression of innate and cellular immunity (T cells) and stimulation of humoral immunity (B cells) [67,68].

TOXIC STRESS AND CLINICAL IMPLICATIONS
Alterations to the nervous, endocrine, and immune systems that stem from a toxic stress response influence multiple organ systems. In adults, these multisystemic changes have been linked to an increased risk of developing chronic disorders, such as metabolic syndrome, cardiovascular disease, allergic and atopic disease, inflammatory diseases, autoimmune diseases, as well as cognitive, mental, and behavioral disorders.

Multisystemic alterations
The prolonged activation of a toxic stress response is associated with systemic alterations because it results in the excessive or deficient secretion of stress-induced hormones (eg, cortisol), catecholamines (eg, norepinephrine and epinephrine), and inflammatory factors (eg, proinflammatory cytokines, CRP) [69]. These alterations impact biological and behavioral functions across systems, including those primarily regulated by the nervous, endocrine, and immune systems.

Neurologic, psychiatric, and behavioral alterations
Promising research suggests that cytokines and altered levels of stress-induced hormones participate in the pathophysiology of developmental, cognitive, mental, and behavioral disorders in children and adults [70–74]. A dysregulation of the HPA axis is associated with behavioral and cognitive changes in the prefrontal cortex, amygdala, and hippocampus. In the prefrontal cortex, chronic exposure to adversities has been shown to cause impairment of executive functions, such as attention, reasoning, self-regulation (eg, impulse control), working memory, and problem solving. In the amygdala, chronic stress response causes alterations in behavioral responses, such as enhanced awareness and responsiveness to potential threats (hypervigilance), an enhanced response to stimuli that elicit a fear response but have not been previously witnessed (unlearned fear), and learned behavioral responses to predicted threats (fear conditioning). In the hippocampus, prolonged stress response can cause behavioral changes such as impaired memory and learning [53].

Early life adversity has also been associated with an increased incidence of adult psychopathology that is linked to a dysregulated HPA axis function. Adolescents exposed to severe adversity have a greater incidence of suicidal ideation, suicide attempts, and dysthymia. A spectrum of other conditions may also be associated with increased and prolonged activation of the HPA axis, including anorexia nervosa, obsessive-compulsive disorder, panic anxiety, excessive exercise, and chronic active alcoholism [40]. In addition, poor caregiving quality can have early effects on HPA axis regulation and is suggested as one of the mechanisms contributing to heightened risk of mental health disorders, such as posttraumatic stress disorder, chronic anxiety, melancholic depression, eating disorders, substance and alcohol abuse, and personality and conduct disorders [75,76].

Similarly, early adversity is frequently associated with disruption of early caregiving interactions, which may alter the development and expression of certain social behaviors. Emerging evidence suggests that failures in regulation of the HPA axis in young children may play a role in shaping the mesocorticolimbic circuits (VTA dopaminergic system) involved in processing threatening experiences encountered later in life, which results in a corresponding labile mesocorticolimbic dopaminergic system and possible dysphoria. These effects, among others, may be mediated via changes in the release of stress-induced hormones such as vasopressin and serotonin. Early social experience can alter concentrations of vasopressin, and serotonin, an essential neurotransmitter for the regulation of emotional and social behaviors, in particular, aggression. Alterations of the release of serotonin have been reported in humans exposed to early adversities such as maltreatment [77]. For example, patients with borderline personality disorder who experienced childhood maltreatment were found to have altered serotonin activity and increased aggressive and impulsive behaviors [78].

Finally, HPA axis dysregulation may also be associated with a peripheral neuroendocrine effect on the gastrointestinal system. In particular, HPA axis activation induces inhibition of gastric acid secretion and emptying while stimulating colonic motor function. The excessive secretion of CRH due to a hyperactive HPA axis may also play a role in the stress-induced colonic hypermotility of patients with irritable bowel syndrome [40].

Endocrine, metabolic, and reproductive alterations

Research continues to link the effects of HPA axis disruption on the immune response with the pathogenesis of metabolic disease and an increase of cardiovascular disease risk [79,80]. In particular, the dysregulation of the HPA axis and the resulting chronically elevated levels of cortisol have been associated with increased tissue sensitivity to glucocorticoids and chronic activation of the glucocorticoid receptors. This chronic and persistent activation is found to be indirectly involved in the pathogenesis of individual components of the metabolic syndrome: obesity, insulin resistance, glucose intolerance, dyslipidemia, and hypertension. Furthermore, glucocorticoids and epinephrine have direct effects on the heart and blood vessels, and high levels of these factors have been found to influence vascular function, early atherogenesis, and vascular remodeling [81–83], increasing the risk for cardiovascular and cerebrovascular diseases.

Thyroid function is also inhibited during stress. Activation of the HPA axis is associated with decreased production of thyroid-stimulating hormone as well as inhibition of peripheral conversion of the relatively inactive thyroxine to the biologically active triiodothyronine. These alterations may be due to the increased concentrations of CRH-induced glucocorticoids and may result in subclinical or clinical hypothyroidism [40,84].

The reproductive system is inhibited at all levels by various components of the HPA axis. HPA axis activation suppresses the secretion of gonadotropin-releasing hormone either directly or indirectly. Glucocorticoids also exert an inhibitory effect on the gonads. During inflammatory stress, for example, the elevated concentrations of cytokines also result in suppression of reproductive function [40,84], which may explain the relationship between high levels of stress and irregularities of the menstrual cycle frequently observed clinically in adolescents.

Immune and inflammatory alterations

A healthy development of the child's immune system depends on a series of essential changes, such as the adaptive immune system response that regulates the immune response toward humoral (B cells and antibodies) or cellular immunity (T cells and T-helper 1 and T-helper 2 response) [85]. Dysregulation of this adaptive response toward an excessive T-helper 2 cell response early in life creates life-long immune hyperreactivity, which increases the risk of developing allergies and asthma [85,86]. Children exposed to early adversity are more likely to develop or report asthma and have poor control of asthma symptoms. In addition, children exposed to early adversity are more likely to have elevated inflammatory markers (eg, cytokines, CRP) and greater inflammatory response to stress as adults, increasing the risk of developing inflammatory and autoimmune diseases [87–90].

Over time, a prolonged stress response has also been associated with impaired cell-mediated acquired immunity due to the combined effects of glucocorticoids and catecholamines, which cause suppression of innate and cellular immunity [67,68]. The effects of stress-related immunosuppression facilitate diseases related to deficiency of the humoral and cellular immune responses, such as common cold, tuberculosis, and certain tumors [91]. In addition to the direct effects of toxic stress, children at highest risk of early adversity are also more likely to be exposed to environmental toxins, such as secondhand smoke and environmental pollution, which increase the risk of developing a hyperreactive immune response [92,93]. Sensitization to these allergens early in life has been correlated with the development of allergic and atopic disease [92].

Fig. 4 summarizes the complex interplay of the mechanisms observed during a chronic toxic stress response and the associated clinical implications.

Genetic factors and epigenetic modifications

The stress response of an individual is determined by multiple factors, many of which are inherited. Genetic polymorphisms, such as those of stress-induced hormones, and their receptors and/or regulators, account for much of the observed variability in the function of the stress response. These polymorphisms are an expression of a complex continuum that ranges from extreme resilience to extreme vulnerability to stress and adversity. Gene-environment interactions likely reflect genetic moderation of the brain and body functional response to stress, including early life stress. It is conceivable that these

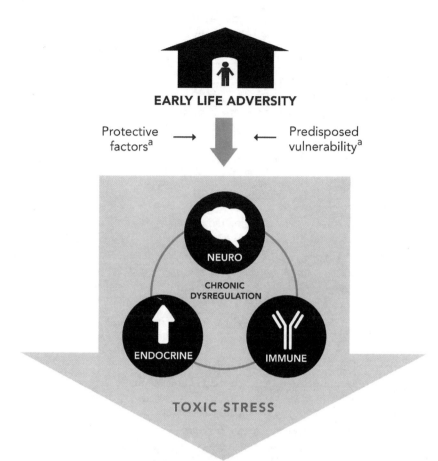

Fig. 4. Overview of toxic stress. ªSocial, biological, genetic factors.

genotype-related alterations underlie individual differences in the susceptibility to develop a toxic stress response.

Additionally, epigenetic regulation in childhood play a role in damaging the systems involved in the organism's future response to stress in adulthood. Epigenetics is defined as heritable changes in gene activity and expression that occur without alteration in DNA sequence. These changes are tightly regulated by 2 major epigenetic modifications: DNA methylation and histone modifications. Epigenetic regulation typically occur in the cells of multiple organ systems, therefore influencing how these structures develop and function. Data suggest that these chemical modifications are highly responsive to early adversity. Some genes can only be modified epigenetically during sensitive periods of development [94–99]. Epigenetic changes that occur early in life, when these organ systems are still developing, can have important effects on long-term physical and mental health outcomes [100]. Therefore, epigenetic regulation caused by a chronically activated toxic stress response during sensitive periods of development affect how the systems respond to stress in adulthood and can result in increased risk of chronic disease.

The brain is particularly sensitive to early life adversity during sensitive periods of development, which influences how its architecture matures and functions. Exposure to severe and prolonged adversity in childhood can lead to long-lasting changes in the brain that may impact how the nervous system responds to future adversity [28]. For example, in animal models and studies with children in foster care, variations in maternal care soon after birth have demonstrated the potent role of epigenetic programming in an offspring's behavioral and neuroendocrine stress responses [29,76,101]. In animals, stressful experiences soon after birth have been shown to cause epigenetic modifications that alter the chemical structure of receptors in the brain, which regulates the activation of the fight-or-flight response. These modifications have been shown to result in prolonged stress responses [101–103].

In addition, in animals, exposure to strong stressors has been correlated with epigenetic changes in brain architecture, brain chemistry, and behaviors that resemble anxiety and depression in humans [104–109]. Human studies have shown associations between severe adverse experiences in children and increased risk for later mental illnesses, including generalized anxiety disorder and major depressive disorder [110–112]. Chronically dysregulated stress responses can also result in epigenetic alterations that have been associated with increased risk of other chronic diseases, such as asthma, hypertension, heart disease, and diabetes [28,110–118].

Conversely, a supportive environment can generate positive epigenetic changes [119]. Recent research demonstrates that even after epigenetic modifications, it may still be possible to reverse negative changes and restore normal physiologic function through positive interactions between child and caregiver [104,120]. In animals, examples of these positive epigenetic modifications are the development of cognitive skills, like learning and memory [121]. Interactions between early adversity, genotype, and epigenetic changes are an important and promising area of future research in humans, due to their it has direct implications for developing new interventions to prevent physical and mental illnesses that are due in part to epigenetic modification.

DISCUSSION
ACEs, including abuse, neglect, household dysfunction, and other early life adversities, have been associated with long-term negative health outcomes. A

toxic stress response has been implicated as a contributing factor to the development of these outcomes. The physiologic response to a stressor is determined by multiple factors, including the duration and severity of the exposure; social, biological, and genetic protective factors and vulnerabilities; and developmental factors. A prolonged stress response can result in the chronic activation of the neuroendocrine immune systems involved in the stress response. If exposure to a stressor is time limited or if the individual has appropriate coping mechanisms, allostatic processes can facilitate an adaptive stress response and return the organism to homeostasis. Prolonged or severe exposure to a stressor, however, can cause a dysregulation in the neuroendocrine immune circuitry, damaging the inhibition feedback and regulation mechanisms and creating a maladaptive, or toxic, stress response. This toxic stress response may produce an excess or deficiency in stress-induced hormones and neurotransmitters, which, when experienced during sensitive periods of development in childhood, can become incorporated into the developing biological systems. This altered availability of hormones and neurotransmitters induces lasting changes that affect multiple organ systems and functions, including brain architecture, endocrine system regulation, and immune response. The alterations of multiple organ systems, in conjunction with genetic vulnerability and epigenetic regulation, place an individual at risk for negative physical, mental, and behavioral health outcomes well into adulthood.

Despite increased awareness of toxic stress, many limitations restrict current understanding of the topic and clinical implications for pediatric health. Because the factors influencing the development of toxic stress and disease are multifactorial, the field has been challenged in defining the precise connections between genetic vulnerability to stress, alterations in the molecular and neuroendocrine immune pathways that modulate the stress response, and the clinical presentation of these alterations. Further clarification of the role that toxic stress plays, either as an effect modifier or as part of the causal pathway for disease, will help practitioners better identify appropriate screening and treatment modalities and ultimately lead to more effective policies that address the effects of ACEs. Another limitation is the lack of information on effective interventions. Evidence from animal models shows that bolstering the child-caregiver relationship can reverse the effects of adversity at both physiologic and epigenetic levels and improve health outcomes [122,123]. Further research on the neurobiology of resilience and protective mechanisms for development is needed to better understand how interventions can both prevent and heal the effects of a toxic stress response.

As researchers work to address the gaps in understanding, policymakers and practitioners are seeking ways to address the effects of adversity and toxic stress in diverse settings. The American Academy of Pediatrics has called on pediatricians to screen for precipitants of toxic stress [124]. Assessing a patient's history of early adversity places the mental and social aspects of an individual's life firmly into the physical health sphere, enabling medical providers to use the biopsychosocial model of health care more effectively. Through this model, providers can raise awareness among patients of the effects of early adversity and stress on children's physical health. Medical providers can also use this patient history to consider modifications to standard prevention or screening advice for various medical conditions. In addition, using the biopsychosocial model of toxic stress to address clinical conditions that are traditionally understood as behavior dependent (eg, obesity) can help shift the stigma of adversity and improve engagement in treatment options for both children and their caregivers.

A critical next step for the field is the development of clinical diagnostic criteria for toxic stress. As the research on toxic stress moves forward, standardized ways of identifying patients at risk using well-defined risk factors and/or biomarkers will help better elucidate the public health challenge that practitioners and policymakers face. Clinical diagnostic criteria will enable researchers, medical practitioners, and policymakers to work together to inform prevention and treatment of health outcomes associated with early life adversity. Standardized criteria will also allow for the development of interventions focused on helping children reduce acute physiologic responses to stressors, develop natural protective mechanisms of resilience and prevent long-term pathogenic processes from initiating or worsening.

Although the intricacies of the physiologic impact of adversity and toxic stress are still being investigated, the science is clear: early adversity dramatically affects health across a lifetime. It is critical for practitioners and policymakers to move forward to prevent, screen, and heal the effects of early adversity and toxic stress.

Acknowledgments

The authors thank Dr Jessica Duvall, Dr Kadiatou Koita, Sukhdip Purewal, Allison Ipsen, and Dr Petra Jerman for their helpful feedback on this article.

References

[1] Shonkoff JP, Garner AS, Committee on Psychosocial Aspects of Child and Family Health, et al. The lifelong effects of early childhood adversity and toxic stress. Pediatrics 2012;129(1):e232–46.
[2] Dahl RE. Adolescent brain development: a period of vulnerabilities and opportunities. Keynote address. Ann N Y Acad Sci 2004;1021:1–22.
[3] Knudsen EI. Sensitive periods in the development of the brain and behavior. J Cogn Neurosci 2004;16(8):1412–25.
[4] Anda RF, Dong M, Brown DW, et al. The relationship of adverse childhood experiences to a history of premature death of family members. BMC Public Health 2009;9:106.
[5] Brown DW, Anda RF, Tiemeier H, et al. Adverse childhood experiences and the risk of premature mortality. Am J Prev Med 2009;37(5):389–96.
[6] Pechtel P, Pizzagalli DA. Effects of early life stress on cognitive and affective function: an integrated review of human literature. Psychopharmacology (Berl) 2011;214(1):55–70.
[7] Smith SM, Vale WW. The role of the hypothalamic-pituitary-adrenal axis in neuroendocrine responses to stress. Dialogues Clin Neurosci 2006;8(4):383–95.
[8] Taylor SE. Mechanisms linking early life stress to adult health outcomes. Proc Natl Acad Sci U S A 2010;107(19):8507–12.

[9] Felitti VJ, Anda RF, Nordenberg D, et al. Relationship of childhood abuse and household dysfunction to many of the leading causes of death in adults. The Adverse Childhood Experiences (ACE) Study. Am J Prev Med 1998;14(4):245–58.

[10] Dube SR, Anda RF, Felitti VJ, et al. Childhood abuse, household dysfunction, and the risk of attempted suicide throughout the life span: findings from the Adverse Childhood Experiences Study. JAMA 2001;286(24):3089–96.

[11] Johnson SB, Riley AW, Granger DA, et al. The science of early life toxic stress for pediatric practice and advocacy. Pediatrics 2013;131(2):319–27.

[12] Wright RJ, Visness CM, Calatroni A, et al. Prenatal maternal stress and cord blood innate and adaptive cytokine responses in an inner-city cohort. Am J Respir Crit Care Med 2010;182(1):25–33.

[13] Fekkes M, Pijpers FI, Fredriks AM, et al. Do bullied children get ill, or do ill children get bullied? A prospective cohort study on the relationship between bullying and health-related symptoms. Pediatrics 2006;117(5):1568–74.

[14] Hutto N, Viola J. Toxic stress and brain development in young homeless children. In: Matto HC, Strolin-Goltzman J, Ballan M, editors. Neuroscience for social work: current research and practice. New York: Springer; 2013. p. 263–77.

[15] Essex MJ, Klein MH, Cho E, et al. Maternal stress beginning in infancy may sensitize children to later stress exposure: effects on cortisol and behavior. Biol Psychiatry 2002;52(8):776–84.

[16] Sacks V, Murphey D, Moore K. Adverse childhood experiences: national and state-level prevalence. Bethesda (MD): Child Trends; 2014. Available at: http://www.childtrends.org/wp-content/uploads/2014/07/Brief-adverse-childhood-experiences_FINAL.pdf.

[17] Pascoe EA, Smart Richman L. Perceived discrimination and health: a meta-analytic review. Psychol Bull 2009;135(4):531–54.

[18] Gilbert LK, Breiding MJ, Merrick MT, et al. Childhood adversity and adult chronic disease: an update from ten states and the District of Columbia, 2010. Am J Prev Med 2015;48(3): 345–9.

[19] Center for Youth Wellness in partnership with Public Health Institute. A hidden crisis: findings on adverse childhood experiences in California. 2014. Available at: http://www.centerforyouthwellness.org/resources. Accessed December 15, 2015.

[20] Bethell CD, Newacheck P, Hawes E, et al. Adverse childhood experiences: assessing the impact on health and school engagement and the mitigating role of resilience. Health Affairs 2014;33(12):2106–15.

[21] Bright MA, Alford SM, Hinojosa MS, et al. Adverse childhood experiences and dental health in children and adolescents. Community Dent Oral Epidemiol 2015;43(3):193–9.

[22] Wing R, Gjelsvik A, Nocera M, et al. Association between adverse childhood experiences in the home and pediatric asthma. Ann Allergy Asthma Immunol 2015;114(5):379–84.

[23] Burke NJ, Hellman JL, Scott BG, et al. The impact of adverse childhood experiences on an urban pediatric population. Child Abuse Negl 2011;35(6):408–13.

[24] Flaherty EG, Thompson R, Dubowitz H, et al. Adverse childhood experiences and child health in early adolescence. JAMA Pediatr 2013;167(7):622–9.

[25] Centers for Disease Control and Prevention. 2013 U.S. mortality multiple cause files. Available at: http://www.cdc.gov/nchs/data_access/Vitalstatsonline.htm. Accessed December 15, 2015.

[26] Karlen J, Ludvigsson J, Hedmark M, et al. Early psychosocial exposures, hair cortisol levels, and disease risk. Pediatrics 2015;135(6):e1450–7.

[27] American Academy of Pediatrics. 2014. The medical home approach to identifying and responding to exposure to trauma. Available at: https://www.aap.org/en-us/Documents/ttb_medicalhomeapproach.pdf. Accessed December 15, 2015.

[28] Shonkoff JP, Boyce WT, McEwen BS. Neuroscience, molecular biology, and the childhood roots of health disparities: building a new framework for health promotion and disease prevention. JAMA 2009;301(21):2252–9.

[29] Ellis BJ, Boyce WT. Biological sensitivity to context. Curr Dir Psychol Sci 2008;17(3): 183–7.

[30] Schneiderman N, Ironson G, Siegel SD. Stress and health: psychological, behavioral, and biological determinants. Annu Rev Clin Psychol 2005;1:607–28.

[31] LeDoux JE. Emotion circuits in the brain. Annu Rev Neurosci 2000;23:155–84.

[32] McEwen BS. Physiology and neurobiology of stress and adaptation: central role of the brain. Physiol Rev 2007;87(3):873–904.

[33] Haggerty RJ, Sherrod LR, Garmezy N, et al, editors. Stress, risk, and resilience in children and adolescents: processes, mechanisms, and interventions. New York: Cambridge University Press; 1996.

[34] Herd JA. Cardiovascular response to stress. Physiol Rev 1991;71(1):305–30.

[35] Chrousos GP. The neuroendocrinology of stress: its relation to the hormonal milieu, growth and development. Growth Genet Horm 1997;13:1–8.

[36] Tsigos C, Chrousos GP. Hypothalamic-pituitary-adrenal axis, neuroendocrine factors and stress. J Psychosom Res 2002;53(4):865–71.

[37] Ulrich-Lai YM, Herman JP. Neural regulation of endocrine and autonomic stress responses. Nat Rev Neurosci 2009;10(6):397–409.

[38] Tarullo AR, Gunnar MR. Child maltreatment and the developing HPA axis. Horm Behav 2006;50(4):632–9.

[39] Habib KE, Gold PW, Chrousos GP. Neuroendocrinology of stress. Endocrinol Metab Clin North Am 2001;30(3):695–728, vii–viii.

[40] Charmandari E, Tsigos C, Chrousos G. Endocrinology of the stress response. Annu Rev Physiol 2005;67:259–84.

[41] Imperato A, Puglisi-Allegra S, Casolini P, et al. Changes in brain dopamine and acetylcholine release during and following stress are independent of the pituitary-adrenocortical axis. Brain Res 1991;538(1):111–7.

[42] Roth H, Tam SY, Ida Y, et al. Stress and the mesocorticolimbic dopamine systems. Ann N Y Acad Sci 1988;537:138–47.

[43] Gray TS. Amygdala: role in autonomic and neuroendocrine responses to stress. In: McCubbin JA, Kaufman PG, Nemeroff CB, editors. Stress, neuropeptides, and systemic disease. New York: Academic Press; 1991. p. 37.

[44] Liu JP, Clarke IJ, Funder JW, et al. Studies of the secretion of corticotropin-releasing factor and arginine vasopressin into the hypophysial-portal circulation of the conscious sheep. II. The central noradrenergic and neuropeptide Y pathways cause immediate and prolonged hypothalamic-pituitary-adrenal activation. Potential involvement in the pseudo-Cushing's syndrome of endogenous depression and anorexia nervosa. J Clin Invest 1994;93(4): 1439–50.

[45] Egawa M, Yoshimatsu H, Bray GA. Neuropeptide Y suppresses sympathetic activity to interscapular brown adipose tissue in rats. Am J Physiol 1991;260(2 Pt 2):R328–34.

[46] McEwen BS. The neurobiology of stress: from serendipity to clinical relevance. Brain Res 2000;886(1–2):172–89.

[47] Sterling P, Eyer J. Allostasis: a new paradigm to explain arousal pathology. In: Fisher S, Reason J, editors. Handbook of life stress, cognition and health. New York: Wiley; 1988. p. 629–49.

[48] Danese A, McEwen BS. Adverse childhood experiences, allostasis, allostatic load, and age-related disease. Physiol Behav 2012;106(1):29–39.

[49] McEwen BS. Protective and damaging effects of stress mediators. N Engl J Med 1998;338(3):171–9.

[50] McEwen BS, Wingfield JC. The concept of allostasis in biology and biomedicine. Horm Behav 2003;43(1):2–15.

[51] McEwen BS. Protective and damaging effects of stress mediators: central role of the brain. Dialogues Clin Neurosci 2006;8(4):367–81.

[52] McEwen BS, Gianaros PJ. Stress- and allostasis-induced brain plasticity. Annu Rev Med 2010;62:431–45.

[53] Cerqueira JJ, Mailliet F, Almeida OF, et al. The prefrontal cortex as a key target of the maladaptive response to stress. J Neurosci 2007;27(11):2781–7.

[54] Miller GE, Chen E, Zhou ES. If it goes up, must it come down? Chronic stress and the hypothalamic-pituitary-adrenocortical axis in humans. Psychol Bull 2007;133(1):25–45.

[55] Heim C, Newport DJ, Mletzko T, et al. The link between childhood trauma and depression: insights from HPA axis studies in humans. Psychoneuroendocrinology 2008;33(6): 693–710.

[56] Raison CL, Miller AH. When not enough is too much: the role of insufficient glucocorticoid signaling in the pathophysiology of stress-related disorders. Am J Psychiatry 2003;160(9): 1554–65.

[57] Blalock JE, Smith EM. Conceptual development of the immune system as a sixth sense. Brain Behav Immun 2007;21(1):23–33.

[58] Granger DA, Granger GA, Granger SW. Immunology and developmental psychopathology. In: Cicchetti D, Cohen DJ, editors. Developmental psychopathology. 2nd edition. New York: Wiley; 2006. p. 677–709.

[59] Bierhaus A, Wolf J, Andrassy M, et al. A mechanism converting psychosocial stress into mononuclear cell activation. Proc Natl Acad Sci U S A 2003;100(4):1920–5.

[60] Kiecolt-Glaser JK, Preacher KJ, MacCallum RC, et al. Chronic stress and age-related increases in the proinflammatory cytokine IL-6. Proc Natl Acad Sci U S A 2003;100(15): 9090–5.

[61] Dantzer R, O'Connor JC, Freund GG, et al. From inflammation to sickness and depression: when the immune system subjugates the brain. Nat Rev Neurosci 2008;9(1):46–56.

[62] Rhen T, Cidlowski JA. Antiinflammatory action of glucocorticoids—new mechanisms for old drugs. N Engl J Med 2005;353(16):1711–23.

[63] Webster JI, Tonelli L, Sternberg EM. Neuroendocrine regulation of immunity. Annu Rev Immunol 2002;20:125–63.

[64] Thayer JF, Sternberg EM. Neural aspects of immunomodulation: focus on the vagus nerve. Brain Behav Immun 2010;24(8):1223–8.

[65] Tolmay CM, Malan L, van Rooyen JM. The relationship between cortisol, C-reactive protein and hypertension in African and Caucasian women: the POWIRS study. Cardiovasc J Afr 2012;23(2):78–84.

[66] Tracey KJ. The inflammatory reflex. Nature 2002;420(6917):853–9.

[67] Cohen S, Tyrrell DAJ, Smith AP. Psychological stress and susceptibility to the common cold. N Engl J Med 1991;325(9):606–12.

[68] Glaser R, Rabin B, Chesney M, et al. Stress-induced immunomodulation: implications for infectious diseases? JAMA 1999;281(24):2268–70.

[69] Sapolsky RM, Krey LC, McEwen BS. The neuroendocrinology of stress and aging: the glucocorticoid cascade hypothesis. Endocr Rev 1986;7(3):284–301.

[70] Gabbay V, Klein RG, Alonso CM, et al. Immune system dysregulation in adolescent major depressive disorder. J Affect Disord 2009;115(1–2):177–82.

[71] Keller PS, El-Sheikh M, Vaughn B, et al. Relations between mucosal immunity and children's mental health: the role of child sex. Physiol Behav 2010;101(5):705–12.

[72] Marsland AL, Prather AA, Petersen KL, et al. Antagonistic characteristics are positively associated with inflammatory markers independently of trait negative emotionality. Brain Behav Immun 2008;22(5):753–61.

[73] Misener VL, Gomez L, Wigg KG, et al. Cytokine genes TNF, IL1A, IL1B, IL6, IL1RN and IL10, and childhood-onset mood disorders. Neuropsychobiology 2008;58(2):71–80.

[74] Raison CL, Capuron L, Miller AH. Cytokines sing the blues: inflammation and the pathogenesis of depression. Trends Immunol 2006;27(1):24–31.

[75] Gunnar M, Quevedo K. The neurobiology of stress and development. Annu Rev Psychol 2007;58:145–73.

[76] Gunnar MR, Quevedo KM. Early care experiences and HPA axis regulation in children: a mechanism for later trauma vulnerability. Prog Brain Res 2008;167:137–49.

[77] Veenema AH. Early life stress, the development of aggression and neuroendocrine and neurobiological correlates: what can we learn from animal models? Front Neuroendocrinol 2009;30(4):497–518.

[78] Rinne T, Westenberg HG, den Boer JA, et al. Serotonergic blunting to meta-chlorophenylpiperazine (m-CPP) highly correlates with sustained childhood abuse in impulsive and autoaggressive female borderline patients. Biol Psychiatry 2000;47(6):548–56.

[79] Bjorntorp P, Holm G, Rosmond R. Hypothalamic arousal, insulin resistance and type 2 diabetes mellitus. Diabet Med 1999;16(5):373–83.

[80] Smith GD, Ben-Shlomo Y, Beswick A, et al. Cortisol, testosterone, and coronary heart disease: prospective evidence from the Caerphilly study. Circulation 2005;112(3):332–40.

[81] Alevizaki M, Cimponeriu A, Lekakis J, et al. High anticipatory stress plasma cortisol levels and sensitivity to glucocorticoids predict severity of coronary artery disease in subjects undergoing coronary angiography. Metabolism 2007;56(2):222–6.

[82] Guder G, Bauersachs J, Frantz S, et al. Complementary and incremental mortality risk prediction by cortisol and aldosterone in chronic heart failure. Circulation 2007;115(13):1754–61.

[83] Lin RC, Wang XL, Morris BJ. Association of coronary artery disease with glucocorticoid receptor N363S variant. Hypertension 2003;41(3):404–7.

[84] Chrousos GP, Gold PW. The concepts of stress and stress system disorders. Overview of physical and behavioral homeostasis. JAMA 1992;267(9):1244–52.

[85] Hertz-Picciotto I, Park HY, Dostal M, et al. Prenatal exposures to persistent and non-persistent organic compounds and effects on immune system development. Basic Clin Pharmacol Toxicol 2008;102(2):146–54.

[86] Hurtado A, Johnson RJ. Hygiene hypothesis and prevalence of glomerulonephritis. Kidney Int Suppl 2005;(97):S62–7.

[87] Chen E, Fisher EB, Bacharier LB, et al. Socioeconomic status, stress, and immune markers in adolescents with asthma. Psychosom Med 2003;65(6):984–92.

[88] Chen E, Miller GE. Stress and inflammation in exacerbations of asthma. Brain Behav Immun 2007;21(8):993–9.

[89] Suglia SF, Duarte CS, Sandel MT, et al. Social and environmental stressors in the home and childhood asthma. J Epidemiol Community Health 2010;64(7):636–42.

[90] Suglia SF, Enlow MB, Kullowatz A, et al. Maternal intimate partner violence and increased asthma incidence in children: buffering effects of supportive caregiving. Arch Pediatr Adolesc Med 2009;163(3):244–50.

[91] Elenkov IJ, Chrousos GP. Stress hormones, Th1/Th2 patterns, pro/anti-inflammatory cytokines and susceptibility to disease. Trends Endocrinol Metab 1999;10(9):359–68.

[92] Gaffin JM, Phipatanakul W. The role of indoor allergens in the development of asthma. Curr Opin Allergy Clin Immunol 2009;9(2):128–35.

[93] Krieger JK, Takaro TK, Allen C, et al. The Seattle-King County healthy homes project: implementation of a comprehensive approach to improving indoor environmental quality for low-income children with asthma. Environ Health Perspect 2002;110(Suppl 2):311–22.

[94] Isles AR, Wilkinson LS. Epigenetics: what is it and why is it important to mental disease? Br Med Bull 2008;85:35–45.

[95] Jirtle RL. Randy L. Jirtle, PhD: epigenetics a window on gene dysregulation, disease. Interview by Bridget M. Kuehn. JAMA 2008;299(11):1249–50.

[96] Nafee TM, Farrell WE, Carroll WD, et al. Epigenetic control of fetal gene expression. BJOG 2008;115(2):158–68.

[97] Sinclair DA, Oberdoerffer P. The ageing epigenome: damaged beyond repair? Ageing Res Rev 2009;8(3):189–98.

[98] Szyf M. Early life, the epigenome and human health. Acta Paediatr 2009;98(7):1082–4.

[99] Szyf M. The early life environment and the epigenome. Biochim Biophys Acta 2009;1790(9):878–85.

[100] Das R, Hampton DD, Jirtle RL. Imprinting evolution and human health. Mamm Genome 2009;20(9–10):563–72.

[101] Weaver IC, Cervoni N, Champagne FA, et al. Epigenetic programming by maternal behavior. Nat Neurosci 2004;7(8):847–54.

[102] McGowan PO, Sasaki A, D'Alessio AC, et al. Epigenetic regulation of the glucocorticoid receptor in human brain associates with childhood abuse. Nat Neurosci 2009;12(3):342–8.

[103] Meaney MJ, Szyf M, Seckl JR. Epigenetic mechanisms of perinatal programming of hypothalamic-pituitary-adrenal function and health. Trends Mol Med 2007;13(7):269–77.

[104] Champagne FA, Curley JP. Epigenetic mechanisms mediating the long-term effects of maternal care on development. Neurosci Biobehav Rev 2009;33(4):593–600.

[105] Champagne FA, Weaver IC, Diorio J, et al. Maternal care associated with methylation of the estrogen receptor-alpha1b promoter and estrogen receptor-alpha expression in the medial preoptic area of female offspring. Endocrinology 2006;147(6):2909–15.

[106] Chen E, Schreier HM. Does the social environment contribute to asthma? Immunol Allergy Clin North Am 2008;28(3):649–64, x.

[107] Moriceau S, Sullivan RM. Maternal presence serves as a switch between learning fear and attraction in infancy. Nat Neurosci 2006;9(8):1004–6.

[108] Rice CJ, Sandman CA, Lenjavi MR, et al. A novel mouse model for acute and long-lasting consequences of early life stress. Endocrinology 2008;149(10):4892–900.

[109] Thompson JV, Sullivan RM, Wilson DA. Developmental emergence of fear learning corresponds with changes in amygdala synaptic plasticity. Brain Res 2008;1200:58–65.

[110] Bradley RG, Binder EB, Epstein MP, et al. Influence of child abuse on adult depression: moderation by the corticotropin-releasing hormone receptor gene. Arch Gen Psychiatry 2008;65(2):190–200.

[111] Gillespie CF, Bradley B, Mercer K, et al. Trauma exposure and stress-related disorders in inner city primary care patients. Gen Hosp Psychiatry 2009;31(6):505–14.

[112] Hovens JG, Wiersma JE, Giltay EJ, et al. Childhood life events and childhood trauma in adult patients with depressive, anxiety and comorbid disorders vs. controls. Acta Psychiatr Scand 2010;122(1):66–74.

[113] Jovanovic T, Blanding NQ, Norrholm SD, et al. Childhood abuse is associated with increased startle reactivity in adulthood. Depress Anxiety 2009;26(11):1018–26.

[114] Krupanidhi S, Sedimbi SK, Vaishnav G, et al. Diabetes–role of epigenetics, genetics, and physiological factors. Zhong Nan Da Xue Xue Bao Yi Xue Ban 2009;34(9):837–45.

[115] Quas JA, Carrick N, Alkon A, et al. Children's memory for a mild stressor: the role of sympathetic activation and parasympathetic withdrawal. Dev Psychobiol 2006;48(8):686–702.

[116] Swanson JM, Entringer S, Buss C, et al. Developmental origins of health and disease: environmental exposures. Semin Reprod Med 2009;27(5):391–402.

[117] Weidman JR, Dolinoy DC, Murphy SK, et al. Cancer susceptibility: epigenetic manifestation of environmental exposures. Cancer J 2007;13(1):9–16.

[118] Wilson AG. Epigenetic regulation of gene expression in the inflammatory response and relevance to common diseases. J Periodontol 2008;79(8 Suppl):1514–9.

[119] Curley JP, Davidson S, Bateson P, et al. Social enrichment during postnatal development induces transgenerational effects on emotional and reproductive behavior in mice. Front Behav Neurosci 2009;3:25.

[120] Szyf M. Epigenetics, DNA methylation, and chromatin modifying drugs. Annu Rev Pharmacol Toxicol 2009;49:243–63.

[121] National Scientific Council on the Developing Child. The timing and quality of early experiences combine to shape brain architecture. Working paper #5. Cambridge (MA): Center

on the Developing Child at Harvard University; 2007. Available at. http://developing-child.harvard.edu/.

[122] Coe CL, Lubach GR, Schneider ML, et al. Early rearing conditions alter immune responses in the developing infant primate. Pediatrics 1992;90(3 Pt 2):505–9.

[123] Shirtcliff EA, Coe CL, Pollak SD. Early childhood stress is associated with elevated antibody levels to herpes simplex virus type 1. Proc Natl Acad Sci U S A 2009;106(8): 2963–7.

[124] Committee on Psychosocial Aspects of Child and Family Health, Committee on Early Childhood, Adoption, and Dependent Care, and Section on Developmental and Behavioral Pediatrics, Garner AS, et al. Early childhood adversity, toxic stress, and the role of the pediatrician: translating developmental science into lifelong health. Pediatrics 2012;129(1):e224–31.

[125] Anda RF, Brown DW, Felitti VJ, et al. Adverse childhood experiences and prescribed psychotropic medications in adults. Am J Prev Med 2007;32(5):389–94.

[126] Anda RF, Brown DW, Dube SR, et al. Adverse childhood experiences and chronic obstructive pulmonary disease in adults. Am J Prev Med 2008;34(5):396–403.

[127] Dube SR, Felitti VJ, Dong M, et al. The impact of adverse childhood experiences on health problems: evidence from four birth cohorts dating back to 1900. Prev Med 2003;37(3): 268–77.

[128] Duke NN, Pettingell SL, McMorris BJ, et al. Adolescent violence perpetration: associations with multiple types of adverse childhood experiences. Pediatrics 2010;125(4):e778–86.

[129] Hillis SD, Anda RF, Dube SR, et al. The association between adverse childhood experiences and adolescent pregnancy, long-term psychosocial consequences, and fetal death. Pediatrics 2004;113(2):320–7.

[130] Hillis SD, Anda RF, Felitti VJ, et al. Adverse childhood experiences and sexually transmitted diseases in men and women: a retrospective study. Pediatrics 2000;106(1):E11.

[131] Kalmakis KA, Chandler GE. Health consequences of adverse childhood experiences: a systematic review. J Am Assoc Nurse Pract 2015;27(8):457–65.

Advances in Pediatrics 63 (2016) 429–451

ADVANCES IN PEDIATRICS

ELSEVIER
MOSBY

Update on Adolescent Contraception

Molly J. Richards, MD[a],*, Eliza Buyers, MD[b]

[a]Section of Adolescent Medicine, Children's Hospital Colorado, University of Colorado School of Medicine, 13123 East 16th Avenue, B025, Aurora, CO 80045, USA; [b]Section of Pediatric and Adolescent Gynecology, University of Colorado School of Medicine, 13123 E 16th Avenue B467, Aurora, CO 80045, USA

Keywords
- Contraception • Adolescents • Sexual history taking
- Long-acting reversible contraception

Key points
- Pediatric providers play a key role in the well-being of adolescents, including their sexual health.
- Pediatric providers can offer or refer for all contraceptive options, educate teens on available methods, and support adolescents to continue contraception.
- The implant and intrauterine devices, referred to as long-acting reversible contraception (LARC), have the highest efficacy and continuation of any methods.
- LARC are recommended as safe, effective, first-line options for adolescents requesting contraception.

ADOLESCENT CONTRACEPTION

Pediatric providers play a key role in adolescent sexual health. Leading medical organizations, such as the American Academy of Pediatrics, recommend that pediatric providers take a sexual history and address contraception with all their adolescent patients to help reduce the negative health consequences related to unintended teen pregnancy. This article outlines important aspects of adolescent health visits, specifically sexual history taking, reviews adolescent development as it relates to sexuality, and discusses contraceptive counseling appropriate to an adolescent's developmental stage. The article also summarizes key information needed to educate teens on available methods, provides

*Corresponding author. E-mail address: molly.richards@childrenscolorado.org

0065-3101/16/$ – see front matter
http://dx.doi.org/10.1016/j.yapd.2016.04.008

up-to-date contraceptive options, and support adolescents to continue contraception in the context of achieving their goals. The topics of menstrual suppression with hormonal methods, contraception with complex medical conditions, and birth control for adolescents with physical and development disabilities are also reviewed.

TEEN PREGNANCY AND CONTRACEPTIVE USE

Primarily owing to increased use of contraception, the teen birth rate in the United States was at a record low in 2013, decreasing by 10% from 2012 and an overwhelming 43% since 1991. However, the US teen pregnancy rate continues to be among the highest in the developed world and a considerable public health problem [1]. Each year, almost 615,000 US women aged 15 to 19 years become pregnant and 82% of these pregnancies are unintended [2]. Teen pregnancy and childbearing affects poorer youth of all races disproportionately. It also carries significant short and long-term impacts for teen mothers and their children [3].

Sexual intercourse is common among adolescents. In 2013, nearly one-half (48%) of those aged 17, 61% of 18-year-olds, and 71% of 19-year-olds reported ever having had sex [4]. Yet, many teens are not using adequate and/or consistent protection against pregnancy and sexually transmitted infections (STIs). One in 4 female teens report using no contraceptive method at last intercourse [5] and only 20% report having used both a condom and a hormonal method [6], although dual method protection is considered the most effective way to prevent pregnancy and STIs.

For decades, pediatric providers and their adolescent patients have been limited in their choice of contraceptive options to barrier and short-acting hormonal methods. Condoms and the pill are still the most common contraceptive methods used by adolescents, despite their dependence on user adherence and high rates of incorrect and inconsistent use. In 2013, almost 60% of currently sexually active high school students reported using a condom during their last sexual intercourse, 19% of females reported the use of the pill, and 4.7% reported the use of depot medroxyprogesterone acetate (DMPA), the patch, or the birth control ring [7]. These short-acting contraceptive methods have low continuation rates and high pregnancy rates in adolescents [8].

Although recommended as first line for contraception, only 4.5% of female teen contraceptive users in 2009 relied on long-acting reversible contraceptives (LARC), including intrauterine devices (IUDs) and implants. This is, however, an increase from only 1.5% in 2007 and just 0.3% in 2002 [9]. The American Academy of Pediatrics and the American College of Obstetricians and Gynecologists recommend the contraceptive implant and IUD as first line for adolescents requesting contraception [10,11] owing to the overwhelming potential for LARC to reduce unintended pregnancy in this population. The IUDs and the etonogestrel implant are safe, acceptable, and highly efficacious methods with continuation rates in teens and young adults of 81% and 82%% at 1 year, respectively [12]. This is in comparison with short-acting methods, such as the pill and the vaginal ring, which have continuation rates of 30% to 40% at 1 year in a similar population [12]. The landmark CHOICE Project, a large contraceptive research study that enrolled more than 9000 women requesting birth control, with 61% between the ages of 14 and 25 years of age, demonstrated that if barriers to use, such as cost and access, are removed, LARC methods are highly preferred in all women, including teens. Furthermore, teens who chose LARC had lower rates of pregnancy, birth, and abortion than those of sexually active teens [13].

ADOLESCENT HEALTH VISITS
Adolescent health care providers are a valuable and trusted resource to teens for accurate information about sexual health and contraception [14]. Medical organizations, including the American Academy of Pediatrics, recommend that adolescent visits include a confidential, one-on-one interview to discuss sexuality and sexual health topics, which include sexual orientation, sexual behaviors, STI prevention, and contraception [15,16].

Talking about sex with an adolescent can be daunting to many providers. However, adolescents are usually candid about their sexual history when asked in a confidential, nonjudgmental manner. There are several key factors in establishing a safe and trusting environment most conducive to adolescent visits.

Adolescent-friendly environment
Pediatric clinics that serve adolescents should make them feel welcome. Waiting and examination rooms can have appropriate reading materials and resources for teens. Clinic providers and staff should be well-versed in policies regarding adolescent visits so that scheduling, communication, which may need to be confidential, and rooming are appropriate. Handouts, including those on sexual health, should be geared to teens and young adults (Fig. 1).

One-on-one relationship between provider and adolescent
From infancy, a child's relationship with their health provider has been mediated by their parent or guardian. However, the transition to adulthood requires that adolescents learn how to manage their own health care needs. The one-on-one interview should be introduced in early adolescence (about age 11–12) as a routine part of all visits.

Providers should focus on establishing rapport and providing anticipatory guidance based on the teen's developmental stage. It is also important for parents to know they are not being excluded from their child's care, but are helping their teen to develop the skills needed to care for themselves as they become older and more independent.

Confidentiality and its limits need to be discussed
Adolescents are more likely to seek health care, provide truthful answers, and ask relevant questions if assured of confidentiality. The Society for Adolescent Medicine's position paper on the subject outlines the essential nature of confidential care for teens [17]. There is a clinical imperative based on adolescents

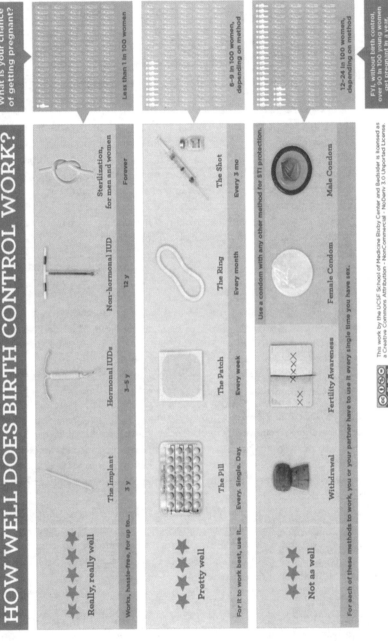

Fig. 1. Teen-appropriate patient handout for contraceptive counseling. IUD, intrauterine device. (*Courtesy of* Bedsider.org; with permission.)

developing autonomy and independence, the need for health screening based on confidential information (STIs, pregnancy), research findings that support better care, as well as the ethical and legal principles that guide providers [17]. Minors' right to confidential care, including contraceptive services, varies by state, with 26 states allowing all minors to consent to contraceptive services. Individual state policies can be accessed at www.guttmacher.org [18].

Despite the need for minors to be able to consent to their own contraceptive care, it is important to consider parental involvement. Parents are highly influential in adolescent sexual and contraceptive decision making. Parental involvement has been shown to improve contraceptive compliance [19] and should be encouraged and facilitated when possible.

ADOLESCENT DEVELOPMENT AND THE SEXUAL HISTORY

Adolescence is a time of rapid change. Although providers commonly focus on the physical changes of adolescence, equally significant are the developmental changes, including emerging and evolving sexuality. Adolescents become very aware of themselves as a gender-specific and sexual human being, even early in adolescence. Adolescent development can be described in 3 stages: early, middle, and late adolescence. Taking a sexual history from an adolescent should be developmentally appropriate, nonassuming, and comprehensive. Sexual histories should be taken in the context of adolescents' age and developmental stage (Table 1).

Early adolescence (age 11–14) is marked by the onset of puberty with accompanying physical and emotional changes. These changes can be embarrassing and confusing for teens. Experimentation, such as masturbation, is common. Although sexual feelings and curiosity may begin in early adolescence, sexual intercourse before age 14 is uncommon and should alert the provider to a potentially risky situation. Cognitive abilities during early adolescence tend to be concrete, so providers should take care to ensure understanding of questions and counseling and clarify if needed. Normalization of a maturing adolescent's physical changes, acknowledgment and acceptance of emerging sexuality, and clear encouragement for sexual abstinence is appropriate. Parents and guardians should be encouraged to communicate with their teens about sexual health topics, such as the adult's values regarding relationships and expectations for healthy, responsible behavior. Discussions at this stage should focus on the formation of healthy and safe relationships with friends, as well as romantic partners.

Middle adolescence (ages 14–17) is characterized by the exploration of identity and independence. Rates of sexual behaviors increase during middle adolescence. Only 16% of teen have had sex by age 15, but this increases to nearly one-half (48%) of those aged 17 years [4]. Despite this, the cognitive ability to think abstractly about future consequences and delay gratification are still being established [20]. Adolescents often revert back to more concrete thinking in stressful or emotionally charged situations. This can make consistent condom and contraceptive use challenging. Access to confidential care may

Table 1
Adolescent stages and sexual health counseling

Cognitive development	Social-emotional development	Counseling	Examples
Early adolescence (ages 11–14)			
• Growing capacity for abstract thought. • Mostly interested in the present.	• Extremely self-conscious. • Tendency to return to "childish" behavior. • Greater interest in privacy.	• Ideal time for anticipatory guidance. • Sexual orientation/preference may be formed. • Provider needs to introduce sexual health topics and explore teen's definition of "sex." Younger teens not likely to bring up on their own. • Encourage patient to apply the same qualities of healthy friendships (mutual respect, communication) to romantic partners.	"It's important for me to discuss sexual health topics with all of my patients, maybe even before they have questions. What does the term "sex" mean to you?" "Tell me about your best friend or what you look for in a friend...It sounds like you would not want to hang out with someone who treated you badly or made you feel badly about yourself."
Middle adolescence (ages 15–17)			
• Greater capacity for setting goals. • Continued growth of abstract thought.	• Intense self-involvement. • Increased drive for independence. • Greater reliance on friends.	• Discussion of peer group may help teen talk more freely and reveal misconceptions about sex and contraception. • Ask what is most important to them about birth control (eg, that it works really well, or does not make them gain weight). • Support *them* to make the decision based on your counseling.	"What are your friends using for birth control? What do they say about it?" "Have your friends or family talked about any birth control methods? What are their thoughts about them?" "It sounds like the most important thing for you is to avoid pregnancy and you said pills are hard to take. What do you think would be the best method for you?

(continued on next page)

Table 1 continued			
Cognitive development	Social-emotional development	Counseling	Examples
Late adolescence (age 18–21)			
• Greater ability to delay gratification and plan for future. • Can reason through problems.	• Increased sense of identity and emotional stability. • Desire for intimacy and serious relationships.	• Ask about future plans. Discuss how having a child now might affect these plans. • Ask what partner thinks about child bearing and birth control. • Discuss that with a long-term, serious sexual relationship comes a higher chance of pregnancy and, if pregnancy not desired, a greater need for effective birth control.	"Do you want to have children in the future and, if so, when?" "It sounds like you do not want to have a child now. What birth control method would work best for you?

also be a barrier and many teens do not seek health care until well after their first sexual intercourse, leaving them at high risk for STIs and unintended pregnancy. All providers should confidentially offer resources, such as medically accurate, teen-friendly websites on sexual health (Table 2), discuss skills such as negotiation for correct and consistent condom use, and explain the options for highly effective contraception.

Table 2 Teen-friendly, medically accurate websites on sexual health	
www.bedsider.org	
Who	What
The National Campaign to Prevent Teen Pregnancy's online birth control support network. No funding from pharmaceutical companies.	• Information and comparison of all contraceptive methods. • Health clinic finder (enter zip code). • Can set up daily, weekly, monthly text message reminders (for short-acting methods).
www.itsyoursexlife.org or www.GYTNOW.org	
Who	What
MTV's public health campaign to support young people to make responsible decisions about their sexual health. Also supported by the Kaiser Family Foundation.	• STI information and prevention. • Talking to partner about sexually transmitted infections. • Links to other trusted sexual health resources including live chat feature.

Late adolescents (age 18–21) have often reached full physical maturity and the majority (71%) have had sexual intercourse by age 19 [4]. Teens of this age are more likely to be involved in serious relationships and condom use often declines as a relationship progresses [21], leaving them at high risk for unintended pregnancy. Despite this, older teens have more capacity to think abstractly and plan for the future. Providers can have more in-depth conversations about healthy and safe relationships, STI prevention and screening, intentions for child bearing, and the importance of contraception in meeting their goals.

Regardless of age, open-ended, inclusive, and clarifying questions are essential to obtain correct information and normalize varying sexual preferences and behaviors. After assessing what the teen understands the term to mean, using the phrase "having sex" is more likely to be understood than "having intercourse" or "being sexually active." Providers also should be cognizant of judgmental questions. Instead of "You don't have unprotected sex, do you?", a provider might ask, "How do you protect yourself from pregnancy and STIs when having sex?" Finally, avoiding leading questions can help to assess where there is an opportunity for intervention. Instead of asking "You are using condoms all the time?", ask "How often do you use condoms?" or "When was the last time you had sex without a condom?"

CONTRACEPTIVE COUNSELING

Contraception should be discussed with all teens. Depending on their age and developmental stage, adolescents are often very curious and willing to discuss contraceptive options, even if they do not intend to imminently engage in sexual activity or initiate contraception. Pediatric health care providers and parents can be reassured that medically accurate information about STI prevention and contraception does not increase rates of sexual activity [22].

Contraceptive counseling does not only include education about available options. Sexually active adolescents may decline contraception because they have concerns about birth control or because they feel they do not need it. Providers need to explore these concerns, address adolescent's ambivalence, and work with the teen to identify the positive influence contraception could have on their life and their future.

Understand patient misconceptions

Many adolescents hold misconceptions that can influence their decision to initiate contraception. Asking adolescents about positive and negative contraceptive experiences among their friends and family members, as well as their own experiences, beliefs, and opinions, can reveal important information for education and counseling. Providers can offer accurate information about contraceptive safety and efficacy, as well as reassurance regarding common concerns such as contraceptives effect on the menstrual cycle (eg, patients may have concern about long-term medical effects of amenorrhea), weight, mood, and future fertility.

Discuss the potential impact of contraception on current and future goals

Asking an adolescent of any age about their plans to start a family and have children of their own can be an effective strategy to start a discussion about contraception. This creates an alliance with the adolescent in supporting their efforts to have children when they are ready. It also provides an opportunity to discuss adolescent's goals before starting a family and how contraception may be useful to them. Because most adolescents will report that they want to delay childbearing for at least 1 year or longer, this question can pave the way for a discussion of the benefits of LARC.

The medical benefits of certain contraceptive methods may be enticing to teens as well. Understanding the noncontraceptive benefits of birth control methods in treating menstrual problems like dysmenorrhea or menorrhagia may encourage teens to initiate or continue birth control, regardless of current sexual activity.

Empower adolescents to choose

Adolescent development is a progression of increased identity formation, autonomy, and independence. It is important for providers to offer accurate and comprehensive information, but then to support the adolescent to decide which method is best for them. Adolescents may be wary of initiating LARCs because they cannot stop the method on their own, which may feel like a threat to their autonomy. They should be assured that they can have the device removed at any time. Studies have shown that when given accurate information about the most effective methods, and removing barriers of cost, access, and confidentiality, the majority of adolescents will choose and continue LARC [23].

Start a contraceptive method on the day of visit

Given the potential consequences of an unintended pregnancy, there should be no delay in initiation once an adolescent decides to use contraception. All methods can be provided immediately, including LARC. If a provider does not offer a certain method, such as the implant or the IUD, the teen can start a bridge method (such as a combined hormonal contraception [CHC] or DMPA) until the visit for their desired method. Counseling on the use of condoms, provision of emergency contraception if indicated, and STI testing should also be performed without delay. Barriers such as cost and confidentiality can be addressed by referrals to federally funded Title X clinics that provide low-cost, confidential family planning services, as well as other community clinics that may serve adolescents and young adults, such as school clinics, health departments, universities, and reproductive health clinics.

CONTRACEPTIVE METHOD SUMMARIES

There are many contraceptive options available to adolescents who want to avoid an unintended pregnancy. LARC, the implant and the IUDs, are the most effective methods and should be discussed first when educating teens on all options. Pediatric providers play an important role in helping teens choose a method, managing common side effects and supporting teens to change methods when requested. Here we summarize the most common available methods. Advantages and disadvantages of these methods can be found in Table 3.

The Contraceptive implant
Key points
- Progestin-only rod. Easy and quick to insert into the arm (Table 4).
- Greatest efficacy of any reversible contraceptive method.
- Primary mechanism of action is prevention of ovulation.

Table 3
Contraceptive methods: advantages and disadvantages

Advantages	Disadvantages
Subdermal implant (contains no estrogen; see Table 4)	
Greatest efficacy.	Uterine bleeding, although not dangerous,
High satisfaction and continuation.	may be frequent and prolonged.
Simple and quick insertion.	Small percent of users (6%–12%) report
Discreet. Immediate reversibility.	weight gain, but unclear if owing to implant
Relief of dysmenorrhea and endometriosis symptoms.	use.
No effect on bone density.	
IUDs (contain no estrogen; see Table 5)	
Very high efficacy.	Pelvic examination required for insertion.
Highest satisfaction and continuation of any method.	
Discreet. Immediate reversibility.	
Levonorgestrel IUDs: Treatment for bleeding, dysmenorrhea, anemia owing to menorrhagia, and relief of endometriosis symptoms.	
Safe for almost all teens, including those with complex medical conditions. No medication interactions.	
DMPA (contains no estrogen)	
High efficacy.	Irregular bleeding common in first 3–9 mo.
Simple and quick injection.	Possible increased appetite and associated
Discreet.	weight gain.
Relief of dysmenorrhea and endometriosis symptoms.	Visit every 11–13 wk.
No medication interactions.	
Combined hormonal contraception: OCPs, patch, ring (contain estrogen + progestin)	
Good efficacy when used correctly and consistently.	Remember each day (pills), week (patch), month (ring).
Widespread familiarity.	Visits to pharmacy for refills.
Many noncontraceptive benefits.	Requires storage of medication.
Easy for user to start (and stop)	Increased contraindications and medication interactions.

Abbreviations: DMPA, depot medroxyprogesterone acetate; IUD, intrauterine device; OCP, oral contraceptive pill.

Table 4
Subdermal implant

Description	4 cm × 2 mm rod inserted into subdermis of upper, inner arm
Contents	Inactive rod: flexible copolymer (no latex)
	Active hormone: the progestin etonogestrel
Duration of use	3 y, but can be removed anytime
Mechanism of action	Prevents ovulation
Provider training requirement	Manufacturer provides Food and Drug Administration–required free, 3-h long course.
	Providers should contact Merck to request training.

- Can cause unpredictable, but not dangerous, uterine bleeding. Counseling in advance about unpredictable bleeding, and reassurance during use increases method satisfaction and continuation. Fifty percent of users will have a decrease in their bleeding, including infrequent, minimal, or no bleeding (amenorrhea).

Mechanism of action
The implant's primary mechanism of action is suppression of ovulation. There may be additional efficacy owing to the thickening of cervical mucus and alterations of the endometrial lining. The implant is the most effective method of any contraceptive method. Only 0.05% out of every 100 women experienced a pregnancy during the first year of typical use [24].

Advantages and method counseling
The implant is the method of choice for many teens, particularly those ages 14 to 17 years [23]. Insertion is quick and easy and can be done in any outpatient or inpatient setting. A teen can easily palpate her implant and be confident about its presence. The implant can be inserted at any time during the menstrual cycle and same-day insertion is recommended (Fig. 2). Adolescents should be reassured that they do not have to "commit" to 3 years of use, because this may feel daunting to them. The implant can be removed at any time when they request.

Managing common, expected side effects
The contraceptive implant causes changes in bleeding patterns that will be unpredictable for the entire duration of use. Episodes of frequent bleeding are more common in the first 3 months, but may continue. When considering a 90-day interval, the bleeding patterns include infrequent bleeding (34%), amenorrhea (22%), prolonged bleeding (18%), and frequent bleeding (8%) [25]. Counseling and education about changes in bleeding patterns before receiving the implant may increase satisfaction and continuation of the method. Because the bleeding pattern in each individual is different, there is no reason to dissuade patients from using this method owing to the possibility of frequent bleeding. In the Contraceptive CHOICE study, 12-month continuation rates for adolescent (14–19 years old) implant users was an impressive 82% [12] despite varying bleeding patterns.

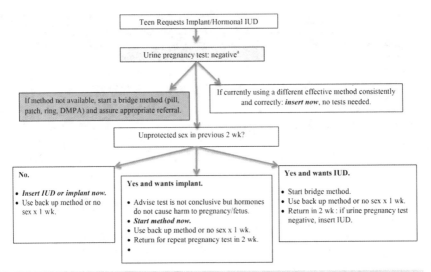

Fig. 2. Same-day start protocol for intrauterine device (IUD)/implant. ° If pregnancy test is positive, provide options counseling. DMPA, depot medroxyprogesterone acetate. (*From* the Committee on Adolescence. Counseling the adolescent about pregnancy options. Pediatrics 1998;101(5):938–40; with permission.)

When irregular or prolonged bleeding occurs with ongoing use, reassurance from the entire health care team is crucial, and is usually all that is necessary. Risk for STIs should be assessed, because infections can cause breakthrough bleeding on any contraceptive method. Some patients and providers feel more comfortable after an assessment of hemoglobin, although it is well-documented that hemoglobin levels will increase with implant use despite irregular bleeding patterns [26]. It is also possible to offer medical treatments to control bothersome bleeding. Although studies are scarce, it is reasonable to consider a trial of (1) nonsteroidal antiinflammatory drugs for 5 to 7 days or (2) combined oral contraceptive pills (OCPs) for 10 to 20 days [27,28]. The Centers for Disease Control and Prevention has created an easy to follow algorithm to manage bleeding irregularities while using contraception (Fig. 3). There does not seem to be any danger in long-term use of oral contraceptives in addition to the implant, either continuously or intermittently, to control bothersome bleeding. It is helpful to advise all patients, especially adolescents, to return and discuss any problems with their provider.

Intrauterine devices

Description and mechanism of action

There are 4 different IUDs now available in the United States, all of which are safe and effective for nulliparous and multiparous women, including adolescents (Table 5). All IUDs produce a sterile foreign body reaction within the uterine cavity that creates a hostile environment for sperm. The contraceptive effects of IUD use occur before fertilization, and therefore IUDs are not

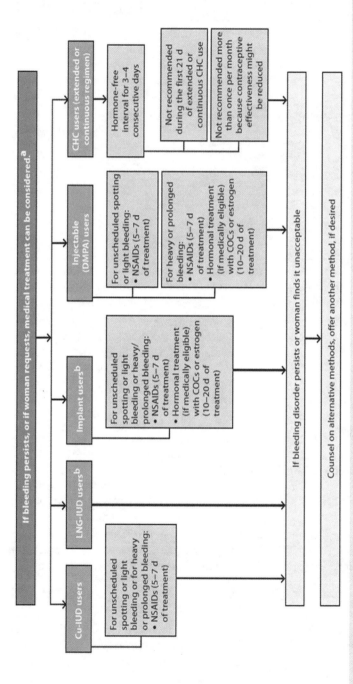

Fig. 3. Management of bleeding irregularities while using contraception. [a] If clinically warranted, evaluate for underlying condition. Treat the condition or refer for care. [b] Heavy or prolonged bleeding, either unscheduled or menstrual, is common. CHC, combined hormonal contraceptive; COC, combined oral contraceptive; Cu-IUD, copper-containing intrauterine device; DMPA, depot medroxyprogesterone acetate; LNG-IUD, levonorgestrel-releasing intrauterine device; NSAIDs, nonsteroidal antiinflammatory drugs. (*From the* US selected practice recommendations for contraceptive use. Bethesda (MD): Centers for Disease Control; 2013. Available at: www.cdc.gov/mmwr/pdf/rr/rr6205.pdf.)

Table 5
Types of intrauterine devices (IUDs) currently available in the United States

IUD name	Mirena	Liletta (generic)	Skyla	Paragard copper T
Hormone	Levonorgestrel 52 mg		Levonorgestrel 13.5 mg	No hormone
FDA-approved duration (y)	5	3ª (5 y approval expected)	3	10
Effect on menstrual bleeding	Decreased bleeding with continued use; 20% with amenorrhea at 1 y. Evidence-based treatment for menorrhagia and dysmenorrhea.		Lighter periods but amenorrhea less likely.	May have heavier and more painful periods, especially in first 6 mo.

Abbreviation: FDA, Food and Drug Administration.
ªLiletta is identical to the Mirena; ongoing trial to achieve similar, 5-year approval.

abortifacients [29]. The copper IUD causes an increase in copper ions, enzymes, white blood cells, and prostaglandins in uterine and tubal fluids, which impair sperm function and prevent fertilization. Levonorgestrel IUDs have a local effect on the endometrium, causing release of foreign body mediators and suppression of the endometrium. Progestin hormone also thickens cervical mucus and inhibits sperm capacitation and survival. Systemic absorption of levonorgestrel is low and most cycles are ovulatory [30]. IUDs are very effective, with failure rates of less than 1%. The levonorgestrel IUDs have slightly lower failure rates than the copper IUD [21] in adolescents and young adults [31].

Method counseling
IUDs are highly acceptable methods of contraception in many adolescents. Time should be taken to educate teens and young adults about their anatomy and the positioning of an IUD in their body. They may have concerns about the IUD "falling out," "being felt during sex," or "moving around the body" and these should be addressed with every patient. Using models and pictures can be helpful in allaying their fears about IUD complications.

An IUD can be inserted at any time in a woman's menstrual cycle as long as the provider is reasonably sure she is not pregnant [27] (see Fig. 2). IUDs can be inserted without a prior pelvic examination and in adolescents who have never been sexually active.

The pain experienced with IUD insertion is rated as tolerable by most women, including teens [32]. Screening for chlamydia and gonorrhea is indicated at least annually for all sexually active teens and can be done at the same visit as insertion even in high-risk adolescents [27]. An IUD does not have to be removed if an STI is detected or even in the case of pelvic inflammatory disease. Treatment can occur with the IUD in place as long as resolution of symptoms is documented [27].

Managing common, expected side effects
In the first days and weeks after IUD insertion, there may be bleeding and cramping related to the procedure itself. The risk of complications such as uterine perforation, expulsion, and infection are very low [33–35]. Heavy bleeding, severe pain, nausea, vomiting, or fevers should be evaluated with a complete history and examination including a speculum examination to look for IUD strings and a bimanual examination to assess for infection. There is an increased risk of pelvic inflammatory disease in the first 20 days after IUD insertion. After this point, the risk for pelvic inflammatory disease is the same as an adolescent without an IUD [34].

Users of the levonorgestrel IUD should expect unscheduled bleeding or spotting in the first 3 to 6 months of use. This bleeding is not harmful and will decrease with continued use. Over time, many women experience only light menstrual bleeding or amenorrhea. Patients may need reassurance that this is a safe, expected benefit of levonorgestrel IUD use and that no treatment is needed. STI testing, pregnancy testing, and/or pelvic examination can be done if warranted by history.

Missing strings
There is no evidence-based recommendation to have patients "check their strings" during IUD use. This may be uncomfortable and anxiety provoking, especially for adolescents. However, providers should be able to palpate and visualize IUD strings on pelvic examination. If strings are not visible, a pregnancy test should be done followed by a pelvic ultrasound that confirms the intrauterine location of the IUD. Patients should be encouraged to use another contraceptive method until the IUD location is confirmed. If the IUD is confirmed to be inside the uterus, no other treatment is needed.

Depot medroxyprogesterone acetate
Key points
- Progestin-only injectable contraception given as a single dose every 11 to 13 weeks.
- Very effective method of contraception.
- Continuation at 1 year in adolescents is low.
- Primary mechanism of action is prevention of ovulation.
- Can cause irregular bleeding especially in first 3 to 9 months. Approximately 80% of women will become amenorrheic after 6 to 9 months of continuous use.

Description and mechanism of action
DMPA is available in the United States in 2 formulations that only differ in their routes of administration: DMPA 150 mg/mL (intramuscular) and DMPA 104 mg/.65 mL (subcutaneously) The primary mechanism of action for DMPA is suppression of ovulation. Progestin methods also cause thickening of the cervical mucus to prevent sperm penetration.

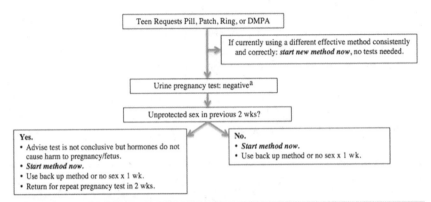

Fig. 4. Same-day start protocol for pill, patch, ring, and depot medroxyprogesterone acetate (DMPA). [a] If pregnancy test is positive, provide options counseling. (*From* the Committee on Adolescence. Counseling the adolescent about pregnancy options. Pediatrics 1998;101(5):938–40; with permission.)

Advantages and method counseling

DMPA injection can be done easily in an outpatient, inpatient, or emergency room setting. DMPA can be initiated anytime during the menstrual cycle after a negative urine pregnancy test is obtained. This same-day, quick start protocol for initiation is an important aspect of reducing barriers to contraceptive use (Fig. 4).

DMPA is a progestin-only method and can be used in patients with medical contraindications to estrogen. It can be safely used immediately postpartum and in lactating women. Noncontraceptive advantages include improvement in dysmenorrhea, menorrhagia, protection against endometrial cancer [36], and induction of menstrual suppression. DMPA may reduce seizure activity in certain women with epilepsy [37] and reduce pain crises in women with sickle cell disease [38].

Managing common, expected side effects

The most common side effects are menstrual irregularities and weight gain. The irregular bleeding associated with DMPA use often occurs in the first 3 to 6 months and can be unpredictable and prolonged in duration. Provider reassurance that irregular bleeding is to be expected and is likely to improve may be helpful.

Weight gain on DMPA is unpredictable and may vary widely among different women [39]. Research on weight gain with DMPA is mixed [40], although the Food and Drug Administration package insert reports an average of 5 pounds in the first year. "Early gainers" (gain of 5% of body weight in first 6 months) may be at greater risk for continued weight gain than other users [41]. Anticipatory guidance about nutrition and exercise as well as close monitoring for rapid weight gain is important in adolescents, especially those at high risk for obesity or related morbidities.

The possible effect of DMPA on bone density has caused much concern and unnecessarily restricted its use in many adolescents despite mounting evidence that these effects are reversible and clinical significance is lacking [42]. The American College of Obstetricians and Gynecologists, along with other leading medical groups, state that the effect of DMPA on bone mineral density should not prevent practitioners from prescribing DMPA or continuing its use beyond 2 years, particularly when DMPA is the adolescent's preferred method [42].

Although DMPA injection is only needed 4 times a year, adolescents often experience problems with continuation. In a recent study looking at use of short-acting birth control methods, only 20% of DMPA users continued this method at 1 year [8]. Adolescents who are having difficulty returning for injections should be strongly encouraged to consider long-acting methods that do not require return visits once inserted.

Combined hormonal contraception
Key points
- CHC (oral pill, transdermal patch, vaginal ring) contains estrogen and progestin.
- Typical use failure rates are often high, especially in adolescents.
- Continuation at 1 year in adolescents is low.
- Primary mechanism of action is prevention of ovulation.
- Safe for most teens. Refer to US Medical Eligibility Criteria for Contraceptive Use for contraindications.

Description and mechanism of action
CHC refers to methods that contain both estrogen and progestin. This includes OCPs, the transdermal patch, and the vaginal ring. All CHC methods prevent pregnancy by suppression of ovulation. The progestin component of combined hormonal methods provides the majority of its contraceptive efficacy by preventing ovulation via negative feedback on the hypothalamic–pituitary system. The estrogen component is added to stabilize the endometrium and allow for better cycle control. Medical eligibility and risks are also similar among all combined hormonal methods and should be discussed with patients. The incidence of venous thromboembolism and stroke are slightly increased among users of CHC [43], but the benefits of use outweigh these risks for most adolescents [27].

Although there are more than 70 different combined OCPs available in the United States, the only major differences are in estrogen dose, progestin type, and packaging regimen of active and placebo pills. Efficacy and side effects among pills are comparable.

The transdermal contraceptive patch is marketed as Xulane, a generic version of the OrthoEvra patch, which is no longer available. It is a thin, beige adhesive patch that contains ethinyl estradiol and the progestin norelgestromin. It can be applied to the torso, buttocks, or upper arms and needs to be changed each week.

The vaginal contraceptive ring (NuvaRing) is a soft, flexible 54-mm diameter ring that releases ethinyl estradiol and the progestin etonogestrel. The ring is inserted by the user into the vagina and needs to be removed and replaced monthly. It is important to assess the adolescent's comfort in insertion and removal before prescribing, and also ensure that the user is aware that the ring is not a barrier method, does not prevent STIs, and needs to be used as directed to be effective.

Extended or continuous cycling can be used with all CHC and may provide contraceptive as well as noncontraceptive benefits. Research suggests that extended cycling may provide greater suppression of the ovaries and the endometrium, leading to better control of gynecologic conditions and increased contraceptive efficacy. Reducing period frequency can also reduce the frequency of estrogen withdrawal symptoms and menstrual associated disorders [44], including premenstrual syndrome, dysmenorrhea, and menstrual migraines. Tables 6 and 7 outline several recommended practices for prescribing CHC.

Managing common, expected side effects
In the first 3 months of CHC use, unexpected bleeding is not uncommon. Providers should confirm correct usage and reassure that the bleeding should resolve with continued and consistent use. Setting a daily alarm on the user's mobile phone, or signing up for a free text message reminder can be helpful for some teens. Providers should consider pregnancy testing and test for STIs if appropriate. Adolescents that have difficulty with consistent use of these methods should be encouraged to consider other methods, specifically LARC.

Progestin in CHC causes thinning of the endometrial lining and can result in amenorrhea for some users. If the teen is using the method correctly and consistently, there is no danger to this side effect and reassurance can be given as long as pregnancy is ruled out. OCP users who would prefer to have a monthly period can try switching to a different brand of pill.

Users of extended or continuous CHC should expect unscheduled bleeding, especially in the first 4 months of use. This can be due to thinning and instability of the endometrial lining. Users can either (1) continue on the method as previously instructed and expect some continued bleeding, (2) take a 5-day break (and then restart) to allow for a withdrawal bleed, or (3) try a 5-day course of nonsteroidal antiinflammatory drugs. These options are outlined in the Fig. 3, an algorithm from the Centers for Disease Control and Prevention.

Table 6
Best practice for prescribing combined hormonal contraception

Dispense	Most insurance companies will dispense a 90-day supply.
Refills	Provide enough refills for at least 1 y.
Getting started	Teen should start pill, patch, ring as soon as she obtains it (see Fig. 4).
Tips for consistent use	Set an alarm on cell phone.
	Sign up for a text message reminder at www.bedsider.org.

Table 7
Options for dosing combined hormonal contraception

	Common dosing	Expected bleeding pattern
Traditional		
OCP	21 active pills (contain estrogen and progestin) + 7 placebo pills	Monthly period during placebo week, mimics "natural" cycle.
Patch	Apply a new patch × 3 wk then remove patch for 1 wk	Bleeding occurs owing to hormone withdrawal.
Ring	Insert ring into vagina × 3 wk then remove × 1 wk	—
Extended or continuous		
OCP	Active pill × 84 d in a row, then 5 d off. Can dose any OCP in an extended or continuous fashion, or use an OCP packaged for extended or continuous use.	Period every 3–4 months depending on timing of withdrawal. May have more unscheduled bleeding then traditional 21/7 dosing at first, but less unscheduled bleeding with continued use.
Patch	Apply a new patch every wk × 9 wk, then 1 wk off.	
Ring	Insert a ring into the vagina every 4 wk × 3 mo, then 1 wk off	

MENSTRUAL SUPPRESSION

Even in the absence of a significant gynecologic condition, many adolescents prefer to have fewer or no periods once they are aware that there are no safety concerns, and specifically no impact on their future fertility. This can be accomplished with many available contraceptive methods.

Adolescents who choose progestin-only methods should be counseled in advance that no bleeding (amenorrhea) or lighter, fewer periods is an expected and common benefit to use, with corresponding lower rates of anemia in users [45]. The levonorgestrel IUD and Depo Provera achieve high rates of amenorrhea with continued use and are ideal methods for patients who would enjoy fewer or no periods. Amenorrhea with the implant is less predictable and only occurs in about 20% of users.

CHC can also be used to induce amenorrhea secondary to the progestin dominant effect on the endometrium. Extended or continuous dosing can be offered based on the patient's preference for frequency of periods along with counseling about the potential for unscheduled bleeding. Table 7 reviews these options and patient instructions for use. About 50% of women will achieve amenorrhea with continuous use of OCPs at 1 year, and an additional 25% will report only light bleeding. Bleeding that occurs after prolonged use of CHC can be treated with a 5-day withdrawal of the medication.

COMPLEX MEDICAL CONDITIONS

A safe and effective contraceptive option exists for all adolescents, including those with complex medical conditions. Sexual activity among teens with

Table 8
Contraception and considerations in adolescents with disabilities

Comments on menstrual regulation with method	
Levonorgestrel IUD	First-line for contraception.
	Very few medical contraindications.
	Placement may require anesthesia.
	Excellent option for menstrual suppression; amenorrhea rates up to 50% at 1 y; decreased flow in almost all users. Initial bleeding/ spotting should be expected for first 3 mo of use.
Copper IUD	First-line for contraception.
	Very few medical contraindications.
	Placement may require anesthesia.
	No reduction in menstruation; may have increased bleeding/ cramping.
Implant	First-line for contraception.
	Very few medical contraindications.
	Placement is quick and easy but does require patient's cooperation.
	Amenorrhea occurs in some (20% at 1 y) but unpredictable bleeding is common and should be expected.
DMPA	Effective contraception.
	Few medical contraindications.
	Efficacy not affected by anticonvulsants
	Concerns about weight gain and bone mineral density may limit use, but are not absolute contraindications if DMPA best option available.
	Injection every 3 mo; patient cooperation necessary.
	Amenorrhea in 50%–80% after 1 y of use, but initial bleeding very common.
OCPs	Effective contraception if taken correctly and consistently
	Refer to the USMEC for contraindications to use. Increased VTE risk in adolescents with limited mobility is a consideration but risks unknown.
	Avoid with certain anticonvulsants owing to decreased contraceptive efficacy.
	Pill must be taken each day. Can be crushed for G-tube.
	Amenorrhea in 50% at 1 y using continuous dosing. Break-through bleeding occurs most often if first 3 mo of use. When bleeding occurs with prolonged use, can often manages with a 5 d break to allow for a withdrawal bleed and then restart.
Patch	Effective contraception if used correctly and consistently.
	Refer to the USMEC for contraindications to use. Increased VTE risk in adolescents with limited mobility is a consideration but risks unknown. Total estrogen exposure is higher with patch than OCP.
	Avoid with certain anticonvulsants owing to decreased contraceptive efficacy.
	New patch applied each week; patient cooperation required so patch is not removed.
	Amenorrhea rates with continuous use comparable with OCPs.

Abbreviations: DMPA, depot medroxyprogesterone acetate; IUD, intrauterine device; OCP, oral contraceptive pill; USMEC, US Medical Eligibility Criteria for Contraceptive Use; VTE, venous thromboembolism.

medical conditions may occur at the same rate as their healthy peers. Furthermore, reproductive health outcomes such as unplanned pregnancy and untreated sexually transmitted disease might have an even greater impact on long-term health.

The US Medical Eligibility Criteria for Contraceptive Use was developed by the Centers for Disease Control and Prevention and the World Health Organization. It provides evidence-based guidance for safe contraceptive use in women, including adolescents, with medical conditions. The US Medical Eligibility Criteria for Contraceptive Use is available on-line at www.cdc.gov and can be downloaded as a free application for mobile devices. This tool is easy to use, and can provide an immediate, direct answer to common clinical questions.

PHYSICAL AND DEVELOPMENTAL DISABILITIES

Similar to their peers, adolescents with physical and developmental disabilities need reproductive health care. Many disabled teens can consent to sexual activity and desire contraception. Furthermore, caregivers may request contraception because of concerns about the risk of sexual abuse or assault. Menstrual suppression or reduction is also a common request from teens with developmental and physical disabilities and their families (Table 8).

Safety of the teen's environment and abuse prevention should be discussed with all teens and their families. Abusers can exploit physical and developmental disabilities, and victims may be less able to communicate that the abuse occurred. Studies show that rates of sexual abuse in children with disabilities are significantly higher than their nondisabled peers, especially those with primary or comorbid behavioral disorders [46]. Disabled teens in a romantic relationship are at greater risk for dating violence than their peers [47]. Pediatric providers who care for adolescents with disabilities are well-equipped to provide appropriate counseling and recommendations for contraception based on the individual adolescents needs.

SUMMARY

Pediatric providers are instrumental in educating adolescents about their contraceptive options and supporting them to obtain and continue their preferred method. LARC has an overwhelming potential to reduce unintended teen pregnancy, which in the United States remains at the highest rate of any developed nation. Contraceptive counseling should be developmentally appropriate, and follow best practices that encourage initiation and continuation of birth control methods.

References

[1] Martin JA, Hamilton BE, Osterman MJK, et al. Births: final data for 2013. Natl Vital Stat Rep 2015;64(1):1–65.
[2] Finer LB, Henshaw SK. Disparities in rates of unintended pregnancy in the United States, 1994 and 2001. Perspect Sex Reprod Health 2006;38(2):90–6.

[3] National Campaign to Prevent Teen and Unplanned Pregnancy, Counting it up: the public costs of teen childbearing. 2013. Available at: http://thenationalcampaign.org/. Accessed May 21, 2014.

[4] Finer LB, Philbin JM. Sexual initiation, contraceptive use, and pregnancy among young adolescents. Pediatrics 2013;131(5):886–91.

[5] Mosher WD, Jones J. Use of contraception in the United States: 1982–2008. Vital Health Stat 23 2010;(29):1–44.

[6] Martinez G, Copen CE, Abma JC. Teenagers in the United States: sexual activity, contraceptive use, and childbearing, 2006–2010 National Survey of Family Growth. Vital Health Stat 23 2011;(31):1–35.

[7] Kinchen KL, Shanklin SL, Flint KH, et al. Youth risk behavior surveillance—United States, 2013. MMWR Suppl 2014;63(4):1–168.

[8] Raine TR, Foster-Rosales A, Upadhyay UD, et al. One-year contraceptive continuation and pregnancy in adolescent girls and women initiating hormonal contraceptives. Obstet Gynecol 2011;117(2 Pt 1):363–71.

[9] Finer LB, Jerman J, Kavanaugh ML. Changes in use of long-acting contraceptive methods in the United States, 2007–2009. Fertil Steril 2012;98(4):893–7.

[10] Committee on Adolescent Health Care Long-Acting Reversible Contraception Working Group, The American College of Obstetricians and Gynecologists. Committee opinion no. 539: adolescents and long-acting reversible contraception: implants and intrauterine devices. Obstet Gynecol 2012;120(4):983–8.

[11] Committee on Adolescence. Contraception for adolescents. Pediatrics 2014;134(4): e1244–56.

[12] Rosenstock JR, Peipert JF, Madden T, et al. Continuation of reversible contraception in teenagers and young women. Obstet Gynecol 2012;120(6):1298–305.

[13] Secura GM, Madden T, McNicholas C, et al. Provision of no-cost, long acting contraception and teenage pregnancy. N Engl J Med 2014;371(14):1316–23.

[14] Melo J, Peters M, Teal S, et al. Adolescent and young women's contraceptive decision-making processes: choosing "The Best Method for Her". J Pediatr Adolesc Gynecol 2015;28(4):224–8.

[15] American Medical Association. Guidelines for adolescent prevention services (GAPS). Chicago: American Medical Association; 1997.

[16] Hagan JF, Shaw JS, Duncan P, editors. Bright futures: guidelines for health supervision of infants, children, and adolescents. 3rd edition. Elk Grove Village (IL): American Academy of Pediatrics; 2008.

[17] Ford C, English A, Sigman G. Confidential health care of adolescents: position paper for the Society of Adolescent Medicine. J Adolesc Health 2004;35(2):160–7.

[18] Guttmacher Institute, Minors' access to contraceptive services, State Policies in Brief. 2013. Available at: www.guttmacher.org/statecenter/spibs/spib_MACS.pdf. Accessed May 20, 2013.

[19] Short MB, Yates JK, Biro F, et al. Parents and partners: enhancing participation in contraception use. J Pediatr Adolesc Gynecol 2005;18(6):379–83.

[20] Hartman LB, Monasterio E, Hwang LY. Adolescent contraception: review and guidance for pediatric clinicians. Curr Probl Pediatr Adolesc Health Care 2012;42(9):221–63.

[21] Fortenberry JD, Tu W, Harezlak J, et al. Condom use as a function of time in new and established adolescent sexual relationships. Am J Public Health 2002;92(2):211–3.

[22] Kirby D, Laris BA, Rolleri L. Impact of sex and HIV education programs on sexual behaviors of youth in developing and developed countries [Youth Research Working Paper, No. 2]. Research Triangle Park (NC): Family Health International; 2005.

[23] Mestad R, Secura G, Allsworth JE, et al. Acceptance of long-acting reversible contraceptive methods by adolescent participants in the Contraceptive CHOICE Project. Contraception 2011;84(5):493–8.

[24] Trussell J. Contraceptive failure in the United States. Contraception 2011;83:397–404.

[25] Mansour D, Korver T, Marintcheva-Petrova M, et al. The effects of Implanon on menstrual bleeding patterns. Eur J Contracept Reprod Health Care 2008;13(Suppl 1):13–28.

[26] Affandi B. An integrated analysis of vaginal bleeding patterns in clinical trials of Implanon®. Contraception 1998;58:99S–107S.

[27] Division of Reproductive Health, National Center for Chronic Disease Prevention and Health Promotion, Centers for Disease Control and Prevention (CDC). U.S. Selected practice recommendations for contraceptive use, 2013: Adapted from the World Health Organization selected practice recommendations for contraceptive use, 2nd ed. MMWR Recomm Rep 2013;62(RR-05):1–60.

[28] Guiahi M, McBride M, Sheeder J, et al. Short-term treatment of bothersome bleeding for etonogestrel implant users using a 14-day oral contraceptive pill regimen: a randomized controlled trial. Obstet Gynecol 2015;126(3):508–13.

[29] Sivin I. IUDs are contraceptives, not abortifacients: a comment on research and belief. Stud Fam Plann 1989;20:355–9.

[30] Xiao BL, Zhou LY, Zhang XL, et al. Pharmacokinetic and pharmacodynamics studies of levonorgestrel-releasing intrauterine device. Contraception 1990;41(4):353–62.

[31] Teal SB, Sheeder J. IUD use in adolescent mothers: retention, failure and reasons for discontinuation. Contraception 2012;85(3):270.

[32] Andersson K, Odlind V, Rybo G. Levonorgestrel-releasing and copper-releasing (Nova T) IUDs during five years of use: a randomized comparative trial. Contraception 1994;49:56–72.

[33] Long-term reversible contraception. Twelve years of experience with the TCu380A and TCu220C. Contraception 1997;56:341–52.

[34] Grimes DA. Intrauterine device and upper-genital-tract infection. Lancet 2000;356:1013–9.

[35] Deans EI, Grimes DA. Intrauterine devices for adolescents: a systematic review. Contraception 2009;79:418–23.

[36] Kaunitz AM. Depot medoroxyprogesterone acetate contraception and the risk of breast and gynecologic cancer. J Reprod Med 1996;41(5 Suppl):419–27.

[37] Herzog AG. Progesterone therapy in women with epilepsy: a 3-year follow-up. Neurology 1999;52(9):1917–8.

[38] Manchikanti A, Grimes DA, Lopez LM, et al. Steroid hormones for contraception in women with sickle cell disease. Cochrane Database Syst Rev 2007;(2):CD006261.

[39] Westhoff C. Depot-medroxyprogesterone acetate injection (Depo-Provera): a highly effective contraceptive option with proven long-term safety. Contraception 2003;68:75–87.

[40] Lopez LM, Edelman A, Chen M, et al. Progestin-only contraceptives: effects on weight. Cochrane Database Syst Rev 2013;(7):CD008815.

[41] Le YC, Rahman M, Berenson AB. Early weight gain predicting later weight gain among depot medroxyprogesterone acetate users. Obstet Gynecol 2009;114(2 Pt 1):279–84.

[42] Committee on Adolescent Health Care and Committee on Gynecologic Practice. Committee Opinion No. 602: depot medroxyprogesterone acetate and bone effects. Obstet Gynecol 2014;123(6):1398–402.

[43] O'Brien SH. Contraception-related venous thromboembolism in adolescents. Semin Thromb Hemost 2014;40(1):66–71.

[44] Gold MA, Duffy K. Extended cycling or continuous use of hormonal contraceptives for female adolescents. Curr Opin Obstet Gynecol 2009;21(5):407–11.

[45] Bahamondes L, Bahamondes V, Shulman LP. Non-contraceptive benefits of hormonal and intrauterine reversible contraceptive methods. Hum Reprod Update 2015;21(5):640–51.

[46] McEachern AG. Sexual abuse of individuals with disabilities: prevention strategies for clinical practice. J Child Sex Abus 2012;21(4):386–98.

[47] Mitra M, Mouradian VE, McKenna M. Dating violence and associated health risks among high school studies with disabilities. Matern Child Health J 2013;17(6):1088–94.

Advances in Pediatrics 63 (2016) 453–471

ADVANCES IN PEDIATRICS

ELSEVIER
MOSBY

Docosahexaenoic Acid and Arachidonic Acid Nutrition in Early Development

Susan E. Carlson, PhD[a],*, John Colombo, PhD[b,c]

[a]Department of Dietetics and Nutrition, University of Kansas Medical Center, MS 4013, 3901 Rainbow Boulevard, Kansas City, KS 66160, USA; [b]Department of Neurology, University of Kansas Medical Center, 3901 Rainbow Boulevard, Kansas City, KS 66160, USA; [c]Department of Psychology, Life Span Institute, 1000 Sunnyside Avenue, University of Kansas, Lawrence, KS 66045, USA

Keywords
- Allergy • Arachidonic acid (ARA) • Cognition • Development
- Docosahexaenoic acid (DHA) • Growth
- Long-chain polyunsaturated fatty acids (LCPUFA) • Programming

Key points
- Docosahexaenoic acid (DHA), an omega-3 polyunsaturated fatty acid, and arachidonic acid (ARA), an omega-6 polyunsaturated fatty acid, are nutrients that were first added to formulas in the United States in 2002.
- DHA intake is low in the US population and this has implications for development.
- Early studies found more mature cortical visual function in infants fed formulas containing DHA and ARA and this led to a claim for improved visual acuity after these fatty acids were added to infant formula.
- Recent studies found positive effects of feeding DHA and ARA in infancy on cognition, brain connectivity, and allergy in early childhood, which provides evidence that these fatty acids program cognitive and immune development.
- The optimal balance of DHA and ARA intake during infancy is still not known, but current best practice suggests that the amount of DHA in infant formula should not exceed the amount of ARA.

Continued

Funding: NIH, HD047315 and P30 NICHD HD 002528.

*Corresponding author. E-mail address: scarlson@kumc.edu

0065-3101/16/$ – see front matter
http://dx.doi.org/10.1016/j.yapd.2016.04.011

Continued

- The effect of DHA and ARA status and supplementation in infancy has been largely evaluated through global developmental assessments focused on attainment of normative milestones, although more granular measures of specific cognitive function may be more sensitive markers of these effects.

INTRODUCTION

Docosahexaenoic acid (DHA; 22:6ω3) is an omega-3 fatty acid with 22 carbons and 6 double bonds (22:6n-3). Arachidonic acid (ARA; 20:4ω6) is an omega-6 fatty acid with 20 carbons and 4 double bonds. These two fatty acids are the predominant long-chain (20 and 22 carbons) polyunsaturated fatty acids (LCPUFAs) in human brain [1,2]. Brain DHA begins to accumulate around 22 weeks' gestation and the absolute amount per gram of brain as well as the weight percent of total fatty acids increases progressively from 22 weeks until at least 2 years of age [3–6]. The absolute amount of ARA per gram of brain also increases in brain but decreases in weight percent of total fatty acids after birth [1].

All human milk contains ARA and DHA to support DHA and ARA requirements for the growing and developing brain as well as other organs and tissue after birth. In human milk, the amount of ARA typically exceeds that of DHA. Milk ARA content is also less varied than DHA and, unlike DHA, does not seem to be linked to maternal intake. Because worldwide DHA intake is variable, milk DHA content is variable across cultures. Reports of milk DHA concentration range from 0.05% of total fatty acids in vegan vegetarians [7] to 2.8% in the marine region of China, where a diet high in seafood is consumed [8]; the median value of DHA in human milk worldwide is ~0.3% [9]. Women in the United States have low milk DHA levels (levels around 0.1% DHA are typical [10]) unless they regularly consume DHA or a supplement during and/or after their pregnancy. Jensen and colleagues [11] found that a supplement of 200 mg of DHA per day in US women could increase milk DHA to ~0.3% of total fatty acids, which is the amount that the European Food Safety Authority (EFSA) requires in infant formula in order to make a claim for support of infant visual development [12].

Red blood cell DHA and ARA levels are lower in infants fed formula without DHA and ARA, compared with infants fed human milk [10,13,14]; this is evidence of lower status. However, autopsy studies find lower brain DHA levels and higher omega-6 LCPUFA levels in infants fed formula without LCPUFA [14–16]. In term infants, frontal cortex DHA level is about 20% [14] lower if fed formulas without DHA and ARA. In preterm infants, who do not have the same opportunity to accumulate DHA from placental transfer, the amount of DHA that accumulates is ~50% less if formula is lacking in DHA and ARA [15].

DHA, ARA, and docosatetraenoic acid (DTA; 22:4ω6) are the major LCPUFAs in brain phosphoglycerides [6,14,15,17]; however, the amount of omega-6 LCPUFAs (ARA, DTA, and docosapentaenoic acid [omega 6 DPA; 22:5ω6]) exceeds the amount of DHA in the brains of humans and nonhuman primates. It is not known what happens to brain composition if human infants are fed only omega-3 LCPUFA (DHA or DHA plus EPA); however, some studies suggest that diets feeding only omega-3 result in major reductions in the omega-6 to omega-3 LCPUFA ratio. Baboon infants fed a formula with a higher proportion of DHA than ARA (0.96% and 0.64%, respectively) were shown to have reduced cortical and hypothalamic omega-6 LCPUFA levels, and omega-3 LCPUFA level exceeded that of omega-6 LCPUFA in the frontal lobe [18]. A recent trial conducted in our laboratory (the DHA Intake and Measurement of Neural Development [DIAMOND] trial, discussed later) included a formula in which omega-3 LCPUFA intake was substantially higher than omega-6 LCPUFA intake, and in which outcomes were somewhat consistent with these animal studies.

It seems advisable and prudent to follow human milk as a model for adding LCPUFA in infant formula given that the optimal balance of these two families of fatty acids in the developing brain is unknown. Infant formulas in the United States have contained both DHA and ARA since 2002, typically in a ratio of ~2:1 of ARA to DHA, although the amounts of DHA and ARA fed vary. Before 2002, all formula-fed preterm and term infants in the United States received formula without DHA and ARA.

Long-chain polyunsaturated fatty acid intake as a source of docosahexaenoic acid and arachidonic acid

As noted previously, human newborns obtain both DHA and ARA from human milk and infant formulas currently contain these fatty acids. However, other foods provide little DHA and ARA in the diet of US infants. Using validated assessments of food intake in 207 infants, the authors estimated DHA intake at 9 and 12 months of age to be on average 4.0 mg (median = 0 mg) and 13 mg (median = 4 mg), respectively. ARA intake from foods other than human milk or formula in the same 207 infants at the same ages was estimated respectively to average 15 mg (median = 4 mg) and 41 mg (median = 20 mg) at 9 and 12 months of age. Fish, chicken, and egg yolk are good food sources of DHA and ARA, but only 3 of 207 children were reported to have consumed these foods on the day of their 12-month, 24-hour dietary recall (Carlson SE, unpublished data, 2016). US infants may depend on human milk or formulas with DHA and ARA for their primary intake of these nutrients in infancy. After infancy, DHA intake in US children is not appreciably higher than is found at 12 months of age [19].

Fetal stores as a source of docosahexaenoic acid

Evidence suggests that DHA accumulated in fetal adipose tissue can support DHA requirements for some time after birth [20]. Beginning around 26 weeks' gestation, DHA accumulation increases progressively in fetal adipose tissue to term birth. However, the amount accumulated depends on maternal DHA intake. Haggarty [20] suggests that there is little to no accumulation of DHA in fetal adipose tissue if maternal intake is less than 90 mg/d; this is significant because the mean reported intake of DHA from food and supplements of US women 19 to 50 years of age is only 53 mg/d [21]. The offspring of US women may accumulate less adipose DHA than the offspring of women in populations with much higher DHA intake.

Long-chain polyunsaturated fatty acid synthesis as a source of docosahexaenoic acid and arachidonic acid

All omega-6 and omega-3 LCPUFAs (including DHA and ARA) can be obtained by synthesis from their 18-carbon precursors. DHA can be synthesized from alpha-linolenic acid (18:3ω3) and ARA can be synthesized from linoleic acid (18:2ω6) through a process of elongation and desaturation. However, none of the many studies to date has found equivalent DHA and ARA status in developing infants fed 18-carbon fatty acids compared with infants fed LCPUFAs, and this is particularly true for DHA. Conversion of alpha-linolenic acid to EPA and DHA is decreased by high dietary intake of linoleic acid, because linoleic acid (an omega-6 fatty acid) competes with alpha-linolenic acid (an omega-3 fatty acid) for the same elongation and desaturation pathway [22]. High linoleic acid intakes and a high ratio of linoleic acid to alpha-linolenic acid are characteristics of most persons in the United States; linoleic acid has increased dramatically in the US food supply in the past 60 years [23]. Adipose tissue concentrations of linoleic acid have increased dramatically as well [24].

Compared with ARA, DHA synthesis requires additional elongation and desaturation steps and involves an additional organelle, the peroxisome [6,25]. As a result, conversion is extremely inefficient and highly variable. Women of reproductive age can convert up to 9% of alpha-linolenic acid to DHA [26]; however, at a typical alpha-linolenic acid intake of 1 g/d, US women could synthesize no more than ~90 mg/d of DHA, although the DHA need during pregnancy approaches 300 mg/d. The usual DHA intake of US women and synthesis meet less than half of this need, thus compromising fetal DHA accumulation [20].

Fatty acid synthesis is also influenced by the fatty acid desaturase genes, FADS1/FADS2. These genes code for the delta-5 and delta-6 desaturase enzymes required to synthesize LCPUFA. Single-nucleotide polymorphisms in FADS1/FADS2 influence both LCPUFA status and response to LCPUFA intake [27–31].

Roles of docosahexaenoic acid and arachidonic acid in the brain

A detailed discussion of the role of DHA and ARA in the central nervous system is beyond the scope of this article; however, several functional roles are plausible based on what is currently known and their concentration in membranes in the central nervous system. Individual phosphoglyceride classes (phosphatidylethanolamine, phosphatidylserine, phosphatidylcholine, and phosphatidylinositol) in brain cerebral gray and white matter have unique LCPUFA profiles. ARA greatly exceeds DHA in inositol phosphoglycerides, whereas DHA exceeds ARA in serine phosphoglycerides [17]. Both of these phosphoglyceride classes are important in signal transduction; for example, inositol phosphoglycerides are key to the phosphatidyl inositol-3-kinase/Akt pathway [32] and phosphatidyl inositol 4,5-bisphosphate signaling [33], whereas serine phosphoglycerides are important for long-term potentiation [34]. It has been shown that animals with lower DHA status have less brain serine phosphoglyceride, and that DHA intake can increase brain serine phosphoglyceride concentration and long-term potentiation (a process critical to memory formation) [34].

In addition to their roles in brain phosphoglycerides, LCPUFAs are precursors for physiologically important metabolites, including prostaglandins, leukotrienes, and more recently discovered families of oxygenated metabolites including resolvins, which reduce inflammation through nuclear factor kappa B signaling [35–37]. DHA and ARA are also precursors of the endocannabinoids N-docosahexaenoylethanolamide and anandamide, respectively, which are modulators of the central and enteric nervous systems [38–40]. For example, N-docosahexaenoylethanolamide has been shown to promote hippocampal development [38] and anandamide to modulate spatial memory after stress [40]. In addition, DHA and AA and their metabolites are ligands for the nuclear receptor, peroxisome proliferator-actvated receptor gamma (PPARγ) [41,42]. All of these metabolites could influence physiologic functions of organs and tissues, and all have the potential for long-term effects on brain function and behavior (programming).

Given the clear role of LCPUFA in the brain, much interest has been generated about the effect of DHA and ARA on brain development and cognition in infancy and early childhood. We posit that these effects may be best assessed and understood from a perspective informed by the principles of early brain development and the nature of early assessment. These issues are addressed later in this article.

Brain development and assessment in infants and children

Brain development occurs in fairly specific stages during early life. By the end of the embryonic period (ie, the first 8 prenatal weeks), the fundamental structures of the brain and central nervous system are fairly well defined [43], and neurogenesis has begun [44]. As neurons are generated, they migrate to their final positions in the brain, guided along distinct pathways by specialized adhesion molecules on cell surfaces, or by crawling along radial glia [45]. Once neurons have finished migrating, 2 processes occur. First, dramatic neuronal growth forces brain surfaces to become contorted within the finite space of the skull; this results in the characteristic ridges (sulci) and folds (gyri) seen in the mature brain. Second, neurons engage in arborization, a process through which the dendrites of an estimated 100 billion neurons [46] form up to 1000 functional connections (synapses) with the axons or terminal branches of other neurons [43]; this rich and dense network of interconnections mediates all forms of behavior and cognition seen in the organism across the life span. This dendritic branching continues to occur postnatally [47]; so much so that neural connections that prove to be redundant or less used during the course of the organism's experience or behavior are "pruned" [48,49] and superfluous neurons die off and are resorbed. The final step in brain development is the emergence of myelin [50], a fatty substance that wraps axons and increases the efficiency of neural transmission. Bundles of myelinated axonal fibers appear as mature white matter tracts or pathways, as opposed to unmyelinated gray-matter fibers [43]; again, myelination occurs at different schedules in different parts of the brain.

Note that although genetic influences contribute in obvious ways to the initiation and organization of the program for brain development, exogenous forces strongly determine much of the ultimate structural and functional characteristics of the central nervous system. Maternal environment can meaningfully affect even the earliest processes of central nervous system development, including neurogenesis [51], neuronal migration [52], and synaptogenesis [53]. Depending on the timing and dose of experiences, the effects of these early maternal or environmental conditions can be powerful in their influence on the long-term developmental outcome of offspring. The disproportionate effects of such influences on early prenatal and postnatal life gave rise to the concept of prenatal and early postnatal life as critical periods [54] for determining later development. In the dietary or nutrition literature, the lasting nature of such effects is often considered to reflect early developmental programming of later cognitive or behavioral outcomes [55–57].

The cycle of neurogenesis, migration, synaptogenesis, and pruning characterizes brain development at the cellular level, but, for understanding behavioral and cognitive development, considerations from a more structural perspective are also critical. Between the third and fifth weeks of prenatal life, the neural tube differentiates structurally into distinct structural components that give rise to the brain stem, midbrain, and cerebral cortex. Most brain stem (eg, pons, medulla) functions are related to the maintenance of vital (respiratory, cardiovascular, sleep-wake, and other autonomic) characteristics. Midbrain (eg, thalamus, hypothalamus, amygdala) functions are related to processing sensory input and motivating behavioral responses related to basic survival and reproductive needs. More complex and flexible forms of behavior and cognition are mediated by integration of controlling cerebral structures with lower-order cognitive functions. However, behavior and cognition are rarely governed by the activity of a single area or structure; behavior and cognition may be best considered as derivatives of interactions among these 3 structural levels. However, because the 3 structural levels have distinct developmental courses, behavioral and cognitive development necessarily reflect the interaction of these systems at different stages of maturity [58]. Furthermore, maturation within structural levels (particularly within cerebral and cortical pathways) also follows distinct and dissociable developmental courses. For example, lower-order (and phylogenetically earlier) senses such as olfaction, taste, and touch emerge earlier than audition, and vision follows after that; vision has a protracted developmental course that extends into the third postnatal year [59]. Following on sensory development, cerebral structures generally mature in a posterior-to-anterior direction with the frontal areas of the cerebrum maturing last [60]. Thus, simple forms of cognitive functions such as attention and memory emerge early but become increasingly interrelated and integrated as the frontal lobes mature, and this integration leads to the emergence of increasingly complex forms of cognition, such as goal-directed behavior, strategic planning, reasoning, and other executive functions [61]. Modern models of the emergence of specific cognitive abilities suggest that repeated use of particular neural circuits (ie, through practice or simple repetition) results in the parcellation of brain areas devoted to those abilities; in turn, this makes such abilities independent and dissociable, thus giving the appearance of cognitive modularity [62,63].

The conceptualization of behavioral development has important implications for how clinicians choose to measure early cognition. A common strategy in quantifying behavioral development in infancy and early childhood involves the assessment of whether the emergence of an individual child's common, global motoric responses (eg, sitting up, crawling, walking) matches with the normal or typical developmental course (as derived from a standardized sample). Slightly more sophisticated assessments may tap whether other, more complex behavioral responses (eg, imitation, word production, following instructions) are behind, at, or ahead of a similar normative schedule. However, given the conceptualization of behavioral and cognitive constructs from the principles of brain development described earlier, these global measures (particularly in infancy, when systems are immature) are unlikely to relate to or signify long-term outcomes, and the global nature of such measures may obscure deficiencies (or, for that matter, advantages) in the function of specific brain systems during development [64].

Over the last several decades [65] developmental scientists have generated strategies for tapping into more targeted and specific measures of cognitive abilities in infancy and early childhood. One of the advantages of this approach is that, if the effects of an environmental or organismic condition/status are more specific, measurement of that specific skill (eg, attention, memory, inhibition) is more likely to reveal an effect. Another important advantage is that measurement of specific cognitive constructs or systems may be more likely to be related to longer-term outcomes than a global measure that conflates the contribution of many systems or cognitive constructs, some of which may be irrelevant to longer-term outcomes. Recent empirical findings implicate specific and targeted cognitive measures taken during infancy in both direct [64,66] and indirect [67,68] prediction models of cognitive outcomes in childhood.

Cortical visual acuity

Cortical visual acuity was the first brain function studied in preterm infants to determine whether DHA would improve development. Both electrophysiologic [69] and behavioral outcomes [70] were measured. Subsequently, several masked clinical studies compared commercially available infant formulas without DHA and ARA with formulas with DHA and ARA and showed higher visual acuity in both term and preterm infants (see Ref. [71] for review).

Most studies stopped assessing visual acuity at 12 months of age or earlier, but Birch and colleagues [72] studied 4-year-old children and found poorer visual acuity in the group that was not fed LCPUFA in infancy, but similar visual acuity in groups fed DHA or DHA plus ARA, compared with the group that was breast-fed. Based on these studies, EFSA allowed the claim that DHA contributes to the visual development of infants from birth to 12 months so long as the formula contained at least 0.3% of total fatty acids as DHA [12]. The most recent study of visual acuity in supplemented infants was from a large dose-response study (0.32%, 0.64%, or 0.96% total fatty acids as DHA and 0.64% as ARA compared with a formula without DHA and ARA). The DIAMOND trial began in 2003 and was conducted at 2 sites in the United States (Dallas, TX, and Kansas City, MO). DHA and ARA supplementation significantly enhanced visual acuity at 12 months of age, confirming earlier studies. The study found similar benefit of LCPUFA-containing formula for visual acuity at 12 months of age compared with formula without LCPUFA regardless of DHA dose [73].

Cognition

In addition to visual acuity, the high accumulation of DHA and ARA in brain has prompted substantial interest in the effects of these LCPUFAs on cognition. The first evidence that DHA could improve cognitive function was reported in 1996 from 2 studies in very low birth weight preterm infants, 1 with DHA and EPA supplementation to 2 months corrected age (CA) and 1 with DHA and EPA supplementation to 9 months CA. In both studies infants had significantly shorter duration looks during a fixed time to test [74,75], which reflects more rapid visual information processing [76]. Shorter duration looks at 12 months CA in infants supplemented only to 2 months CA was also the first evidence that improving DHA status during early development could program higher cognitive function long after supplementation is discontinued [74]. Shorter duration looking was also later observed in monkeys fed a standard nursery diet with alpha-linolenic acid compared with a diet deficient in omega-3 fatty acids.

Children from the Kansas City cohort of the DIAMOND trial had lower heart rates when fed formula with DHA and ARA compared with formula without DHA and ARA, but no dose-response effect was observed [77]. The groups of infants fed 0.32% and 0.64% DHA showed higher quality attention, spending more time engaged in active stimulus processing (sustained attention) than the group fed the control formula. The group fed 0.96% DHA had a response that was intermediate between the control and 0.32%/0.64% groups and did not differ significantly from these groups [77]. The authors then conducted age-appropriate tests of development on the children in each group every 6 months from 18 months to 6 years of age [78]. Positive effects of DHA and ARA supplementation were observed on rule-learning and inhibition tasks when the children were between 3 and 5 years of age, and on standardized tests of vocabulary and verbal intelligence quotient (IQ) at 5 and 6 years of age (Peabody Picture Vocabulary Test and Weschler Primary Preschool Scale of Intelligence) [78]. With the exception of 1 task (requiring the child to inhibit a prepotent response to a stimulus), the group fed 0.96% DHA/0.64% ARA performed less well than the 0.32% and 0.64% DHA groups but better than the control group (although not significantly different from either). A 6-country study in Europe of formula-fed infants also found cognitive benefit (faster information processing) at 6 years of age in children who were fed formula with 0.2% DHA and 0.35% ARA for only 4 months in infancy compared with a control formula without LCPUFA [79]. These results in young children are consistent with several earlier reports showing advantages of early developmental exposure to higher DHA intake during pregnancy and/or with human milk feeding that also provided ARA to the developing fetus/newborn [80,81].

In general, the results of studies show benefit or no effect on cognitive function at school age of early exposure to higher DHA or DHA plus ARA. However, a Danish study that supplemented lactating women who were low fish consumers with a high-dose fish oil compared with olive oil found poorer performance in the fish oil group at age 7 years: processing speed was slower overall and a measure of prosocial behavior was lower in boys [82]. However, the investigators did not publish the results of the human milk fatty acid composition; it would be interesting to know whether DHA was present in great excess relative to ARA.

Several studies of the effects of DHA or DHA plus ARA supplementation on cognition have been conducted in very low birth weight infants at school age. A study in Norway that provided DHA and ARA supplementation to human milk until discharge from the hospital found no effect of the randomization on several tests at 20 months [83] or on cognitive function or brain macrostructure on MRI at age 8 years [84]. A large cohort from the Australian DHA for the Improvement of Neurodevelopmental Outcome in Preterm Infants (DINO) trial compared neurodevelopment at 7 years of age in children who were fed ∼0.35% DHA compared with 1% DHA until term CA and found no evidence of benefit; however, group mean scores on the Wechsler Abbreviated Scale of Intelligence were high, ranging from 98.0 to 98.8 for both the primary and secondary assessments of IQ [85]. A study from the United Kingdom found some positive results at 10 years of age for infants fed 0.5% DHA in formula from birth to 9 months of age for verbal IQ, full-scale IQ, and memory; and benefits for literacy in girls [86]. With the exception of Isaacs and colleagues [86], the studies were of short duration and the control groups were receiving the same LCPUFA as the intervention group, making it impossible to conclude that these infants did not benefit from DHA or DHA plus ARA. The control groups in 2 of these studies seem to have been provided adequate LCPUFA.

Not all cognitive domains tested in the Kansas City cohort of the DIAMOND trial showed behavioral effects of DHA and ARA. For example, spatial memory and advanced problem solving were not influenced by early DHA and ARA intake. Neither were early tests of global development such as the Bayley Scales of Infant Development (BSID) and the MacArthur-Bates Communicative Developmental Inventory [78], which were designed to determine whether infants and young children are meeting normal milestones of development. In contrast, DHA-supplemented and ARA-supplemented children from the Dallas cohort of the DIAMOND trial, with different demographics, scored 5.7 points higher on the BSID Mental Developmental Index at 18 months [87], but had poorer receptive vocabulary at 2 years (although not at 3.5 years) [88]. Global tests of development generally have similar null findings to ours and serve as the main basis for 4 systematic reviews that conclude either (1) that there is no benefit of LCPUFA supplementation in infancy to cognitive development, or (2) that there is insufficient evidence to conclude that an effect exists (see Ref. [89] for commentary). However, there are fewer studies that have assessed targeted tasks so these do not lend themselves to systematic reviews.

Brain electrophysiology and studies in childhood

In addition to measuring behavior, this article has discussed brain electrophysiology in the DIAMOND cohort, measuring evoked response potentials (ERPs) during a Go–No-go task at 5.5 years in which children were asked to press a button only if a fish appeared but to inhibit button press if a shark appeared. Children fed DHA and ARA during infancy compared with the control group showed a distinct N2 amplitude response to No-go versus Go trials before the button press that the authors interpret as engagement of more mature inhibitory control [90]. Children fed DHA and ARA also showed a unique microstate during No-go trials that was consistent with involvement of frontal structures on the inhibition of a response. More recently, the authors have studied about half of the cohort at 9 years of age using structural, functional, and metabolic studies of brain: MRI, magnetic resonance spectroscopy, and magnetoencephalography (manuscript in preparation). In both ERP and subsequent brain imaging studies at 9 years, the 0.64% DHA/0.64% ARA group consistently has the most mature brain performance and differs most from the control group.

Grayson and colleagues [91] recently reported that cortical interconnectivity in the brain of adult rhesus macaques exposed to a lifetime of omega-3 fatty acids intake was similar to organization in healthy human brain but different from that of macaques exposed to a lifetime of an omega-3–deficient diet.

Single-nucleotide polymorphisms and cognition

As mentioned earlier, there are genetic differences in ability to synthesize ARA and DHA from the18-carbon essential fatty acid precursors. An intriguing possibility suggested by the recent work of Peters and colleagues [92] is that individuals with fatty acid desaturases (FADS) minor alleles have poorer quality brain white matter development, which affects brain function. Martinez and Vazquez [93] first showed a link between brain DHA accumulation and myelination in children with peroxisomal disorders who are unable to synthesize DHA, so differences in LCPUFA synthesis could theoretically decrease brain myelination. Limitations in LCPUFA synthesis could thus indirectly affect brain myelination.

Three studies have investigated the relationship between 1 FADS2 polymorphism (rs174575) and IQ in cohorts of children or adults who were fed either human milk (which contains cholesterol as well as omega-3 and omega-6 LCPUFAs) or formula in infancy (before the addition of DHA and ARA to infant formula) [94–96]. In all 3 studies the groups that carried 1 or both major alleles had higher IQs if they were fed human milk compared with infant formula. Rizzi and colleagues [96] were the only group of investigators to control for parental education, which attenuated the effect of human milk on IQ. If there is an advantage of human milk feeding for major allele carriers, both dietary LCPUFA and cholesterol could be invoked and neither can be ruled out. In contrast, none of these studies showed enough difference among the FADS allele groups fed formula to suggest an effect of FADS allele on IQ. What is intriguing is that in 2 of these studies there is no obvious increase in IQ with human milk feeding in individuals homozygous for the minor allele [94,96], whereas Steer and colleagues [95] found that minor allele homozygotes had the lowest IQ with formula feeding and the highest IQ when fed human milk. The data available at this time are difficult to interpret and may depend on a better understanding of how LCPUFA synthesis is controlled; for example, it has been reported recently that FADS2 contains a sterol regulatory element [97]. There may be undiscovered links between LCPUFA and cholesterol that influence the response of the developing brain to variations in LCPUFA and cholesterol intake.

Allergy and immunity

Higher omega-3 LCPUFA intake is associated with lower allergy incidence in several studies, including those of Duchen and colleagues [98,99]. A recent Scandinavian study linked minor allele carriers of several FADS alleles associated with lower blood ARA with reduced risk of atopic eczema but not respiratory allergy at age 13 years [100]. Several studies have looked at immune function or allergy in groups of infants randomly assigned to different LCPUFA intakes. Field and colleagues [101] found that infants fed formula with DHA and ARA had immune cells and cytokine profiles more similar to infants fed human milk and different from infants fed formula without LCPUFA. Two US studies show lower allergy incidence in young children randomly assigned to formula with DHA and ARA compared with formula without LCPUFA during infancy [102,103]. Birch and colleagues [102] analyzed combined studies of formulas containing ~0.3% DHA and 0.6% ARA that were fed for varying periods of time during infancy. They found fewer medically documented allergic illnesses in the first 3 years of life in children receiving formula with compared with without LCPUFA. Similarly, the authors recently reported fewer medically documented allergies in the first 4 years of life with formulas containing DHA (0.32%–0.96%) and ARA (0.64%) compared with formula without LCPUFA [103]. When the authors assessed predictors of skin allergy and wheeze/asthma, we found an interaction with maternal allergy: LCPUFA protected against skin allergy in children of women who did not report allergy and against wheezing/asthma in children of women who reported allergy [103]. There is a need to determine when in development LCPUFA is important for reducing allergy [104–106].

Body composition

It is well known from animal and cell models that the omega-6 fatty acids, linoleic acid, and ARA are adipogenic [107,108]. Casado-Diaz and colleagues [41] reported that ARA, but not omega-3 LCPUFA (DHA and eicosapentae-noic acid [EPA; 20:5ω3]) induce adipogenesis of human mesenchymal stem cells. In addition to serving as a reservoir for DHA, adipose tissue DHA accumulation in the fetus may play a role in programming body composition in childhood by counteracting the effects of omega-6 fatty acids. Moon and colleagues [109] reported an association between pregnancy DHA status and higher lean mass in childhood; and higher ARA status and higher fat mass in childhood using DXA. Using Bod Pod assessments, the authors found significantly higher fat-free mass in 5-year-old children (n = 78) whose mothers were randomly assigned to a DHA supplement of 600 mg/d during pregnancy compared with children of women assigned to a placebo of soybean and corn oils (n = 75) (presented at the ninth World Congress of the Developmental Origins of Health and Disease, Cape Town, South Africa, 2015).

The Imact of Nutritional Fatty Acids During Pregnancy and Lactation for Early Human Adipose tissue Development (INFAT) study conducted in Germany provided 1200 mg of omega-3 LCPUFA to pregnant women during the last 2 trimesters of pregnancy and the first 4 months of lactation. The supplement dramatically increased omega-3 LCPUFA exposure of the fetuses/infants [110]. Much and colleagues [110] found a significant positive relationship between the sum of 4 skinfold measurements at 1 year and maternal milk omega-3 LCPUFA at 6 weeks postpartum, in apparent contrast with the reports discussed earlier. The authors recently reported that children fed formula with DHA and ARA compared with no LCPUFA had higher length/stature and weight-for-age percentiles from birth to 6 years of age, but no increase in body mass index [111]. We speculate that increased DHA intake during pregnancy and infancy in populations with low DHA intake, such as the US population, may program early lineage of fetal mesenchymal stem cells resulting in higher fat-free mass relative to fat mass in the offspring. More work in this area is needed, including research using validated measures of body composition to understand how body composition in infancy influences body composition in childhood.

Assessment of the literature on docosahexaenoic acid and arachidonic acid and infant development

This assessment of the importance of DHA and ARA in infancy is biased toward US studies of infants randomly assigned to formula with DHA plus ARA compared with formula without LCPUFA. There are few such studies and US studies are overrepresented. As noted earlier, meta-analyses do not support benefits of DHA and ARA addition to infant formula, consequently it is not universally accepted that infants benefit from the addition of DHA and ARA to infant formula. The focus is on US studies in this article because (1) systematic reviews of published results rely heavily on a single test of global neurodevelopment designed to determine whether infants are meeting normal milestones of development, rather than on specific and more granular measures of cognitive constructs in infancy and early childhood [89]; (2) most studies of DHA and ARA supplementation have been conducted in countries where adults, including presumably women in their reproductive years, consume significantly more DHA than do women in the United States; and (3) few trials have followed children to ages at which the results of sophisticated tests of cognition or brain structure/function tests can be and are obtained.

DHA and ARA are nutrients, and a strong case can be made that DHA intake is inadequate in the US adult population [112]. As well, the positive effects of DHA and ARA supplementation on cognition, allergy incidence, growth, and body composition noted here for US children exposed to higher DHA or DHA plus ARA during development could not be found in an LCPUFA-sufficient population. There is no reason to suspect that studies that find no effect of LCPUFA supplementation are wrong; however, the authors do not regard meta-analyses as an ideal way to determine whether a nutrient deficiency needs correcting in a given group for DHA any more than, for example, for iron. The case for studying the effects of DHA in populations that are deficient in DHA has already been made [113].

In the past 10 years, there have been numerous articles published on the FADS alleles. It is now understood that among individuals there is a range in ability to synthesize LCPUFA, and this is an important advance. However, this article does not focus much on FADS alleles even though they probably play a role in some of the inconsistencies in individual and group responses to LCPUFA supplementation found in the studies discussed here.

Researchers now have access to techniques to measure brain electrical interconnectivity and brain structure and function; these techniques were not used in the early studies of DHA and ARA supplementation. Positive effects of perinatal DHA and ARA exposure were observed in the DIAMOND study cohort that suggest that early DHA and ARA exposure in infancy resulted in more coherent and engaged brain function long after children were weaned to a standard US diet that was, incidentally, low in DHA [90]. More recent results from a subset of this cohort who underwent studies of brain structure, function, and metabolism show persistent positive effects of supplementation at 9 years of age (manuscript in preparation). The authors think that there is great potential for more direct studies of the brain because even the most targeted behavioral tests of cognition may underestimate the true effects of proper LCPUFA balance on brain functioning. We hope others will study older children and young adults from cohorts exposed to DHA and ARA early in development. Such studies should involve interdisciplinary teams of investigators, including investigators with expertise in brain structure, function, electrophysiology, and metabolism.

References

[1] Svennerholm L, Vanier MT. The distribution of lipids in the human nervous system. 3. Fatty acid composition of phosphoglycerides of human foetal and infant brain. Brain Res 1973;50(2):341–51.

[2] Martinez M. Tissue levels of polyunsaturated fatty acids during early human development. J Pediatr 1992;120(4 Pt 2):S129–38.

[3] Martinez M, Mougan I. Fatty acid composition of human brain phospholipids during normal development. J Neurochem 1998;71(6):2528–33.

[4] Clandinin MT, Chappell JE, Leong S, et al. Intrauterine fatty acid accretion rates in human brain: implications for fatty acid requirements. Early Hum Dev 1980;4(2):121–9.

[5] Clandinin MT, Chappell JE, Leong S, et al. Extrauterine fatty acid accretion in infant brain: implications for fatty acid requirements. Early Hum Dev 1980;4(2):131–8.

[6] Martinez M. Developmental profiles of polyunsaturated fatty acids in the brain of normal infants and patients with peroxisomal diseases: severe deficiency of docosahexaenoic acid in Zellweger's and pseudo-Zellweger's syndromes. World Rev Nutr Diet 1991;66:87–102.

[7] Sanders TA, Ellis FR, Dickerson JW. Studies of vegans: the fatty acid composition of plasma choline phosphoglycerides, erythrocytes, adipose tissue, and breast milk, and some indicators of susceptibility to ischemic heart disease in vegans and omnivore controls. Am J Clin Nutr 1978;31(5):805–13.

[8] Ruan C, Liu X, Man H, et al. Milk composition in women from five different regions of China: the great diversity of milk fatty acids. J Nutr 1995;125(12):2993–8.

[9] Brenna JT, Varamini B, Jensen RG, et al. Docosahexaenoic and arachidonic acid concentrations in human breast milk worldwide. Am J Clin Nutr 2007;85(6):1457–64.

[10] Putnam JC, Carlson SE, DeVoe PW, et al. The effect of variations in dietary fatty acids on the fatty acid composition of erythrocyte phosphatidylcholine and phosphatidylethanolamine in human infants. Am J Clin Nutr 1982;36(1):106–14.

[11] Jensen CL, Voigt RG, Prager TC, et al. Effects of maternal docosahexaenoic acid intake on visual function and neurodevelopment in breastfed term infants. Am J Clin Nutr 2005;82(1):125–32.

[12] Scientific Opinion of the Panel on Dietetic Products, Nutrition and Allergies. DHA and ARA and Visual Development: Scientific substantiation of a health claim related to docosahexaenoic acid (DHA) and arachidonic acid (ARA) and visual development pursuant to Article 14 of Regulation (EC) No 1924/2006. EFSA J 2009;941:1–14.

[13] Sanders TA, Naismith DJ. A comparison of the influence of breast-feeding and bottle-feeding on the fatty acid composition of the erythrocytes. Br J Nutr 1979;41(3):619–23.

[14] Makrides M, Neumann MA, Byard RW, et al. Fatty acid composition of brain, retina, and erythrocytes in breast- and formula-fed infants. Am J Clin Nutr 1994;60(2):189–94.

[15] Farquharson J, Cockburn F, Patrick WA, et al. Infant cerebral cortex phospholipid fatty-acid composition and diet. Lancet 1992;340(8823):810–3.

[16] Byard RW, Makrides M, Need M, et al. Sudden infant death syndrome: effect of breast and formula feeding on frontal cortex and brainstem lipid composition. J Paediatr Child Health 1995;31(1):14–6.

[17] Svennerholm L. Distribution and fatty acid composition of phosphoglycerides in normal human brain. J Lipid Res 1968;9(5):570–9.

[18] Hsieh AT, Anthony JC, Diersen-Schade DA, et al. The influence of moderate and high dietary long chain polyunsaturated fatty acids (LCPUFA) on baboon neonate tissue fatty acids. Pediatr Res 2007;61(5 Pt 1):537–45.

[19] Minns LM, Kerling EH, Neely MR, et al. Toddler formula supplemented with docosahexa-enoic acid (DHA) improves DHA status and respiratory health in a randomized, double-blind, controlled trial of US children less than 3 years of age. Prostaglandins Leukot Essent Fatty Acids 2010;82(4–6):287–93.

[20] Haggarty P. Fatty acid supply to the human fetus. Annu Rev Nutr 2010;30:237–55.

[21] Papanikolaou Y, Brooks J, Reider C, et al. U.S. adults are not meeting recommended levels for fish and omega-3 fatty acid intake: results of an analysis using observational data from NHANES 2003-2008. Nutr J 2014;13:31.

[22] Gibson RA, Neumann MA, Lien EL, et al. Docosahexaenoic acid synthesis from alpha-linolenic acid is inhibited by diets high in polyunsaturated fatty acids. Prostaglandins Leukot Essent Fatty Acids 2013;88(1):139–46.

[23] Blasbalg TL, Hibbeln JR, Ramsden CE, et al. Changes in consumption of omega-3 and omega-6 fatty acids in the United States during the 20th century. Am J Clin Nutr 2011;93(5):950–62.

[24] Guyenet SJ, Carlson SE. Increase in adipose tissue linoleic acid of US adults in the last half century. Adv Nutr 2015;6(6):660–4.

[25] Sprecher H, Chen Q. Polyunsaturated fatty acid biosynthesis: a microsomal-peroxisomal process. Prostaglandins Leukot Essent Fatty Acids 1999;60(5–6):317–21.

[26] Burdge GC, Wootton SA. Conversion of alpha-linolenic acid to eicosapentaenoic, docosa-pentaenoic and docosahexaenoic acids in young women. Br J Nutr 2002;88(4):411–20.

[27] Schaeffer L, Gohlke H, Muller M, et al. Common genetic variants of the FADS1 FADS2 gene cluster and their reconstructed haplotypes are associated with the fatty acid compo-sition in phospholipids. Hum Mol Genet 2006;15(11):1745–56.

[28] Koletzko B, Lattka E, Zeilinger S, et al. Genetic variants of the fatty acid desaturase gene cluster predict amounts of red blood cell docosahexaenoic and other polyunsaturated fatty acids in pregnant women: findings from the Avon Longitudinal Study of Parents and Chil-dren. Am J Clin Nutr 2011;93(1):211–9.

[29] Xie L, Innis SM. Genetic variants of the FADS1 FADS2 gene cluster are associated with altered (n-6) and (n-3) essential fatty acids in plasma and erythrocyte phospholipids in women during pregnancy and in breast milk during lactation. J Nutr 2008;138(11):2222–8.

[30] Lattka E, Illig T, Koletzko B, et al. Genetic variants of the FADS1 FADS2 gene cluster as related to essential fatty acid metabolism. Curr Opin Lipidol 2010;21(1):64–9.

[31] Scholtz SA, Kerling EH, Shaddy DJ, et al. Docosahexaenoic acid (DHA) supplementation in pregnancy differentially modulates arachidonic acid and DHA status across FADS geno-types in pregnancy. Prostaglandins Leukot Essent Fatty Acids 2015;94:29–33.

[32] Nguyen TL, Kim CK, Cho JH, et al. Neuroprotection signaling pathway of nerve growth factor and brain-derived neurotrophic factor against staurosporine induced apoptosis in hippocampal H19-7/IGF-IR [corrected]. Exp Mol Med 2010;42(8):583–95.

[33] Zhou Y, Wong CO, Cho KJ, et al. SIGNAL TRANSDUCTION. Membrane potential modu-lates plasma membrane phospholipid dynamics and K-Ras signaling. Science 2015;349(6250):873–6.

[34] Kim HY, Huang BX, Spector AA. Phosphatidylserine in the brain: metabolism and function. Prog Lipid Res 2014;56:1–18.

[35] Northstone K, Emmett PM. Are dietary patterns stable throughout early and mid-childhood? A birth cohort study. Br J Nutr 2008;100(5):1069–76.

[36] Northstone K, Emmett P. Multivariate analysis of diet in children at four and seven years of age and associations with socio-demographic characteristics. Eur J Clin Nutr 2005;59(6):751–60.

[37] Allan K, Devereux G. Diet and asthma: nutrition implications from prevention to treatment. J Am Diet Assoc 2011;111(2):258–68.

[38] Kim HY, Moon HS, Cao D, et al. N-Docosahexaenoylethanolamide promotes development of hippocampal neurons. Biochem J 2011;435(2):327–36.

[39] Trautmann SM, Sharkey KA. The endocannabinoid system and its role in regulating the intrinsic neural circuitry of the gastrointestinal tract. Int Rev Neurobiol 2015;125:85–126.

[40] Morena M, De Castro V, Gray JM, et al. Training-associated emotional arousal shapes endocannabinoid modulation of spatial memory retrieval in rats. J Neurosci 2015;35(41): 13962–74.

[41] Casado-Diaz A, Santiago-Mora R, Dorado G, et al. The omega-6 arachidonic fatty acid, but not the omega-3 fatty acids, inhibits osteoblastogenesis and induces adipogenesis of human mesenchymal stem cells: potential implication in osteoporosis. Osteoporos Int 2013;24(5):1647–61.

[42] Spencer-Smith MM, Spittle AJ, Lee KJ, et al. Bayley-III cognitive and language scales in preterm children. Pediatrics 2015;135(5):e1258–65.

[43] Stiles J, Jernigan TL. The basics of brain development. Neuropsychol Rev 2010;20(4): 327–48.

[44] Kostovic I, Jovanov-Milosevic N. The development of cerebral connections during the first 20-45 weeks' gestation. Semin Fetal Neonatal Med 2006;11(6):415–22.

[45] Nadarajah B, Alifragis P, Wong RO, et al. Neuronal migration in the developing cerebral cortex: observations based on real-time imaging. Cereb Cortex 2003;13(6):607–11.

[46] Pakkenberg B, Gundersen HJ. Neocortical neuron number in humans: effect of sex and age. J Comp Neurol 1997;384(2):312–20.

[47] Maravall M, Koh IY, Lindquist WB, et al. Experience-dependent changes in basal dendritic branching of layer 2/3 pyramidal neurons during a critical period for developmental plasticity in rat barrel cortex. Cereb Cortex 2004;14(6):655–64.

[48] Huttenlocher PR, de Courten C, Garey LJ, et al. Synaptogenesis in human visual cortex–evidence for synapse elimination during normal development. Neurosci Lett 1982;33(3): 247–52.

[49] Paolicelli RC, Bolasco G, Pagani F, et al. Synaptic pruning by microglia is necessary for normal brain development. Science 2011;333(6048):1456–8.

[50] Brody BA, Kinney HC, Kloman AS, et al. Sequence of central nervous system myelination in human infancy. I. An autopsy study of myelination. J Neuropathol Exp Neurol 1987;46(3): 283–301.

[51] Lemaire V, Koehl M, Le Moal M, et al. Prenatal stress produces learning deficits associated with an inhibition of neurogenesis in the hippocampus. Proc Natl Acad Sci U S A 2000;97(20):11032–7.

[52] Murmu MS, Salomon S, Biala Y, et al. Changes of spine density and dendritic complexity in the prefrontal cortex in offspring of mothers exposed to stress during pregnancy. Eur J Neurosci 2006;24(5):1477–87.

[53] Coe CL, Kramer M, Czeh B, et al. Prenatal stress diminishes neurogenesis in the dentate gyrus of juvenile rhesus monkeys. Biol Psychiatry 2003;54(10):1025–34.

[54] Colombo J. The critical period concept: research, methodology, and theoretical issues. Psychol Bull 1982;91(2):260–75.

[55] Armitage JA, Taylor PD, Poston L. Experimental models of developmental programming: consequences of exposure to an energy rich diet during development. J Physiol 2005;565(Pt 1):3–8.

[56] Langley-Evans SC. Developmental programming of health and disease. Proc Nutr Soc 2006;65(1):97–105.

[57] Taylor PD, Poston L. Developmental programming of obesity in mammals. Exp Physiol 2007;92(2):287–98.

[58] Colombo J. The development of visual attention in infancy. Annu Rev Psychol 2001;52: 337–67.

[59] Boothe RG, Dobson V, Teller DY. Postnatal development of vision in human and nonhuman primates. Annu Rev Neurosci 1985;8:495–545.

[60] Chugani HT, Phelps ME, Mazziotta JC. Positron emission tomography study of human brain functional development. Ann Neurol 1987;22(4):487–97.

[61] Colombo J, Cheatham CL. The emergence and basis of endogenous attention in infancy and early childhood. Adv Child Dev Behav 2006;34:283–322.

[62] Jacobs RA. Computational studies of the development of functionally specialized neural modules. Trends Cogn Sci 1999;3(1):31–8.

[63] Johnson MH, Vecera SP. Cortical differentiation and neurocognitive development: The parcellation conjecture. Behav Processes 1996;36(2):195–212.

[64] Colombo J. Infant cognition: predicting later intellectual functioning. Newbury Park (CA): Sage Publications; 1993.

[65] Colombo J, Fagen J, editors. Individual differences in infancy: reliability, stability, prediction. New York: Psychology Press; 1990. p. 2014.

[66] Bornstein MH, Sigman MD. Continuity in mental development from infancy. Child Dev 1986;57(2):251–74.

[67] Bornstein MH, Hahn CS, Bell C, et al. Stability in cognition across early childhood. A developmental cascade. Psychol Sci 2006;17(2):151–8.

[68] Bornstein MH, Hahn CS, Wolke D. Systems and cascades in cognitive development and academic achievement. Child Dev 2013;84(1):154–62.

[69] Birch EE, Birch DG, Hoffman DR, et al. Dietary essential fatty acid supply and visual acuity development. Invest Ophthalmol Vis Sci 1992;33(11):3242–53.

[70] Carlson SE, Werkman SH, Rhodes PG, et al. Visual-acuity development in healthy preterm infants: effect of marine-oil supplementation. Am J Clin Nutr 1993;58(1):35–42.

[71] Uauy R, Hoffman DR, Peirano P, et al. Essential fatty acids in visual and brain development. Lipids 2001;36(9):885–95.

[72] Birch EE, Garfield S, Castaneda Y, et al. Visual acuity and cognitive outcomes at 4 years of age in a double-blind, randomized trial of long-chain polyunsaturated fatty acid-supplemented infant formula. Early Hum Dev 2007;83(5):279–84.

[73] Birch EE, Carlson SE, Hoffman DR, et al. The DIAMOND (DHA Intake and Measurement of Neural Development) Study: a double-masked, randomized controlled clinical trial of the maturation of infant visual acuity as a function of the dietary level of docosahexaenoic acid. Am J Clin Nutr 2010;91(4):848–59.

[74] Carlson SE, Werkman SH. A randomized trial of visual attention of preterm infants fed docosahexaenoic acid until two months. Lipids 1996;31(1):85–90.

[75] Werkman SH, Carlson SE. A randomized trial of visual attention of preterm infants fed docosahexaenoic acid until nine months. Lipids 1996;31(1):91–7.

[76] Reisbick S, Neuringer M, Gohl E, et al. Visual attention in infant monkeys: effects of dietary fatty acids and age. Dev Psychol 1997;33(3):387–95.

[77] Colombo J, Carlson SE, Cheatham CL, et al. Long-chain polyunsaturated fatty acid supplementation in infancy reduces heart rate and positively affects distribution of attention. Pediatr Res 2011;70(4):406–10.

[78] Colombo J, Carlson SE, Cheatham CL, et al. Long-term effects of LCPUFA supplementation on childhood cognitive outcomes. Am J Clin Nutr 2013;98(2):403–12.

[79] Willatts P, Forsyth S, Agostoni C, et al. Effects of long-chain PUFA supplementation in infant formula on cognitive function in later childhood. Am J Clin Nutr 2013;98(2):536s–42s.

[80] Helland IB, Smith L, Saarem K, et al. Maternal supplementation with very-long-chain n-3 fatty acids during pregnancy and lactation augments children's IQ at 4 years of age. Pediatrics 2003;111(1):e39–44.

[81] Jensen CL, Voigt RG, Llorente AM, et al. Effects of early maternal docosahexaenoic acid intake on neuropsychological status and visual acuity at five years of age of breast-fed term infants. J Pediatr 2010;157(6):900–5.

[82] Cheatham CL, Nerhammer AS, Asserhoj M, et al. Fish oil supplementation during lactation: effects on cognition and behavior at 7 years of age. Lipids 2011;46(7):637–45.

[83] Westerberg AC, Schei R, Henriksen C, et al. Attention among very low birth weight infants following early supplementation with docosahexaenoic and arachidonic acid. Acta Paediatr 2011;100(1):47–52.

[84] Almaas AN, Tamnes CK, Nakstad B, et al. Long-chain polyunsaturated fatty acids and cognition in VLBW infants at 8 years: an RCT. Pediatrics 2015;135(6):972–80.

[85] Collins CT, Gibson RA, Anderson PJ, et al. Neurodevelopmental outcomes at 7 years' corrected age in preterm infants who were fed high-dose docosahexaenoic acid to term equivalent: a follow-up of a randomised controlled trial. BMJ Open 2015;5(3):e007314.

[86] Isaacs EB, Ross S, Kennedy K, et al. 10-year cognition in preterms after random assignment to fatty acid supplementation in infancy. Pediatrics 2011;128(4):e890–8.

[87] Drover JR, Hoffman DR, Castaneda YS, et al. Cognitive function in 18-month-old term infants of the DIAMOND study: a randomized, controlled clinical trial with multiple dietary levels of docosahexaenoic acid. Early Hum Dev 2011;87(3):223–30.

[88] Drover JR, Felius J, Hoffman DR, et al. A randomized trial of DHA intake during infancy: school readiness and receptive vocabulary at 2-3.5 years of age. Early Hum Dev 2012;88(11):885–91.

[89] Colombo J, Carlson SE. Is the measure the message: the BSID and nutritional interventions. Pediatrics 2012;129(6):1166–7.

[90] Liao KMB, Carlson SE, Colombo J, et al. Long-chain polyunsaturated fatty acid supplementation in infancy: response inhibition in childhood. Dev Sci, 2016. in press.

[91] Grayson DS, Kroenke CD, Neuringer M, et al. Dietary omega-3 fatty acids modulate large-scale systems organization in the rhesus macaque brain. J Neurosci 2014;34(6):2065–74.

[92] Peters BD, Voineskos AN, Szeszko PR, et al. Brain white matter development is associated with a human-specific haplotype increasing the synthesis of long chain fatty acids. J Neurosci 2014;34(18):6367–76.

[93] Martinez M, Vazquez E. MRI evidence that docosahexaenoic acid ethyl ester improves myelination in generalized peroxisomal disorders. Neurology 1998;51(1):26–32.

[94] Caspi A, Williams B, Kim-Cohen J, et al. Moderation of breastfeeding effects on the IQ by genetic variation in fatty acid metabolism. Proc Natl Acad Sci U S A 2007;104(47):18860–5.

[95] Steer CD, Davey Smith G, Emmett PM, et al. FADS2 polymorphisms modify the effect of breastfeeding on child IQ. PLoS One 2010;5(7):e11570.

[96] Rizzi TS, van der Sluis S, Derom C, et al. Genetic variance in combination with fatty acid intake might alter composition of the fatty acids in brain. PLoS One 2013;8(6):e68000.

[97] Reardon HT, Zhang J, Kothapalli KS, et al. Insertion-deletions in a FADS2 intron 1 conserved regulatory locus control expression of fatty acid desaturases 1 and 2 and modulate response to simvastatin. Prostaglandins Leukot Essent Fatty Acids 2012;87(1):25–33.

[98] Duchen K, Yu G, Bjorksten B. Atopic sensitization during the first year of life in relation to long chain polyunsaturated fatty acid levels in human milk. Pediatr Res 1998;44(4):478–84.

[99] Duchen K, Casas R, Fageras-Bottcher M, et al. Human milk polyunsaturated long-chain fatty acids and secretory immunoglobulin A antibodies and early childhood allergy. Pediatr Allergy Immunol 2000;11(1):29–39.

[100] Barman M, Nilsson S, Torinsson Naluai A, et al. Single nucleotide polymorphisms in the FADS gene cluster but not the ELOVL2 gene are associated with serum polyunsaturated fatty acid composition and development of allergy (in a Swedish birth cohort). Nutrients 2015;7(12):10100–15.

[101] Field CJ, Van Aerde JE, Robinson LE, et al. Effect of providing a formula supplemented with long-chain polyunsaturated fatty acids on immunity in full-term neonates. Br J Nutr 2008;99(1):91–9.

[102] Birch EE, Khoury JC, Berseth CL, et al. The impact of early nutrition on incidence of allergic manifestations and common respiratory illnesses in children. J Pediatr 2010;156(6):902–6, 906.e1.

[103] Foiles AM, Kerling EH, Wick JA, et al. Formula with long chain polyunsaturated fatty acids reduces incidence of allergy in early childhood. Pediatr Allergy Immunol 2016;27(2): 156–61.

[104] Furuhjelm C, Jenmalm MC, Falth-Magnusson K, et al. Th1 and Th2 chemokines, vaccine-induced immunity, and allergic disease in infants after maternal omega-3 fatty acid supplementation during pregnancy and lactation. Pediatr Res 2011;69(3):259–64.

[105] Jenmalm MC, Duchen K. Timing of allergy-preventive and immunomodulatory dietary interventions - are prenatal, perinatal or postnatal strategies optimal? Clin Exp Allergy 2013;43(3):273–8.

[106] Best KP, Gold M, Kennedy D, et al. Omega-3 long-chain PUFA intake during pregnancy and allergic disease outcomes in the offspring: a systematic review and meta-analysis of observational studies and randomized controlled trials. Am J Clin Nutr 2016;103(1):128–43.

[107] Hutley LJ, Newell FM, Joyner JM, et al. Effects of rosiglitazone and linoleic acid on human preadipocyte differentiation. Eur J Clin Invest 2003;33(7):574–81.

[108] Massiera F, Saint-Marc P, Seydoux J, et al. Arachidonic acid and prostacyclin signaling promote adipose tissue development: a human health concern? J Lipid Res 2003;44(2):271–9.

[109] Moon RJ, Harvey NC, Robinson SM, et al. Maternal plasma polyunsaturated fatty acid status in late pregnancy is associated with offspring body composition in childhood. J Clin Endocrinol Metab 2013;98(1):299–307.

[110] Much D, Brunner S, Vollhardt C, et al. Breast milk fatty acid profile in relation to infant growth and body composition: results from the INFAT study. Pediatr Res 2013;74(2):230–7.

[111] Currie LM. Long chain polyunsaturated fatty acid supplementation in infancy increases length- and weight-for-age but not BMI to 6 years when controlling for effects of maternal smoking. Prostaglandins Leukot Essent Fatty Acids 2015;98:1–6.

[112] Murphy RA, Yu EA, Ciappio ED, et al. Suboptimal plasma long chain n-3 concentrations are common among adults in the United States, NHANES 2003-2004. Nutrients 2015;7(12):10282–9.

[113] Forsyth S. Why are we undertaking DHA supplementation studies in infants who are not DHA-deficient? Br J Nutr 2012;108(5):948.

Advances in Pediatrics 63 (2016) 473–480

ADVANCES IN PEDIATRICS

ELSEVIER
MOSBY

Using Shared Decision-Making Tools to Improve Care for Patients with Disorders of Sex Development

Kathleen Graziano, MD[a],*, Mary E. Fallat, MD[b]

[a]Reproductive Anomalies/DSD Clinic, Phoenix Children's Hospital, 1920 East Cambridge Avenue, Suite 201, Phoenix, AZ 85006, USA; [b]Hiram C. Polk Jr Department of Surgery, Kosair Children's Hospital, University of Louisville, Louisville, KY, USA

Keywords

- Disorder of sex development • DSD • Shared decision making
- Complete androgen insensitivity syndrome • CAIS
- Congenital adrenal hyperplasia • CAH
- Mayer Rokitansky Kuster Hauser syndrome

Key points

- Disorders of sex development (DSD) are complex conditions and require a different and comprehensive approach to assure adequate education for the patient and caregivers.

- Patient/family values must be considered when discussing sensitive issues regarding the body and sexual activity, regardless of patient age.

- Controversies in the care of these patients should be shared with the age-appropriate patients and/or caregivers in an up-to-date and unbiased manner.

- Informed consent involves a complete understanding of the expected outcomes. All questions must be answered thoroughly before irreversible surgery, especially regarding gonads or other reproductive organs.

INTRODUCTION

Disorders or differences of sex development (DSD) is a broad term that encompasses a wide range of diagnoses affecting infants, children, and adolescents [1]. Patients with DSD can have genetic abnormalities, anatomic differences, or a combination of the 2 (Table 1). The families of DSD patients are faced with

*Corresponding author. E-mail address: kgraziano@phoenixchildrens.com

0065-3101/16/$ – see front matter
http://dx.doi.org/10.1016/j.yapd.2016.04.004

Table 1
Types of disorders of sexual differentiation

46,XX DSD	46,XY DSD	Gonadal ambiguities or absence	Anatomic/ developmental anomalies

CAH
  21-hydroxylase def.
  11-hydroxylase def.
  3β-hydroxysteroid
    def.
Aromatase def.
	Androgen insensitivity
	  syndrome (AIS)
	  Partial AIS
	  Complete AIS
	Insufficient
	  testosterone
	  production
	  P450scc defect
	  P450c11 defect
	  P450c17 defect
	  P450c21 defect
	Inability to convert
	  testosterone to
	  dihydrotestosterone
	  3β-hydroxysteroid
	    dehydrogenase
	  17-ketosteroid
	    reductase def.
	  5α-reductase def.
		Mixed gonadal
		  dysgenesis
		  (45,X/46,XY)
		Pure gonadal
		  dysgenesis
		  (46,XX or 46,XY)
		Ovotesticular DSD
		  (46,XX or 46,XY)
			Cloacal
			  abnormalities
			Bladder exstrophy
			Caudal regression
			  syndrome
			VACTERL syndrome
			Persistent Mullerian
			  duct syndrome
			MRKH/vaginal
			  agenesis
			Distal vaginal
			  agenesis
			Persistent urogenital
			  sinus

Abbreviation: def, deficiency.

important decisions regarding medical, surgical, and psychological care. There is active research focused on improving the long-term outcomes for these patients and their families. In the setting of that research, the concept of shared decision making has played an increasingly important role [2,3]. The barriers that the patient and family can face include value systems that conflict with those of the providers, a lack of understanding of these complex diagnoses, an ever-changing environment with regards to the controversies and evolution of care, and more basic concerns, such as lack of access to care due to cost or distance.

In this overview, the authors discuss the concept of shared decision-making tools for patients with DSD and their family members. They highlight the controversies in care that led to the development of these checklists, and the intended results regarding optimization of informed consent and expected outcomes.

MANAGEMENT GOALS
History of the care of children with disorders of sex development
A major shift in the care of these complex patients has happened in the last decade as a result of collaboration between medical providers and patient advocates. A Consensus Statement on Management of Intersex Disorders by

the Lawson Wilkins Pediatric Endocrine Society and the European Society of Paediatric Endocrinology was published in 2006 [4]. Fifty international experts in various fields convened to suggest needed changes in nomenclature, diagnosis, medical and surgical management, psychosocial care, and the approach to informed consent and improving long-term outcomes. These efforts fostered what is now a broad clinical research focus in this field, and a recommendation that patients with DSD be cared for in a longitudinal manner within a comprehensive, multidisciplinary clinic. The spotlight is not on surgical correction of anatomic differences but on the medical care of the patient and the psychosocial outcome that is desired. Progress has been slow, but the commitment to improving care has not wavered. Decision-making tools are a natural way for providers to help patients and families who are facing varied treatment options.

Importance of shared decision making for patients with disorders of sex development

Shared decision making has been advocated for any diagnosis in which care can involve a decision tree with multiple possible pathways. Patients and families cannot be expected to know how to navigate care when there are multiple options, and providers need to be careful to avoid spinning crucial information to bias the patient toward a particular treatment pathway when data are lacking as to the best practice. Providers who specialize in bioethics have become part of the local and national teams taking care of DSD patients [5,6]. The historical paternalistic approach has been replaced with patient and family autonomy, and DSD teams can learn how to tailor the approach to care by asking for input from patient advocacy groups. Advocacy groups of affected individuals and/or family members are an important resource for providing input for decision-making tools. Some established support groups are listed in Box 1. When asked what they wish they would have known when going through the process, these sophisticated family members are able to articulate the important details that new patients should understand [7].

DSD diagnoses are complex. In gathering all pertinent information in one tool using tenets that extend from diagnosis and treatment in infancy all the way to adolescence or adulthood, providers can aim to cover a range of

---

Box 1: Advocacy groups for disorders of sex development patients and families

Advocates for Informed Choice (AIC)

AIS-DSD (Androgen Insensitivity Syndrome)

Beautiful You (MRKH)

Cares (CAH)

DSD families/DSD teens

HEA (Hypospadias and Epispadias Association)

anticipatory guidance and help the patient and family gain enough knowledge to avoid or lessen decisional regret [8–10]. These tools need to remain dynamic and must be updated when new management strategies are developed.

Legal aspects of disorders of sex development care with regard to informed consent

In the United States, parents are automatically given the right to make decisions for their children. That includes decisions regarding gender of rearing in cases of complex DSD. It also includes the right to decide whether reconstructive surgery is performed in the newborn period. The consensus statement of 2006 stated that it is reasonable to perform reconstructive genital surgery before 2 years of age because there are not adequate data to determine if early surgery or late surgery (after puberty) results in superior outcomes. Conflicting with that sentiment is the recent fact sheet published by the United Nations calling for providers to prohibit normalizing genital surgery on infants in the absence of medical necessity. Because some patients have a urogenital sinus and may be prone to trapping urine in the vagina and chronic leaking or have obstruction of menstrual flow at puberty, reconstructive surgery may be indicated and necessary in these cases. In general, there are no informed consent documents that are specific to patients with DSD. The concept of informed consent includes allowing families to gather unbiased and complete information, to make decisions without pressure, and to hear options that include risks of surgery, benefits of surgery, and alternatives to the proposed therapy. This process can be lengthy when much is at stake in a rapidly changing field and when there are also external social and psychological factors.

The role of shared decision making in managing expectations

It is difficult to study expectations when patients and families may wish to be "normal," and providers may have a different definition of what that means. For providers, adequate function and relief of obstruction are the most important measures of success, but families may define success in other ways that may or may not be realistic. A goal for both families and the medical team is to help define and accept what will be normal for an individual. One way to alert patients/families to this disparity is to give them an honest assessment of what they can expect but also let them know that "perfect outcomes" are rare. One method is to implement a consent readiness document that asks the patient or family to repeat what they are hearing the provider say regarding the procedure, the recovery time, the follow-up requirements, and their knowledge of whether additional surgeries will be needed over time [11]. Even in the best of circumstances, expectations may be difficult to meet. There are ways to make these patients feel more "normal," and one piece of advice from the advocacy groups is that each patient or family with a new DSD diagnosis should meet another person with the same diagnosis. This advice achieves the goal of lessening the sense of shame that comes with being told something is different about the reproductive organs of a child or adolescent. Then, smaller goals regarding medical and surgical management can be addressed.

How to implement the shared decision-making tools

Part of the multidisciplinary approach is to have a new patient and family of the patient with a DSD meet all appropriate members of the team in order to gather consensus on the particular diagnosis and address any urgent concerns. A family might meet a social worker or clinical coordinator, an endocrinologist, a geneticist, a psychologist, and members of the surgical team, including a urologist, gynecologist, or pediatric surgeon. The amount of new and possibly conflicting information from various providers can be overwhelming. Decision-making tools are divided into sections that help organize this information; important components are listed in Box 2. A section on basic information, such as how the patient or family found out about their diagnosis and the extent of their current knowledge base, can help set the stage for the work that needs to be done. The values the family has regarding information and dialogue about future sexual function and the reproductive tract and the body are important, and different cultures will have a different approach to discussing these topics with the providers. In some cultures, the father will be the main or only spokesperson. If the patient is an age-appropriate adolescent and the parents resist disclosure, this can present a different challenge for the medical team. Another section on nomenclature that asks about the preferred terms a patient or family would like to use helps set the groundwork for more in-depth discussion about function. Another section lists the various topics that should be covered over time, both medical and social, to facilitate a complete working knowledge of the condition and how it affects the body. Every patient and family should have a list of questions that need to be answered before any irreversible surgery is considered so another section of the decision-making tool lists those questions. Many patients would not know what to ask, so providing a list is empowering. A final section lists specific treatment options and allows that patient/family member to consider the pros and cons for each with the provider. Decision-making checklists for each diagnosis have similar sections. It

---

Box 2: Components of decision-making checklists for disorders of sex development patients

Components

1. Overview/introduction of goals/review of patient's values

2. Preferred words/review of nomenclature

3. List of short-term and long-term topics

4. List of questions that need to be addressed by providers

5. Management options including nonsurgical options

Updated checklists can be found at http://turl.ca/dsdcklist. Pediatric Surgeons of Phoenix DSD diagnoses checklists, last updated December 1, 2015.

should be expected that the tools will not be completed in a single visit but rather in multiple visits with the team.

Special concerns for specific diagnoses

Congenital adrenal hyperplasia

Congenital adrenal hyperplasia (CAH) is a disorder of sex development where a child is born with "normal" chromosomes but due to a deficiency in an enzyme in the steroid pathway, the child is exposed to excess androgens. Infant girls can have an enlarged clitoris and/or a urogenital sinus (a common channel for the urethral and vaginal openings), and the severity of the anatomic abnormality is on a wide spectrum. Some CAH babies are thought to be male gender prenatally because of the size of the clitoris; this can cause considerable distress for the family, who may have chosen a male name for the baby. Having decision-making tools for parents helps them gain knowledge of the condition and can lead them through decisions regarding reconstructive surgery. Involving patient advocates in the development of these tools helps ensure that providers are not biasing families toward any given surgical or social outcome; this is particularly difficult because of the shift that has taken place in the overall approach to "normalizing" genital surgery. Use of a checklist can make it mandatory to review nonsurgical options with the family, encourage them to use support resources other than physicians, and can lead to more families choosing to delay procedures until the children themselves can use the age-appropriate decision-making tools.

Mayer Rokitansky Kuster Hauser syndrome

Mayer Rokitansky Kuster Hauser syndrome (MRKH), or vaginal agenesis, is most often diagnosed in teenagers who have primary amenorrhea and are found on examination to have a vaginal dimple but no vaginal opening, no vagina, and usually no functional uterine tissue. These patients have functioning ovaries and secondary sex characteristics consistent with the female gender. Their chromosomes are 46,XX. The use of a decision-making checklist with this population allows a better understanding of the diagnosis. Most patients have a very limited knowledge of the reproductive organs and their function and have difficulty grasping what it means when some of the organs failed to form. The checklist helps go through options for therapy and helps highlight nonsurgical options, including serial dilation to form a vaginal canal. The surgical options themselves are quite varied, and the decision-making tool allows the patient to understand all the options and what the pros and cons would be to choosing any reconstructive surgery. The checklists help organize the thoughts of these stressed patients and families and help to slow down the process. Families need to come to terms with the diagnosis, and the checklists help ensure that this happens. Meeting another woman with MRKH and/or using online advocacy resources becomes important as part of the process for patients and families to fully understand treatment options.

Complete androgen insensitivity syndrome and other XY disorders of sex development
Patients with XY DSD can be classified into a broad category of diagnoses in which there is a mismatch between chromosomal sex and phenotypic sex. Patients are sometimes diagnosed after puberty when they present with amenorrhea and are found to have a normal introitus and distal vagina but no uterus. In some cases, the gonads are intra-abdominal and consist of functional testicular tissue. In other cases, the gonads failed to form and the patients have decreased sex hormone production, possibly due to an enzymatic deficiency. Parents often have difficulty understanding the diagnosis, and this is partly because there are many diagnoses that can be classified into the category of XY DSD, a wide variety of anatomic differences, and each requires a different approach. The decision-making tools are helpful with this group in order to reassure the patients and the family that nothing has changed about their personality and gender just because there is new information regarding their genetic makeup. Patients often do not have any external evidence of an abnormality so confusion arises when providers who are not familiar with the diagnosis use routine care such as ordering a urine human chorionic gonadotropin for pregnancy testing and attempting vaginal examinations in the office, creating stress for the patient and family and adding to the mistrust they may have regarding the medical community. There is a robust support community for patients with androgen insensitivity, and the checklists help connect families to those groups and help them explore issues such as gonad preservation.

DISCUSSION
DSD are complex and require a different and comprehensive approach to assure adequate education for both patient and caregivers. The use of an organized but fluid and frequently updated checklist helps providers stay up-to-date on the latest concepts, therapies, and controversies for each of these diagnoses. Patients respond well to a patient-centered approach and are capable of exercising autonomy in decision-making when given the right tools.

Patient/family values and cultural competency must be considered when discussing sensitive issues regarding the body and sexual activity. What works for a Caucasian family may not work for a Native American family or a Hispanic family. The age of consent for decision making varies among groups as well, and providers need to focus on the individual family dynamic and help in a way that meshes with the cultural context. An age-appropriate child or adolescent should participate in the decision-making process whenever appropriate.

Controversies in the care of these patients should be shared with the patients/caregivers in an up-to-date and unbiased manner. These issues can be met head-on, and together the team and the patient and/or family can come up with a customized plan. Informed consent involves a complete understanding of the expected outcomes. All questions must be answered thoroughly before irreversible surgery, especially regarding gonads or other reproductive organs; this is increasingly important when reconstructive surgeries may later be perceived as personal violations of autonomy. Each patient and family needs to be treated using a compassionate and empathetic approach, remembering that decision trees provide guidance, but the same guidance will not work with every patient despite similarities. Providers need to be aware of this, use a team approach to families, but also remain flexible regarding the decision-making process.

Surgical reconstruction of the genital tract of infants will inevitably over time become less common, although deferring surgery will also present a host of new challenges for families, such as explaining to siblings and to caregivers and to relatives and ultimately to the involved child why the child "looks different." As practitioners, a secondary goal is to help the family accept this "new state of normal." This new state of normal will not always be straightforward and checklists will by design become very important. Routinely implementing these tools will help educate patients and families, decrease stress, and lead to a better quality of life and less decisional regret for both the parents of infants and small children and the adolescents who have never had surgical intervention.

References

[1] United Nations Office of the High Commission for Human Rights (UN OHCH). Available at: http://www.ohchr.org/.
[2] Karkazis K, Tamar-Mattis A, Kon AA. Genital surgery for disorders of sex development: implementing a shared decision-making approach. J Pediatr Endocrinol Metab 2010;23: 789–805.
[3] Siminoff LA, Sandberg DE. Promoting shared decision making in disorders of sex development (DSD): decision aids and support tools. Horm Metab Res 2015;47:335–9.
[4] Lee PA, Houk CP, Ahmed SF, et al. Consensus statement on management of intersex disorders. International consensus conference on intersex. Pediatrics 2006;118:e488–500.
[5] Lipstein EA, Dodds CM, Britto MT. Real life clinic visits do not match the ideals of shared decision making. J Pediatr 2014;165:178–83.
[6] Kon AA. Ethical issues in decision-making for infants with disorders of sex development. Horm Metab Res 2015;47:340–3.
[7] What we wish our parents knew. Available at: inter.act@aiclegal.org.
[8] Lorenzo AJ, Pippi Salle JL, Zlateska B, et al. Decisional regret after distal hypospadias repair: single institution prospective analysis of factors associated with subsequent parental remorse or distress. J Urol 2014;191:1558–63.
[9] Streuli JC, Vayena E, Cavicchia-Balmer Y, et al. Shaping parents: impact of contrasting professional counseling on parents' decision making for children with disorders of sex development. J Sex Med 2013;10:1953–60.
[10] Brehaut JC, O'Connor AM, Wood TJ, et al. Validation of a decision regret scale. Med Decis Making 2003;23:281–92.
[11] Liao LM, Doyle J, Crouch NS, et al. Dilation as a treatment for vaginal agenesis and hypoplasia: a pilot exploration of benefits and barriers as perceived by patients. J Obstet Gynaecol 2006;26:144–8.